CLINICAL BIOSTATISTICS

CLINICAL BIOSTATISTICS

Alvan R. Feinstein, M.D.

Professor of Medicine and Epidemiology,
Yale University School of Medicine,
New Haven, Conn.

The C. V. Mosby Company

SAINT LOUIS   1977

The C. V. Mosby Company
11830 Westline Industrial Drive, St. Louis, Missouri 63141

Library of Congress Cataloging in Publication Data

Feinstein, Alvan R
    Clinical biostatistics.

    Originally appeared as essays in the journal Clinical pharmacology and therapeutics.
    Includes bibliographies.
    1. Medical statistics—Addresses, essays, lectures.
2. Medical research—Statistical methods—Addresses, essays, lectures. I. Title. [DNLM: 1. Biometry.
2. Epidemiologic methods.   HA29 F299c]
RA409.F36   610'.1'5195   77-3703
ISBN   0-8016-1563-1

CB/CB/CB   9   8   7   6   5   4   3   2   1

*For my mother, Bella, and my wife, Linda,
who have given me
roots, wings, and love*

PREFACE

When I began writing the series of essays called "Clinical biostatistics" in 1970, I thought I would run out of material in about a year. I knew I had some unorthodox things to say and some unconventional viewpoints to develop, but I believed the development would require only six or seven essays. As I became more deeply immersed in biostatistical ideas, however, I constantly found more to do. At every level of contemplation—ranging from the massive logistics of large-scale clinical trials, to the elaborate complexities of "retrospective case-control" studies, to such apparently simple questions as how (and why) to calculate a standard deviation—the world of biostatistics seemed beset with scientific problems that had received unsatisfactory solutions because the -*statistics* had been given more attention than the *bio-*. As I began grappling with those challenges, the essays continued to proliferate, until almost 40 of them have now appeared.

While the essays were making their bimonthly and later trimonthly appearances in *Clinical Pharmacology and Therapeutics*, readers of the journal were highly complimentary; and many urged me to publish the series as a book. At first I resisted this suggestion, mainly because I have never liked this type of autoanthology. The author of a book, I thought, should prepare a suitably renovated text, not just an unaltered collection of previously published papers. My resistance to the suggestion eventually collapsed, however, under two sets of pressures: time and audience. As I kept wanting to prepare that new text while never finding the necessary time to do so, I realized that the only hope for achieving a book in the imminent future was to preserve the original essays. Furthermore, many readers kept assuring me that the original essays should remain intact—that their "spirit" might be lost in a revision and that the book would be more enjoyable to read if it preserved the informality of the original prose. Adding to these incentives for an "anthology" format were the fiscal concerns of The C. V. Mosby Company, publishers of the journal where the "Clinical biostatistics" essays have appeared. The cost of publishing the book could be substantially reduced if the essays were maintained in their original form, with each text and bibliography unchanged.

Accordingly, this book contains a collection of original essays from the "Clinical biostatistics" series. They have been rearranged as chapters, into a logical pattern that differs from the chronologic sequence in which they first appeared. A few of the original titles and many of the identifying numbers of the essays have been changed to conform with the current sequence of chapters. Otherwise, the texts and lists of references for each essay remain intact. To keep the book from being too large, I have omitted a few of the essays that contained quantitative surveys of the medical and statistical literature, digressions into the ethics of research and the teaching of statistics, or specific critiques of individual clinical investigations. The remaining 29 essays have been divided into an introductory chapter that is followed by five major sections, each preceded by a brief commentary.

The essays are intended for people who have already developed an interest in biostatistical issues. The interest may have arisen spontaneously; it may have been necessitated by the demands or comments of a manuscript reviewer; or it may have been provoked by the efforts needed to understand the many mathematical machinations that are used in published reports of current research. I assume that the reader is aware of rudimentary statistical tactics, but is otherwise not particularly adept in mathematics and is possibly frightened by it. With that assumption, the goal is to enlighten and perhaps to entertain with the style of an essay, not to educate with the formality of a textbook.

Conventional textbooks and courses in biostatistics are usually devoted to the theoretical processes that produce such mathematical calculations as P values, confidence intervals, correlation coefficients, and regression equations. Amid the mathematical emphasis, almost no attention has been given to the basic scientific procedures used for planning research, obtaining data, and analyzing results. The aim of these essays is to provide supplemental reading for the many important topics that are omitted from conventional textbooks, and also some remedial reading for topics that usually receive inadequate consideration.

Because of the way the book has been assembled, it contains three features for which I apologize. The first is that the text regularly contains references to previous or forthcoming essays in the originally published series. Although useful liaisons for essays that were dispersed in time, many of the references will now appear in the wrong places in the rearranged series. Since the current text is identical to what originally appeared in the journal publications, these references could not be changed. The second flaw is that the original bibliographic citations have also, of necessity, been preserved at the end of each essay. This process, while making the citations easy to find, produces frequent redundancy in some of the listings. The third infelicitous feature is that certain ideas are mentioned repeatedly in different locations of the text. The repetition seemed desirable in a succession of individual essays spread over a 6-year period, but may be less appealing if the essays are read contiguously. I hope that readers will find these sporadic repetitions instructive rather than irritating.

In discussing the various challenges and imperfections of biostatistics, I have tried to keep the prose lively and have occasionally made it deliberately provocative. Most readers have said they enjoy this approach, but it has sometimes led to the accusation that I am antistatistical. This accusation has probably been received by anyone who has ever been discontent with the defects of any status quo. Like the established tenets of clinical medicine and epidemiology, the established creeds of statistics contain many infirmities. In pointing out the infirmities, I have always tried to offer constructive suggestions for improvement; and I would hardly want to spend so much effort working in the domain of clinical biostatistics if I did not respect both the *clinical bio-* and the *-statistics* portions.

To do the kind of thinking and writing that have produced these essays, I have had many sources of support for which I want to express thanks. The Veterans Administration, at its hospital in West Haven, provided research aid for many years while I was Chief of the Eastern Research Support Center and, later, of the Cooperative Studies Program Support Center. For my activities at the Yale University School of Medicine, the National Center for Health Services Research and Development supplied grants for several projects from which many of these essays emerged as by-products. During a highly productive period from 1971-1973, as a visiting professor, I received professional hospitality and illuminating stimulation from the Department of Clinical Epidemiology and Biostatistics at McMaster University Medical Center in Hamilton, Ontario, Canada. For the past few years, the essays have been composed in my work as Director of the Yale Clinical Scholar Program, which is sponsored by the Robert Wood Johnson Foundation.

In addition to this institutional aid, I have been greatly helped by human talents and contributions. Before submitting the prepared essays for publication, I have relied on thoughtful appraisal and stringent evaluation from critics who are clinicians, epidemiologists, statisticians, or computer experts. In acknowledging my gratitude for their valuable help, I also herewith absolve them of any responsibility for the contents. They are Linda Marean Feinstein, Michael Gent, Charles A. Goldsmith, Moreson H. Kaplan, Donald Mainland, Walter A. Ramshaw, David L. Sackett, Helen L. Smits, Walter O. Spitzer, and Carolyn K. Wells. I am also especially grateful to Dr. Walter Modell, Editor of *Clinical Pharmacology and Therapeutics*, for his constant encouragement and for the editorial freedom he has provided. For excellent performance in the tasks of typing the difficult combinations of prose and mathematical symbols, I thank Elizabeth Tartagni, Carrol Ludington, and Pamela Rowe.

Finally, I want to thank my wife, Linda, and our children, Miriam and Daniel, who have gently tolerated the many hours in which I was absent or secluded while working on these essays, and who have filled the nonwriting hours with warmth, affection, and joy.

Alvan R. Feinstein
New Haven, 1977

CONTENTS

CLINICAL BIOSTATISTICS

CHAPTER 1

Introduction and rationale

*The "Clinical biostatistics" series began when I was invited to succeed Dr. Donald Mainland,
who had retired from writing a bimonthly "column" on statistics for* Clinical Pharmacology
and Therapeutics. *The first essay in the series contains my tribute to Dr. Mainland's many
previous contributions to biostatistics and also describes the background philosophy with
which the new series would be approached. The text was as follows.*

—ARF

Donald Mainland can be succeeded but not replaced. His training, timing, and temperament have made him a unique figure in the domain of medical statistics, and a tough act to follow.

In training, he was graduated in medicine with honors in 1925 at Edinburgh, where he was later awarded the Doctor of Science degree for his research in embryology and histology. After finishing medical school, he taught anatomy at Edinburgh for several years and then went to Canada. He worked at Manitoba from 1927 to 1930, when he left to become Professor and Chairman of the Department of Anatomy at Dalhousie University. His first publication in 1927—dealing with an uncommon abnormality in a muscle[13] —was a harbinger of his subsequent concern with frequency distributions in biology. Within the next two years, he was evaluating the accuracy of techniques for estimating irregular anatomic areas.[14] Later on, during various embryologic in-

vestigations, he contemplated methods for assessing the size and volume of cellular structures.[15-19] Over the next few years, he applied his quantitative interests to measuring the forces of muscles[20-21]; and then, in 1934, with a paper on "Chance and the blood count,"[22] the quantitative anatomist started his metamorphosis into medical statistician. By 1936, after some additional research on blood cells and blood counts, he had begun to write on "Problems of chance in clinical work."[23] In 1938, he produced his first book on quantitative medicine,[24] and twelve years later, after continuous productivity in both biologic research and medical statistics, he accepted New York University's invitation to become Professor of Medical Statistics. From that position, with persistent intellectual growth and enormous practical experience, he has continued to provide enlightenment to his colleagues, students, consultees, and readers.

In timing, Dr. Mainland became interested in biologic statistics during an era when the analytic techniques were in primitive stages of conception and dissemination. He knew many of the early

*This chapter originally appeared as "Clinical biostatistics—
I. A new name and some other changes of the guard."
In Clin. Pharmacol. Ther. 11:135, 1970.*

heroes in the contemporary statistical pantheon, and he became a pioneer physician in developing the modern relationship between statistics and medicine. After the first edition of his classic book, *Elementary Medical Statistics*[25] in 1952, he continued to produce a powerful array of creative, didactic, expository, and polemic publications on the use of statistics in medicine. With his textbook, now in its second edition,[26] and his many other writings, he has probably contributed as much as any single person to the statistical sensibility of clinical investigators in North America today.

In temperament, he has managed to preserve the extraordinary virtue of common sense, despite his constant exposure to the abstract concepts, arcane models, and intellectual folderol that lurk in the statistician's world. Part of this virtue is attributable to Mainland's firm rooting in the realities of medical biology. He has not merely preached about biostatistical research; he has practiced it. During the development of his statistical interests, he maintained his activities in biologic investigation—contributing, among other items, a textbook on anatomy[27]—and he currently continues an active role in several large-scale clinical research projects, chiefly in rheumatoid arthritis.

But the greater part of Mainland's virtue is probably attributable to the man himself. Now near the age of retirement, he remains young in mind, in spirit, and in outlook. What other "older man," venerated and respected as he nears completion of his major work, is ready to recognize that "repetition of this theme during two or three decades, by others as well as myself, has had very little effect"[31]; to confess that he is "technically unsophisticated"[32]; to solicit disagreement and rebuttals to all of his comments; and to be constantly receptive to new approaches for old problems. How many established "authorities" are brave enough to appraise their previous work with comments like these: "Grading all four items together

today, I would award a C, or perhaps a C+, but nothing higher,"[28] or "I sometimes wonder how many more instances of stupidity I might dig up from the days when I was hypnotized by statistical techniques applied to pooled data."[30]

My own first encounter with Mainland came in about 1960, when I discovered his publications entitled "Notes from a Laboratory of Medical Statistics"—a group of documents still cherished by the recipients who were lucky enough to learn about the "Notes," and to satisfy Mainland's hardy standards for the mailing list. ("There is a limit of 3,000 to the number of 'Notes' that can be issued. . . We are sorry that we can no longer replace 'Notes' that have disappeared after they have been received . . . Agencies that require formal invoicing are also too much trouble to deal with.") These "Notes," which Mainland issued periodically whenever he found time to do so, were the ancestors of the more recent "Statistical ward rounds" in this JOURNAL, and the "Notes on Biometry in Medical Research," which have appeared under the sponsorship of the Veterans Administration.

I still remember the enchantment of discovering those early "Notes." For several years previously, my own clinical research had brought me increasingly in contact with statistical procedures, and my manuscripts were being frequently sent to statisticians for review. Since many of the reviewers' comments were either clinically absurd or statistically incomprehensible, I had begun, in self-defense, to read textbooks on statistics. Like Mainland's, my education in statistics is largely self-acquired; but unlike most physicians, I was not intimidated by the arithmetic, since I had done graduate work in pure mathematics before entering medical school. What I found in the textbooks was sometimes enlightening, but more often appalling.

From my previous activities in pure mathematics and in biologic science, I had become accustomed to a rigorous type of either logical or empirical documentation for any assertion. In pure mathematics, such an assertion was called a *theorem,* and the rigorous documentation was a sequence of logically cohesive statements called a *proof.* In biologic science, the assertion was called a *hypothesis,* and the rigorous documentation was a collection of empirical data called *observed evidence.* But most of the statistical textbooks seemed to contain neither a logical nor an empirical documentation for the assertions. The texts were often like cookbooks, containing a series of instructive recipes on how to tabulate data and perform certain "tests of significance." These instructions were seldom accompanied by a proof of their validity, by any references to where a proof might be found, or by any empirical data to demonstrate that the procedures would remain valid when their prerequisite conditions were violated. From time to time, I would explore the literature of mathematical statistics, looking for either the rational logic or the scientific evidence to support what appeared in the "cookbooks," but I was seldom successful. Even with a mathematical background, I could not understand many of the esoteric formulations; and my biologic background made me wary of the unrealistic assumptions that underlay many of the mathematical arguments.

I did not know at the time that some of these mathematical defects were so commonplace as to arouse public lament by distinguished statisticians. Said Harold Hotelling[11] in 1960:

The custom of omitting proofs, which would not be tolerated in pure mathematics beyond a very limited extent, is common in the teaching of statistics, and is excused on the grounds that the students do not know enough mathematics to understand the proofs. Perhaps in some cases a better reason is that the teachers, and the authors of the textbooks, do not understand the proofs. In some instances no proofs exist, and in some instances no genuine proofs can exist, because the methods taught are demonstrably wrong.

Aware of some of the many intellectual problems that pervade work in clinical medicine, I had expected to find that the cerebral grass would be greener in the statistician's yard. To my dismay, I found many weeds being cultivated and labeled as flowers. Apart from my dissatisfactions with the absence of proofs for didactic assertions, I was disturbed by the lack of real attention to the consequences of the biologic component of "biostatistics." Here were men of high professional and intellectual competence. How could they so blithely ignore the effects of their erroneous assumptions that most clinical data came from "random samples" with "normal distributions" and "continuous variables"? How could they discuss the design of clinical experiments by extrapolating from a brewery vat or an agricultural field to a human population? How could they give so much emphasis to procedures for purely statistical analysis, while showing so little rigorous concern for such basic issues in scientific logic as specifying the fundamental question, determining whether the research would answer that question, choosing an appropriate control group, checking the reliability of the data, establishing reproducible criteria for subjective evaluations, and ascertaining whether the investigated population was both homogeneous enough for everyone to be "lumped" together and selected in a manner that justified the idea of "randomness"?

Wandering among statistical doctrines that often seemed neither mathematically validated, biologically cogent, nor intellectually challenged, I came upon Mainland's "Notes." The man seemed to know that biostatistics ought to pertain to biology, and he seemed to know about biology. He sounded like someone who had learned about research not by agglomerating theories of probability, or massaging data whose origins he had never observed, but by actually feeling a tissue, handling an animal, calibrating an instrument, looking through a microscope, or talking to a patient. An effective stimulant for the intellectual torpor of the textbooks, Mainland's "Notes" made biostatistics vivid, vital, and exciting. He brought into open view many of the critical issues that lay hidden beneath glib traditional preconceptions; he helped demonstrate that many statistical models were inappropriate and misleading for biology; and he provided a medium in which biologic scientists—insecure and anxious in their heretical suspicions about conventional statistical dogmas—could take comfort from seeing that other scientists and statisticians shared the same heresies. Here, at last, was a statistician who could talk sensibly about clinical research. (He could also sometimes talk too long, but verbosity is an accepted occupational hazard of biostatisticians. Mainland was readily forgiven for occasional ventures into prolix prose, and his successor in these columns hopes that future readers will be equally tolerant.)

Mainland was the first medical statistician I had encountered who acted as though "bio" were an integral part of "biostatistics," instead of a prefix attached casually to "statistics" for the sake of an occasional teaching exercise or a book intended for graduate students in biologic domains. Since that time, I have met a few other statisticians who have truly become biostatisticians, but Mainland remains a pioneer both in migrating in the unusual profession direction from biology to statistics, and in exemplifying the modern fusion of biology with statistics. Clinical investigators today owe him an inestimable debt of gratitude for the contributions he has made to our domain by preserving thoughtful realism in our statistical outlook. Many people believe that his book, *Elementary Medical Statistics,* could benefit from tighter organization and greater succinctness, but it is still the only such publication that gives at least as much attention to the medical issues of medical statistics as to the statistical maneuvers. As clinical investigators be-

come increasingly involved in biostatistics, and as we begin to appreciate its scope, accept its challenges, educate our statistical co-workers in its problems, and contribute creative solutions to those problems, Donald Mainland will remain one of our honored "founding fathers." He is a physician who helped establish the basic concept on which we must now build— the concept that biostatistics can best be developed neither from abstract theory in statistics nor from imprecise anecdotage in biology, but from a coordinated integration of perceptive observation and thinking in both.

In succeeding Dr. Mainland as master of ceremonies for these columns, I hope to preserve his basic outlook and philosophic standards, although I shall undoubtedly introduce some deviations of my own, because our specialized interests and training have been so different. His prestatistical domain was anatomy; mine has been clinical medicine. His basic work for almost two decades has been centered in a department of medical statistics; mine has been (and remains) centered in a department of internal medicine. He became intimately familiar with many aspects of the basic mathematical precepts of statistical tactics; my acquaintance with some of these precepts is tenuous, and I shall regularly ask my statistical colleagues for help when the discussions get into issues with which I am relatively unfamiliar. Since Dr. Mainland's packs of cards and barrels of discs have not been transmitted as a legacy of this job, I shall probably use a computer for many of the exercises in random number selection that he would have consigned to his trusty manual companions. I shall probably also call upon the computer for certain new activities that it now makes possible in modern biostatistics.

One of the main challenges will be to keep the column as least as interesting, informative, and provocative as Mainland made it. Connoisseurs of the Mainland style will recall that he often goads his readers deliberately, hoping to elicit further discussion. (Example: "I hope that . . . I have trodden on some official corns hard enough to initiate a foot-to-brain-to-hand reflex that will produce a defense of their . . . methodology."[29]) My own tactics in provocation may be somewhat different and occasionally inadvertent, but I hope to preserve the principle that all of us need vigilant prodding to avoid or destroy complacency. The pace of science and technology has become too rapid for anyone to maintain prolonged intellectual comfort about any established axioms, concepts, or other beliefs that have not been regularly subjected to intensive scrutiny and skeptical reappraisal.

To help augment the role of this column as a medium of vigorous communicative exchange and intellectual growth, I plan to invite various guests, either as proponents of their views or in rebuttal of mine, to become the "columnist" from time to time. The columns will be titled in a numbered sequence for my own papers, but a different designation will be used to accommodate other authors. I also hope that readers will frequently write to express their agreement or dissent about anything that appears here, and I would plan to have the letters (with the author's name omitted, if so desired) become a source of lively discourse in future columns. The medical statistical problems with which we struggle are too numerous and too important to be resolved without an abundance of argument. I hope that the arguments from all the people who contribute to these proceedings will be responsible, thoughtful, clearly written, and prepared in an atmosphere of light rather than heat —but arguments nonetheless.

Readers are invited not only to express opinions about what has appeared, but also to make suggestions about topics for future discussion. My ideas about choice of topics will come from several sources: (1) personal adventures during my own research activities; (2) review and occasional revival of ideas expressed pre-

viously by Dr. Mainland and by other people who have written about clinical biostatistics; (3) new stimulation from projects encountered in work at the Veterans Administration Research Support Centers, which are currently asked to help prevent or remedy biostatistical maladies in hundreds of biomedical research tasks each year; and (4) comments from readers. Those first three sources of input have already provided the topics planned for discussion in the next few columns, but the slots are open thereafter, and suggestions will be happily received.

One immediately obvious change is in the title of this column. Many leaders are "done in" by their successors, and Dr. Mainland should not have to worry about being blamed for my mistakes, misconceptions, or mischief. To give him that freedom of responsibility, and also to allow him to use "Statistical ward rounds" as a title for a possible book, the name of these essays has been changed to "Clinical biostatistics." I know that many readers will prefer the older title; the new one seems more formal, somber, and sesquipedalian, but it was the least of the available evils in nomenclature, and I hope that these new "rounds" will retain the appealing informality and free-wheeling intellectual fun of their ancestors.

● ● ●

There are more profound reasons, however, for a change that brings *clinical* into juxtaposition with *biostatistics*. In quantitative nomenclature, the *statistics* part of *biostatistics* occupies ten letters and the *bio* only three; the addition of eight *clinical* letters to the total phrase may help restore nominal as well as conceptual balance. More importantly, however, the domain of biostatistics is currently beset with many intellectual maladies that I believe can be remedied only if clinical biologists begin to make active contributions to the domain. These maladies, which arise not in the contents of statistical thinking but in the way statistical concepts are applied to other disciplines, have recently become subjects of public comment by leading statisticians:

John W. Tukey[38]—

A teacher of biochemistry does not find it intolerable to say, "I don't know." Nor does a physicist. . . . Why should not . . . statisticians do the same? . . . Far better an approximate answer to the *right* question, which is often vague, than an exact answer to the *wrong* question, which can always be made more precise.

J. G. Skellam[37]—

. . . Valuable information which affects common-sense judgments tends to be ignored when formal statistical tools are employed along conventional lines. . . . Surprisingly little attention is normally given to what is often a much more serious source of error and deception, the defects of the model itself. . . . There is an important difference of emphasis between the application of mathematics to biology, and the mathematization of biology, and it is the latter which needs the most encouragement, for it is here that the real difficulties lie. . . . I am somewhat disturbed by the thought that the exalted status of mathematics . . . might possibly . . . exercise . . . (an) unintentional brand of tyranny over other ways of thinking.

William Feller[5]—

I do not criticize statistical theory as such or the proper uses of statistics. . . . The trouble is that these methods are often used thoughtlessly and routinely by researchers for purposes for which they were not intended. . . . In biologic experimental work, for instance, a . . . common abuse is to use a statistical test to try to "prove" a hypothesis. . . . The scandal is that the "significant" results are published as though they had meaning. . . . All too frequently statisticians impose all kinds of nonsensical conditions on the poor biologist or psychologist—conditions which, although they produce unequivocal statistical results, actually hinder him in his research.

Complaints about the status quo have also come from computer experts trying to implement some of the existing mathematical approaches and models. Said R. W. Hamming[10]:

I have been repeatedly shocked to find out how often I thought I knew what I was talking about; but that in the acid test of describing explicitly to a machine what was going on I was revealed to have been both ignorant and extremely superficial. It is this many-times-repeated experience that has led me to assert that mathematics has often chosen to ignore the careful examination and exposition of the methods it uses.

Other discontents have recently been expressed by statisticians about the methods used to prepare consultants for the role they have been playing for more than 40 years, ever since R. A. Fisher's[6] epochal book made biologists begin the frequent search for statistical advice. Among the comments have been the following:

J. G. Skellam[37]—

I attribute this (undesirable) attitude largely to the way that statistics is usually taught—as a mathematical discipline of great intrinsic interest imparted to talented students who unfortunately have rarely had proper training in natural science or first hand experience of scientific research.

M. Zelen[39]—

The statistical design of experiments . . . as taught in most schools, seems so far removed from reality, that a heavy dose may be too toxic with regard to future applications. . . . It is absolutely vital that the future biometrician spend part of his training as a biometrician-in-residence at an institution or laboratory where active scientific work is being conducted.

C. P. Cox[1]—

If the discipline of statistics is to retain its identity . . . the inter-connections of statistics and research in "user" disciplines must be continually developed. . . . Besides training in statistics, an aspirant statistical consultant should receive complementary and systematized, as distinct from casually acquired, training in the disciplines in which he is expected to consult. . . . All the scientists concerned may be advantageously encouraged to scrutinize and clarify their ideas on scientific method and to challenge purely statistical inferences whenever these are unconvincing.

The direction of communication

What is surprising about all these critical comments is that they have come from statisticians rather than from clinicians or other recipients of the statistical consultations. In an era in which patients have been increasingly vocal in complaints about the services received from their clinical consultants in problems of medicine, clinicians have been notably silent in commenting on the "quality of care" in the interchange that occurs when the clinician* is a "patient" coming to a "doctor" who is a statistical consultant in problems of research.

Clinicians have had many of these consultative encounters. Courses on statistics are now offered in the curricula of most medical schools. Editors of many medical, psychologic, and other journals will routinely request that suitable manuscripts be passed by a statistical censor. Proposals for large-scale clinical trials are not only often designed by statisticians, but also must be approved by statisticians before the project is funded.

During these many interplays of statistics and medicine, however, the path of consultative enlightenment has remained unidirectional. Thus, although the manuscripts and contents of medical journals are regularly subjected to critical statistical appraisal, almost no evidence of exposure to clinical reviewers can be found in the many medically oriented papers that regularly appear in such periodicals as *Biometrics, Biometrika,* and the *Journal of the American Statistical Association.* Many critiques have been published on the unsuitable or incorrect statistical

methods used for papers that have appeared in the medical literature,[2-4, 8, 33-35] but I am not aware of any comparable critiques of the inappropriate or sometimes bizarre medical assumptions contained in papers that appear in the statistical literature. Innumerable books have been written on the general topic of elementary statistics for clinicians, but no one has written a clinical primer for statisticians.

It is time that clinicians began to widen this narrow path of communication and to inform our colleagues of the statistically pertinent knowledge that was learned during those many years in hospital wards and clinical practice. Although the statistician has spent many years in graduate school getting his Ph.D. degree, and can tell us a great deal about what he discovered during that time and afterward, the clinician has spent many years getting not only his M.D. degree, but also such additional postdoctoral "degrees" as F.A.C.P. or F.A.C.S. If clinicians need to know about the mystic statistic, statisticians might benefit from discovering the clinical pinnacle. We all have much to teach each other.

The composition of "statistics"

One of the main first steps in this process of mutual education is to recognize that "statistics" is a composite domain, containing at least two distinctly different intellectual activities: (1) the acquisition, logical organization, and numerical presentation of data, and (2) the analysis of the data to arrive at decisions about degrees of variation, interrelation, and difference. The first type of activity is often called *descriptive statistics*; it produces the collections of data that appear in baseball batting averages, in financial charts, in the birth rates and death rates of "vital statistics," and in the many graphs, tables, and other numerical expressions of biomedical projects ranging from molecular explorations to therapeutic surveys. The second type of activity,

---

*To avoid ambiguity, let me define a clinician as a member of one of the healing professions—such as medicine, osteopathy, and clinical psychology—who takes direct responsibility for the care of living patients, or who has spent substantial amounts of postgraduate time (more than an internship) in developing his skillful knowledge of such activities. The clinician may be in private practice, academic research, or administrative work, but his distinguishing characteristic is a background of observational and therapeutic experience in dealing with sick people. Although an M.D. degree is sometimes regarded as the hallmark of a clinician, many M.D's— such as anatomists, biochemists, "clinical" pathologists, epidemiologists, microbiologists, pathologists, pharmacologists, and physiologists—may have neither the training nor the functional responsibilities of clinicians. This definition is intended only to clarify what I am talking about, and has no pejorative connotations in any direction.

sometimes cited as "inferential statistics," will here be called *inductive statistics;* it is responsible for such calculations as correlation coefficients and multivariate linear regression, and it provides the P values, t tests, confidence intervals, chi square techniques, analysis of variance, and other procedures used to test "statistical significance."

Although these two activities are regularly intermingled in biostatistics, there are drastic differences in the content of each activity, and in the prerequisite background for its performance. In content, descriptive statistics deals with observations of actual substances and phenomena, classified with concepts derived from previous observations, and prepared for the sake of direct information, comparison, and application. In this real world, the descriptive statistician organizes his tabulations, histograms, averages, rates, and other numerical statements that summarize the observed facts. Inductive statistics, in contrast, is based on idealized assumptions about continuity of variables and linearity of relationships; on theoretical concepts of probability; and often on the abstract idea of taking random samples an indefinite number of times from a vast uninspected population whose distribution is deemed but not demonstrated to be "normal," and whose true "parameters" are estimated but never known. In this imaginary world, the inductive statistician develops models that are used in the world of reality to express the association of events and to quantify the contributions of chance.

In prerequisite educational background, descriptive statistics requires no particular scholastic training in "statistics" and is regularly performed by intelligent people whose main statistical skill is only the ability to keep careful records. For example, automobile drivers engage in descriptive statistics whenever they check their gasoline mileage. For complex scientific domains, such as clinical biology, the

procedures of descriptive statistics have become an integral part of the domain and are often learned concomitantly, without conscious effort, as one learns the contents of the domain. Inductive statistics, on the other hand, requires intensive deliberate study; and for most people who take courses in "statistics," the main motive is to learn the various analytic maneuvers and tests. Most elementary courses in statistics contain a brief homage to the medians, means, standard deviations, frequency polygons, and other numerical tactics of descriptive statistics, but the instructor thereafter usually concentrates on the theories of probability, inferential strategies, and various analytic procedures that are considered the major domain of the trained statistician. Thus, most 12-year-old boys in the United States could state the descriptive statistical methods for determining baseball batting averages, but few boys (or grown men) would know how to decide statistically that one player's average is significantly higher than another's.

The antipodal differences between these two types of activity—the apparent ease of learning and understanding the real world data of descriptive statistics, in contrast to the theoretical training and mathematical efforts necessary to comprehend the methods of inductive statistics— can be held responsible both for the consultative role of statisticians in modern biologic science, and also for the many intellectual failings of contemporary biostatistics. Familiar with methods of producing descriptive statistics in biology, the clinical investigator tends to disregard their importance and take them for granted. When he seeks statistical advice, he usually wants management of the analytic procedures that he does not comprehend. Unfamiliar with the basic logic and data of the descriptive medical statistics, mathematically unchallenged by their contents, and somewhat awed by the associated mystique, the statistician often accepts the clinician's request, performs the tests, and hopes the clinician will be sensible enough to ignore results that are inappropriate.

During this collaboration, both men engage in the self-delusions that create the major fallacies of biostatistics. The clinician, forgetting the importance of his own contribution to the logic and data of the research, becomes mesmerized by what he does not understand: the statistical analyses. He assumes that the statistical computations will somehow validate the more basic activities, rectifying errors in observation and correcting distorted logic. The statistician, believing that problems in the basic logic and data have already been resolved or are unresolvable, becomes oblivious to what he does not understand: the clinical background of the descriptive statistics. He accepts the data as presented, and he concentrates on the way he will fit them into his array of analytic statistical maneuvers. The ensuing results may satisfy the clinician, the statistician, the editor, the granting agency, and the reader—but what really emerges is often an elaborately analyzed "statistically significant" collection of bad logic and bad data whose scientific deficiencies are not merely neglected but actually embellished and convoluted amid the mass of numbers and statistical tests.

Let us consider a nonmedical illustration. Suppose the administrative advisor of a major league baseball team must decide what salaries should be offered to the team next year. He searches for a way of evaluating the worth of the players and chooses the batting average as a useful index. An enlightened man, he knows that chance may enter into a batter's success, and so he performs statistical analyses of the differences among players. He finds that Player A's average was higher than Player B's, with a P value of <0.001, and that Player B's average was higher than Player C's, but with a P value of only < 0.2. The first of these statistical differences is "highly significant"; the second is not. What should the advisor conclude about the relative value of these three players to the team?

The answer, of course, is that he should draw no conclusions. The statistical analysis was silly, because batting averages alone are not an appropriate test of a player's worth, no matter what the P values show. To make a really sound decision would require attention to many other features of the players and of their batting activities. How much does each player contribute to the general spirit and morale of the team? Are they "colorful" players who will lure spectators to the box office? Is B a relief pitcher who has saved many important games, whereas A is an outfielder? These and many other questions would immediately be contemplated by any connoisseur of baseball who is asked to evaluate players. The P values produced by the statistical analysis would be dismissed as unimportant, and the main judgment would depend on many items of descriptive data that are statistically omitted from the batting averages.

Suppose, however, that our administrative advisor is not a connoisseur of baseball and, in fact, does not understand the game at all. His reputation as a consultative wizard in athletics may have been based on his previous success in a sport like horse racing, where the horse's performance can always be quantitatively evaluated from such numerical indexes as time and finishing position in races. Upon asking a connoisseur of baseball for "instructive" (i.e., numerical) help about evaluating players, the advisor may be greatly disappointed to receive such nonquantitative phrases as "spirit," "colorful," and "saving games." Knowing that the analysis of dimensional information has worked so well in his previous sporting activities, the advisor decides to ignore the "soft" verbal descriptions and to base his evaluations on the "hard" numerical data of the batting averages. The owner and manager of the team may be somewhat queasy about the idea, but they go along with it and say nothing because they do not want to seem ignorant about P values, and besides, they are reluctant to doubt the word of an eminent consultant who has been widely acclaimed for his success in applying statistical analysis to athletics.

The situation just described would probably never happen in baseball. The game is too well known to too many people, and even if the owner and manager were foolish enough to entrust their evaluation of players to this type of statistical analysis, they would probably soon rescind the action because of the roars of outrage, laughter, and protest that would ensue from sportswriters and baseball fans. But the activities of biomedical research, alas, are not so well known, and counterparts of the foolishness just described constantly occur, although less obviously, in the activities of modern biostatistics.

Violations of scientific principles

The situation just cited contained violations of three elementary principles of scientific analysis: (1) the neglect of heterogeneity of a population during the process of comparing its members; (2) the use of a single property as the main index for assessing a phenomenon expressed in multiple manifestations; and (3) the application of a statistical test to prove a "significance" that may be meaningless or unimportant. These and many other departures from sound scientific reasoning constantly occur during biostatistical work because an infatuation with inductive statistics has overwhelmed a careful appraisal of the descriptive statistics. Examples of these violations are so abundant in biomedical statistics that the singling out of any specific situation would be unfair to the many outstanding candidates for selection. The illustrations here will be confined to problems that often occur in the evaluation of therapeutic trials.

1. Neglected heterogeneity. In many statistically designed trials of therapy for major chronic diseases, all the patients with that disease are regularly "lumped" together for the allocation of treatment. When the results are later reported for the total group of patients, the clinician has no way of knowing whether the compared therapeutic agents had the same effects in the good prognostic risks as in the bad, or whether patients with different degrees of clinical severity responded differently. Because heterogeneous patients have been statistically managed as homogeneous, the results of an elaborate, expensive trial may have little or no value for future clinical application.

2. Univariate responses. Since the performance of statistical tests requires that a specific index be chosen for evaluation, the response to treatment in a clinical trial is regularly expressed in terms of a single property (or "variate"), such as survival time or white blood count. When treatment is evaluated in the real world by a clinician, of course, the assessment of response is based on a multitude of properties, including the patient's pain or incapacitation and the treatment's side effects and inconvenience. These clinical properties, however, are often unattractive to a statistician because they represent subjective appraisals expressed in qualitative verbal phrases. Even if these "soft" clinical data were to be accepted for analysis, however, the importance of each property could not be easily "weighted" for combination into a single index. If the properties were not combined, and were analyzed separately as individual indexes of therapeutic response, the statistical results would contain an array of many tabulations, tests, and P values, instead of a single neat answer. The reader would have to review the reports of the diverse responses, and might have to make his own decision about which variates are important, based on clinical and biologic values, rather than statistical tests. To avoid this type of messy imprecision, the statistician opts for the neatness of analyzing a single univariate response; the investigator agrees;

and another clinical trial produces simplistic results that have little pertinence to the complex world of reality.

3. *Spurious significance.* The biostatistical malpractice committed with tests of "significance" has become, as noted earlier,[5] a scandal, and the phrase "statistical significance" has become such a malignant mental pathogen that major efforts to excise it will be undertaken here in a future discussion. Let it suffice for the moment to note that a test of statistical significance tells nothing about the quality of thought, planning, or execution in the work; nothing about the biologic or clinical meaning of the difference in numbers; and nothing about whatever has allegedly caused the difference. Too often, however, the inappropriate word *significance* has served to intoxicate a research worker with the belief that his preconceptions have been confirmed, to divert an editor or reviewer from carefully contemplating the logic and data, and to delude a reader into believing that the value, importance, and meaning of the research have somehow been authenticated because the results are "statistically significant." In the planning of clinical trials, the number of patients needed for "statistical significance" has currently become a major focus in the thoughts devoted to "design," and the calculation of this number is sometimes the acme of the biostatistician's contribution. To manipulate the α and β levels of "significance," of course, the biostatistician must often neglect the heterogeneity of the patients and must base his calculations on univariate appraisals of response—but the disregard of science and of clinical applicability seems unimportant as long as the number that emerges from the calculations holds the glittering promise of "statistical significance."

Sources of difficulty

No single simple cause can be blamed for the lamentable state of affairs that produces the cited violations and many other biostatistical infractions of scientific principles of research. The statistician is not really responsible for the difficulties. He is doing the best he can with what he knows, but he often makes the false assumption that what he does not know about the subtleties of clinical biology will be amply managed by his clinical colleagues. The clinical investigator is not really responsible, either. He has been told that his complex clinical problems will be solved by statistical help, so he gets it, but he often makes the false assumption that inductive statistical sagacity eliminates the need for interpretive clinical wisdom. The consequence of this *folie à deux* is a mutual belief that the main targets of clinicostatistical research are the rigid digits of statistical analysis, rather than the valid facts of biologic science. Instead of giving basic scientific attention to the logic and data of the research, the collaborators become obsessed with the quantitative lure of the statistics.

How can the situation be improved? The problems have obviously not been solved by statisticians' many efforts to educate clinicians. As a result of these and other efforts, clinical investigators now regularly use such statistically approved procedures as control groups, random allocations, and double-blind techniques. But the "controls" are often chosen inadequately; the random allocations are often meaningless; and the double-blind techniques often yield amaurotic results from which no one can discern what has been accomplished. Perhaps the educational efforts of the past few decades have been too unidirectional. Perhaps clinicians, instead of being purely passive recipients of statistical consultation, should now become active contributors in a process of intellectual exchange that enlightens both the statistical and clinical participants. What contribution can clinicians make to help convert statistical art into biostatistical science? Since the greatest knowledge at the clinician's disposal is his familiarity with the data and patterns of events that describe the biologic realities of nature, the clinician can teach the artful inductive statistician about the science of descriptive statistics.

Most creative mathematicians and many statisticians properly regard themselves as artists,[9] since they seek their challenges not in nature but in abstract systems or "spaces" conceived as acts of artistic imagination. The theories created in this statistical art are not a part of science unless they relate to nature, with concepts and tactics that either emerge from nature, or that are compatible with the events of nature. As discussed earlier, the statistician's customary education has given him little or no direct observational experience with which to develop his perception of these natural realities. His postgraduate activities may also not expand his scientific vision, because he may persist in playing the Procrustean role for which he was trained—a role of choosing and altering the data to fit his tests, instead of choosing or altering his tests to fit the data.

Anyone who doubts that last remark should review the taxonomic arrangement of topics in textbooks on statistics. If an investigator has a problem that requires testing the difference between two collections of nominal, ordinal, or metric data, he will be unable, with rare exception,[7, 36] to find a statistical textbook that arranges its topics according to the types of data. The topics are almost all arranged according to the available statistical tests, not according to the characteristics of the data. Thus, if the investigator already knows what test to choose for a particular problem, he can find the test. (An analogous type of backward logic occurs in the organization of many textbooks on "physical diagnosis" and other aspects of diagnostic medicine. Students often find the textbooks frustrating because they are organized according to "disease," although a student begins his diagnostic search by observing symptoms and signs.

To read about the diagnostic significance of the symptoms and signs, the student is forced to begin by knowing what diagnoses to look under.)

Since the statistician has seldom been trained or provoked to enter the natural world of scientific observation, he has really had no way of becoming familiar with the complex data and intricate logic that describe that world. He has had to rely on clinical biologists to make the observations, to arrange their logic, and to explain their significance. And we have not done so. If the statistician has built castles in the air, he is not to blame; clinicians have not only failed to put the castles on a sound foundation, but have often moved into the illusive castles and extolled the architecture.

Plans for the future

In future columns of "Clinical biostatistics," I hope we can provide some solid ground on which clinicians and statisticians can join to build a better structure for the future. If an inductively oriented statistician (or a perceptively realistic clinician) believes that *descriptive statistics* is an unsatisfactory title for this activity, let us call it something else. One of the most distinguished contemporary statisticians, John W. Tukey, has proposed an excellent new term, *data analysis.* Tukey[37] has also proposed some excellent rules and plans for the new meeting ground:

We should seek out wholly new questions to be answered. . . . We need to tackle old problems in more realistic frameworks. . . . We should seek out unfamiliar summaries of observational material, and establish their useful properties. . . . It can help, throughout this process, to admit that our first concern is with "data analysis". . . . To the extent that pieces of *mathematical statistics* fail to contribute, or are not intended to contribute, even by a long and tortuous chain, to the practice of data analysis, they must be judged as pieces of *pure* mathematics, and criticized according to its purest standards. Individual parts of mathematical statistics must look for their justification toward either data analysis or pure mathematics. Work which obeys neither master . . . cannot fail to be transient, to be doomed to sink out of sight. And we must be careful that, in its sinking, it does not take with it work of continuing value.

. . . Finally, we need to give up the vain hope that data analysis can be founded upon a logico-deductive system like Euclidean plane geometry . . . and to face up to the fact that *data analysis is intrinsically an empirical science*. . . . It will still be true that there will be aspects of data analysis well called technology, but there will also be the hallmarks of stimulating science: intellectual adventure, demanding calls upon insight, and a need to find out "how things really are" by investigation and the confrontation of insights with experience. . . . The future of data analysis . . . (depends on) our willingness to take up the rocky road of real problems in preference to the smooth road of unreal assumptions, arbitrary criteria, and abstract results without real attachment.

At our next meeting, two months from now, the topic for discussion will be the design of experiments. In this domain of experimental design, which has long been regarded as the province of inductive statistics, clinical biologists can make major contributions to the scientific future of data analysis.

References

1. Cox, C. P.: Some observations on the teaching of statistical consulting, Biometrics **24**:789-801, 1968.
2. Douglas, A. S.: Anticoagulant therapy, Philadelphia, 1962, F. A. Davis Company.
3. Feinstein, A. R.: Standards, stethoscopes, steroids and statistics. The problem of evaluating treatment in acute rheumatic fever, Pediatrics **27**:819-828, 1961.
4. Feinstein, A. R., and Spitz, H.: The epidemiology of cancer therapy. I. Clinical problems of statistical surveys, Arch. Intern. Med. **123**:171-186, 1969.
5. Feller, W.: Are life scientists overawed by statistics? Scientific Research **4**:24-29, 1969.
6. Fisher, R. A.: Statistical methods for research workers, Edinburgh, 1925, Oliver & Boyd, Ltd. (Ed. 13, 1963.)
7. Freeman, L. C.: Elementary applied statistics, New York, 1965, John Wiley & Sons, Inc.
8. Gifford, R. H., and Feinstein, A. R.: A critique of methodology in studies of anticoagulant therapy for acute myocardial infarction, New Eng. J. Med. **280**:351-357, 1969.
9. Halmos, P. R.: Mathematics as a creative art, Amer. Scientist **56**:375-389, 1968.
10. Hamming, R. W.: Numerical analysis vs. mathematics, Science **148**:473-475, 1965.
11. Hotelling, H.: The teaching of statistics, chap. 3, *in* Olkin, I., editor: Contributions to probability and statistics (Essays in honor of Harold Hotelling), Stanford, Calif., 1960, Stanford University Press.
12. Mahon, W. A., and Daniel, E. E.: A method for assessment of reports of drug trials, Canad. Med. Ass. J. **90**:565-569, 1964.
13. Mainland, D.: An uncommon abnormality of the flexor digitorum sublimis muscle, J. Anat. **62**:86-89, 1927.
14. Mainland, D.: The technique of estimating small irregular areas in biological research, with notes on the tests of accuracy, J. Anat. **63**:345-351, 1929.
15. Mainland, D.: A study of the sizes of nuclei in ovarian stroma, Anat. Rec. **48**:323-340, 1931.
16. Mainland, D.: The measurement of ferret pronuclei, Trans. Roy. Soc. Canad., 3rd series, **25**: Section V, 9 pages, 1931.
17. Mainland, D.: A quantitative study of the polar body of the ferret, with a note on the second polar spindle, Amer. J. Anat. **47**:195-240, 1931.
18. Mainland, D.: The sizes of ferret pronuclei, Anat. Rec. **49**:103-120, 1931.
19. Mainland, D.: The volumes of ferret ova, with special reference to the methods of determination, Anat. Rec. **50**:53-83, 1931.
20. Mainland, D.: The forces exerted by individual human muscles, with special reference to errors in muscle measurement, Trans. Roy. Soc. Canad., Section V, pp. 265-276, 1933.
21. Mainland, D.: Forces exerted on the human mandible by the muscles of occlusion. J. Dent. Res. **14**:107-124, 1934.
22. Mainland, D.: Chance and the blood count, Canad. Med. Ass. J. **31**:656-658, 1934. (Edit.)
23. Mainland, D.: Problems of chance in clinical work, Brit. Med. J. **2**:221-224, 1936.
24. Mainland, D.: The treatment of clinical and laboratory data: An introduction to statistical ideas and methods for medical and dental workers, Edinburgh and London, 1938, Oliver & Boyd, Ltd.
25. Mainland, D.: Elementary medical statistics: The principles of quantitative medicine, Philadelphia, 1952, W. B. Saunders Company.
26. Mainland, D.: Elementary medical statistics, ed. 2, Philadelphia, 1963, W. B. Saunders Company.
27. Mainland, D.: Anatomy as a basis for medical and dental education, New York, 1945, Paul B. Hoeber, Inc., Medical Book Division of Harper & Row, Publishers.

28. Mainland, D.: Notes from a laboratory of medical statistics. Note 20, pp. 8-9, October 24, 1961.

29. Mainland, D.: Notes from a laboratory of medical statistics. Note 104, p. 3, March 16, 1965.

30. Mainland, D.: Notes from a laboratory of medical statistics. Note 116, p. 4, May 13, 1965.

31. Mainland, D. Notes on Biometry in Medical Research. Veterans Administration Monograph 10-1, Suppl. 7, p. 1, June, 1969.

32. Mainland, D.: Statistical Ward Rounds—16, CLIN. PHARMACOL. THER. 10:576-586, 1969.

33. Saiger, G. L.: Errors of medical studies, J. A. M. A. 173:678-681, 1960.

34. Schor, S.: Statistical reviewing program for medical manuscripts, Amer. Statis. 21:28-31, 1967.

35. Schor, S., and Karten, I.: Statistical evaluation of journal manuscripts, J. A. M. A. 195:1123-1128, 1966.

36. Siegel, S.: Nonparametric statistics for the behavioral sciences, New York, 1956, Mc-Graw-Hill Book Company, Inc.

37. Skellam, J. G.: Models, inference, and strategy, Biometrics 25:457-475, 1969.

38. Tukey, J. W.: The future of data analysis, Ann. Math. Statist. 33:1-67, 1962.

39. Zelen, M.: The education of biometricians, Amer. Statis. 23:14-15, 1969.

SECTION ONE

THE ARCHITECTURE OF COHORT RESEARCH

Although most statistical interpretations of research depend on the idea of an experiment, most medical research is not experimental. The people assembled for the research are almost never chosen randomly from the groups they allegedly represent; the "causal" agents under comparison are seldom contrasted concurrently; and the agents are not assigned according to a suitable prearranged plan. Because most clinical and epidemiologic investigations are conducted as surveys, not experiments, major problems of bias or distortion can occur when the compared groups are assembled and when their results are analyzed. Even when the research is experimental, however, such problems can still appear because of flaws in chronologic aspects of design or because of vicissitudes in the action of fate during random choices or random assignments.

Although diverse mathematical models have been developed for the statistical analysis of research data, no corresponding models have been available for the scientific architecture of the research itself. The first few essays in this section are concerned with the establishment of an appropriate scientific model for showing the research structure of a cause-effect relationship. An entity in some defined baseline condition or initial state is exposed to a principal maneuver, which is the causal agent or effector. The outcome is then observed in the subsequent state. For contrast, another entity, in a similar initial state, is exposed to a comparative (or "control") maneuver.

The model is quite simple and direct, since it takes the exact form of the normal "anatomy" and "physiology" of an experiment. The model is directly applicable to any form of cohort research—whether etiologic or therapeutic, survey or experiment—in which the observed groups are followed forward in time (or "longitudinally"), being investigatively pursued in the customary scientific direction from imposition of a "cause" to occurrence of an "effect."

If the groups consist of people, however, diverse features of human and medical life can produce biases that create "pathology" in the research structure. As people traverse the pathway from anonymity at home to immortality as biostatistical units, the biases may distort the comparison of the maneuvers by altering the baseline equality of the compared groups, the performance of the maneuvers, the detection of the outcome events, or the chronologic duration of persistent observation. The act of allocating the compared maneuvers by a randomization process is often helpful, but it provides no guarantee that these difficulties will be avoided. In fact, randomized allocation can sometimes increase the problems by lulling the investigator into a state of false serenity.

All of the cited hazards of cohort research can occur when the research format is altered, so that the groups are pursued in a "cross-sectional" or "retrospective" rather than forward direction. The changes in direction, however, also introduce some separate additional problems that will be discussed in Section Two.

CHAPTER 2

Statistics versus science in the design of experiments

The design of experiments has been a favorite concern of statisticians ever since R. A. Fisher,[16] after emphasizing the importance of statistics in research, published a second book in 1935, entitled *The Design of Experiments*,[17] and stated that "a clear grasp of simple and standardized statistical procedures will . . . go far to elucidate the principles of experimentation." Fisher's book, now in its eighth edition,[18] has been followed by many other statistical texts and papers on this topic. With minimal effort, I was able to find 16 current statistical books,[1, 3-7, 15, 18, 24, 26, 28, 30, 31, 35-37] written in English, with "experimental design" or some congener in their titles. In a recent bibliographic review[23] of the topic, the authors cited about 800 items published since 1957.

After inspecting the names of these 800 publications and the tables of contents in the textbooks, a clinical investigator might wonder about the kind of knowledge necessary to plan scientific experiments dealing with sick people and human populations. The topics in the statistical texts are generally devoted to randomized blocks, Latin squares, Graeco-Latin squares, Youden squares, lattice arrangements, partial confounding, analysis of variance, analysis of covariance, and tests of "significance." The papers in the bibliographic review are classified in such groups as factorial designs, response surface designs, designs for nonlinear models, and serial designs. The books and papers are thus concerned mainly with statistical tactics in analyzing data, and little or no attention is given to such clinical biologic problems as defining the goal of the experiment, choosing the experimental material, and validating the results.

Amid the intensely statistical discussions contained in this literature on experimental design, there occasionally appears a modest scientific warning, such as "uniformity is the only requisite between the objects whose response is to be contrasted,"[20] but the warning is not accompanied by a description of scientific methods for assessing "uniformity" or appraising "response." One writer even makes the experimenter's role wholly subservient to the statistician's by stating that "the purpose of an experiment is to produce a sample of observations which will furnish estimates of the parameters of the population together with measures of the uncertainty of these estimates."[34]

Many years of exposure to these purely mathematical ideas about experimental work may have obscured the realization that for most scientists the purpose of experiments is to get answers to questions. A scientist's main concern is not the idealized elegance of a mathematical design, but a realistic plan for asking an important question in a way that will yield a reliable an-

With the same name, this chapter originally appeared as "Clinical biostatistics—II." In Clin. Pharmacol. Ther. 11:282, 1970.

swer. The object is to get scientific validity, not just statistical "significance"; and meaningful answers, not just magisterial numbers.

The designs discussed in statistical literature provide splendid examples of mathematical art in the imaginary world for which they were created. They may even be scientifically satisfactory for the agricultural fields or chemical vats in which the models have often been applied. But they do not focus on the basic problems of design in most activities of clinical biostatistics. The statistical concepts do not provide methods for attaining the documentation, precision, validity, and reproducibility that characterize scientific research; and the statistical designers have seldom had either the training or the experience needed to discern subtle scientific distinctions about human populations. Because a group of people has neither the homogeneous uniformity nor the simple responses of a field or vat, investigators cannot properly design and comprehend experiments on people merely by contemplating mathematical principles or by extrapolating statistical theories that may have worked for nonhuman material. Such scientific issues as the choice of hypothesis, appropriateness of sampling, suitability of control, selection of maneuver, stratification of prognosis, and criteria for response are critical principles of design in clinical biostatistics—but these principles are generally overlooked, neglected, or glossed over in most statistical discussions of "design."

When Sir Ronald Fisher inaugurated the campaign for statistical attention to the planning of experiments, clinical biologists needed to be persuaded that the anecdotal doctrines of the past were no longer acceptable, and that medical science required the confirmation of quantitative experiments. After more than three decades, the campaign has generally been quite successful. Clinical investigators now use control groups, randomization, and quantification in many designs of biomedical re-

search, and the medical literature contains an abundance of statistical surveys and experimental trials of therapy. Unfortunately, however, many of these projects have been designed according to abstract strategies of statistical principles, rather than realistic methods of clinical science. The control groups are often chosen improperly, and are not truly comparable; the randomization is usually performed promiscuously, with no concern for prognostic heterogeneity; and the quantification is often spurious, because the wrong variables were measured. Fisher's complaint about the clinical practices of 35 years ago was that "The liberation of the human intellect must . . . remain incomplete so long as it is free only to work out the consequences of a prescribed body of dogmatic data, and is denied the access to unsuspected truths, which only direct observation can give."[19] The pendulum has now swung far enough so that the same complaint is once again cogent, but its target today would be the dogmas of current statistical theories.

As direct observers of experimental phenomena in people, clinical investigators owe statistical colleagues an access to a methodologic description of important biologic principles that are unsuspected, ignored, or minimized in the current infatuation with statistical designs. My object in this paper is to outline the diverse structures that are considered or created in the experiments of clinical research, and to indicate some of the reasons why these structures cannot be adequately designed with current statistical models. Using these structures as a new basis for the architecture of clinical research, subsequent papers in this series will be devoted to operational principles and other details of scientific methods for the constructions.

The structure of clinical experiments

The basic structure of any experiment consists of a temporal sequence in which a preparation is exposed to a maneuver, and undergoes a response. The preparation is described according to its initial state, and the response is determined by noting the subsequent state either alone or in comparison to the initial state. For the clinical biologic experiments that will be considered here, the "preparation" is a person,* who is healthy or diseased in either the initial state, or the subsequent state, or both. The maneuver performed in the experiment can be chosen by nature, by the investigator, or by the person who acts as the experimental preparation.

In this sequence of

Initial State	Maneuver	Subsequent State
	$\longrightarrow$	

the crucial scientific issues in designing and analyzing the experiment depend on why the experiment was done, what maneuver was used, who chose the maneuver, and what was the state of the preparation before and after the maneuver.

The experiments of nature. Nature performs at least three different experiments that are of clinical interest.[9] The structure of these experiments is shown in Table I. As an ontogenetic activity, nature allows a healthy person to change as he grows older. As a pathogenetic activity, nature makes a healthy person diseased, or creates a diseased newborn. As a pathogressive activity, nature takes a diseased person through the clinical course of the disease. In most of these events, nature chooses the experimental maneuver, but in other activities, the choice is made by the affected person. Such choices occur, for example, when someone drinks polluted water, or when two people with sickle cell trait decide to marry and produce children.

These experiments of nature receive scant attention in statistical concepts of design, probably because the investigator does not choose the maneuver, and hence engages in no "experimental design." Nevertheless, these experimental activities

---

*In many activities of contemporary "clinical research," the basic material is an animal, a substance derived from a person or animal, or an inanimate system.[12] The discussion here is limited to the types of clinical research in which the "material" under surveillance is a person, or group of persons.

Table I. *The experiments of nature*

Initial state	Maneuver	Subsequent state	Type of experiment
Healthy	Normal growth	Healthy	Ontogenetic
Healthy	Development of disease	Diseased	Pathogenetic
Diseased	Clinical course of disease	Healthy, diseased, or dead	Pathogressive

of nature are constantly studied with statistical methods. Tabulations of these natural experiments are the basis for all of the birth rates, death rates, geographic distributions of disease, and other data of "vital statistics"; and for all of the statistical epidemiologic studies of causes of disease.[10] Such tabulations are also used to determine the "range of normal" for various types of clinical and laboratory data in the conditions created by nature, and to establish the diagnostic concepts for identifying diverse diseases. Moreover, statistical accounts of the clinical course of disease are the basis for the extraordinary activities, described in the next section, in which clinicians impose therapeutic intervention on the events begun by nature.

For investigating these natural phenomena, the researcher's main challenge is not to create an experimental design, but to devise a plan for discerning the design created by nature. He engages in planned observation rather than experimentation, and his activity is usually given the "passive" name of *survey*, rather than the "active" name of *trial* or *experiment*.

The experiments of man. In the observational activities just described, the investigator wants to determine what nature has done, and he accepts nature's "maneuver" as the basic force that connects the initial and subsequent state of each person who forms a statistical unit in the research. In what is usually regarded as an "experiment," however, the main maneuver is

Table II. *The interventional therapeutic experiments of man*

Initial state	Maneuver	Planned subsequent state	Type of experiment
Healthy	Prevention of disease	Healthy	Contrapathic
Diseased	Alteration of disease	Improved or cured	Remedial
Diseased	Prevention of adverse progress	Not worse	Contratrophic

chosen by man. For the activities of clinical investigation, the purpose of this maneuver can be either to change the course of nature, to explain the way nature works, or to provide better methods for collecting and interpreting the investigative data.

Interventional experiments. Clinical therapy is a unique type of experimental activity because it contains the events of two simultaneous experiments, one imposed on the other: an act of man intervening in an act of nature. The purpose of ordinary clinical therapy is to change the course of nature by preventing what nature may do, or altering what nature has already done. According to the patient's initial state and the target chosen to be altered or prevented, therapeutic activities can be classified as remedial, contrapathic, or contratrophic,[9] as shown in Table II.

In remedial treatment, such as the relief of pain, the clinician tries to modify or remove a symptom, lesion, or other target that already exists in a diseased patient. In contrapathic treatment, such as immunization against poliomyelitis, the clinician tries to prevent a healthy person from becoming diseased. In contratrophic treatment, such as rigorous regulation of diet and blood sugar for diabetes mellitus, the object is to prevent adverse progress of an established disease.

Although each act of ordinary clinical therapy contains the temporal sequence of an experiment,[8] the procedure is not usually regarded as an "experiment" because the maneuver for each patient is chosen in an arbitrary *ad hoc* manner by the attending clinician. No fixed protocol is established for the allocation of treatment within a group of individual patients, and the comparative "controls" depend on results obtained in similar situations of the past. When the results of such individual adventures in ordinary treatment are collected and analyzed, the research is called a *therapeutic survey.* Unlike the activities studied in an observational survey, routine treatment involves a maneuver of man imposed on a maneuver of nature, and the purpose of a therapeutic survey is to discern what man's intervention has done to the course of nature. When this same experimental sequence and purpose are carried out with a prearranged plan for choosing comparative groups and for allocating treatment to each patient, the activity is regarded as truly experimental and is called a therapeutic trial.

Explanatory experiments. In the therapeutic activities just described, the maneuver was planned to create a permanent change in the patient's condition. An existing initial state was to be remedied, or an expected subsequent state was to be prevented. In many other clinical experiments, however, the motive is not to change the course of nature, but to explain the way in which natural phenomena are created or altered. In such experiments, the maneuver is used as a stimulus for transient reactions that are analyzed as the "response," but the patient returns to the initial state after the experiment is completed.

PROBATIVE EXPERIMENTS. The response to an experimental maneuver is often used for identifying the patient's capacities in his initial state, or for differentiating his condition from the initial state encountered in other patients. Thus, the electrocardiographic changes after a burst of exercise will sometimes distinguish healthy people from those who have coronary artery disease; the response of serum and urine in a glucose tolerance test is often used for the diagnosis of diabetes mellitus; and various types of climatic and other physical stimuli may be employed to determine the range of physiologic response in normal people.

These procedures are an active experimental counterpart of the more passive observational activities, described earlier, that are used to determine the range of normal and diagnostic boundaries for various conditions of health and disease. Although the procedures can be called experiments, because the investigator chooses the maneuver and uses control groups, each experiment is really conducted as a "probe" to identify what was created during the antecedent "experimental" activities of nature. A design is prepared for these clinical experiments, but the basic aim of the design is to discern what happened in the original "design" prepared by nature.

MANEUVERAL EXPERIMENTS. In this type of experiment, the goal is to determine whether a particular maneuver can elicit a specified response, or to assess the effects of different degrees of the maneuver. An example of such an experiment is the attempt to induce disease by inhalation or injection of microbial substances. More characteristic examples of these experiments are the procedures performed in "phase II" therapeutic investigations for appraising the mode of action and optimal dosage of pharmaceutical agents. Unlike the probative type of explanatory experiments, which are intended to elucidate a stimulus and response created by nature, maneuveral experiments are intended to clarify the operation of an agent of man.

CONJUNCTIVE EXPERIMENTS. Certain experiments are prepared as a conjunction of one or more of the two types of experimental activities just described. For example, as the first part of the total experiment, a healthy volunteer may have malaria deliberately induced so that the second part of the experiment can be used for testing the antimalarial therapeutic properties of a new pharmaceutical agent. A combined probative and maneuveral experiment is conducted when healthy and diseased patients are exposed to varying doses of a pharmaceutical agent to determine whether the patients with different clinical states respond differently, and whether the responses depend on the doses employed in the maneuver.

Methodologic experiments. The last main type of clinical experiment is intended neither to change the course of nature nor to explain it, but rather to investigate the methods used for the other types of activities. Examples of such methodologic explorations would be a study of observer variability in the interpretation of roentgenograms, or a comparison of a patient's history obtained by a computer "interview" versus that obtained by a physician.

In such procedures, the "material" investigated in the "experiment" is the human or mechanized observational apparatus; the "maneuver" is the exposure of this "apparatus" to the film or patient; and the "response" is the roentgenographic interpretation or history that emerges from the exposure. These methodologic explorations are seldom regarded as truly experimental because they are based on "passive" observations of the phenomena used in obtaining and interpreting data, and no "active" attempt is made to probe or treat the state of the patients used in the "maneuver." Nevertheless, investigations of this type are critical prerequisites for the scientific validity of the data obtained in any other form of clinical research.

The inadequacies of statistical design

Most of these scientific structures in clinical research cannot be adequately planned with the concepts described in current statistical writings about experimental design. Randomized blocks, Latin squares, lattice arrangements, and other statistical strategems can often be used successfully in research whose scientific architecture has already been well designed. But the statistical models are not pertinent for many of the types of clinical investigation just cited, and, when pertinent, are too superficial for the fundamental demands of scientific rigor. The statistical tactics of "design" depend on the basic assumptions that the research is being performed as an experiment, that the experimental material and its responses can be reproducibly identified, that "random samples" can be readily obtained, and that "random allocations" will provide satisfactory solutions to problems in "control"—but all of these assumptions are either too naive or too erroneous for scientific design in clinical investigation.

The concept of an experiment. Statistical principles of experimental design are not pertinent for the many observational surveys, therapeutic surveys, and methodologic explorations that provide the fundamental data of clinical science. Since these surveys and explorations are neither designed nor conducted as "experiments," their intellectual construction is not considered in statistical descriptions of "experimental design."

Furthermore, for the therapeutic trials and probative experiments that can truly be regarded as experiments, statistical tactics in design are scientifically superficial because they are based on a model that is oversimplified. These clinical investigations contain the profound complexity of a simultaneous dual experiment, in which a design of man is imposed on a "design" of nature for the purpose of explaining or changing nature's activities, but the statistical models are planned to manage only one major experimental activity, not two.

Reproducible identification of material. Statistical models also begin with the assumption that the experimental material can be reproducibly identified, but this elementary necessity of science cannot be taken for granted in clinical epidemiologic research, and its achievement is one of the most difficult challenges in planning the research.

In the diverse epidemiologic surveys that depend on occurrence rates of disease at different times and places, a widespread contemporary fallacy is the belief that sta-

tistical tabulations of a disease represent that disease. What these tabulations represent, of course, is the rate of diagnosis of that disease, rather than its actual occurrence. Because "disease" is a wholly intellectual concept of nosology, and because both the nosography and diagnostic technology of disease are constantly changing, statistical enumerations of rates of "disease" cannot be scientifically satisfactory unless accompanied by a satisfactory assessment of the diagnostic procedures extant at the time and geographic locale for each item of the reported statistics.[10]

Another common fallacy in epidemiologic research based on "vital statistics" is the belief that the occurrence rate of a particular disease becomes scientifically validated if the available evidence has been reviewed to confirm the diagnosis whenever that disease was recorded on a death certificate. This type of confirmation can only eliminate "false positive" diagnoses; it does not detect the "false negative" situations in which the disease occurred without being diagnostically reported.

These errors are so ubiquitous and their scientific effects are so virulent that they cast major doubt on the validity of any of the massive epidemiologic tabulations dealing with changing rates of incidence, prevalence, and mortality for diverse diseases, and with statistical conclusions about causes of disease. The main scientific challenge in the design of this type of research is not in using statistics, but in discerning the changes created in "disease" by changes in the standards, dissemination, and application of nosologic and technologic principles of diagnosis.[10]

In surveys and trials of therapy, the clinical problems of diagnosis are different from the epidemiologic difficulties just cited. In treatment, the main diagnostic sources of variability are not the diverse techniques used to identify "disease" in different eras and geographic locales, but the diverse ways in which a particular set of techniques is applied by different physicians. Consequently, a scientific necessity in any investigation of therapy is a clear, precise statement of the criteria used for diagnosis of the disease under treatment. Despite all the recent attention given to statistical methods of therapeutic design, such criteria are frequently absent from the clinical literature. For example, adequate diagnostic criteria were omitted in 24 of 32 prominent clinicostatistical studies of anticoagulant therapy for acute myocardial infarction[22]; the pretherapeutic criteria of "operability" were described inconsistently and nonreproducibly in 26 prominent clinicostatistical reports of surgery for carcinoma of the lung.[14]

The concept of "random sampling." One of the most pernicious scientific delusions now prevalent in the world of medical research is the idea that concepts of "random sampling" can be readily applied to clinical populations. This idea is completely vitiated by the use of patients as the "material" of clinical investigation, because a patient—unlike an agricultural field, chemical vat, or the material of any other type of experimentation—chooses the investigator, rather than vice versa. Before a person can become a statistical unit in a study of disease, he must traverse a long and intricate series of directional transitions that lead him from his medical anonymity at home to his statistical inclusion in a collection of data. After nature has created the disease, the diseased person must be provoked, by symptoms or by other events, to see a doctor and to become a patient. According to the iatrotropic[8, 10] and other stimuli, the doctor may or may not suspect the existence of that disease in the patient. According to the intensity of the doctor's suspicions and his available diagnostic procedures and criteria, he may or may not be able to diagnose that disease. If the disease is suspected or diagnosed, the patient may then be referred to various other consultant doctors, who in turn may select the hospital to which he is referred for further "work-up." According to the consultants,

the hospital, the diagnostic facilities of the hospital, a variety of socioeconomic features, the presence of a suitable investigator at that hospital, and the patient's willingness to participate in both the initial plans of his doctors and the subsequent plans of the investigator, the patient may then appear as a unit of data in a statistical series.

None of these activities can possibly be regarded as "random." Each of them is strongly motivated (or biased) by the many decisions made at each transition that moved the patient from one part of the spectrum[8, 10] of the disease into another. Unless these decisions are carefully identified and classified, the statistical collection of patients with that disease will be scientifically meaningless because the results cannot be extrapolated. The patients represent no one except themselves; they are a "sample" of a larger population that cannot be specified because of the many alterations created by such determinant features as iatrotropic stimuli, fashions in medical "work-ups," diagnostic criteria, pretherapeutic criteria, the effects of coexisting diseases, the patients' acceptance of the doctors' proposals, and the chronologic "date-marks" used for tabulating statistics.[13] Nevertheless, clinicians and statisticians seldom classify or tabulate these determinant features, and persist in analyzing the statistical data with concepts based on "random sampling."

In most enumerated surveys or probative experiments designed to demonstrate the characteristics of hospitalized patients with a particular disease, these determinant features are rarely cited. Upon this scientifically defective description of the collection of patients, there is then imposed the statistical absurdity of calculating "standard errors" and "95 per cent confidence intervals" to estimate the "true parameters" of the mythical "base population" of which this polygenous collection of the disease is assumed to be a "random sample." Worse yet, a "control" group of people who do not have the disease is generally selected, by even more defective methods, from the rest of the patients in the hospital, and the "parameters" are then estimated for the mythical "base population" of the "controls."

The problem of choosing suitable control groups for this type of "retrospective" or "cross-sectional" study of etiology and pathogenesis of disease will be considered in a later paper of this series. The main point to be noted here is that if hospitalized patients with a particular disease are "random" representatives of nothing, hospitalized "controls" represent even less. Nevertheless, statistical "tests of significance" are constantly performed upon the differences of the populational "parameters" estimated in the fallacious science and bizarre mathematical imagery of these "random samples." The statistical problems of inappropriate "parametric estimations" can be avoided with nonparametric tests, quantile methods, and other suitable techniques,[2, 27, 33] but these statistical alternatives do not affect the basic scientific error of using the poorly identified "disease" and "control" groups for extrapolations to a more general population.

The concept of "random allocation." A different facet of the *random* problem occurs in allocating treatment for a therapeutic trial. In the types of research described in the previous section, the investigator wants to compare a group of diseased patients with other people who do not have the disease, and one of his main scientific problems is to ascertain that the compared groups are properly representative of the external population of diseased or nondiseased people. In a trial of treatment, however, the investigator deals only with people who have the disease. His choice of a "control" group can depend on his own maneuver in assigning therapeutic agents, rather than on nature's maneuver in creating disease. In this situation, one of the investigator's main scientific concerns is that the "control" group and the "treated" groups be selected without bias. Statistical techniques of "random alloca-

tion" seem to fulfill this requirement because they offer the opportunity to assign treatment randomly (as well as to estimate the "parameters" of the treated populations).

Unfortunately, however, in order for the therapeutic maneuver to be the main variable in the "design," the statistical concepts require that the initial experimental material be "homogeneous." This requirement cannot be achieved in the many clinical trials, particularly in chronic disease, in which the patients are extremely heterogeneous in their prognosis for whatever target is under treatment. By conducting a pathogressive "maneuver" in the outcome of disease concomitant with the clinician's maneuver in therapy, nature creates the complex dual experiment that invalidates simplistic statistical designs based on a single maneuver alone.

Unless the prognostic differences of the patients are appropriately identified and classified, the treatment will be allocated indiscriminately to "good risk" and "bad risk" cases whose basic differences are left unrecognized. This type of promiscuous randomization may remove bias in the assignment of treatment, but it also removes clinical sense in the evaluation of results. The results will be clinically meaningless because a clinician will not know how to apply them in the future; he cannot determine whether "good risk" and "poor risk" patients responded the same way to each therapeutic agent. The results may even be clinically misleading because, as discussed elsewhere,[11] agent A and agent B may have exactly the reverse therapeutic effects in "good risk" and "bad risk" patients, but the differences will be obscured when all the results are added up in a grand statistical conglomeration that ignores prognostic differences.

Aware of prognostic heterogeneity in patients, some statisticians attempt to stratify the treated population into "comparable" groups. The trouble with most of these stratifications is that the "comparable" groups are usually selected according to the demographic features of age, race, and sex, instead of the clinical and paraclinical phenomena that are harbingers of prognosis. The problems of a suitably correlated prognostic stratification have been described elsewhere[11] and are beyond the scope of the discussion here; they currently constitute one of the major scientific obstacles that impede statistical and clinical progress in the design of therapeutic trials.

Reproducible identification of response and other pertinent data. The last item to be contemplated here is a common type of statistical advice that actually hinders the clinical investigator's quest for science. Because of the concepts that underlie most statistical theories, a statistician generally likes to deal with continuous rather than categorical variables, and because of his desire for precise information, he generally prefers "hard" rather than "soft" data. A *continuous* variable—such as age, height, and serum cholesterol—can be expressed numerically as a dimension on an established scale that permits "continuous" gradations. A *categorical* variable—such as occupation, ability to work, and severity of chest pain—is expressed either as a titular name or an ordinal rank in a category that does not have continuous values on a numerical scale. "Hard" data consist of objective facts like age, sex, serum cholesterol, and death; whereas "soft" data contain subjective statements and judgments such as severity of pain and functional quality of life.

To avoid categorical expressions and subjective information, a statistician giving advice about the design of clinical surveys and trials will often concentrate on "hard" data, and particularly on data expressed in continuous variables. This choice of data seems desirable because it avoids the scientific problems of using subjective information that is unstandardized and possibly unreliable, and it avoids the statistical problems of developing suitable methods for analyzing categorical rather than continuous data. Unfortunately, however, this choice also avoids the clinical and scientific

necessity for getting meaningful results.

For the sake of this apparent scientific and statistical convenience, the data used to assess post-therapeutic response may be "hard" and continuous, but inappropriate. For example, the treatment of disabling angina pectoris is often expressed not in terms of what happened to the patient's chest pain or incapacitation, but in terms of his serum cholesterol or electrocardiographic waves; the "palliation" of cancer is usually reported according to survival time, white blood count, and roentgenographic abnormalities instead of the true palliation of the patient's discomfort, distress, and functional status.

The persistent focus on these inappropriate choices of crucial variables serves to enhance and perpetuate scientific deficiencies in clinical procedures. Clinicians could improve the quality of clinical science by preserving their attention to the important information contained in "soft data," establishing rigorous criteria for "dissecting" judgmental decisions into component parts,[8] and performing suitable studies to remove or minimize observer variability in collecting the data needed for those decisions. Instead, however, clinicians and statisticians often accept the reasoning of "clinical judgment" as a mystique that is beyond the reach of analytic science, and ignore crucial judgmental information in favor of "hard" data that may be statistically satisfying but clinically and scientifically useless.

The architecture of clinical biostatistics

Not all statisticians have become obsessed with a purely statistical approach to experimental design, and thoughtful biostatisticians have pointed out its follies[25] and dangers.[38] When experienced biostatisticians analyze the plan of a research project, they generally concentrate on judging the basic scientific principles that must be managed before any statistical theories of design can be applied. In a recent paper describing "misleading medical research," Stanley Schor[32] emphasized the need for careful statistical judgment in at least five basic prerequisites to scientific research:

Did the researcher choose the right people to question or experiment on?

Did the researcher choose a statistical unit that made his problem solvable?

Did the researcher use a control group and choose and use it properly?

Are the groups compared truly comparable?

Did the researcher guard against a probable bias in the people he was testing?

Each of these five issues as well as many of the other scientific principles cited here and elsewhere[8] are constantly mismanaged in clinical investigation, because a distinct methodologic discipline has not been established for this type of research. A clinical or epidemiologic investigator who wants advice about suitable ways to choose control groups, define statistical units, avoid bias, establish criteria, arrange comparability, and perform many of the other prerequisites to scientific research cannot find published specifications for the activities. The statistical literature contains many precise instructions for tests that quantify the operations of chance, but almost no instructions for the judgment needed to make decisions of science.

Clinical biostatistics has thus been obscured in the mystiques of two types of nondescript "judgment"—an artful clinical "judgment" whose rational characteristics are omitted from clinical publications dealing with medical science, and a scientific statistical "judgment" whose operational details are omitted from statistical publications dealing with artful design. An able clinician constantly uses clinical judgment in his investigative decisions but does not describe its components; and an able statistician engages in an analogous occultation of the statistical judgment used to plan research.

"Mathematics," said Prof. P. G. H. Gell,[21] "has now matured into a sacred cow which as often as not gets in the way of scientific traffic." The current collection of abstract statistical models for the design of experiments has not been and cannot become satisfactory for the realistic scientific architecture of clinical biostatistics.

The difficulty has been well summarized by a mathematician[29]:

A frequent cause of incompatibility between the model and reality is the neglect or confusion among influential variables or the imposition of unrealistic bounds on variables. . . . A proof within a mathematical model proves nothing in biology. . . . The choice or design of a valid mathematical model is . . . dictated by what is needed to describe the real situation. . . . This requires a well-structured imagery, based on deep knowledge and understanding of the real situation, and it is precisely here that the major influence of workers in biology must be felt. . . . My choice of the term imagery . . . was not accidental. It was chosen to connote the imaginative, interpretive, even poetic outlook which biologists must provide.

A methodologic research discipline in clinical biostatistics will require a "well-structured imagery" that represents the fusion of realistic science and poetic art. Since this fusion is better suggested by the term *architecture* than by the existing name *design*, the surveys, trials, experiments, and explorations discussed in this paper can be regarded as an outline of the structures produced in the *architecture of clinical research*. The next few papers in this series will be devoted to operational principles and other details of this biostatistical architecture.

References

1. Baird, D. C.: Experimentation: An introduction to measurement theory and experiment design, Englewood Cliffs, N. J., 1962, Prentice-Hall, Inc.
2. Bradley, J. V.: Distribution-free statistical tests, Englewood Cliffs, N. J., 1968, Prentice-Hall, Inc.
3. Chapin, F. S.: Experimental designs in sociological research, revised ed., New York, 1955, Harper & Row, Publishers.
4. Cochran, W. G., and Cox, G. M.: Experimental designs, New York, 1950, John Wiley & Sons, Inc.
5. Cox, D. R.: Planning of experiments, New York, 1958, John Wiley & Sons, Inc.
6. Edwards, A. L.: Experimental design in psychological research, ed. 3, New York, 1968, Holt, Rinehart & Winston, Inc.

7. Federer, W. T.: Experimental design, New York, 1955, The Macmillan Company.

8. Feinstein, A. R.: Clinical judgment, Baltimore, 1967, The Williams & Wilkins Company.

9. Feinstein, A. R.: Clinical epidemiology: I. The populational experiments of nature and of man in human illness, Ann. Intern. Med. **69:**807-820, 1968.

10. Feinstein, A. R.: Clinical epidemiology: II. The identification rates of disease, Ann. Intern. Med. **69:**1037-1061, 1968.

11. Feinstein, A. R.: Clinical epidemiology: III. The clinical design of statistics in therapy, Ann. Intern. Med. **69:**1287-1312, 1968.

12. Feinstein, A. R., Koss, N., and Austin, J. H. M.: The changing emphasis in clinical research. I. Topics under investigation. An analysis of the submitted abstracts and selected programs at the annual "Atlantic City Meetings" during 1953-1965, Ann. Intern. Med. **66:**396-419, 1967.

13. Feinstein, A. R., Pritchett, J. A., and Schimpff, C. R.: The epidemiology of cancer therapy. II. The clinical course: Data, decisions, and temporal demarcations, Arch. Intern. Med. **123:**323-344, 1969.

14. Feinstein, A. R., and Spitz, H.: The epidemiology of cancer therapy. I. Clinical problems of statistical surveys, Arch. Intern. Med. **123:**171-186, 1969.

15. Finney, D. J.: Experimental design and its statistical basis, Chicago, 1955, The University of Chicago Press.

16. Fisher, R. A.: Statistical methods for research workers, Edinburgh, 1925, Oliver & Boyd, Ltd.

17. Fisher, R. A.: The design of experiments, Edinburgh, 1935, Oliver & Boyd, Ltd.

18. Fisher, R. A.: The design of experiments, ed. 8, Edinburgh, 1966, Oliver & Boyd, Ltd.

19. Fisher, R. A.: The design of experiments, ed. 8, Edinburgh, 1966, Oliver & Boyd, Ltd., p. 9.

20. Fisher, R. A.: The design of experiments, ed. 8, Edinburgh, 1966, Oliver & Boyd, Ltd., p. 33.

21. Gell, P. G. H.: Research and imagination, *quoted in* Lancet **1:**273, 1969.

22. Gifford, R. H., and Feinstein, A. R.: A critique of methodology in studies of anticoagulant therapy for acute myocardial infarction, New Eng. J. Med. **280:**351-357, 1969.

23. Herzberg, A. M., and Cox, D. R.: Recent work on the design of experiments: A bibliography and a review, J. Royal Statist. Soc. (Series A) **132:**29-67, 1969.

24. Hicks, C. R.: Fundamental concepts in the design of experiments, New York, 1964, Holt, Rinehart & Winston, Inc.

25. Hogben, L.: Statistical theory; The relationship of probability, credibility and error, London, 1957, George Allen & Unwin.

26. Kempthorne, O.: The design and analysis of experiments, New York, 1952, John Wiley & Sons, Inc.

27. Mainland, D.: Elementary medical statistics, ed. 2, Philadelphia, 1963, W. B. Saunders Company.

28. Mendenhall, W.: Introduction to linear models and the design and analysis of experiments, Belmont, Calif., 1968, Wadsworth Publishing Company, Inc.

29. Nooney, G. C.: Mathematical models, reality, and results, J. Theor. Biol. **9:**239-252, 1965.

30. Peng, K. C.: The design and analysis of scientific experiments, Reading, Mass., 1967, Addison-Wesley International Division.

31. Quenouille, M. H.: The design and analysis of experiment, London, 1953, Charles Griffin & Company, Ltd.

32. Schor, S. S.: How to evaluate medical research reports, Hosp. Physician **5:**95-109, 1969.

33. Siegel, S.: Nonparametric statistics for the behavioral sciences, New York, 1956, McGraw-Hill Book Company, Inc.

34. Snedecor, G. W.: The statistical part of the scientific method, Ann. N. Y. Acad. Sci. **52:**792-799, 1950.

35. Vajda, S.: The mathematics of experimental design: Incomplete block designs and Latin squares, London, 1967, Charles Griffin & Company, Ltd.

36. Winer, B. J.: Statistical principles in experimental design, New York, 1962, McGraw-Hill Book Company, Inc.

37. Wortham, A. W., and Smith, T. E.: Practical statistics in experimental design, Dallas, 1960, Dallas Publishing House.

38. Zelen, M.: The education of biometricians, Amer. Statis. **23:**14-15, 1969.

CHAPTER 3

Components of the research objective

Because the scientific fundamentals of clinical research are omitted in most statistical discussions of the "design of experiments,"[5] a new scientific architecture must be developed as a methodologic discipline for planning clinical investigations. These investigations can be constructed in several different ways, according to the events, problems, and challenges contained in the clinical experiments of nature and of man. In the previous paper of this series,[5] I outlined those diverse investigative structures, which include the following: surveys of nature's activities in preserving health, or in creating and evolving human disease; surveys and experimental trials of man's therapeutic attempts to intervene in the course of nature; explanatory experiments that probe a maneuver of nature or delineate a maneuver of man; and exploratory efforts to assess and improve the methodology used in the foregoing research activities.

This paper and its two successors in this series are concerned with the "architectural" operations used in constructing those projects. The last of the research structures just cited—the methodologic exploration—

is arranged quite differently from the other activities and will not be considered further in this discussion, which is confined to the construction of clinical surveys and experiments.

The operational concepts that are described here are not original. They have been expressed, in whole or part, in various treatises on scientific methods of research,[1-3, 7, 9-11, 13, 14, 16, 18-20] and although given scant attention in conventional statistical texts, the principles have received extensive discussion in the first half of Donald Mainland's *Elementary Medical Statistics*.[12] My own contribution is to arrange these principles in a different way, based on the sequential events of an experiment. This sequence occurs as

$$\text{Initial State} \xrightarrow{\text{Maneuver}} \text{Subsequent State} ,$$

and its investigative architecture is designed during ten operations that are introduced or combined at various stages in the contemplation of the sequence. The first operation is outlined in this paper; the other nine operations will be outlined in the next two papers of this series; and further details of the operational structures and processes will be discussed subsequently.

This chapter originally appeared as "Clinical biostatistics— III. The architecture of clinical research." In *Clin. Pharmacol. Ther.* 11:432, 1970.

1. Objective

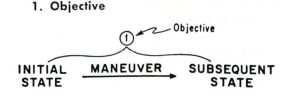

The first operational principle in planning a research project is to stipulate the objective of the research. Although this principle seems obvious, or perhaps because it is so obvious, it is often managed ineffectually in proposals or reports of clinical investigation. In meeting with a biostatistical consultant, an investigator may expansively describe the background for his proposed research, the reasons he wants to do it, and its presumptive importance, but he often does not specify the components or the logic of what he wants to do. The specifications are also often omitted when a completed project is reported in the literature. The investigator's failure to make a clear, precise statement of the objective of the research is detrimental both to the biostatistician who helps design a project, and to the reader-reviewer who later decides whether the work is worth doing or who appraises its completed results, because all of the detailed planning and analysis of the research depend on the original stipulation of the objective.

An adequate description and logic for the initial state, the maneuver, and the subsequent state of the observed population are prerequisite to both the scientific methods and the artistic taste that enter into the architecture of a research project. The scientific methods are used to achieve the investigator's objective, and the work will inevitably become misdirected or incomplete if the objective is not suitably specified. The artistic taste is needed for evaluating the general importance and worth of the research, and for making intermediary decisions during the choice of methods and procedures. This discussion is concerned mainly with logical issues in scientific method, because the issues can be readily defined and described. The many crucial roles of "artistic" judgment will be noted when they appear, but the performance of the judgments involves complexities that are beyond the scope of this discussion. Among such judgments are the "common sense" used for intermediate decisions during the architectural construction, and the basic original decision that the research project is worth doing. If we agree that the work should be done, we can then proceed to its plans.

At the onset of design for a clinical investigation, the objective is usually stated in the form of a question. "What happens," the investigator may say, "when something X is done to something Y?" In this original statement of the research question, the investigator almost always indicates the principal maneuver under surveillance, and he usually also mentions or implies the initial state of the population. Regardless of how well the question has been stated, however, it almost never contains all the details needed to implement the objective of a research project. Consequently, the first main principle of biostatistical architecture is to expand the investigator's original statement into adequate specifications of the initial state and subsequent state of the population, and to establish the necessary distinctions of the principal and subsidiary maneuvers that may be employed.

A. Initial state. The initial state of a population requires two different specifications —a diagnostic account of the existing conditions of health or disease, and a prognostic anticipation of the likelihood of achieving the subsequent state. For the illustrations that follow, let us consider a mythical new drug, Excellitol.

1. Diagnostic demarcation. Suppose an investigator asks the question, "Is Excellitol good for angina pectoris?" From the wording of this question, we do not know the initial state of the population. We cannot tell whether the purpose of the therapeutic maneuver is remedial, to relieve angina pectoris whenever the pain occurs; or contrapathic, to prevent angina in people who have never had it; or contratrophic, to prevent an adverse course of coronary artery disease in patients who have had angina.

Another unsatisfactory wording of a research question would be: "Does Excellitol retard the growth of normal children?" Aside from the later problems of defining what is meant by "retard" and "growth," this question does not indicate what kind of normality is sought in the initial state of the children. Are they to be "normal" in general physical health, or must they also be free of any mental, psychic, or biochemical abnormalities?

As the first step in architectural specifications, therefore, the initial state must be diagnostically demarcated according to the types of healthy or diseased people that are to be assembled for the investigation.

2. Prognostic stratification. In the type of problem just cited, the state of the initial population was diagnostically imprecise. A more subtle and more common difficulty occurs when an investigator asks the question, "Does Excellitol lower the fatality rate in patients with acute myocardial infarction?" In this situation, the initial diagnostic state of the population is specified and the purpose of the therapeutic maneuver is clearly noted as contratrophic, since it is intended to prevent death in diseased patients. Nevertheless, the question is imprecise because it does not specify the types of patients to be considered within the broad clinical spectrum of acute myocardial infarction.

Because of nature's underlying "maneuvers" in producing and evolving the course of a myocardial infarction, the disease has a diverse clinical spectrum of patients with major differences in their prognostic anticipations. The fatality rate, although quite low in "good-risk" patients who have had no symptoms other than transitory chest pain, is quite high in "bad-risk" patients with shock, pulmonary edema, and/or significant arrhythmias.[15, 17] Although both types of patients share the diagnosis of "acute myocardial infarction," their anticipated outcomes are so disparate that the patients are not comparable. They represent two different "experiments" instigated by nature, and they must be separated into two different groups within which therapy can be assessed.[3, 4]

The stratification performed to divide these prognostically disparate groups is thus used not to create different "factorial blocks" in the same experiment, but to establish the initial populations for different experiments, within each of which the same therapeutic maneuvers may then be imposed. Because of these distinctions, groups of patients with contrasting prognoses should not be statistically mingled in an analysis of variance as though they had "interactive variables." The "good-risk" population forms one experiment; the "bad-risk" forms another; and their statistical appraisals must be planned accordingly.

B. Subsequent state. The subsequent state of the population serves as the target of the experimental maneuver. In a survey of the ontogenetic, pathogenetic, or pathogressive activities of nature, this target represents nature's production of various states of health or disease. In a survey or trial of man's therapeutic activities, this target represents the remedial or prophylactic goal to be achieved by the treatment. In an explanatory experiment, the target is selected as a particular response to be evoked by the chosen maneuver. To plan the architecture of a clinical research project, the targets in the subsequent state must be identified, differentiated, and prognostically correlated.

1. Identification of targets. Since a person can change or react in innumerable ways while under observation, and since an investigator could not assemble detailed information about all of these possible responses, the targets of the research must be identified to denote the basic observations that are to be performed and analyzed. In all of the examples that follow, the primary target of the research maneuver is inadequately cited in the expressed question, and the reasons are noted in the associated parenthetical question:

"Is Excellitol hazardous to health?" (What kind of hazard?)

"What is the optimal dose of Excellitol?" (Optimal for what goal?)

"Is Excellitol a good analgesic agent?" (For what type of pain?)

"Is Excellitol good for angina pectoris?" (To prevent angina or to relieve it?)

In addition to a clear identification of the primary target, all of the other possible targets of the maneuver must be specified, so that suitable plans can be made for observation of the subsequent state.

2. *Differentiation of targets.* Although the maneuver of an experiment has a primary target, many other events can be studied as ancillary targets, and additional phenomena may be noted as incidental targets. For example, although the primary target of Excellitol therapy may be the relief of angina pectoris, the investigator may also want to examine such ancillary targets as the palatability of the medication, the convenience of administration, and the occurrence of symptomatic side effects. Furthermore, although Excellitol may not be expected to affect the white blood count or blood urea nitrogen, these entities may be chosen for observation to ensure that they have not incidentally received an adverse effect from the drug.

Thus, in listing all the properties that are to be observed as possible targets in the subsequent state, the investigator must differentiate the primary, ancillary, and incidental role of the targets in the research.

3. *Correlation of prognostic strata.* One of the main reasons for differentiating the targets of an investigated maneuver is to provide an appropriate correlation for performing the prognostic stratification of the initial state. Since members of the same population will have different prognoses for different targets, the selection and classification of the variables used for a particular prognostic stratification will depend upon the chosen target. Thus, the same group of healthy women might be classified in one way according to their likelihood of becoming pregnant, and in another way according to their risk of developing thrombophlebitis; similarly, in patients with acute myocardial infarction, the prognostic classifications for the duration of chest pain are different from the classifications that demarcate 30-day survival.

Because of these distinctions, a prognostic stratification cannot be designed arbitrarily according to age, race, sex, etc., and must, instead, be planned in direct correlation with the particular target under surveillance.[4] If the primary target of a particular maneuver is to prevent event A, the initial population should be stratified according to their risk of achieving event A. If a different event, B, is encountered as a "side effect" of the maneuver, the proper evaluation of the results requires that the population receive a completely separate stratification according to the risk of achieving event B.

C. Maneuver. All of the features just cited refer to a suitable identification and classification of the population before and after the maneuver. The next step in architectural design deals with the logic needed to ensure that the maneuver is suitably applied and evaluated. This logic is based on the maneuver's potency and on the comparison, multiplicity, and concurrence of additional maneuvers.

1. *Potency.* The potency of a maneuver refers to its capacity to achieve the desired target state. This capacity may depend on the dose or intensity of the maneuver, and on its manner of administration. For example, if we wish to test whether cigarette smoking causes a particular disease, what will be the acceptable quantity of cigarettes for someone to be regarded as a "smoker"? Should the classification of *nonsmoker* or *stopped-smoker* be used for a person who has not smoked for decades after having consumed a total of several packages at diverse times during adolescence? Should we distinguish cigarette smokers who "inhale" the smoke from those who do not?

A more subtle problem in potency of the maneuver deals with pharmaceutical agents—such as digitalis, aspirin, anti-coagulants, and insulin—that may require a different dosage in different people to produce the desired effect. If these agents are given at a fixed dosage to all the patients in an investigation of therapy, the clinical activity is improper because some patients will receive too much of the drug and others will receive not enough. On the other hand, if the agents are given in variable dosage, the statistical analysis may seem to be confounded by the necessity to evaluate the many different dosages of the same treatment.

An analogous type of problem arises if we want to compare surgical versus medical therapy of a particular disease, but find that each surgeon may want to perform the operative procedure in a slightly different way, according to his own particular skills and judgment. If the surgeons are denied the opportunity to employ their own minor variations in performing the operation, the general surgical procedure may not be carried out in an optimum manner by each of the individual operators.

In the first type of situation (choice of an appropriate "dose" and "inhalation" of cigarettes), there is no scientific solution for the problem. The decision must be made according to whatever seems sensible to the investigator and acceptable to the people who review the results. In the second and third type of situation (dealing with variable doses of drugs or minor modifications of a surgical procedure), the most scientifically appropriate decision is to recognize that we want to test the drug or the surgical operation at its optimal "potency"; therefore, we would choose a flexible dosage for the drug and allow individual modifications in the surgical procedure, because this flexibility provides the best way of performing the selected maneuvers. The statistical appraisals are not confounded by this decision, because our objective is to test a particular type of maneuver, rather than each of its minor variations. Accordingly, we would combine

the results of the different dosages or operative procedures, and we would regard the administered spectrum of the drug or operation as a single form of treatment that has been given in optimal "potency."

2. Comparison. When an investigation is performed for purely descriptive purposes—as for example, in surveys of the growth, development, or treatment of a state of health or disease—no comparative maneuver need be considered. Examples of research containing no comparative maneuvers are the investigations conducted to answer the following questions: "Does blood pressure increase as healthy people grow older?"; "What is the incidence of pulmonary embolism in hospitalized patients?"; and "What have been the results of cardiac transplantation?"

In many other types of clinical research, however, a comparative maneuver is employed as part of the necessary scientific logic of the experiment. We could not demonstrate, for example, that Excellitol is hazardous to health unless we had data for the comparative maneuver of not taking Excellitol. Nor could we assess the value of Excellitol in relieving angina pectoris unless some other mode of relief was compared. For many investigative situations, therefore, the complete architecture of the "maneuver" involves the choice of comparative maneuver(s) as well as the particular one under prime consideration.

The scientific logic used in choosing comparative maneuvers is a crucial feature in the design of research, and requires careful consideration of the relativity, constituents, and environment of the comparison.

A. RELATIVITY. The comparative maneuver must be specifically related to the question to be answered in the research. If the question deals with *efficacy* of the experimental maneuver, the appropriate comparison should contain essentially no maneuver or a placebo, but if the question deals with *efficiency*, the comparative procedure should contain a deliberately comparable maneuver. For example, if we want to know whether Excellitol is capable of relieving headache, its efficacy is under question, and it should be compared against a placebo; but if we want to know whether Excellitol works better than existing anti-headache preparations, its efficiency should be compared against an established agent, such as aspirin.

B. CONSTITUENTS. The internal surroundings of the main maneuver represent its "constituents." For a surgical procedure, the constituents include such features as the associated anesthesia; for a pharmaceutical agent, the constituents include the medium in which the active ingredient is conveyed; for a maneuver such as cigarette smoking, the constituents include the paper in which the tobacco is wrapped.

Since the scientific purpose of comparison is to expose the compared groups to maneuvers that are identical in every way except for the "active ingredient," the constituents of the main maneuver must be considered when its comparative maneuver is planned. For example, a sham surgical procedure is not adequately comparable to the real surgical procedure if the sham is performed with a different anesthetic agent; if Excellitol is dissolved in some special solution before being administered intravenously, the comparative placebo should also be dissolved in that same solution.

C. ENVIRONMENT. The external surroundings of the main maneuver represent its "environment." In a maneuver of clinical therapy, the environment would include: the home, hospital, or other setting in which the treatment is given; the ancillary treatment that may be employed in addition to the main maneuver; the personal efforts necessary for the patient to adhere to the treatment; and the frequency and intensity of the interchange between the doctor and patient. Thus, even if the comparative maneuver has a composition essentially identical to that of the main maneuver, the two maneuvers are not truly comparable

unless they are administered in similar environmental surroundings.

For example, one of the main roles of placebo treatment is to ensure that both patient and physician are exposed to the medicinal ritual, personal meetings, and therapeutic expectations that would not occur if the comparative maneuver were simply "no treatment" rather than a placebo. An example of inappropriate comparisons that ignored the environmental differences of ancillary therapy occurred in surveys of anticoagulant treatment for myocardial infarction.[8] The patients who received "no treatment" in the pre-anticoagulant era were usually kept at prolonged bed rest, whereas the patients who received anticoagulants also often received chair rest, early ambulation, and elastic stockings.

A more subtle problem in the analysis of environment occurs when an extraordinary personal effort is necessary for a patient to adhere to the assigned maneuver. Thus, a patient's maintenance of oral medication ordinarily creates no psychic difficulties or discomfort except for his remembering to take the medication, but adherence to an unappetizing or displeasing diet may require a heroic resolution that is seldom found in most people. When such heroic efforts are required to comply with a maneuver, the persons who are willing or able to make the special effort may have other distinct characteristics that will make their postmaneuver state different from the state of people who cannot adhere to the prescribed maneuver—but the different results in the adherers and nonadherers may then be fallaciously ascribed to the maneuver. For example, suppose it is true that life is prolonged by such "healthful" patterns of living as regular amounts of sleep and exercise, and suppose that people who are compulsive enough to adhere to an unappealing diet will also assiduously maintain "healthful" patterns of living. Now suppose we want to test whether continued use of a low-sulfate diet, although extremely distasteful, can lower mortality rates. The results of the research may show that people who maintain this diet live longer than those who do not adhere to the diet, but what may really have happened is that the compulsively "healthful" people, who would live longer anyhow, were the only persons capable of adhering to the diet over long periods of time. To avoid this problem, a strictly comparable maneuver would involve the use of an equally distasteful diet that is not low in sulfate.

3. Multiplicity. The next issue to be considered is the number of maneuvers that will be contrasted. In most research projects, the investigator wants to compare two maneuvers—a presumably active agent versus a presumably inert one, or a new agent versus an old one—but in certain types of research, more than two maneuvers are examined. Such situations occur when the investigator seeks to find a "best" or "worst" among several agents; when the experiment is performed to explain the action of a particular maneuver; or when the research project is particularly difficult to execute, so that the investigator wants it to answer as many questions as possible.

An example of the search for a best agent would be the comparison of Excellitol, aspirin, buffered aspirin, and placebo in the relief of headache; another such example would be a test of Excellitol given at five different dose levels to determine which dose produces the best results. An example in which multiple maneuvers are employed to explain a mechanism of action would be the comparison of various ingredients of Ringer's solution, given alone or in diverse combinations, to determine which of the ingredients is necessary to produce an effect noted after administration of the intact composite solution. In a large-scale cooperative study of the treatment of a chronic disease, involving many years of observation for hundreds of patients at different hospitals, the investigators might want to test several different diets and drug regimens in order to gain as much information as possible from the

efforts needed to carry out the execution of the long, complicated project.

The use of multiple maneuvers creates subtle problems in the scientific logic used for assessing the results of the comparison. If we are interested in only one subsequent target, the compared maneuvers are relatively easy to assess, no matter how many are used. This ease is due to the simplicity of ratings when only a single target is considered. Without any subtle decisions, the effect of each maneuver on the single target can be ranked as highest down to lowest, or "best" through "worst." When more than one target is under scrutiny, however, the analysis of results becomes complicated by the different ratings that each maneuver can achieve for its individual effect on the different targets.

Suppose that the primary target of our maneuver is to relieve headache, but we also intend to assess such ancillary targets as speed of relief, cost of drug, palatability of drug, and adverse side effects. If we are comparing only two drugs—Excellitol versus aspirin—we might find that Excellitol acts somewhat more rapidly and tastes somewhat better than aspirin, but costs ten times as much and has many more adverse side effects. Since neither science nor statistics provides a method for deciding which of these results is most desirable or how they counterbalance one another, we must make the decision as an act of judgment or clinical "common sense." Because only two maneuvers are involved, the judgment is not particularly difficult. We can readily compare and "weigh" the effects of the two maneuvers on each of the multiple targets, and, in this case, we might conclude that aspirin is the better agent because the increased costs and side effects of Excellitol outweigh its slight advantages in other features.

On the other hand, if the research involved a simultaneous comparison of five different antiheadache preparations rather than two, we would have much greater difficulty in making a similar judgment because each agent might rank differently for each of the four targets under consideration. In trying to make decisions that involve multiple concomitant "weighings," the standard judgmental procedures we use for "common sense" are confronted by a complexity seldom encountered in our ordinary acts of thinking, where we usually restrict our *simultaneous* comparisons to two alternatives rather than a multitude. For this reason, multiple maneuvers can be used most advantageously only when a single target is to be assessed. In large-scale clinical surveys and trials of therapy, where many different effects and side effects must be evaluated in the target state, the use of multiple maneuvers may often be unavoidable, but will greatly increase the difficulty and complexity of the subsequent analysis of data.

Another problem in multiple maneuvers arises because the comparisons may be either *equivalent* or *additive*. Equivalent maneuvers are expected to act in essentially the same way or to produce the same type of effect, and can be used as replacements for one another. Thus, in the previous example of a four-way test of Excellitol, aspirin, buffered aspirin, and placebo in the relief of headache, each of the four maneuvers might be regarded as equivalent, and the "winner" of the test would then be preferred instead of the others. On the other hand, additive maneuvers contain agents that are expected to act differently or to produce different results, so that the maneuvers may be combined. Thus, if we want to compare Excellitol versus whisky in the relief of headache, we might assume that these two agents act differently, and we might also want to assess the effects of a combination of Excellitol and whisky.

When additive maneuvers are employed, the choice of appropriate comparisons is made difficult by the need to establish a suitable comparison for each of the different maneuvers, alone or in combination. For example, in the Excellitol-whisky test that was just described, each of the following maneuvers would require consideration if all possible comparisons were to be checked:

> Excellitol alone
> Whisky alone
> Excellitol and whisky
> Excellitol and whisky placebo
> Excellitol placebo and whisky
> Excellitol placebo and whisky placebo
> Excellitol placebo only
> Whisky placebo only
> No treatment

Since the above array contains too many maneuvers for the practical realities of clinical research, the number of comparisons must be sharply reduced, and, since no rules of science or statistics are available for the reducing procedure, another act of logic is needed to choose the maneuvers that are most cogent for the specific question of interest to the investigators. If the objective is to determine which of the two agents or both is the most effective, the comparison in the above example might be reduced to:

> Excellitol and whisky
> Excellitol and whisky placebo
> Excellitol placebo and whisky

4. Concurrency. The last issue to be considered here is the concurrency of the compared maneuvers. In most experimental situations, the maneuvers are tested concurrently in people who receive the compared maneuvers during essentially the same period of time. In certain circumstances, however, the maneuvers may be administered serially. The serial situations occur in "crossover" therapeutic trials, where the same person is successively exposed to different maneuvers, or in "conditional" experiments where maneuver B will follow maneuver A provided that maneuver A has elicited a certain result. An example of a "conditional" situation is the use of preoperative radiotherapy for certain cancers: The surgery is performed afterward only if the patient has remained "operable" at the conclusion of the radiotherapy. The most common type of clinical research involving nonconcurrent maneuvers is in the "dystemporal" surveys of treatment that compare the results of a new therapeutic agent with the results obtained many years earlier in a group of patients treated with older methods.

For the scientific validity of comparison, all of these nonconcurrent maneuvers create hazards that arise not from the maneuvers, but from differences in the initial population or in the ancillary maneuvers employed at the different times when the compared maneuvers were actually administered.

A. SERIAL MANEUVERS. A "crossover" trial of therapy is based on the assumption that the patient has the same initial state each time he is exposed to the next maneuver. This assumption is seldom valid in clinical reality because of "carry-over" effects created in the target by the agents used in the previous maneuver, or because the patient's clinical state may have been changed by the preceding treatment or by the evolving course of his disease. For this reason, the various Latin, Graeco-Latin, or other "squares" that are so popular in statistical discussions of "experimental design" are frequently not applicable in clinical research. A "crossover" trial can be valid only when a long enough "wash-out" period elapses between the successive therapeutic agents, and when the patient returns to the same initial clinical state after each treatment is completed. Examples of possibly suitable populations for crossover trials are essentially healthy people who are persistently asymptomatic, or who have a predictively recurrent symptom, such as dysmenorrhea.

B. CONDITIONAL MANEUVERS. In studies of conditional maneuvers, major bias may be created by the demand that the patient attain a particular state before the second maneuver can be given. Because of this bias, the combination of two maneuvers may be given mainly to patients whose prognostic anticipations are significantly better or worse than the patients who receive only one of the two. For example, in surveys of the treatment of lung cancer, the maneuver of surgery alone may be compared against the two maneuvers of surgery followed by radiotherapy. This comparison is obviously not valid because radiotherapy is usually ordered after surgery only when the operation disclosed intrathoracic metastases. The patients without metastases are seldom given postoperative irradiation, but also have better prognoses than those who receive it. A converse example is provided by trials of preoperative irradiation for lung cancer. The patients who can go through the time required for the radiotherapy, while still keeping their tumors anatomically operable, may have slower growing cancers, and hence better prognoses, than the patients with diverse rates of growth who receive surgery immediately. A more suitable comparison for preoperative radiotherapy might be a group of patients who remain "operable" and receive surgery after a time delay equal to that consumed by radiotherapy.

C. DYSTEMPORAL MANEUVERS. When a treatment used during one period of time is compared, in a therapeutic survey, with another treatment used at a later era, the dystemporal comparison may create two different types of bias, unless the two populations exposed to the maneuvers are carefully checked for prognostic stratification and environmental effects. Because the passage of time may bring improvements both in diagnosis and in ancillary aspects of therapy, these temporal improvements, rather than the differences in the main treatment, may be responsible for the better results found in the group treated at the later date. In comparison to the earlier population, the later group may contain milder cases of the disease (with better prognoses) and may also be exposed to better methods of ancillary treatments that were disregarded in the environmental assessment. Examples of this type of dystemporal comparison were cited earlier during the discussion of therapeutic surveys of anticoagulants in myocardial infarction.[8]

• • •

In his introduction to the *Design of Ex-*

periments, Sir Ronald Fisher[6] makes the following remarks:

> The authorative assertion, "His *controls* are *totally* inadequate" must have temporarily discredited many a promising line of work. . . . This type of criticism is usually made by what I might call a heavyweight *authority* (who has) . . . prolonged experience, or at least the long possession of a scientific reputation. . . . Technical details are seldom in evidence. . . . Such an authoritarian method of judgment must surely continue, human nature being what it is, so long as theoretical notions of the principles of experimental design are lacking. . . .

Fisher's scorn for imprecise standards of criticism was unfortunately not followed by the development of technical details about the logical structure of scientific research. Although stating that "statistical procedure and experimental design are only two different aspects of the same whole," Fisher created a magnificent set of strategies for mathematical analysis of scientific experiments, but neither he nor his statistical successors established a rigorous set of principles to be used for analyzing the logic of the design.

The procedures just described for delineating the objective of a clinical research project require a thorough knowledge of clinical science rather than theoretical statistics, and the cited distinctions require much more attention than any of the subsequent operations in planning the architecture of a clinical investigation. The initial state of the population must be diagnostically demarcated and prognostically stratified; the targets of the subsequent state must be identified, differentiated, and correlated with the prognostic stratification; and the maneuver(s) must be properly chosen for potency, comparison, multiplicity, and concurrency. After these principles of scientific logic and precision have been fulfilled in specifying the objective of the research, the rest of the design can continue.

The next two papers of this series will be concerned with the nine remaining operational principles that are used to complete the basic architecture of a clinical investigation.

References

1. Beveridge, W. I. B.: The art of scientific investigation, New York, 1950, Random House, Inc.
2. Cox, K. R.: Planning clinical experiments, Springfield, Ill., 1968, Charles C Thomas, Publisher.
3. Feinstein, A. R.: Clinical judgment, Baltimore, 1967, The Williams & Wilkins Company.
4. Feinstein, A. R.: Clinical epidemiology. III. The clinical design of statistics in therapy, Ann. Intern. Med. 69:1287-1312, 1968.
5. Feinstein, A. R.: Clinical Biostatistics. II. Statistics versus science in the design of experiments, CLIN. PHARMACOL. THER. 11:282-292, 1970.
6. Fisher, R. A.: Design of experiments, ed. 8, Edinburgh, 1966, Oliver & Boyd, Ltd.
7. Freedman, P.: The principles of scientific research, London, 1949, MacDonald & Co. (Publishers), Ltd.
8. Gifford, R. H., and Feinstein, A. R.: A critique of methodology in studies of anticoagulant therapy for acute myocardial infarction, New Eng. J. Med. 280:351-357, 1969.
9. Hamilton, M.: Lectures on the methodology of clinical research, Edinburgh, 1961, E & S. Livingstone, Ltd.
10. Handy, R.: Methodology of the behavioral sciences, Springfield, Ill., 1964, Charles C Thomas, Publisher.
11. Jevons, W. S.: The principles of science, London, 1900, The Macmillan Company.
12. Mainland, D.: Elementary medical statistics, ed. 2, Philadelphia, 1963, W. B. Saunders Company.
13. Northrop, F. S. C.: The logic of the sciences and the humanities, New York, 1959, Meridian Books, Inc.
14. Plutchik, R.: Foundations of experimental research, New York, 1968, Harper & Row, Publishers.
15. Schnur, S.: Mortality and other studies questioning evidence for and value of routine anticoagulant therapy in acute myocardial infarction, Circulation 7:855-868, 1953.
16. Stone, K.: Evidence in science, Bristol, 1966, John Wright & Sons, Ltd.
17. Tillman, C.: Acute myocardial infarction: Ten-year study of consecutive cases managed and evaluated by same physician, Arch. Intern. Med. 111:77-82, 1963.
18. Wilson, E. B.: An introduction to scientific research, New York, 1952, McGraw-Hill Book Company, Inc.
19. Witts, L. J., editor: Medical surveys and clinical trials, London, 1964, Oxford University Press.
20. Wolf, A.: Essentials of scientific method, London, 1925, The Macmillan Company.

CHAPTER 4

Intake, maintenance, and identification

In the biostatistical architecture of clinical research, the first operational principle is to specify the components and choose the logic of the objective of the research. As discussed in the previous paper of this series,[11] the components consist of a sequence of *initial state, maneuver,* and *subsequent state.* The logic consists of suitable scientific judgment in the decisions made to demarcate the diagnostic and prognostic conditions of the initial state of the population; to identify, differentiate, and prognostically correlate the diverse targets of the subsequent state; and to choose maneuvers that are satisfactory in potency, comparison, multiplicity, and concurrency.

After the objective of a research project has been specified, its implementation is planned in nine subsequent architectural operations whose principles are outlined here and in the next paper of this series.

2. Intake

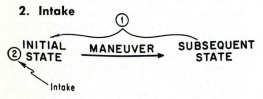

This chapter originally appeared as "Clinical biostatistics—IV. The architecture of clinical research (continued)." In Clin. Pharmacol. Ther. 3:432, 1970.

Before a group of people can be studied in a clinical investigation, each person must undergo a series of transfers that bring him from his home to his position as a unit in the research. The diverse decisions that determine the transfers can greatly alter the population available to form the "initial state." Consequently, the second operation of biostatistical architecture is to delineate the role of these decisions in providing the populational "intake" for the research. Because the people under investigation make so many of the crucial choices, the word *intake* seems more appropriate for this procedure than the conventional term, *sampling,* which does not connote the important effects of self-selection in the populational "samples" studied in clinical research.

The judgments that govern these transfers are the product of decisions made by the people who are studied, by various sources of referral, and by the investigators or their professional colleagues.

A. *Personal decisions.* The individual members of a population under investigation must make several types of personal decision before becoming units in the research.

1. Iatrotropic stimuli. The iatrotropic stimulus has been defined as the reason that a patient seeks medical attention.[5, 6] This attention must be solicited as the first step in the process that ultimately brings the patient into a research project conducted at a medical setting. The stimulus can arise from symptoms of a disease or can come from such features as anxiety over death of a friend, a pre-employment physical examination, or the incentives created by public health campaigns urging various types of "checkups." Because of differences in iatrotropic stimuli, a group of patients with the "same" disease may be found at different stages of the disease, and may therefore have different prognostic anticipations.[5]

In certain types of research projects, the motivation for the subjects' entry is not the desire to visit a doctor for specific medical attention. Instead, the subjects are solicited directly by the investigator via a mailed questionnaire or a public call for volunteers. The populational response elicited by a mailed questionnaire will be greatly affected by the recipient's attitudes toward the topic, the kinds of questions that are asked, and the difficulty or inconvenience encountered in answering the questions.[3] The composition of a group of "volunteers" may strongly depend on the monetary or other incentives offered by the investigator or on the psychic state of the potential "volunteers."[17]

2. Iatric attractions. After a person decides to become a patient, his choice of a doctor or hospital will be affected by his reactions to such features as reputation, cost, geographic location, technologic facilities, and ethnic or religious considerations. A particular doctor or hospital may therefore receive a collection of patients with the same "disease" seen by other doctors and hospitals, but the prognostic severity and other aspects of the population may be strikingly different.

3. Acceptance of proposals. After reaching medical attention, the patient may accept or reject the various referrals, diagnostic "work-ups," or therapeutic procedures that are offered to him. If he rejects one of these offers, he may receive an alternative proposal, and he must then decide about accepting the alternative.

None of these personal decisions is made randomly, and all of their effects must be carefully considered when the results of a research project are analyzed. The effects may greatly alter the initial state of the population either prognostically, confounding the assessment of the maneuvers, or diagnostically, impeding attempts to extrapolate the results or to employ statistical concepts based on "random sampling."

B. Referral decisions. The investigator is seldom the first physician to see the patients whom he studies, and the population available for research at a medical setting will have been altered by many antecedent decisions made by the investigator's medical colleagues.

1. Interiatric referrals. Just as a patient can have diverse reasons for his original choice of a medical setting, doctors or hospitals can have varied patterns of practice that lead to transfer of the patient from one doctor to another, from one hospital to another, or from one service to another within the same hospital.

In addition to these interiatric referrals, another aspect of iatric decision depends on the willingness of an attending physician to "release" his patient for entry into a therapeutic trial in which treatment for a particular disease is to be assigned by randomization. If the attending physicians at an individual medical setting are unenthusiastic about one or more of the therapeutic agents in the trial, the physicians may not allow certain types of patients to be subjected to the randomization. The collection of patients "referred" for the therapeutic trial may thus become a distorted version of the general spectrum of the disease seen in regular clinical practice.

2. Retrieval of medical records. When a survey is performed by reviewing the records of patients at a medical center, the investigator must beware of bias that can enter during the retrieval of the records from their storage locations.[10] For example, an investigator may not receive all the records he requests from the medical record librarian because some other investigator may have sequestered some of the records for a research project of his own; and the absence of those records may then create a significant bias in the population available for the first investigator's scrutiny.

Another kind of bias may arise if the investigator uses the medical record library as his only source of diagnostic retrieval. The diagnoses that are made in specialized out-patient settings (such as the emergency room, the radiotherapy and chemotherapy clinics, or even the general medical and surgical clinics) may not be recorded in the diagnostic files maintained in the library; and, in many hospitals, information about out-patients is not included among the in-patient records.[10] By confining his population to the in-patient group available from the files of a medical record library, the investigator may thus limit his spectrum of a disease to the more severe instances in which the patients required hospitalization, ignoring the many other patients who were treated in ambulatory settings by doctors in other parts of the hospital or in the community. In both of the instances just cited—sequestration of records and limitations of source—the investigator may receive a distorted picture of the patients associated with the therapeutic maneuvers in a survey of treatment for a particular disease.

C. Eligibility decisions. After the basic populational intake has been brought to the site of an investigation, a series of eligibility decisions will reduce the population to the group of people who will constitute the *initial state*. These decisions—which may be made by the investigator, by his colleagues, or by both—involve the choice of diagnostic criteria, co-morbidity criteria, and pretherapeutic criteria[8, 14] that determine a patient's eligibility for a particular activity of ordinary clinical management or of research.

1. Diagnostic criteria. A population may be greatly altered by the criteria used for diagnosis of "health" or "disease." For example, if protracted chest pain is demanded as a criterion for "acute myocardial infarction," the population will exclude patients who had only milder forms of thoracic pain or more severely ill patients whose infarction was manifested only by sudden onset of arrhythmias or congestive heart failure.

Outside of a medical setting, the population may have reached the investigator directly by "volunteering" for a project or by answering a questionnaire. Nevertheless, the investigator must still decide which questionnaires or volunteers will be used for the research. He may exclude questionnaires that have been smudged or filled out improperly, or he may reject volunteers who seem unattractive in appearance or in personality. He must then be concerned about the way that these selections have altered the population that becomes the group of research subjects.

2. Co-morbidity criteria. The presence of major associated diseases may create problems in establishing diagnosis for a particular disease[14] and in choosing or excluding patients for therapy. If too many co-morbid patients are excluded from an investigation, the resultant "pure" population with the main disease may not represent the true state of that disease in clinical reality. In a study of therapy, co-morbid diseases may have major prognostic effects that create unrecognized sources of bias in the post-therapeutic results.

3. Pretherapeutic criteria. In addition to co-morbidity, other kinds of pretherapeutic criteria may be used to include or exclude patients from an investigation of therapy. These criteria may depend on such features as age, economic and geographic status, and severity or extent of the main disease under treatment.

For example, in order to be regarded as having "operable cancer," a patient must have *suitable* diagnostic evidence of the disease; he must be free of associated co-morbid ailments that might *impair* his tolerance of the operative procedure or his subsequent survival; and the cancer must be *appropriately* localized in an anatomic position that permits resection. Thus, the collection of two groups of patients with "operable cancer" can vary greatly according to the criteria chosen to define the concepts of "suitable" diagnostic evidence, "impairing" co-morbid ailments, and "appropriate" anatomic localization. Moreover, a patient with "inoperable" cancer may be "inoperable" because he refused a proposed operative resection, or because the physician decided that the tumor was unresectable, or because death occurred before any of these decisions could be made. Since these three kinds of "inoperable" patients have major differences in prognostic anticipation,[4] they cannot be regarded as comparable in their initial state.

An additional problem in pretherapeutic criteria—particularly in long-term trials—is the investigator's frequent decision to restrict admission to "compliant" people who appear particularly likely to maintain the assigned maneuver and to continue under investigation. The absence of the "noncompliant" candidates, however, may create a serious bias in the spectrum of the observed disease.

As a result of these diverse decisions by patients and doctors about iatrotropy, acceptance of proposals, iatric referrals, eligibility, and other transfer mechanisms, two groups of people who apparently have the same "initial state" may differ in many characteristics that can greatly affect the outcome in the subsequent state. Major differences in people with an apparently similar initial state may thus arise if the medical setting is urban or rural, large or small, American or British. Within the same academic hospital center, great diversities may exist in populations chosen from private or ward services, surgical or medical services, and "university" or "VA" services. A population that is not at a medical setting may be significantly altered by its selection through replies to a mailed questionnaire rather than through personal interviews.

The neglect of populational bias caused by these transfer decisions is one of the main sources of nonreproducible data and defective scientific logic in contemporary biostatistics.

3. Maintenance

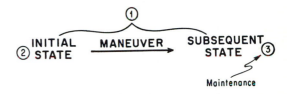

The next step in planning a research project is to decide about the methods that will be used to maintain the population long enough for the subsequent state to occur and to be observed. When the objective of a research project is specified, the investigator creates the concepts that determine whether the project is worth doing; when the maintenance of the population is contemplated, the investigator determines whether the project is feasible and can be carried out. The ability to maintain the population is particularly important in research dealing with the cause, course, or treatment of chronic disease, since a long time may elapse between the initial and subsequent states. No matter how well the rest of the research project is planned, the plans may be wasted if the population cannot be adequately preserved and examined.

Many different issues in maintenance* must be considered: duration and frequency of examinations; opportunity for detection of target; adherence to maneuvers; and preservation of protocol, data, and investigators.

A. *Duration and frequency of examinations.* Members of an investigated popula-

---

*The complex issues of *ethics* in clinical research are beyond the scope of this outline.

tion must be encouraged to remain in the project for a duration suitable for the conditions and maneuvers under investigation. For example, a much longer duration of observation will usually be required when the maneuver provides treatment for a cancer than for the common cold. The encouragement to a patient's continued participation, particularly in a long-term study, will depend on many aspects of the interchange among patient, doctor, and investigative setting. For example, to achieve persistent attendance of patients at a clinic, the investigator may need to make many special arrangements for such features as efficiency of staff, location and timing of clinics, and transportation of patients.

The frequency of examination will also depend on the circumstances of the investigation. Routine periodic examinations may be needed to obtain evidence about phenomena that would be missed if not sought often enough. For example, if one of the main targets in the subsequent state is the occurrence of a streptococcal infection, the patient may need to be examined at monthly or bimonthly intervals for the performance of suitable tests. On the other hand, monthly observations would not be needed to determine the occurrence of death.

Other important reasons for periodic examinations are the regulation of medications (when appropriate), the preservation of the patient's interest and morale, and the maintenance of communication to learn about incidental events and changes in the patient's clinical or geographic status. In experiments conducted by double-blind techniques (in which neither the patient nor the examining physician knows the identity of the maneuver), a "fail-safe" procedure must be established for the potential occurrence of disastrous clinical events. The procedure should include suitable arrangements for learning the identity of the maneuver in emergency situations, for discontinuing or modifying maneuvers that have led to major adversities, and for

instituting appropriate types of ancillary or replacement therapy.

B. Opportunity for detection of target. If the "target" in the subsequent state is the development of an event that was not present in the initial state, the compared populations should have equal opportunities for that target to be detected when it occurs. The opportunities will be equal if all the people exposed to the different maneuvers are also exposed to the same thoroughness and frequency of subsequent examinations, but inequalities will commonly be produced by various characteristics of the initial state, the maneuver, or the target. The subsequent comparison of data may then be fallacious because different conditions of observation made the target more likely to be detected in one group of people than in another.

One obvious source of such disparities is the population's access to medical examination. People who can see doctors easily and conveniently may appear to have higher rates of minor or even major diseases than people for whom medical supervision is less prevalent. Once a treatment has been suspected of causing adverse side effects, the occurrence rate of those effects may increase spuriously because they are sought with increased attention in people receiving the treatment. The patients themselves may become fearful, so that they solicit medical attention more often and for lesser reasons than usual, or the doctors may become particularly diligent about detecting the side effects. For example, the high rate of phlebitis found in nurses (with or without "the pill") may merely reflect their propensity both to note the condition and to seek medical attention for it.

A second cause of difficulty arises when a maneuver itself requires techniques of administration or observation that differ from the procedures used in maintaining another maneuver. For example, patients receiving long-term anticoagulants must receive periodic examinations for the dosage of anticoagulants to be regulated, and at these examinations, the physician also has the opportunity to detect minor intercurrent illnesses. The subsequent rate of such illnesses may then be falsely higher in the anticoagulant group than in a "placebo" or untreated group who did not receive equally frequent examinations.

Another source of disparity is the population's access to medical technology. If certain technologic procedures (such as electrocardiography, roentgenography, and laboratory tests) are more consistently available for one population than for another, the two populations will have different rates of identification for diseases whose diagnoses require these technologic procedures for confirmation or exclusion. For example, facilities for prompt, inexpensive identification of streptococcal infections have recently been made available to practitioners by the health departments of several states. The rates of streptococcal infection in those states have subsequently soared. Similarly, a major "epidemic" of lupus erythematosus has occurred in the past two decades after the introduction of effective laboratory tests for identifying the disease.

The last source of disparity to be noted here is the performance of routine "screening" examinations in the two populations. The rates of disease in a certain region of the body for two populations will inevitably differ if one population has that region examined only when appropriate symptoms appear, whereas the other population receives routine periodic examinations regardless of symptoms.

The neglect of these problems has been a major source of intellectual blunders in contemporary biostatistics, and has greatly impaired the validity of many epidemiologic surveys of the occurrence rates and therapy of disease. Berkson[2] has demonstrated the statistical fallacies of studying the rates of concomitant diseases in hospital populations, but egregious statistical fallacies are just as likely to occur for single diseases in non-hospital populations with unequal opportunities for detection of target. Some of the fallacies can be illustrated as follows:

1. If women receiving contraceptive pills are examined more closely or more often than women who use mechanical types of contraception, the "pill" group may have a rate of subsequent thrombophlebitis or cervical cancer that is spuriously higher than the rate found in the "controls," whose medical state was not checked with equally careful attention.

2. The executive personnel in an industrial population may be found to have a higher rate of coronary artery disease than the laborers, but the difference may not be due to any characteristics inherent in the executives. They may have been subjected to routine cardiac "screening" examinations that enabled all of their symptomatic and asymptomatic coronary disease to be diagnosed before death, whereas much of asymptomatic coronary disease in the "unscreened" laborers may not have been detected during life.

3. In comparison to people who have not had chronic constipation, people with this symptom are more likely both to have used suppositories and to have received barium enema examinations. If an epidemiologic statistician discovers that suppository users have a higher rate of colonic polyps than non–suppository users, he may then regard the suppositories as a probable cause for the polyps, with no attention given to the unequal exposure of the two populations to the barium enemas needed for detecting the polyps.

4. A different variant of this problem occurs in epidemiologic research in which the subsequent state is described by entries on a death certificate. If the development of disease X is under survey, the investigators will often check the patient's premortem data to eliminate false positive diagnoses of disease X, but the false negative side of the diagnostic issue is almost never explored to see whether disease X might have occurred without being listed on the death certificate.[7] In this way, many epidemiologic studies based on death certificate diagnoses of arteriosclerosis or cancer provide inaccurate results that differ significantly from the data found by necropsy or by thorough methods of premortem examination.

5. To illustrate misleading therapeutic results produced by a maneuver's distortion of equal opportunities for target detection, consider the following example. Suppose we want to test the hypothesis that large daily doses of aspirin will be useful prophylaxis for preventing streptococcal infections, and suppose our method of detecting the infections is to perform a throat culture whenever a febrile illness occurs. In this experimental situation, with these techniques of target detection, the "treated" group, which has its fever suppressed by the aspirin, will have a much lower

rate of streptococcal detection than the untreated "controls," and we might then falsely conclude that aspirin is an effective antistreptococcal agent.

6. A final example of "detectional bias" occurs in a situation, quite different from those just cited, in which detection of the target creates an additional clinical hazard for one populational group but not for the other. Suppose we are testing medical therapy versus vascular-implant surgery for coronary artery disease. Both groups of patients receive coronary arteriography to delineate their initial state, but the surgical group later receives repeat arteriograms to test the patency of the coronary vasculature after the operation. The morbidity and mortality rates associated with the second arteriographic procedure for the surgical group create an additional investigative hazard that is not present in the medically treated patients. Either the experimental plan or the subsequent analysis would require suitable modifications to avoid the bias thus imposed, after the main experimental maneuver, on the patients treated surgically.

C. Adherence to maneuvers. When an oral drug, diet, or other activity (such as exercise) is to be maintained by the patient at home, away from the site of the investigation, the patient must be encouraged to adhere to the assigned maneuver. Moreover, regardless of whether the maneuver was assigned by the investigator or chosen by the patient, the assessment of the patient's adherence to the maneuver is a critical feature of the subsequent evaluation, and depends on suitable information about adherence, obtained by means of direct questions to the patient or with more objective procedures. The evaluation of such data will be discussed at a later stage of the architecture.

D. Preservation of protocol, data, and investigators. When a long period elapses between the maneuver and the subsequent state, or when many examinations, patients, and investigators are involved in a research project, the principal investigator must establish satisfactory methods for ascertaining that the research protocol is properly carried out by the diverse participants, for coordinating the collection and analysis of data, and for suitable replacement of collaborating investigators who have discontinued participation in the

project or who participate ineffectually. These issues have been thoroughly discussed by Mainland[18] and will not be further considered here.

4. Initial identification

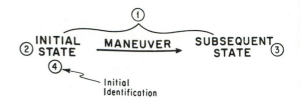

Identification is a core problem in scientific research. Unless the entities under investigation have been suitably identified, the work cannot be reproduced; the data cannot be assessed; the results cannot be validated. In clinical research, the problems of identification are much greater than in any other form of investigation, because the clinician must cope with many human attributes that are not encountered in animals, animate fragments, or inanimate substances.[5] These human attributes are not only different from the isolated variables studied in nonclinical research; they are also much more abundant and they must be assessed before, during, and after the experimental maneuver. Despite these distinctions in identification, most traditional discussions of "experimental design" contain little or no attention to the problems of choosing, observing, and classifying the basic evidence.

The identification stage of research architecture is intended to provide implementation for the ideas expressed in the objective of the project. All of the general concepts that described the objective of the research, and the intake and maintenance of the population, must now be expressed operationally in terms of the observed evidence. For example, the diagnostic and prognostic requirements of the population may have been stated in such categorical phrases as "healthy," "anemic," "angina pectoris," or "good risk," but none of these phrases indicates the actual items of evidence that will be examined and interpreted.

A. Types of evidence. Each property (or "variable") to be used in an investigation depends on the observation of certain basic evidence. Thus, the presence of anemia may be assessed from measurements of blood hemoglobin or hematocrit; the presence of angina pectoris may be noted from history taking; and anatomic metastases of a cancer may be sought with clinical examination, roentgenography, endoscopy, biopsy, cytology, surgical exploration, or necropsy. The characteristics of the basic evidence in an investigation must be thoughtfully considered, because the quality of the raw data can not only affect the elemental facts but also distort the variables chosen to represent the elemental facts.

The raw data obtained in a clinical investigation can be verbal or numerical. Thus, a particular person can be described verbally as a *red-haired American laborer with chest pain,* and numerically as *68 inches tall,* and *the father of 4 children,* with a *serum cholesterol of 260 mg. per cent.* Regardless of whether the basic evidence is verbal or numerical, the term "hard" is often applied to data—for such variables as age, sex, weight, serum cholesterol, and death—whose observation and interpretation require few or no subjective judgments. The term "soft" is often applied to data—such as statements about the existence of angina pectoris, severity of dyspnea, or ability to work—that require many subjective activities in observation and interpretation. Since hard data are obviously more reliable than soft data, the clinico-statistical collaborators who design a research project will usually prefer, whenever possible, to work with hard data as the main source of evidence.

B. Types of variables. The raw data of an investigation can be preserved intact or converted into the values for four different types of variables. A *metric* variable is expressed in dimensionally ranked values that have measurably equal inter-

vals between adjacent ranks. Examples of such values are *0, 1, 2, 3 . . .* for number of children, and *. . . 67, 68, 69, 70 . . .* for inches of height.

The other three types of variables are expressed with categorical rather than dimensional values. An *ordinal* variable has semiquantitative values that can be ranked in a graded order, but the intervals between any two adjacent ranks are not measurably equal. Examples of such values are *0, 1+, 2+, 3+,* and *4+* for briskness of reflexes, and *none, mild, moderate,* and *severe* for severity of dyspnea. A *nominal* variable has values that cannot be ranked in a graded order. Examples of such values are *red* for color of hair, *American* for nationality, and *laborer* for occupation. For an *existential* variable, the scale of values consists of *present* and *absent,* or *yes* and *no.* Examples of existential variables are *presence of chest pain* and *survival for at least 6 months.* The values for existential variables can sometimes be semiordered in a scale such as *definitely absent, probably absent, uncertain, probably present,* and *definitely present.*

The procedures used for converting raw data into values for these different types of variables have been described elsewhere.[12]

C. Selection of indexes. From the diverse data collected in an investigation, certain variables or combinations of variables may be used as indexes to delineate particularly important properties in the research. These are the properties used for any of the graphs, tabulations, or other decisions in the "admission" of people to the project, or in the analysis of results. Although the investigators may have assembled information about a great many variables, the *index* variables are the ones that actually become used in including or excluding people from the project and in the appraisal of the data. Thus, data for such topics as *name, address, occupation, height,* and *serum calcium value* might have been obtained during the research, but might never be used thereafter in the subsequent analyses, whereas information about such topics as *existence of disease X, severity of cardiac decompensation, prognostic risk,* and *serum cholesterol value* might become index variables.

As the "key" data from which critical investigative conclusions will be drawn, the index variables require careful selection.

1. Form of expression: Dimensional versus categorical. Despite the mathematical appeal of dimensional data, many variables may become scientifically or clinically more meaningful when their numerical values are converted into categorical expressions. For example, although a person's hematocrit can be measured quantitatively, the result is often more meaningful when stated in one of the ordinal categories: *anemic, normal,* or *polycythemic.* Similarly, such measurements as temperature, serum cholesterol, and streptococcal antibody titer are often best classified not in their original dimensions but in the converted ordinal categories of *high, normal,* and *low.*

The conversion of dimensions to categories may be particularly valuable for assessing the importance or meaning of a change in a variable. For example, suppose "statistical significance" has been noted for the comparison of an average decrement of 5 in one group of patients, with an average of 2 in the other group. Regardless of the "statistical significance," this difference would not be meaningful clinically if the changes were "falls" of 5 mm. per hour and 2 mm. per hour from an initial Westergren sedimentation rate that averaged 180 mm. per hour in both groups. In this situation, the common sense judgment would depend on the categorical decision that both 5 mm. per hour and 2 mm. per hour were too small a change for the transition to be regarded as a significant *fall.* In many analogous situations, categorical distinctions are invaluable for making decisions about whether a "statistically significant" difference is clinically meaningful.

*2. Chronologic components: Unitempo-*ral *versus multitemporal.* The value used for an index variable at a particular single state in time may be chosen from one or more temporal values. A unitemporal index is based on the patient's state at a single point in time, whereas a multitemporal index involves consideration of more than one temporal state.

For example, before administering an agent intended to lower blood pressure, we might obtain a series of "base-line" or "control" values by measuring the patient's blood pressure daily for two weeks. When we later analyzed the patient's response to the antihypertensive agent, we would use a unitemporal index for the initial state of blood pressure if the value depended only on a single reading just before the therapeutic agent was given; and the index would be multitemporal if the single value for initial state depended on a mean, median, or mode of the two-week series of "base-line" readings. Furthermore, if the values in the base-line series were initially high and then fell to a "plateau" just before the onset of therapy, we would have to decide whether to choose the initial state index from all of the base-line readings, or only from those contained in the "plateau." The way this choice is made might have major effects on the magnitude of the blood pressure available for "lowering" by the therapeutic agent.

Another type of multitemporal index consists of a sum of units rather than an average of measurements. Thus, as an index of response to pharmaceutical treatment of angina pectoris, we might count the total number of episodes of angina or the number of nitroglycerine tablets consumed during the period of treatment.

If the index consists of a discrete event, rather than a measurement, the investigator may need to distinguish repetitive or persistent events from those that are single or sporadic. For example, in their initial state before treatment of primary lung cancer, two patients may both have had hemoptysis that first occurred three months previously, but one patient may have had a single episode of hemoptysis, with no repetition, whereas the other may have had recurrent daily episodes. Similarly, a patient who had a severe bout of chest pain that lasted for one day, two weeks previously, is different from a patient whose chest pain has persisted unchanged for two weeks, but the difference would not be stipulated if the index variable were expressed merely as *existence of chest pain during present illness.*

3. *Number of constituents: Elemental versus composite.* An elemental index is based on a single variable in the investigation, whereas a composite index contains data from two or more variables. A particular index may be elemental or composite according to the types of variables used for its creation. For example, *severity of dyspnea* would be an elemental index if based on a single "global" assessment of dyspnea, and composite if it includes specific contributions from such variables as the metric *respiratory rate,* the existential *presence of orthopnea,* and the ordinal *amount of exertion needed to produce respiratory distress.*

For reproducibility of results, an index that contains many constituents should be prepared in a specifically composite manner, so that each constituent can be identified. If an index with many complex ingredients is derived in an elemental manner, as a global act of "judgment," the procedure cannot be reproducible, because the ingredients will not be stipulated. Thus, as a single variable, *existence of thromboembolic phenomenon* can be rated as *present* or *absent,* but the ingredients of the rating will depend on the presence or absence of such constituent variables as pain in leg, circumference of calf, hemoptysis, and roentgenographic abnormalities. If *thromboembolic phenomenon* were to be used as an index variable, its existence would require definition with specific diagnostic criteria established for the appraisal of the constituent evidence.

4. *Form of aggregation: Boolean clusters versus additive scores.* The constituents of a composite index can be aggregated in at least two different ways. A "Boolean cluster" consists of a group of individual categories that are present or absent together in various combinations. For example, the condition of a patient with acute myocardial infarction could be called *good,* if he has neither shock nor pulmonary edema; *fair,* if he has one of these complications but not both; and *poor,* if he has both. An "additive score" is prepared by assigning an arbitrary score (or "weight") to each constituent variable; and the value of the composite index is the sum of these scores. For example, dyspnea might be given 20 points, and tachycardia, peripheral edema, or a large liver, might each be given 10 points, so that a patient who has all four of these manifestations would receive a score of 50 points.

The two methods of aggregation are as different as logic and arithmetic. In the "Boolean cluster" procedure, the categories of each constituent variable are either present or absent, and the values of the index itself are chosen as arbitrary names for simultaneous combinations of categories. In the "additive score" procedure, each category is assigned an arbitrary dimensional value, and the index is the sum of those values. Both the Boolean and the additive techniques may sometimes be combined in a single index. For example, to fulfill the modified Jones criteria[1] for diagnosis of rheumatic fever, a patient is required to have a combination of "major" and "minor" features. The combination is satisfied by any two features of the "major" group together with one of the "minor" features, or vice versa.

5. *Degree of artifice: Natural versus contrived.* The collection of variables in a composite index is "natural" if the variables have a reasonably homogeneous frame of physiologic or clinical reference, and are ordinarily joined in clinical reasoning. Thus, in an earlier example, the index for thromboembolic phenomenon was based on a

natural combination of variables, such as symptoms and physical signs in the legs and chest. On the other hand, if we established a "thromboembolism index" that included such features as age, height, weight, serum sodium, serum potassium, and prothrombin time, as well as the features already cited, the new index would be contrived, because its heterogeneous components do not have a common physiologic frame of reference. They are not combined in ordinary clinical reasoning, and their conjunction in the index was purely arbitrary.

Some of the problems of heterogeneously contrived indexes have been discussed by Mainland.[19] One of the main problems of such contrivances is that diverse entities may be combined in a manner that makes the individual entities unrecognizable, particularly when the indexes are used to assess responses to an experimental maneuver. Thus, in some of the contrived indexes used in rheumatoid arthritis,[16] a patient who has a major improvement in joint symptoms while his sedimentation rate remains persistently elevated could not be distinguished from a patient who remains physically incapacitated while his sedimentation rate declines. A heterogeneous contrived index may sometimes be highly effective for purposes of diagnostic identification, although it may not be applicable to the evaluation of therapy and may obscure the diagnostic constituents. For example, the Jones criteria have provided a highly successful heterogeneous contrived index for the diagnosis of rheumatic fever.[1] The criteria cannot be used, however, for assessing a patient's response to treatment, and moreover, after learning that a patient fulfills these criteria, a physician would not know whether the patient had congestive heart failure alone, chorea alone, or only arthritis.

Two other types of contrived indexes, created in a somewhat less arbitrary and less heterogeneous manner, are commonly used in clinical research. A *homologous index* is one in which the main variable that is to be assessed is deliberately replaced by a second variable with which the main one appears to be correlated. For example, the hematocrit measurement might replace the hemoglobin value, or the thyroid uptake of radioactive iodine might replace the measurement of serum protein-bound iodine. A *substantive index* is a test or score created to give substantive identification to an intellectual concept that does not have a tangible identity. The various psychologic tests for intelligence or anxiety are examples of substantive indexes. Another example is the use of central venous pressure as an index of congestive heart failure.

6. Application of indexes. The single variables or complex combinations that are used as indexes can be employed at many different stages of investigative architecture. In the stage under general consideration here, the indexes are used for identifying the initial state of the population, and they provide the data for such necessities of research as diagnostic criteria, prognostic strata, and eligibility requirements. At later stages of the research architecture, other indexes will be used to identify targets in the subsequent state, and transitions from the initial to the subsequent state.

D. Displacement of Objective. Perhaps the greatest intellectual hazard in choosing indexes for a research project is that the investigator may displace the objective of the research. He may elect to use indexes for phenomena that are scientifically attractive because they can be assessed easily and reliably, but the selected phenomena may not accurately indicate the original goals of the research.

For example, suppose we wanted to study the effect of Excellitol in improving the respiratory distress of patients with chronic pulmonary disease. One of the variables we would want to identify in the initial state is *severity of dyspnea*, but its rating depends on a patient's subjective perception of dyspnea and on a doctor's subjective classification of degrees of severity. Because of this double "softness" in the data, we might decide to replace *severity of dyspnea* with "harder" information, such as the patient's *timed vital capacity*. We have now achieved a more "reliable" measurement, but we have also displaced the phenomenon we wanted to assess. Although a good general correlation may exist between *severity of dyspnea* and *timed vital capacity*, an individual patient's ad hoc performance on a test of vital capacity does not necessarily reflect the respiratory distress he experiences outside the laboratory in the conditions of his daily life.

1. Reliability versus relevance. Analogous displacements of the objective occur when an investigator, while giving treatment to prevent vascular complications of diabetes mellitus, studies change in glucose tolerance test or mortality rate, instead of clinical evidence of vascular complications; or when the relief of angina pectoris is assessed from serum cholesterol, electrocardiographic evidence, or arteriographic evidence, but not from an evaluation of the clinical severity of the angina. The displacements may increase the reliability of the indexes used in the investigation, but they may also displace the objective so greatly that the results do not answer the main question that was the reason for doing the research. These tactics in index displacement are the source of the "substitution game" that Yerushalmy[20] has so forcefully indicted in modern biostatistics.

The problem of reliability versus relevance of data is a constant cause of inadequate design in clinical investigation, and the problem occurs in choosing variables that define not only the initial state of the population but also (as noted later) the targets of the subsequent state. When the quest for science makes the designers displace critically important data with data that are more reliable but less cogent, the research project may emerge with the right answers to the wrong questions. The solution to this problem is not to continue

rejecting crucial soft data, but to "harden" the soft data. When the variables that are necessary to a well-designed investigation are based on soft data, an additional aspect of proper design for the research is the development of better methods of observation and classification to improve the reliability of the essential data.

2. Validation of contrived indexes. In the examples just cited, the indexes chosen for assessment of a particular entity were displaced into another, obviously different entity. The solution to this problem is simple, and requires only that appropriate attention be given to the correct entity. When a contrived index contains a motley mixture of heterogeneous elements, it can be "decomposed" into a series of separate indexes that are individually homogeneous and meaningful. In other circumstances, however, a contrived index that seems plausibly or directly related to the desired entity may be acceptable if its effectiveness has been validated by thoughtful judgment or by actual data.

Examples of such contrivance are the substantive indexes often used in psychologic research. Since no contrived test can provide an exact assessment of intelligence, anxiety, or personality, the investigator must always decide whether the test really measures what he wants it to measure. Is a conventional I.Q. test a "true" measurement of the type of intelligence needed for creativity? Are "anxiety" and "personality" really well measured by some of the tests or "inventories" used for these purposes? In nonpsychologic research, does the substantive index of *central venous pressure* provide an adequate assessment of congestive heart failure? In all of the situations just cited, there is no statistical method for "validating" the index, and its acceptance or rejection depends on the scientific judgment of the investigator.

When the contrived index is created by homologous substitution, the index can sometimes be validated from actual data showing the correlation between the entity under consideration and its homologous index. The investigator must always beware, however, of a correlation that seems satisfactory in an abstract sense, but that may be misleading for the objective of the research. For example, although there is a generally good correlation between height and weight at different ages in a human population, the repeated measurement of height would be a silly index of progress in a study of dieting to reduce obesity. Similarly, the enumerated consumption of nitroglycerine tablets would be an analogous but unsatisfactory index of the total severity of angina pectoris. The number of tablets used by a patient may generally correlate with the severity of the angina, but does not indicate other important functional aspects of "severity," such as the patient's ability to walk, work, or engage in other acts of physical exertion.

3. Computer distortions. As computers become used increasingly for storage and analysis of data in modern research, an additional new cause of the "displaced-objective" problem is not the goal of scientific reliability, but the convenience of computer compatibility. For processing by computer, the basic evidence must first be converted into "machine-readable language." In designing the formats needed for these conversions, the computer personnel may omit or displace many kinds of crucial information for which a suitable format can not be easily prepared at the beginning of the research project, because an appropriate taxonomy does not exist for the general topics and specific categories of the coding.[12, 13] A suitable format could be prepared later, after enough raw data have been collected for the topics and categories to be discerned and coded, but by that time the investigators may have become infatuated with the analysis of what is already in the computer. They may thus ignore crucial raw evidence that remains uncoded and unanalyzed, or they may confine their assessments to the constricted collection of data that could readily be expressed in "machine-readable language".

E. Methods of observation. After all these decisions have been made about the indexes, the variables, and the basic evidence, the investigator can contemplate the acquisition of the basic evidence. If he can establish his own methods of observation for each item of evidence, he must ascertain that the observational procedure is standardized and reliable. The ascertainment may require calibration of equipment, appraisal of observer variability, attempts to remove observer bias by "double-blind" procedures, and other techniques that deal with *quality control* of the primary data. If the investigator cannot establish his own methods, he must contemplate the flaws that might have been present in the procedures by which the available data were collected.

The methodologic issues of quality control are too numerous and complex for the scope of this outline of biostatistical architecture. They have been discussed elsewhere[5, 19] and will be considered again in greater detail in subsequent papers of this series.

F. Methods of classification. After the primary data have been obtained, they must often receive further classification before they can perform their role as variables and indexes. For example, if anemia is a variable to be specified as *present* or *absent*, a description of the method for measuring hematocrit does not indicate "anemia" until the hematocrit values receive classifications that assign ranges of values for *anemia* and *nonanemia*. The taxonomic methods of classifying data are also beyond the scope of this discussion, but two aspects of the problems can be briefly cited with regard to imperfect data and intermediate criteria.

1. Management of imperfect data. The management of imperfect data requires decisions about information that is missing or that creates ambiguity because of disagreements or contradictions. For example, will angina pectoris be diagnosed as present if the patient is said to have a "chest pain" that is not further described, or if the patient tells one examiner that the symptom is present but denies it in discussion with another examiner? Will anemia be diagnosed if the hemoglobin is low but the hematocrit is normal? Since these problems have no statistical solution, the decisions require scientific judgment, and the main issue is to establish reproducible consistency in the methods used for making the decisions.[9]

2. *Intermediate criteria.* The major criteria established for diagnostic, prognostic, or eligibility decisions are often not stated in terms that enable their specific application. For example, criteria for a diagnosis of myocardial infarction may require "abnormal Q waves" in the electrocardiogram but may not indicate what is meant by an "abnormal Q wave." The role of intermediate criteria is to provide all of the specifications for the decisions that transfer the observational evidence from its expression in the primary data to the various categories of designation, appraisal, and inference that constitute the major criteria[12] for the variables and indexes used in the investigation. Although often unspecified in many research projects, these intermediate criteria are necessary for the scientific reproducibility of the results. They are a crucial part of the methodologic process used to "harden" important soft data and to make hard data meaningful.

5. Subsequent identification

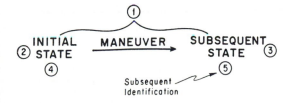

When the objective of the research project was specified, a series of targets in the subsequent state were cited and differentiated. At this fifth stage in bio-

statistical architecture, our concern is with the methods to be used for identifying those targets. The methods will include many of the same procedures just described for choosing, acquiring, and classifying observational evidence in data of the initial state. In addition to containing many of the same methodologic challenges present in the initial identification, however, the subsequent identification may include new kinds of data, criteria, and problems.

A. Additional data. Many of the variables encountered in the subsequent state may not have been present in the initial state and will require suitable arrangements for observation and interpretation. For example, if asymptomatic healthy people are being given a new drug to assay its dosage, their initial state contains no symptoms that need examination, but symptoms may occur as "side effects" in the subsequent state. Additional examination procedures may be needed for laboratory and other tests of new phenomena that first appear after the maneuver.

B. Additional criteria. The diagnostic and other criteria established for the initial state may not provide for many situations that occur subsequently. For example, a target that is to be prevented by a maneuver will not be present in the initial state, and its diagnostic criteria will need stipulation as part of the subsequent identifications. When a particular disease is under treatment, special criteria of "diagnostic co-morbidity"[14] may be necessary to decide whether a new manifestation is diagnostically attributable to the original disease, to the maneuver, or to the development of a co-morbid disease. Another group of distinct criteria will often be necessary to separate the untoward "side effects" of a maneuver from the expected or desired effects.

In the types of criteria that have just been described, an index is provided that describes the condition of a particular entity at a single state in time. An additional challenge in many research projects is to distinguish the change that may occur in the index from one temporal state to another. The criteria required for comparing two states of the same variable involve such concepts as *higher* or *lower*, rather than *high* or *low*, and *better* or *worse*, rather than *good* or *bad*. The appraisal of such transitions, particularly from the initial state to the subsequent state of the investigated population, will be contemplated separately later as the eighth operation of biostatistical architecture.

C. Displacement of target. The logical hazard of "displacing" important soft data variables, described earlier in the initial identification of the population, constitutes an even greater problem when the target variables are chosen. The displacement of target has become a common defect in many "statistically designed" trials of therapy. For example, although anticoagulant treatment is given to prevent thromboembolism in patients with myocardial infarction, the target used in many studies of anticoagulants was mortality rate, rather than thromboembolism.[15] The objective of palliative treatment for patients with inoperable cancer has often been displaced into hard data targets, such as changes in size of tumor, with inadequate attention given to soft data targets, such as discomfort or functional ability in daily life, that would truly indicate whether clinical "palliation" has occurred.[4]

The inappropriate selection of hard data endpoints may not only lead to the types of displacement just cited, but may also, as noted later, create a substantial and sometimes overwhelming increase in the number of patients needed for "statistical significance" in a research project.

• • •

At this advanced point in biostatistical architecture, after completing the first five of the ten major operational principles used in planning clinical research, we have not yet encountered any problems that required a skillful knowledge of statistics. All of the issues that needed thoughtful analysis and decision could have been man-

aged effectively by a sensible clinical scientist who knew nothing of the specialized concepts or theories subsumed under the name of "statistics."

Statistical principles will begin to appear in the next stage of the architecture, however, and in several other stages thereafter. These principles and the associated scientific logic needed to complete the five remaining operations of design in clinical research will be discussed at our next meeting.

References

1. Ad Hoc Committee to revise the Jones criteria (modified) of the Council on Rheumatic Fever and Congenital Heart Disease of the American Heart Association: Jones criteria (revised) for guidance in the diagnosis of rheumatic fever, Circulation **32**:664-668, 1965.
2. Berkson, J.: Limitations of the application of fourfold table analysis to hospital data, Biomet. Bull. **2**:47-53, 1946.
3. Deming, W. E.: Some theory of sampling, New York, 1966, Dover Publications.
4. Feinstein, A. R.: Clinical and intellectual causes for defective statistics for the prognosis and treatment of cancer, Med. Clin. N. Amer. **51**:549-562, 1967.
5. Feinstein, A. R.: Clinical judgment, Baltimore, 1967, The Williams & Wilkins Company.
6. Feinstein, A. R.: Clinical epidemiology: I. The populational experiments of nature and of man in human illness, Ann. Intern. Med. **69**:807-820, 1968.
7. Feinstein, A. R.: Clinical epidemiology: II. The identification rates of disease, Ann. Intern. Med. **69**:1037-1061, 1968.
8. Feinstein, A. R., Pritchett, J. A., and Schimpff, C. R.: The epidemiology of cancer therapy. II. The clinical course: Data, decisions, and temporal demarcations, Arch. Intern. Med. **123**:323-344, 1969.
9. Feinstein, A. R., Pritchett, J. A., and Schimpff, C. R.: The epidemiology of cancer therapy. III. The management of imperfect data, Arch. Intern. Med. **123**:448-461, 1969.
10. Feinstein, A. R., Pritchett, J. A., and Schimpff, C. R.: The epidemiology of cancer therapy. IV. The extraction of data from medical records, Arch. Intern. Med. **123**:571-590, 1969.
11. Feinstein, A. R.: Clinical biostatistics. III. The architecture of clinical research, CLIN. PHARMACOL. THER. **11**:432-441, 1970.
12. Feinstein, A. R.: Taxonorics. I. Formulation of criteria, Arch. Intern. Med., 1970. (In press.)

13. Feinstein, A. R.: Taxonorics. II. Format and coding systems for data processing, Arch. Intern. Med., 1970. (In press.)
14. Feinstein, A. R.: The pre-therapeutic classification of co-morbidity in chronic disease, J. Chron. Dis., 1970. (In press.)
15. Gifford, R. H., and Feinstein, A. R.: A critique of methodology in studies of anticoagulant therapy for acute myocardial infarction, New Eng. J. Med. **280:**351-357, 1969.
16. Lansbury, J.: Methods for evaluating rheumatoid arthritis, *in* Hollander, J. L., editor: Arthritis and allied conditions, Philadelphia, 1966, Lea and Febiger, Publishers, chap. 18, pp. 269-291.
17. Lasagna, L., and von Felsinger, J. M.: The volunteer subject in research, Science **120:** 359-361, 1954.
18. Mainland, D.: The clinical trial—some difficulties and suggestions, J. Chron. Dis. **11:** 484-496, 1960.
19. Mainland, D.: Elementary medical statistics, ed. 2, Philadelphia, 1963, The W. B. Saunders Company.
20. Yerushalmy, J.: On inferring causality from observed associations, *in* Ingelfinger, F. J., Relman, A. S., and Finland, M., editors: Controversy in internal medicine, Philadelphia, 1966, The W. B. Saunders Company, pp. 659-688.

CHAPTER 5

Subsequent implementation of the objective

In considering the design of a project in clinical research, we have thus far passed through five stages of biostatistical architecture. The first stage, concerned with the paramount principles of specifying the objective of the investigation,[19] contained the components and logic used for planning the sequence of *initial state, maneuver,* and *subsequent state.* The next four stages contained procedures for implementing the stated objective by delineating the intake, maintenance, initial identification, and subsequent identification of the population.[20] This paper begins with the sixth stage of the design and continues through the remaining four operational principles that conclude this outline of biostatistical architecture for clinical research. Subsequent papers in this series will be devoted to additional methodologic issues that have been raised during the architectural discussions.

6. Allocation

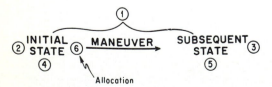

At this sixth stage in the architecture,

This chapter originally appeared as "Clinical biostatistics— V. The architecture of clinical research (concluded)." In Clin. Pharmacol. Ther. 11:755, 1970.

the selected maneuvers are allocated to the populations receiving those maneuvers. The allocation is done in a survey by determining and classifying what happened and, in an experiment, by making the assignment directly. In both types of research, the investigator must beware of problems in priority of maneuvers. For example, patients who are in their second course of treatment for a particular disorder are not necessarily comparable to patients who are receiving a first course of treatment. Beyond this issue of prior maneuver, however, the "allocation" problem in surveys and experiments has major distinctions that will be discussed separately.

A. Surveys. In a survey of clinical therapy or of nature's ontogenetic, pathogenetic, or pathogressive activities,[18] the investigator has not assigned the maneuvers received by the population. Consequently, his first problem is to ascertain the maneuver to which each person was exposed. In addition, he encounters major logical hazards when he classifies maneuvers involving a prolonged passage of time, and when he attempts certain types of contrived comparisons for the premaneuveral initial state.

1. Ascertaining the maneuver. An investigator usually has no problem in verifying the administration of a maneuver given in a hospital or elsewhere under direct medical supervision, and in a "prospective" investigation of maneuvers maintained outside the hospital, the investigator can establish various methods for checking the patient's adherence.

If the maneuver occurred before the research project began, however, the problems of ascertainment are particularly difficult. A person may not accurately recall details of antecedent medications, food habits, alcohol ingestion, or smoking, or he may give distorted answers to questions about them. Thus, in surveys dealing with the effects of such maneuvers as food, alcohol, or smoking, the investigator is confronted with determining not only the initial (pre-maneuver) state of the population but also the population's exposure to the maneuver.

2. *Problems in chronology.* If a maneuver involves the prolonged passage of time for a particular population, the population should be followed "longitudinally" to see what happens to its individual members. Because such research is often difficult to carry out, however, the investigator may instead perform a "cross-sectional" study of different populations at different times. The main logical hazard of such "longitudinal cross-sections" is that the "subsequent population" may have been significantly distorted in emerging from its sources in the unexamined "base population."

This problem is illustrated by a project in which an investigator wants to determine what happens to serum cholesterol as healthy people advance from age 40 to age 70. Instead of longitudinally following a group of healthy 40-year-old persons for 30 years, the investigator may compare the results of a group of healthy 70-year-olds with those of a 40-year-old group. Any differences found in these groups may be misleading because the average values in the 70-year-olds might have been significantly lowered by the earlier deaths of people who had particularly high cholesterol values at age 40.

A different type of example is provided by cross-sectional surveys in which the rates of cardiac damage were much higher in populations with recurrent attacks of rheumatic fever than in populations with first attacks. The fallacious epidemiologic conclusion was that recurrences of rheumatic fever create cardiac damage in many patients who were initially free of it. When this issue was later examined longitudinally,[24, 47] however, the rheumatic patients who already had cardiac damage were found to be particularly susceptible to developing recurrences. Thus, although patients free of carditis in a first rheumatic attack generally do not develop it in a recurrence, a population of "recurrences" nevertheless contains higher proportions of people with cardiac damage than a group of "first attacks."[24]

A separate type of chronologic problem occurs in using the data of "vital statistics" to compare the mortality rate of patients with the "same" disease in different eras. One of the main issues here is whether the compared populations have had equal opportunity for detection of target. For example, although the mortality rate for coronary heart disease in the United States was much higher in 1965 than in 1935, the change may not reflect increasing lethality for this disease, because altered diagnostic procedures during the 30-year interval have greatly increased the opportunities for the disease's detection.

These problems in chronologic logic have not been managed well during the past few decades of biostatistical research in clinical epidemiology.[16] The occurrence rates of disease at different times and in different geographic localities have often been compared without regard to the different opportunities for diagnostic detection. The rates of an alleged cause of disease have been compared "cross-sectionally" or "retrospectively" in people who already have the disease and in "control" groups who were usually chosen from a population conveniently available to the investigator, rather than from a population adequate for scientific validity in comparison. The development of subsequent complications of a disease has often been studied in such restrictive cross-sections as the populations composed of 5-year survivors of that disease, or of people subjected to necropsy. In most of these circumstances, the devotion to statistical analysis and etiologic speculation has usually exceeded the attention to satisfactory data and scientific logic. The methodologic issues of populational "spection"—retrospection, prospection, and cross-sectional "spection"—are too complex for further consideration in this architectural outline, and, like several other methodologic problems, will be reserved for discussion in subsequent papers of this series.

3. *The hazards of contrived comparisons.* A favorite tactic in statistical surveys

is to manipulate the observed populations into certain types of contrived comparison. The rates of an observed event may be "standardized" to make them "age-adjusted" or "sex-adjusted" according to what was found in some "standard population." A "control" group, chosen retrospectively from a conveniently accessible population, may be divided into "paired matchings" with members of the "experimental" group.

These tactics may be satisfactory for certain types of analysis, but they contain many hazards in logic. What constitutes a "standard population"? Are its constituents comparable enough and its data reliable enough for use in the current comparison? How are the properties chosen for a retrospective "matching"? Do they really exert an important influence on the event under scrutiny, or are they often chosen, like age and sex, merely because the data are "hard" and readily available?

The problems of logic in these contrived comparisons are extraordinarily complex, particularly in surveys intended to demonstrate causes of disease, and are beyond the scope of this discussion. Despite the frequency and apparent assurance with which many "adjusted" or "matched" rates appear in the literature, however, the biologic validity of the procedures remains unproved, and the tactics are still in a state of controversial dispute.[8, 35, 36, 39, 42, 48, 50]

B. Experiments. If an investigator can choose the maneuvers, as in a therapeutic or explanatory experiment, the main challenge of allocation is to develop a suitable method of assigning patients to the selected maneuvers. The principal decisions involve judgments about premaneuver stratification, numerical equality of populations, size of total population, and allocation procedure.

1. Pre-maneuver stratification. If m different maneuvers are to be studied, the people entered into the experiment must obviously be divided into m groups. Before the m manuevers are assigned, however, at least two other distinctions may be used to stratify the population further.

One of these distinctions, which is commonly employed in large-scale cooperative studies, involves assigning the maneuvers separately to the patients at each of the cooperating institutions. Thus, if c institutions participate, $c \times m$ groups are established, with plans that allocate patients to each maneuver at each institution. Although the data for each maneuver are usually combined afterward, the interinstitutional stratification may be helpful both in evaluating possible biases in the institutional populations, and in keeping each institution informed of its own results.

A second type of premaneuver stratification is based on prognostic distinctions described previously.[19] If s prognostic strata can be defined before an experiment begins, the maneuvers can be assigned within these s strata, so that the research project becomes essentially a series of s experiments rather than one. If m maneuvers are being studied, each of the s strata will be divided into m parts, so that $m \times s$ groups will be present. If each of these groups is dispersed among c cooperating institutions, a total of $m \times s \times c$ groups will participate in the multicenter study. For example, if we plan to compare Excellitol versus a placebo in treating good-risk, fair-risk, and poor-risk patients during a collaboration of 10 medical centers, we would deal with 60 (= 2 × 3 × 10) distinct groups.

A prognostic stratification is commonly omitted in planning the design of clinical experiments, because the best arrangement of prognostic strata for the main target is seldom clearly known before the experiment begins, and, besides, as discussed previously,[19] many different stratifications might be needed for each of the diverse ancillary targets of the maneuver. The omission of such a pre-allocation stratification, however, does not absolve an investigator of the need for appropriate prognostic divisions afterward. Unless the patients are suitably divided into groups with different "risks" for each target, the investigator may ignore fundamental differences in the natural events upon which his experiment was imposed. He may mix moribund and asymptomatic patients improperly in evaluating the outcome and in performing analyses of variance or other statistical procedures.[17, 19] These analyses may produce misleading results that remain uncorrected because the investigator has failed to discover that certain maneuvers may have had antipodal effects on different prognostic groups[15, 17] or that the allocation procedures, even though "randomized," may have created major prognostic disproportions among the patients assigned to the compared manuevers.

Nevertheless, appropriate prognostic stratifications are constantly neglected in the analysis of clinical experiments. The consultant statistician and principal investigator may convince each other that the stratification is either unnecessary, because the randomized allocation "took care of everything," or inappropriate, because of the *post hoc* timing of the analysis. In other instances, investigators attempting a *post hoc* stratification may discover that some of the necessary data were not obtained as part of the description of the initial state. For example, many computerized collections of information about the treatment of cancer, diabetes, or other major chronic diseases cannot now be thoroughly analyzed because the coded information about the initial state does not include enough details of symptoms, chronometry, co-morbidity, or other important prognostic features.[22, 23]

As discussed later, the process of randomization is an excellent way of allocating experimental treatment in an unbiased manner. But if an appropriate prognostic analysis is not performed either beforehand or afterward, the experimenter may find that he has removed statistical bias with the randomization, but has also removed clinical sense. To avoid making this paper unduly long, the strategy and tactics of *post hoc* prognostic stratification will be reserved for discussion at a later date.

2. Number of patients per maneuver. In most experimental plans, equal numbers of patients are assigned to each of the maneuvers under comparison, since equal divisions usually provide the best statistical opportunity for demonstrating a significant numerical difference among the maneuvers.[37]

In at least two circumstances, however, the numerical assignments to different maneuvers may be deliberately unequal. In one such circumstance, the investigators intend to test two separate maneuvers whose results will later be combined for comparison against a third maneuver. For example, placebo might be compared against two dosage levels of Excellitol, with the Excellitol results later consolidated if desired. In such a situation, each of the two "combinatorial" maneuvers could be assigned half the number of patients assigned to the third maneuver; and when the results of the two maneuvers are later combined, the numbers will equal those of the third.

An unequal number of patients may be assigned in a different type of circumstance when a maneuver suspected of being distinctly inferior must be tested in a therapeutic trial in order for the suspicion to be proved. In this situation, the suspectedly inferior maneuver is sometimes allocated to a smaller number of people than the other maneuvers.

3. Size of the population. At least three different methods can be used for determining the total size of the population entered into an experiment. In the "calendar" method, a fixed period of time is used for populational intake, and the ultimate size of the population depends on the number of people assembled during that calendrical interval. In the "fixed-size" method, a fixed number of people is chosen for admission, and the intake of population continues until that number is reached. The number can be chosen arbitrarily or from statistical formulas based on the magnitude of difference that the investigator hopes to demonstrate.[14, 46] In the "sequential" method,[2] pairs of patients for the two compared maneuvers continue to be successively entered into the experiment until the results reach boundaries of statistical "significance" or "nonsignificance."

Each of these three methods of choosing populational size has its own advantages and disadvantages. In the "calendar" method, the number of patients admitted during the chosen time interval may turn out to be too small for "statistically significant" results. The project might have to be either concluded without attaining statistical proof or extended over a longer time interval to get more patients. In contrast to these hazards of the "calendar" method, both the "fixed-size" and "sequential" methods offer the attraction of assuring "statistical significance." Both of the latter two methods, however, also have the logical handicap of being based on a single target of response. Consequently, the calculated numbers that might yield "significant" differences for the single target may not be adequate for analyzing the many other targets that often require attention in a clinical experiment. In addition, the "sequential" procedure is limited to a comparison of two maneuvers, and the target state must be an entity that can be assessed promptly after the maneuvers, to enable decisions about admitting the next pair of patients.

An additional hazard of the "fixed-size" method occurs when the target of the investigation has been displaced, as described previously,[20] into a hard data "endpoint" that has a much lower rate of occurrence than the "endpoint" for the appropriate entity of soft data. In this situation, the sample size estimated to give "statistical significance" may be a number that is massively higher than what would have been required with the "softer" target.

Suppose, for example, that our objective is to test a treatment intended to improve the severity of angina pectoris, and we want the incremental results (or θ value) in the treated group to be at least 30 per cent better than in the "controls." For our "endpoint" we decide to reject the soft data target of "clinical improvement of severity" and instead we choose the hard data of "fatality rate." This decision will greatly alter the number of patients needed for "significant" results in the experiment. If "clinical improvement" can be expected in 70 per cent of the control group, we would have demanded (according to the θ specification of 30 per cent) that 91 per cent of the treated group "improve"; but if the expected fatality rate in the control group is 10 per cent, we shall demand that this rate be reduced to 7 per cent in the treated group. With these specifications, and with $\alpha = 0.05$ and $\beta = 0.05$, we would have needed a total of 86 patients to get "statistical significance" with the "soft data" endpoint, but with the "hard data" endpoint we shall need 2,240 patients in the trial.* Even if we became more "liberal" and raised the β level to 0.10 while preserving α at 0.05, the "hard data" endpoint would still require 1,811 patients

while the "soft" endpoint would need only 70.* Confronted with the huge amount of extra patients and associated labor required to get numerical "significance" with the "hard" endpoint, the investigator may be so discouraged that he abandons his plans to conduct the experiment.

Despite the cited problems in both numbers and logic, the calculations of "sample size" according to "fixed" or "sequential" methods has become a prerequisite ritual of "statistical design" for contemporary clinical trials.[10, 27, 43] The maneuvers chosen for comparison may be inadequate or illogical; the investigators may not know how to perform a suitable prognostic stratification beforehand and may neglect it afterward; the eligibility criteria may vitiate any numerical anticipations based on previous experience and may preclude admission of the diverse types of patients needed for the trial to be clinically meaningful; and the initial variables or targets of response may be chosen inappropriately and assessed improperly; but the statistician, undaunted by these imprecisions, may marshal his α, β, and θ values and calculate the *exact* number of patients needed for "statistical significance."

Although an estimate of the number of patients and length of time is always desirable for a large-scale investigation, particularly for cooperative studies at multiple institutions, the lamentable aspect of the current "numbers game" is that the intensive planning given to these statistical desiderata is often the main focus of the activities in "statistical design." While the numbers are being meticulously calculated, however, many of the fundamental necessities of scientific logic and data may be ignored.

4. Method of assignment. Regardless of how the numbers of groups and patients are determined, the investigator must choose a method of assigning patients to each maneuver. The main scientific ob-

---

*These calculations were based on the formulas cited in pp. 221-222 of reference 46. I am indebted to Mrs. Elizabeth C. Wright for checking the calculations.

ject of this method is to avoid bias in the assignment. A "double-blind" procedure, which is helpful in preventing bias when subsequent examinations are performed, would also help avoid bias when maneuvers are allocated. In addition, when one maneuver is initially suspected to be distinctly better than another, a double-blind allocation has the further advantage of freeing the investigator from "moral" qualms that may arise if he knows which patients have been assigned to the "inferior" maneuver. For example, in the first large-scale field trials of a poliomyelitis vaccine,[26] a double-blind technique helped avert the ethical quandaries that arose about assignment of patients to the vaccine or to the "control" preparation.

Although a double-blind method of allocation would solve the scientific and ethical problems just cited, it does not solve the practical problem of establishing an order for the assignments. A specific sequence must be chosen for allocating the maneuvers, even though the person who later administers each maneuver may not know its identity. This sequence is best selected by the statistical procedure of randomization. A full description of randomization is beyond the scope of this outline, but its value can be summarized as follows: randomization averts the bias that may arise when maneuvers are assigned in an alternate manner or in any other "systematic" manner (such as patients' unit numbers); it guards against the bias that may occur when double-blind techniques cannot be used; and it provides mathematical legitimacy for the subsequent assessment of results with statistical tests based on "random sampling."

The technique of randomization is one of the major contributions made by inductive statistics to modern clinical research, and the frequent scientific abuse of the procedure, as described here and elsewhere,[17] should not detract from its great value when properly employed. Despite the importance of randomization, however, it does not appear as a cogent principle of research design until this sixth step in the architecture—and then only for research projects that are experiments, rather than surveys. Although many clinicians have been inordinately slow to accept the need for randomization in planning clinical trials and experiments, many statisticians have been overly zealous in promulgating randomization as a panacea for flaws in "experimental design." As an adjunct to well-planned experimental architecture, randomization makes a powerful contribution to modern science; as a substitute for suitable scientific logic, randomization serves to perpetuate defective research, performed and often accepted in the complacent delusion that a satisfactory "statistical design" is alone adequate for valid experimental science.

7. Intrusion

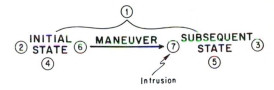

After a maneuver has begun, the pathway from initial state to subsequent state may be interrupted in several ways. The maneuver itself may be abandoned by the patient; the maneuver or the observation period may be altered by an untoward event; the necessary subsequent examinations may not be performed; or the patient may stop participating in the project. The various intrusions that can appear between maneuver and subsequent state are considered in this stage of the architecture.

A. Nonadherence to maneuver. A person may not faithfully adhere to a maneuver that must be maintained over a long period of time. Oral or injectable medication, or such maneuvers as cigarette smoking, may be taken erratically or discontinued entirely by patients who nevertheless continue to be observed in the project.

In stage three of the research architecture (dealing with maintenance of the population[20]), arrangements were made to obtain data about adherence to maneuvers. In this seventh stage of the architectural design, the main challenges are to classify the fidelity of the adherence and to decide about the way in which the results obtained in poor adherers will be ascribed (or not ascribed) to the associated maneuver.

Suppose a patient is assigned to take one oral tablet twice daily, on awakening and at bedtime. How many and what kind of deviations from this prescription will constitute different degrees of fidelity to the regimen, and how many classes of fidelity should be established? Should we simply rate the adherence for all patients as either *good* or *not good,* or should there be four categories of adherence, such as *excellent, good, fair,* and *poor?* What will be the specific criteria for classifying deviations in the intra- and interdiurnal patterns? Will we be satisfied if the patient takes his two tablets each day, but both at one time, or if he ingests one tablet at lunch and the other at supper? Suppose he forgets one tablet on one day and takes three the next? If he omits the tablets for three days in the course of a month, does it make a difference whether the three days occur consecutively or sporadically? No statistical answers are available for any of these questions, which require arbitrary judgments individualized for each research project.

Another tricky problem occurs in ascribing the results obtained in persons who have not maintained the maneuver faithfully. Suppose daily doses of Excellitol were given to lower blood cholesterol, and suppose the adherence to the regimen can be classified as *good, fair,* and *poor.* At the end of the project, we would not be surprised if the cholesterol were significantly lower in the *good* adherers than in the *poor,* but how would we interpret an even lower result in patients with only *fair* adherence? Suppose the placebo patients with *good* and *fair* adherence had substantially lower values for cholesterol than the *poor* adherence Excellitol group? Again, these questions cannot be answered with statistical or scientific theories, and each decision must be made with a logic appropriate to the problem.

B. Untoward events. The patient's ability to maintain an on-going maneuver, such as a diet or medication, may be impaired by the development of an adverse clinical condition not present in the initial state. Beyond any effect on maintenance of the maneuver, each subsequent clinical event or other manifestation must be analyzed

for its diagnostic attribution. For example, during long-term treatment of a chronic disease, the attending physician (or the investigator) must decide whether each posttherapeutic manifestation is due to the treatment itself, or to features associated with either the evolving main disease or co-morbid ailments. Thus, for appropriate classification of anorexia that develops after chemotherapy of a cancer, the investigator must attribute the anorexia to functional effects of the cancer, to a reaction (i.e., a "side effect") produced by the chemotherapeutic agent, to an associated co-morbid disease that was present before or after treatment, to a psychic depression evoked by the patient's emotional response to his illness, to combinations of these factors, or to other causes.

The way that these "co-morbidity" decisions are made can profoundly affect statistics about the target of a research project. For example, in pathogressive surveys of patients with cancer, fatality rates are usually based on all patients who died, regardless of cause of death. Thus, a patient in whom a cancer had been successfully removed but who later died because of a myocardial infarction or in an automobile accident is often statistically counted in the same way as a patient who died of disseminated cancer. Another example of this problem is the misleading rates of disease created from using mortality data of the Bureau of Vital Statistics, where each patient's death is attributed to a single cause, regardless of how many major diseases were present.[16]

The results of two recent large-scale investigations also illustrate some of the difficulties that can occur in evaluating deaths and associated treatments. In comparison with the "control" group, patients with prostatic cancer who were treated with estrogens had fewer deaths "due to cancer" but more deaths ascribed to "other causes," so that the total fatality rates in the two groups were essentially the same.[49] Domiciliary patients receiving a low fat diet had fewer cardiovascular deaths than the "control" group but more noncardiovascular deaths, so that the total fatality rates in the two groups were similar.[13]

The problems of "attribution" in "diagnostic co-morbidity" have been discussed elsewhere,[21] and are beyond the scope of this outline. The main point to be noted here is that no thoroughly satisfactory statistical procedures have been developed for these problems. Their management currently depends on the sensible use of scientific judgment.

C. Displacement of examinations. A third type of intrusive problem occurs in the patient's or the investigator's adherence to the planned examination procedures. A particular examination that was scheduled for repetition at specified intervals may not have been done; it may have been performed on dates other than the ones planned for it, or it may have been "displaced" by some other test.

For example, if serum antibodies are to be tested every two months for detection of intercurrent group A streptococcal infections, should we regard a particular patient as adequately tested if a particular examination was delayed so that a three-month interval elapsed between specimens? If the test after a three-month interval shows that an infection has occurred, in what period does the infection get counted: the previous two-month period, or the next one? What about the situation in which the timing of the test was satisfactory, but a different test was done? Thus, would we regard a patient as adequately examined for group A streptococci if the tests were based on throat cultures rather than serum antibodies? And what about the type of "displacement" in which a particular test produces an "outlyer" result—a value that is extraordinarily higher or lower than the general range of expected values for the test? Should this "outlyer" be rejected from consideration or accepted and included among the other data?

Conventional statistical tactics[30, 37, 40] for dealing with missing data and with "outlyers" are seldom suitable for the circumstances just described. The tactics usually apply to situations in which a group of objects have all received the same test at the same time in a single performance. No provision is made for the problem of interpreting repetitive tests and for managing the other logical difficulties in displacement of data.

If the compared maneuvers have been allocated by randomization, the investigator may take false comfort from the belief that subsequent displacements of data will also occur randomly and that almost any rational method of analyzing them will be satisfactory, since the randomization prevented bias. The flaw in this belief is that the maneuver itself—as described earlier[20]—may create unequal opportunities for detection of the target state. The subsequent displacements of data may thus reflect some of the bias caused, after randomization, by administration of the procedure used in the maneuver.

Suppose oral daily penicillin and monthly injections of long-acting penicillin have been randomly allocated in an experimental trial of their capacity to prevent subsequent streptococcal infections in young patients who have had rheumatic fever, and suppose streptococcal infections will be detected via comparison of antibody titers in bimonthly specimens of sera. If the patients assigned to monthly injections must appear at the research clinic in order to receive the injections, the bimonthly specimens of sera can be obtained as part of the circumstances surrounding the administration of the prophylactic therapy. On the other hand, if the patients taking the oral medication can receive their monthly supply by mail, the routine acquisition of serum specimens will require a special visit to the clinic for an examination that is therapeutically unnecessary. According to the way this inequality of "maintenance" is managed by the investigators, the serologic specimens may be obtained with greater diligence and regularity in the "injection" group than in the "oral" group, or vice versa. A difference in the rate of streptococcal infections in the two groups may thus arise from these problems of intrusion, rather than from the therapeutic maneuvers.

The difficulties just described, which can occur despite randomized allocation of maneuvers in an experimental trial, must be especially guarded against when the research is conducted as a survey. As noted previously,[20] unequal opportunities for detection of the target may cause women taking oral contraceptive pills to have a falsely higher incidence of thrombophlebitis or cervical cancer than women using mechanical devices. Similarly, since people with a chronic cough are more likely to have chest x-rays taken than people without a cough, and since smokers are more likely to have a chronic cough than nonsmokers, some of the higher rate of lung cancer in smokers may be due to their greater opportunity for having lung cancer detected when it occurs.

D. Displacement of patients. The last intrusive problem to be cited here is the loss of patients during an investigation in which the target state occurs long after the initial state. Suppose the main target of investigation is a discrete event—such as death. When we tabulate the frequency of the target event (in such expressions as "5-year survival rates"), what shall be done about patients known to be alive at an earlier date, but later "lost to follow-up" at the 5-year interval selected for analysis?

The usual statistical approach to this problem is the use of an "actuarial" or "life-table" analytic procedure.[4, 11, 38] In this procedure, a numerator and denominator population are counted at periodic intervals, such as 1 year, from the onset of the maneuver. The denominator for each interval consists of an appropriate count of the people who began that interval; the numerator consists of all people in whom the target event occurred during that interval. A rate of the target event is calculated from the numerator and denominator for each successive interval, and the "final" rate for the most advanced time period is the product of the rates calculated for each antecedent interval. Thus, the five-year survival rate would be obtained by first finding the one-year survival rate in people who have been followed for one year; this rate is then multiplied by the survival rate during the second year in people who were followed for a second year; the product of the first two yearly rates is then multiplied by the survival rate during the third year; and so on, until the fifth-year rates are multiplied by the product of the four preceding rates to yield the final result.

The life-table approach is particularly valuable for analyzing data in a research project in which populational intake occurs serially over an extensive calendar interval. Since not all the patients will enter the study at the same time, they will have different lengths of follow-up at the calendar dates on which the investigator prepares "progress reports." Thus, about four years after the project has begun, the investigator may want to calculate 3-year survival rates, but many patients who entered the project only 18 months ago have not yet had the opportunity to survive for three years. For this kind of "serial intake" problem, the life-table method offers an excellent adjustment for duration of follow-up.

The life-table method is much less satisfactory, however, if the problem is one of "serial drop-out" rather than "serial intake." When "losses to follow-up" occur during a particular interval in the life-table calculations, the denominator for the interval is created as the sum of all the patients who were followed throughout the interval, together with half the number of those who were lost; and the "drop-outs" do not appear in the numerator. For example, suppose that death is the target event and occurs in 5 of 90 people who were followed throughout an interval during which 20 other people were "lost." The denominator would be 100 [=90 + 10], and the death rate for the interval would be 5 per cent [=5/100].

Regardless of the theoretical statistical support for this "half-life" procedure, a scientist will feel uneasy that unproved assumptions have been made about the fate of the "lost" patients. A more effective scientific approach to this problem would be to obviate any guesswork based on statistical theories or scientific logic, and to establish adequate epidemiologic methods for following the population carefully enough to provide information about the actual state of all members, thus eliminating the need for conjectural assumptions. If the investigators make vigorous efforts to "trace lost persons," the logical hazard of a "serial drop-out" life-table can be managed by avoiding it.

8. Transition

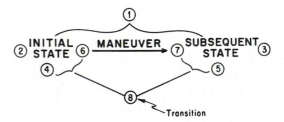

After suitable provision has been made for the types of intrusion just described, standards must be established for assessing the transition that has occurred from the initial to the subsequent state of each person in the population and for the transition in each population group.

A. *Types of change.* The assessment of change involves subtle issues in chronology. As noted previously,[20] the single value of an index for a particular state in time can depend on unitemporal or multitemporal contributions. (For example, the initial-state or subsequent-state value for blood pressure can each be a single reading or the average of a series of readings.) Regardless of the number of temporal contributions included in the index value for a single state, the assessment of a change may involve values for one, two, or more states. According to the number of values that are compared for the delineation, a change can be monadic, polyadic, or dyadic.

1. Monadic changes. In a monadic change, the person's initial state is not really a constituent of the data evaluated for delineating the "transition." There is no actual comparison of a "before" and "after" condition, because the "after" event may not have been present initially, or the subsequent state may be assessed exclusively on the basis of what happened during or after the maneuver. For example, the development of poliomyelitis is the monadic change used as the target to be prevented in contrapathic vaccination of healthy people; death is the monadic change to be prevented as a target of contratrophic treatment for many people with cancer.

Monadic indexes are commonly established as the score of a particular test used to describe a person's condition after the main "maneuver" has already occurred. For example, an I.Q. test may be given to a group of well-nourished and poorly-nourished children, and the investigator, on the basis of the monadic scores, may attempt "retrospectively" to compare the influence of nutrition on intelligence.

Another type of monadic index is used for situations in which the target in the "subsequent state" is an entity that can occur repetitively during the course of an on-going maneuver. In this circumstance, the entire period of time that the maneuver was maintained represents a single monadic "subsequent state." Examples of such indexes are the number of attacks of angina pectoris or the number of nitroglycerin tablets ingested during maintenance of an antianginal drug regimen. In the examples just cited, the indexes were individually multitemporal, because they contained contributions from several points in time; but their sum constituted a monadic description of "change," because the pretreatment state of the patients did not enter into the calculations.

2. Polyadic changes. In contrast to monadic changes, polyadic and dyadic changes represent distinct "transitions" because a value for the initial state is contained in the assessment of the "change." A polyadic change is based on the value of a quantitative variable at three or more different points in time, and the index of change depends on the line or curve that connects those points. For example, if a person initially weighed 130 pounds at age 15, and then weighed 160 pounds at age 18, 190 pounds at age 21, and 220 pounds at age 24, the weight curve has been linear, with an upward slope of 10 pounds per year. A polyadic change is commonly expressed as a "trend," and determined with statistical procedures that find the best-fitting straight line (or nonlinear curve) for the collection of different temporal points. When a linear model is used for "fitting" the line, the trend is usually expressed as the "slope" of the line. Quadratic or other models can be used to fit trends that have distinctly curved shapes or that go up and then down, or vice versa.

3. Dyadic changes. Dyadic transitions are constantly used in therapeutic research for evaluating either remedial treatment, intended to make a patient's condition "better," or contratrophic treatment, intended to keep him from becoming "worse." Unlike the monadic and polyadic changes just described, a dyadic change contains a direct comparison of two temporal states: before and after the maneuver.

The variable used for determining a dyadic change must be expressed in values that have graded ranks. The ranks can be measured or counted dimensions (such as *13, 14, 15, . . .*) or semiquantitative ordinal ratings (such as *high, medium,* or *low*). For dimensional ranks, the transition between the initial and the subsequent state can be expressed as a subtracted increment (or decrement) or as a percentage increase (or reduction). Thus, if the sedimentation rate was 50 mm. per hour before the maneuver and 30 mm. per hour afterward, the change can be expressed as a fall of 20 mm. per hour or as a 40 per cent reduction. For ordinal ranks, the transition is expressed in such comparative categories as *higher, same,* or *lower*.

An interesting aspect of dyadic transitions is their capacity for converting qualitative or quantitative data into semiquantitative categories based on concepts of clinical or biologic desirability. Thus, the ordinal rating scale of *better, same,* or *worse* for dyadic changes can be applied both to quantitative phenomena, such as a reduction in temperature, or to such qualitative alterations as a disappearance of symptoms, or a change in color of urine.

To manage the problems of dyadic transition, the research architect, who has already established sets of criteria for identifying entities in the initial state and subsequent state, must now establish a special new set of criteria for the changes between the two states. These "transition criteria" will require many scientific judgments beyond those that have already been necessary. One set of judgments deals with the conversion of dimensional data into transitional categories. Thus, an initial Westergren sedimentation rate of 180 mm. per hour and a subsequent value of 175 mm. per hour might each be called *markedly elevated* in their single states, but would the decrement of 5 mm. per hour in the two states warrant being called a *fall?* A second set of judgments deals with the magnitude of transition in semiquantitative ordinal categories. For example, if cardiac enlargement is graded as *none, slight, moderate,* and *extreme,* what pairings of categories will be used to denote such transitions as *much smaller, smaller, unchanged, larger,* and *much larger?*

B. Population indexes. Using one of the procedures just cited for describing a change, the investigator can establish an individual index of transition for each important variable in each member of a population. Although a change in the selected variable can thereby be expressed for individual people in the group, additional decisions become necessary in choosing a populational index that can summarize the results of the individual indexes in the entire group.

1. Types of populational indexes. A populational index can be derived from individual indexes in at least two ways. If the individual index is expressed in categories, the proportionate frequency of categories can be enumerated in the population; if expressed dimensionally, its average value can be calculated. For example, the categorical response to treatment of congestive heart failure in a group of 78 patients can be cited proportionately as *excellent* in 9 per cent, *good* in 65 per cent, *fair* in 14 per cent, and *poor* in 12 per cent; the survival time in 112 patients with cancer can be averaged as a median value of 8.3 months, or as mean of 9.1 months. When the individual index has been expressed dimensionally, the populational index can still be expressed categorically. Thus, in the 112 patients just cited, the populational survival could have been categorically stated as a rate of 42 per cent at 6 months. (In the latter expression, the "categories" of survival were *alive at 6 months* and *dead at 6 months.*)

When individual transitions have been expressed in a dimension that was measured repetitively, rather than only at the two times of initial state and subsequent state, the populational performance can be calculated with a "trend" equation, using some of the mathematical models described previously for determining trend in an individual person.

2. Problems in denominators. A group index expressed in proportionate categories consists of a ratio: the numerator is the frequency of occurrence of the selected category within the population of people or events enumerated in the denominator. (Thus, in the earlier example, the 9 per cent *excellent* response rate in congestive heart failure was based on 7 such responses among 78 treated patients.)

The denominator of such expressions may sometimes be displaced inappropriately into what Mainland has called "wrong sampling units" or "spurious replication."[37] As an example of the problem, Mainland cites the attempt to measure personal resistance to new caries by counting the number of carious teeth in a group of people, and dividing this number by the total number of teeth that were counted, instead of dividing the number of people with carious teeth by the total number of people.

The choice of an appropriate denominator is particularly subtle when the numerator consists of k events and when the data available for the denominator consist of m episodes in n people. For example, suppose we know that evidence of new carditis occurred 54 times in 105 recurrent attacks of rheumatic fever in 78 patients. Is the rate of new carditis 54/105 or 54/78? The answer to this question depends on whether we want to know the risk of new carditis in a recurrent attack of rheumatic fever, or in a patient who has a recurrent attack. The risk per attack would be 54/105, but the risk per patient cannot be determined from these data because we would need to know, as numerator, the number of patients who had had new carditis rather than the 54 recurrences in which new carditis had been observed.

When the numerator consists of an event that can occur repetitively, such as streptococcal infections or episodes of angina pectoris, the denominator is often converted to the total time period of observation for the persons in the population. Thus, the occurrence of 40 streptococcal infections in 100 patients observed for a total of 200 patient-years is often reported as an attack rate of "20 per cent per patient-year" rather than "40 per cent per patient." This type of person-time denominator can be useful for many situations, but it carries the hazard of possible distortion by the way the unit of time is chosen and by major disparities in length of the observation period for individual members of the population. Thus, the 20 per cent just cited per patient-year would have seemed miniscule if expressed as 0.55 per cent per patient-day and gigantic if expressed as 200 per cent per patient-decade. Furthermore, 200 patient-years could be obtained by observing each of the 100 patients for about 2 years, or by observing 9 people for about 20 years and the remaining 91 people for about 2 months each. In the latter circumstance, a denominator based on "200 patient-years" would be misleading.

3. Strategies in transstratification. There are no statistical criteria for deciding whether a populational index is best expressed as a curvilinear trend, a categorical ratio, or a dimensional average. For averages, there are also no criteria for preferring the mean or the median as the choice of expression. All of these decisions must be made judgmentally according to the logic of each situation. An example of the considerations is presented elsewhere,[22] in the expression of survival in cancer, where the median is usually preferable to the mean and where the categorical "rate" may be preferable to both the "average" measurements.

A critical aspect of these indexes is not just their selection but their correlation with the strata of population to which they refer. Suppose a population contains 50 people whose value for a particular index in the initial state is *high* and 50 people whose value is *low*. Suppose further, in the transition results, that the value has become *higher* for 50 people and *lower* for 50 people. Did these changes occur throughout both groups or did the high results become higher and the low ones lower, or vice versa? Unless the results are transstratified, we might fail to detect the major differences between one treatment that raises high values and lowers low values and another treatment that has just the reverse effects, making high values low and low values high.

9. Induction

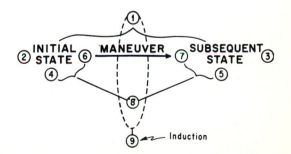

At this next-to-last stage in the architectural operations, we have finally reached a major activity that requires knowledge of what is generally regarded as "statistics." The data having been expressed for the populations exposed to each maneuver, we can now use inductive statistical procedures for analyzing the results and making inferential decisions.

A. Analytic procedures. In statistical analysis, various tests are employed to determine trends (or correlations) and to compare numerical distinctions in the differences among groups or events. The strategy of selecting these tests is beyond the scope of this outline and will depend on such characteristics of the research project as the types of data, the distributions of data, the number of groups, and the number of events. In seeking guides to the choice of analytic statistical procedures, clinical investigators may find certain books or articles[6, 28, 32, 33, 37, 45] particularly valuable because the characteristics of the research data, rather than the innate distinctions of the statistical tests, are used as a basis for taxonomic arrangement of the text.

Despite the many excellent procedures available for statistical analyses, certain fundamental problems in statistical logic remain unresolved and are generally ignored or glossed over in most textbooks.

One of the problems is the validity of applying, to populations that are not at all randomly chosen, statistical tests based on "random sampling." Since the intake of people in a survey, as discussed previously,[20] is seldom if ever "random," investigators could not apply most statistical tests to survey data if we insisted on "random sampling." To allow statistical tests, therefore, we conveniently ignore our constant violations of the basis for the test.

Another problem is created by the modern inversion of the concept of *variance* so that it can refer to the measured objects as well as to the system of measurement. The idea of "variance" was originally created in reference to repeated measurements, and each deviation from the mean contributed to the "error variance."[34] In many modern applications, however, variance refers not to mensurational precision in multiple measurements of a single object, but to populational dispersion in single measurements of multiple objects. "Quality control" and "range of normal" can thus become admixed in the same conceptual procedure, so that either the measuring devices or the people who deviate from a mean become associated with different magnitudes of "error variance."

Two other traditional problems in analytic statistical procedures have acquired new solutions in recent years:

1. Parametric violations. Since most of the dimensional data encountered in clinical research do not have a Gaussian (or "normal") distribution, we may not be justified in using t tests, F ratios or other "parametric" tests that depend on Gaussian distributions. The effect of violating the assumptions of "normality," although seldom mentioned in most statistical books aimed at biologists, has recently been thoroughly discussed in texts devoted to "distribution-free"[6] or "nonparametric"[45] statistics.

2. Validity of transformations. Attempts are often made to "normalize" a non-Gaussian distribution by using logarithms, square roots, or other transformations of the original variables. Since investigators generally decide about meaningful importance by comparing the data they have observed, rather than arbitrary transformations of the data, the scientific logic of these changes is uncertain. Are they preferable to using the alternative "nonparametric" or "distribution-free" tests that rank the observed data without altering the basic values? Suppose we have found that the cube root of the arc tangent of serum cholesterol is "significantly" lower in one group of patients than in another? Is a "significance" based on such a peculiar conversion of data really more meaningful than what could be found by ranking the results in a "nonparametric" or "distribution-free" test?

B. Inferential decision. In all of the procedures just cited, a statistical strategy had to be adopted for choosing the test that would be followed by an inferential decision about "significance." The strategy depends on the following act of contrapuntal logic: We assume, according to the "null hypothesis," that there is no difference among the groups being compared. With this assumption, we determine the probability (or P value) that the observed difference arose by chance. If this probability is at or below a selected α level, such as 0.05 or 0.01, we reject the null hypothesis and proclaim the observed difference to be "significant" at the calculated value for P. This statistical strategy of "hypothesis testing," although sanctified by tradition and worshipped by investigators and editors, is not entirely trouble free, however.

1. Uncertainties of P value strategies. The use of P values has been severely criticized in recent years.[3, 5, 34, 44] Some writers have proposed that P values and "significance" concepts be dropped entirely and replaced by estimations based on "confidence intervals"[5, 25] or "maximum likelihood ratios."[25, 31] In the avant garde today, many statisticians advocate procedures of Bayesian analysis, which replaces conventional quantifications with subjective estimates of numerical probabilities.[9, 31, 34] Partisan theorists are still debating the respective merits of all these proposals,[7, 9, 29] and a "winner" has not yet emerged. Clinical investigators, beset with insecurities about their ignorance of statistical procedures, may be relieved to learn that statisticians are beset with doubts about the basic "security" of the procedures themselves. For example, in one recent "biometrics seminar,"[12] conducted after almost three decades of dissemination and general acceptance of the doctrine that clinical trials required statistical "hypothesis testing," eight statisticians spent 25 pages discussing the charge, made by another statistician,[1] that "the concept of error probabilities . . . has no direct relevance to experimentation."

2. The restrictions of univariate targets. Regardless of the strategy used for a statistical decision about "significance," the decision must be based on a univariate target. Although able to manage multiple variables in the *initial state* of the patient, statistical techniques of "multivariate analysis" are not suitable for multiple clinical targets in the subsequent state. In some of the "multivariate" techniques, the target must be a single variable; in others, multiple target variables are accepted but are given the same relative "weights" or importance. Thus, a thoughtful clinician, appraising the results of treatment, might want to give separate evaluation to such multiple targets as symptomatic response, functional changes, laboratory results, side effects, convenience of treatment, and cost of treatment. The statistical decision procedure, however, is geared either to regarding all targets as having equal importance or to using only one target variable. To get a *single* answer about "statistical significance," clinical investigators usually abandon a judgmental evaluation of separate decisions for each target, and, instead, compress multiple targets into a single variable. This compression is the source of many of the "contrived indexes" whose scientific defects were described previously.[20]

3. Problems of the null hypothesis. Although the two sides of a coin are often used to illustrate concepts of probability, only one side of a two-sided biologic issue is explored in statistical inference based on the null hypothesis, which is used to "prove" a difference but never a similarity. If we wanted to show that two drugs were essentially the same, rather than different, we could not do so directly with the α levels and P value statistics of the "null hypothesis." We would have to modify the basic concepts by using confidence intervals and by applying the ideas of β error introduced by Neyman and Pearson[41] to supplement the unilateral scope of α errors. The modifications may enable the null-hypothesis procedure to be serviceable but do not alter the basic intellectual restrictions[34, 37] that arise in the absence of a specifically formulated procedure for testing "non-null" hypotheses.

4. Procrustean categories of decision. The method of making statistical decisions about "significance" creates one of the most devastating ironies in modern biologic science. To avoid using categorical data, a clinical investigator will usually go to enormous efforts in mensuration. He will get special machines and elaborate technologic devices to supplant his old categorical statements with new measurements of "continuous" dimensional data. After all this work in getting "continuous" data, however, and after calculating all the statistical tests of the data, the investigator then makes the final decision about his results on the basis of a completely arbitrary pair of dichotomous categories. These categories, which are called "significant" and "nonsignificant," are usually demarcated by a P value of either 0.05 or 0.01, chosen according to the capricious dictates of the statistician, the editor, the reviewer, or the granting agency. If the level demanded for "significance" is 0.05 or lower and the P value that emerges is 0.06, the investigator may be ready to discard a well-designed, excellently conducted, thoughtfully analyzed, and scientifically important experiment, because it failed to cross the Procrustean boundary demanded for statistical approbation.

The widespread acceptance of these rigid

categories of "statistical significance" is a lamentable demonstration of the credulity with which modern scientists will abandon biologic wisdom in favor of any quantitative ideology that offers the specious allure of a mathematical replacement for sensible thought.

10. Extrapolation

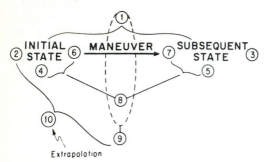

Extrapolation

Now we have reached the last stage. We have made decisions about the numerical distinctions of the data, and we would like to draw conclusions that will enable the results to be extrapolated and used elsewhere. This is the time for reviewing all the previous steps:

Was the objective of the research clearly specified? Was the stated objective implemented by procedures that carried out those specifications? Were the comparative maneuvers properly chosen and allocated? Was the population adequately identified and assessed for bias in intake? Were the data obtained by suitable methods, classified with stipulated criteria, and analyzed appropriately? Were the various forms of "intrusion" recognized and accounted for in the analyses? Were the results suitably stratified for prognostic distinctions of the population? What else might have gone wrong?

If all of these questions receive satisfactory answers, we have probably performed a valid, reproducible act of scientific research. If not, we may have performed yet another exercise in statistical numerology, and the next stage in the work should be not an extrapolation, but an architectural return "to the drawing board."

• • •

Although this outline of biostatistical architecture has now been concluded, many loose ends still remain. No attention has been given to research projects that are performed as methodologic explorations, rather than as clinical surveys and experiments. Such projects include studies of observer variability, establishment of criteria, choice and validation of indexes, and implementation of "double-blind" techniques in circumstances where "blindness" seems either difficult or impossible to attain. Important methodologic issues in logic or in management of data have received only minimal attention. Such issues include: tactics in prognostic stratification, chronologic arrangement of "spection," appraisals of "intrusion," and strategies of transstratification. The uncertainties about many inductive statistical procedures have been but briefly mentioned, and only scant discussion has been given to the many intellectual "pollutants" contained in statistical vocabulary. Although some of the linguistic or intellectual inadequacies of the words *sample, error variance,* and *significance* have already been cited, many other terms have been omitted. Among other statistical phrases that are often designated improperly in name or concept are: *normal, control, regression, negative result, standard error,* and *sampling error.*

All of these topics are available for consideration (and may ultimately appear) in our future sessions here.

References

1. Anscombe, F.: Sequential medical trials; a book review, J. Amer. Statist. Ass. **58**:365-383, 1963.
2. Armitage, P.: Sequential medical trials, Oxford, 1960, Blackwell Scientific Publications.
3. Bakan, D.: The test of significance in psychological research, Psychol. Bull. **66**:423-437, 1966.
4. Berkson, J., and Gage, R. P.: Calculation of survival rates for cancer, Mayo Clin. Proc. **25**:270-286, 1950.
5. Boen, J. R.: P values versus means and standard errors in reporting data, J. A. M. A. **208**:535-536, 1969. (Letter to editor.)
6. Bradley, J. V.: Distribution-free statistical tests, Englewood Cliffs, N. J., 1968, Prentice-Hall, Inc.
7. Bross, D. J.: Applications of probability:

Science vs. pseudoscience, J. Amer. Statist. Ass. **64**:51-57, 1969.

8. Cochran, W. G.: Matching in analytical studies, Amer. J. Public Health **43**:684-691, 1953.

9. Cornfield, J.: The Bayesian outlook and its application. Discussions by Geisser, S., Hartley, H. O., Kempthorne, O., and Rubin, H.: Biometrics **25**:617-657, 1969.

10. Clark, C. J., and Downie, C. C.: A method for the rapid determination of the number of patients to include in a controlled clinical trial, Lancet **2**:1357-1358, 1966.

11. Cutler, S. J., and Ederer, F.: Maximum utilization of the life table method in analyzing survival, J. Chron. Dis. **8**:699-712, 1958.

12. Cutler, S. J., Greenhouse, S. W., Cornfield, J., and Schneiderman, M. A. (with discussion by Ederer, F., Zelen, M., Shaw, L. W. and Beebe, G. W.): Biometrics seminar: The role of hypothesis testing in clinical trials, J. Chron. Dis. **19**:857-882, 1966.

13. Dayton, S., Pearce, M. L., Hashimoto, S., Dixon, W. J., and Tomiyasu, U.: A controlled clinical trial of a diet high in unsaturated fat in preventing complications of atherosclerosis, Circulation **40**:(Suppl. 2) 1-63, 1969.

14. Dixon, W. J., and Massey, F. J., Jr.: Introduction of statistical analysis, ed. 3, New York, 1969, McGraw-Hill Book Co., Inc.

15. Feinstein, A. R.: Clinical judgment, Baltimore, 1967, The Williams & Wilkins Company.

16. Feinstein, A. R.: Clinical epidemiology. II. The identification rates of disease, Ann. Intern. Med. **69**:1037-1061, 1968.

17. Feinstein, A. R.: Clinical epidemiology. III. The clinical design of statistics in therapy, Ann. Intern. Med. **69**:1287-1312, 1968.

18. Feinstein, A. R.: Clinical biostatistics. II. Statistics versus science in the design of experiments, CLIN. PHARMACOL. THER. **11**:282-292, 1970.

19. Feinstein, A. R.: Clinical biostatistics. III. The architecture of clinical research, CLIN. PHARMACOL. THER. **11**:432-441, 1970.

20. Feinstein, A. R.: Clinical biostatistics. IV. The architecture of clinical research (continued), CLIN. PHARMACOL. THER. **11**:595-610, 1970.

21. Feinstein, A. R.: The pre-therapeutic classification of co-morbidity in chronic disease, J. Chron. Dis., 1970. (In press.)

22. Feinstein, A. R., Pritchett, J. A., and Schimpff, C. R.: The epidemiology of cancer therapy. II. The clinical course: Data, decisions, and temporal demarcations, Arch. Intern. Med. **123**:323-344, 1969.

23. Feinstein, A. R., and Spitz, H.: The epidemiology of cancer therapy. I. Clinical problems of statistical surveys, Arch. Intern. Med. **123**:171-186, 1969.

24. Feinstein, A. R., and Stern, E.: Clinical effects of recurrent attacks of acute rheumatic fever: A prospective epidemiologic study of 105 episodes, J. Chron. Dis. **20**:13-27, 1967.

25. Fisher, R. A.: Statistical methods and scientific inference, ed. 2, Edinburgh, 1959, Oliver & Boyd, Ltd.

26. Francis, T., Korns, R. F., Voight, R. B., Boisen, M., Hemphill, F. M., Napier, J. A., and Tolchinsky, E.: An evaluation of the 1954 poliomyelitis vaccine trials summary report, Amer. J. Public Health **45**:(Part 2) 1-63 (Suppl.), 1955.

27. Fredrickson, D. S.: The field trial: Some thoughts on the indispensable ordeal, Bull. N. Y. Acad. Med. **44**:985-993, 1968.

28. Freeman, L. C.: Elementary applied statistics, New York, 1965, John Wiley & Sons, Inc.

29. Good, I. J.: A subjective evaluation of Bode's law and an 'objective' test for approximate numerical rationality, J. Amer. Statist. Ass. **64**:23-49, 1969.

30. Grubbs, F. E.: Sample criteria for testing outlying observations, Ann. Math. Stat. **21**:27-58, 1950.

31. Hacking, I.: Logic of statistical inference, Cambridge, England, 1965, Cambridge University Press.

32. Heath, H.: Elementary statistics, Springfield, Ill., 1968, Charles C Thomas, Publisher.

33. Hill, G. B.: The statistical analysis of clinical trials, Brit. J. Anaesth. **39**:294-310, 1967.

34. Hogben, L.: Statistical theory: The relationship of probability, credibility and error, London, 1957, George Allen & Unwin.

35. Lilienfeld, A. M., Pedersen, E., and Dowd, J. E.: Cancer epidemiology: Methods of study, Baltimore, 1967, The Johns Hopkins Press.

36. MacMahon, B., Pugh, T. F., and Ipsen, J.: Epidemiologic methods, Boston, 1960, Little, Brown & Company.

37. Mainland, D.: Elementary medical statistics, ed. 2, Philadelphia, 1963, W. B. Saunders Company.

38. Merrell, M., and Shulman, L. E.: Determination of prognosis in chronic disease, illustrated by systemic lupus erythematosus, J. Chron. Dis. **1**:12-32, 1955.

39. Miettinen, O. S.: Matching and design efficiency in retrospective studies, Amer. J. Epidem. **91**:111-118, 1970.

40. Mosteller, F., and Tukey, J. W.: Data analysis, including statistics, *in* Lindzey, G., and Aronson, E., editors: Handbook of social psychology, ed. 2, Reading, Mass., 1968, Addison-Wesley, Inc.

41. Neyman, J., and Pearson, E. S.: On the problem of the most efficient tests of statistical

hypotheses, Philos. Trans. Roy. Soc., A **231**: 289-337, 1933.

42. Pike, M. C., and Morrow, R. H.: Statistical analysis of patient-control studies in epidemiology, Brit. J. Prev. Soc. Med. **24**:42-44, 1970.

43. Remington, R. D.: How many experimental subjects? Or, one good question deserves another, Circulation **39**:431-434, 1969.

44. Rozeboom, W. W.: The fallacy of the null-hypothesis significance test, Psychol. Bull. **57**: 416-428, 1960.

45. Siegel, S.: Nonparametric statistics for the behavioral sciences, New York, 1956, McGraw-Hill Book Co., Inc.

46. Snedecor, G., and Cochran, W.: Statistical methods, ed. 6, Ames, Iowa, 1967, Iowa State University Press.

47. Taranta, A., Kleinberg, E., Feinstein, A. R., Wood, H. F., Tursky, E., and Simpson, R.: Rheumatic fever in children and adolescents: A long-term epidemiologic study of subsequent prophylaxis, streptococcal infections, and clinical sequelae. V. Relationship of the rheumatic fever recurrence rate per streptococcal infection to pre-existing clinical features of the patients, Ann. Intern. Med. **60**:(Suppl. 5) 58-67, 1964.

48. Taube, A.: Matching in retrospective studies; sampling via the dependent variable, Acta Soc. Med. Upsal. **73**:187-196, 1968.

49. Veterans Administration Co-Operative Urological Research Group: Treatment and survival of patients with cancer of the prostate, Surg. Gynec. Obstet. **124**:1011-1017, 1967.

50. Yerushalmy, J., and Palmer, C. E.: On the methodology of investigations of etiologic factors in chronic diseases, J. Chron. Dis. **10**: 27-40, 1959.

CHAPTER 6

Sources of 'transition bias'

The idea of a *cohort* is constantly used as a basic tactic in biostatistics. When we contemplate statistics derived from epidemiologic studies of cause of disease, from clinical studies of the course and treatment of disease, or from ontogenetic studies of normal growth, the fundamental scientific logic depends on the investigation of a cohort. A cohort is presumably the source of statistical data dealing with such phenomena as the appearance of lung cancer in cigarette smokers, the occurrence of thrombophlebitis in recipients of the "pill," the survival rates after different forms of treatment for acute myocardial infarction, the development of vascular complications in diabetes mellitus, or the anticipated weight gain in the first year of life. In all of these circumstances, we follow a group of people to see what happens to them after they have been exposed to something: an alleged cause of disease, the action of an established disease, the intervention of a therapeutic agent, or the course of time itself.

Despite the many concepts that depend on this type of scientific reasoning and biostatistical interpretation, the idea of a *cohort* is usually undefined or defined inconsistently in most statistics textbooks. In many books[1, 6-10, 23, 27, 28, 32, 36, 37] that are often used for teaching or for reference in medical activities, the word *cohort* does not appear in the index, and seems absent from the text. In two new biostatistical textbooks, cohorts are described with verbal illustrations but are undefined, and the illustrations are based, in one instance[34], on a life-table analysis of mortality, and in the other instance,[35] on a study of weight gain. During a nonexhaustive search of the literature, I was able to find the term *cohort* defined in only two books that had "statistics" (or some congener) in the title. An additional set of definitions was available (as might be expected) in several textbooks of epidemiology. The diverse concepts expressed in these six sources of definition are noted in Table I.

What seems to be consistent in all these definitions is the principle of longitudinal observation of a group of people, followed forward (or "prospectively") in time. What seems inconsistent are the purposes for which the group is being followed, the specifications for inclusion in the group, and the reference date from which the follow-up period begins. In two definitions, the use of a cohort is limited to studies of cause of disease, but in other definitions the purpose of the research is unrestricted.

This chapter originally appeared as "Clinical biostatistics— X. Sources of 'transition bias' in cohort statistics." In Clin. Pharmacol. Ther. 12:704, 1971.

Table I

Author	Definition of a cohort
Doll[11]	"In the prospective or cohort study, a record is made of the occurrence of an event, suspected of being the cause of the lesion, and the subject is followed forward to see whether the effect is or is not produced." (p. 73)
Fox, Hall, and Elveback[21]	Three definitions are offered or implied: "Groups of persons born in the same year or five-year period" (p. 191) "Related persons (comprising two or three generations) whose past disease experience can be well documented and where future disease experience can be observed" (p. 197) "Population segments born at the same time" (p. 261)
MacMahon, Pugh, and Ipsen[29]	"The investigation over time of an identified group of individuals" (p. 46)
MacMahon and Pugh[30]	(The cohorts) are defined in terms of characteristics manifest prior to the appearance of the disease under investigation . . . (and) are observed over a period of time to determine the frequency of the disease among them. (p. 207)
Mainland[31]	"Groups of individuals born in the same year or within a few years of each other" (p. 142)
Morris[33]	At least two definitions are offered: "The clinical follow-up, over many years if necessary, of whole 'populations' of suitable individuals" (p. 131) "A group of people born in a defined period is called a cohort; and a study of the future history of such a group, of what happens to them, is called 'cohort analysis'." (p. 232)

Several definitions require that the cohort members be similar in age, but other definitions contain no such chronologic demands.

Since the textbooks of statistics and epidemiology have either failed to define a cohort or have offered discordant definitions, we should not be surprised to find that the cohort concept has been used with many logical discrepancies. My object in this discussion is to consider the principles of scientific logic that are suitable for cohort statistics, and to note some of the scientific errors that may occur when the principles are violated.

A. Objectives in cohort research

Since the validity of biostatistical data may be destroyed by bias in the initial selection or subsequent examination of a population, a crucial feature of a cohort is the way it is chosen and maintained. When a single cohort is appraised for general extrapolation, or when two cohorts are compared for the effects of the maneuvers to which they were exposed, the investigator (or reader) must constantly beware of unrecognized bias in the procedures used to assemble the members and to obtain the data of the cohorts.

We can contemplate some of the necessary logic and potential sources of bias if we recall the sequence of

INITIAL MANEUVER SUBSEQUENT
STATE $\longrightarrow$ STATE

that was previously described[17] as a basic guide to the architecture of clinical research. With this sequence in mind, we can consider the purposes for which cohorts are assembled, and the ways in which bias can enter the results.

A cohort can be assembled to investigate at least four different types of maneuver:

ontogenetic, pathogenetic, pathogressive, and interventional. In an ontogenetic survey, the maneuver is time itself, and the effect to be noted is the growth or development of a normal person during a selected period of time. In a pathogenetic survey, the maneuver is exposure to an agent that allegedly causes a disease, and the effect is the development of that disease. The maneuver can be selected by the exposed person (as in cigarette smoking), imposed by "nature" (as in airborne infection, natural disasters, and "normal" or degenerative changes with age), or derived from medical experiences (as in diverse "iatrogenic" ailments). In a pathogressive survey, the maneuver is exposure to an established disease, and the effect is the change in the affected person's condition as the disease takes its course.

The activity that is called *therapy* consists of an interventional maneuver intended to change what might happen after exposure to a causal agent or during the course of a disease. The effect is determined by noting, in prophylactic therapy, whether an anticipated occurrence is prevented, and in remedial therapy, whether an observed manifestation is altered. Thus, in a survey of therapy, the investigator determines what happened to a cohort of patients who have already been treated according to the ad hoc decisions of individual clinicians and patients; and in a trial of therapy, the investigator can assign the treatment according to a prearranged experimental plan.

One of the main purposes of therapeutic surveys is for investigators to discern the appropriate types of data, indexes, and stratifications needed for satisfactory design and evaluation of experimental therapeutic trials.[12, 15] Although an ideal cohort for such surveys would consist of "untreated" people in whom "natural history" could be observed, such "untreated" cohorts are seldom attainable, particularly for the major chronic diseases that constantly receive diverse forms of treatment, includ-ing the decision to give "no treatment." Accordingly, a modern investigator studies natural history by making a *nil hypothesis*. He assumes that no mode of treatment may have been effective; he then combines the results of all patients, regardless of treatment; and he studies the "clinical course" in the cohort obtained by the combination.[10] Having determined indexes of accomplishment and demarcations of different prognostic strata for the entire group of patients, regardless of treatment, the investigator can then appraise the results of treatment within the strata, and can use the results for designing future trials.

A cohort can thus be studied for the observation of cause, course, or intervention, For a cause-cohort, the objective is to determine whether a particular disease develops after exposure to an agent allegedly causing the disease. For a course-cohort, the objective is to determine the path of nature in the normal development of a healthy person or in the outcome of an established disease, with or without treatment. For an intervention-cohort, the objective is to determine whether a particular maneuver alters what would otherwise occur in the course of normal growth, exposure to disease, or course of disease.

The key issue of scientific logic in cohort research is the validity of the comparisons that are performed internally and externally. In studies of *cause* or *intervention*, where the effects of different maneuvers are contrasted, the main comparison takes place "internally" among the cohorts who receive those maneuvers. At least two cohorts must be assembled—one that is exposed to the particular causal or interventional maneuver under consideration, and another cohort that remains either unexposed or exposed to some alternative maneuver. Thus, in patients with disease D, if treatment T_A for cohort C_A gives better results than treatment T_B for cohort C_B, we would first want to be sure that the two cohorts were similar enough so that the treatment, rather than a difference in cohorts, could be held responsible for the difference in the results. After this "internal" comparison is completed, we would want to perform an "external" comparison to extrapolate the results to the larger population from which the cohorts were derived. For this purpose, we would want to ascertain the similarity of cohorts C_A and C_B to other patients with disease D. If the cohorts were sufficiently representative of the diseased population, we might be able to conclude that T_A is better treatment for people with disease D, and not just for the group of patients who constituted cohort C_A. This type of external projection is often the only form of "comparison" in studies of *course*, where maneuvers are not compared and only a single cohort is observed.

B. Sources of bias in cohort statistics

The results of an observed cohort are usually expressed statistically as a ratio, or rate.* The denominator of this ratio contains the number of people initially in the cohort. The numerator contains the number of those people in whom the chosen target event occurred at a later date. For example, if thrombophlebitis develops in 3 of 1,500 women receiving the "pill," the thrombophlebitis rate is 3/1,500 or 0.2%; if 60 of 200 people with a particular cancer survive for three years, the three-year survival rate is 60/200 or 30%. As a general expression, if n_A is the number of people in cohort C_A, and if the target event later occurs in e_A people, the rate of the target event, R_A, is e_A/n_A.

Because of the forward way in which a cohort is followed, this statistical ratio has unique logical distinctions that are not present in any other types of statistical data. For the ratios in all other types of statistical "samples," the numerators and denominators can be assembled in diverse manners and can be related to each other in a variety of ways. In cohort statistics,

however, the people whose target events are counted in the numerators are a temporally delayed subset of the same people who were previously counted in the denominators. The numerators "evolve" from the denominators.

This temporal-subset distinction of cohort statistics provides a role not merely for the numerator and denominator of the statistical ratio, but also for the virgule (or "fraction line") that separates numerator from denominator. The virgule "contains" the time interval that elapses from initiation of the maneuver in the denominator population until the appearance of the target events counted in the numerator. The virgule thus "includes" several crucial features of a cohort: the initiation of the maneuver, the performance of the maneuver, and the observation of the population thereafter.

When these biological and logical distinctions are violated, the temporal changes implied by cohort statistics can become distorted or biased. One fundamental type of bias, which can be called "chronology bias," arises when the cohort is assembled as a cross-section of people in whom the maneuver may have begun at different times in their clinical course, so that the virgule does not represent the inception of the maneuver for each member of the cohort. This type of bias is so important and widespread in cohort statistics that it will receive a separate discussion in the next paper of this series. A second fundamental type of bias, which can be called "transition bias," arises from problems in various aspects of the way that people are transferred from their anonymity in a general population to their prominence in the data for a statistical cohort. The diverse sources and difficulties of transition bias are the topic for the rest of the discussion here.

C. The problems of transition bias

In order to contribute to the statistics of a cohort, each of its members must undergo six major populational transfers: from the general population to the base popula-

---

*I shall not attempt to differentiate among the terms *ratio*, *rate*, and *proportion*. The distinctions are seldom honored, even by people who know the differences, and the three terms are used interchangeably, with *rate* being most popular.

tion of people with the particular condition under study in the denominator; from that base population to the parent population from which the cohort (or cohorts) is (are) derived; from the parent population to the candidate population that is eligible for "admission" to the cohort; from the candidate population to the particular cohort that has been exposed to a maneuver and that becomes counted in the denominator; from the state before inception of the maneuver to a postmaneuveral state in which the target event may occur; and from occurrence of the target event to the detected target that is counted in the numerator.

The first three of these transfers occur before the cohort is assembled, and are not expressed in the cohort data. The members of a general population must have or must develop the particular condition that brings them into the base population under consideration. If the condition is a state of health, as in studies of cause of disease, then the base population consists of those members of the general population who are in the appropriate state of health. If the condition is a state of disease, as in studies of pathogressive course or therapeutic intervention, the base population consists of those members of the general population who have developed the appropriate state of disease. Thus, if the maneuver under study is the effect of cigarette smoking on healthy adults, the base population consists of those people in the general population who are healthy adults. If the maneuver under study is the effect of surgical treatment for angina pectoris, the base population consists of the anginal members of the general population.

Since an entire base population can seldom be studied, investigators usually choose cohorts from a parent population. The parent population contains those members of the base population who reach a milieu that provides the opportunity for the members to be investigatively observed. This milieu is often a clinical setting, such as a hospital, but it also can be the type of epidemiologic setting achieved with a field survey or with mailed questionnaires. Thus, if the cohort statistics are based on treatment of a disease at a particular hospital, the parent population consists of the hospitalized patients with that disease; if the cohort is obtained by mailing questionnaires to a group of healthy adults to ask about their smoking habits, the parent population consists of the people who have been sent the questionnaire.

Not all members of a parent population enter into cohort statistics. Because of various types of eligibility criteria, some or many members of a parent population may be excluded from the candidate population that enters the cohort(s). Thus, in choosing treatment for a particular disease, physicians may exclude patients who are too sick, too uncooperative, or otherwise unsuitable for the proposed therapy. In studies of cause of disease, the people who have received a questionnaire determine their own eligibility for the candidate population by deciding to complete and to return the questionnaire. After these exclusions have been completed, the members of the general population have successively negotiated the various transfers that lead them to the candidate population that enters a cohort. The maneuvers associated with an intervention-cohort are usually assigned ad hoc by a physician or planned by an investigator; the maneuvers associated with a cause-cohort have often been chosen by the members of the cohort and are noted from their responses in a questionnaire or interview.

Since the denominator of cohort statistics is not demarcated until the candidate population has been associated with the maneuver, the transfers from general population to base population to parent population to candidate population are not accounted for in cohort data. Nevertheless, these transfers profoundly affect the extrapolation of the results noted in cohort statistics. Unless the candidate population adequately represents its antecedent populations, the cohort data may not be validly applicable to any group of people beyond the particular persons who were observed. The "internal" comparison of the cohorts may be valid within the candidate population, but a bias in the assembly of the candidate population may prevent the results from being extrapolated to any members of the "external" population in the world beyond the immediate cohorts. For this reason, the final interpretation of cohort statistics depends on crucial features of populational transfers that are not noted or contemplated in any of the numerical data that constitute the statistical results. The problems entailed in detecting and reducing the bias created by these pre-cohort transfers will be reserved for discussion later in this essay.

After the candidate population has been assembled, the remaining types of populational transfer are cited in the statistical ratios, and can be contemplated directly. These transitions can be biased by factors affecting the denominator, the numerator, or the virgule of the statistical ratios. In the denominators, bias is created unless the cohorts compared to assess the effects of a maneuver are shown to have equal susceptibility to the target event before the maneuver begins. In the virgule, bias is created unless the cohorts have equal performance of the compared maneuvers. In the numerators, bias is created unless the cohorts have equal opportunity for the target event to be detected when it occurs. Major disparities in any of these three features—susceptibility to target, performance of maneuver, and detection of target—can produce a transition bias that will impair the scientific validity of the comparisons.

1. Equal susceptibility to the target event. Suppose the expected three-year survival rate for patients with a particular cancer is 70% in those with a localized tumor, and 20% in those with metastatic disease. Now suppose we wanted to compare the results of surgical treatment versus radiotherapy. If the surgical cohort consisted exclusively of patients with localized cancer, and if the radiotherapy cohort consisted exclusively of patients with metastases, we would immediately recognize the comparison as unfair. The contrast of treatment would be biased because the two cohorts had unequal prognostic expectations before treatment was applied.

Now suppose we had a mixture of localized and metastatic patients in the two cohorts. The cohorts would still be biased unless the mixture was proportionately equal in the two strata (or subgroups) that compose the cohorts. For example, let us assume that neither surgery nor radiotherapy has any effect on the natural course of the cancer, but suppose the surgical cohort contained 85% localized patients and 15% metastatic patients, whereas the radiotherapy cohort contained 40% localized and 60% metastatic patients. The survival rates in the two cohorts would be as follows:

Surgery cohort: $(.85)\ (.70) + (.15)\ (.20) =$
$.595 + .030 = 62.5\%$
Radiotherapy cohort: $(.40)\ (.70) + (.60)\ (.20)$
$= .28 + .12 = 40\%.$

Thus, although the two treatments had no effect on the course of the cancer, the disproportionate mixture of localized and metastatic patients would make the survival rate in the surgery cohort seem more than 1½ times higher than that in the radiotherapy cohort. If we were unaware of prognostic differences between localized and metastatic patients, and if we were unaware of the disproportionate mixture of these two groups of patients in the cohorts, we would conclude erroneously that surgery was substantially better treatment than radiotherapy.

The hazard of this type of error is the reason for recognizing prognostic stratification[15] as a crucial feature of cohort research. If a cohort can be divided into strata of people with distinctly different prognoses (i.e., susceptibility to the target event), then the compared cohorts will be biased unless they have similar proportions of the prognostically disparate strata.

The mathematics of this situation can be demonstrated, with the aid of some simple algebra, as follows: Suppose that people with a condition or disease, D, can be divided into two strata, S_1 and S_2, with corresponding expected rates, r_1 and r_2, for the target event. (An example would be the division of cancer patients into a localized group, with expected 70% survival, and a metastatic group, with expected 20% survival.) Now suppose that we assemble cohorts A and B as a mixture of patients from the two strata, S_1 and S_2. In cohort A, let k_A be the proportion of patients from S_1; $1-k_A$ will then be the proportion of patients from S_2. For cohort B, the corresponding proportions for S_1 and S_2 will be k_B and $1-k_B$. The expected rate of occurrence of the target event in cohort A will then be

$$R_A = k_A r_1 + (1-k_A)r_2 = k_A(r_1-r_2) + r_2.$$

For cohort B, the rate will be

$$R_B = k_B r_1 + (1-k_B)r_2 = k_B(r_1-r_2) + r_2.$$

If the proportionate distribution of the two strata were the same in both cohorts, so that $k_A = k_B$, the two cohorts would have similar expectations, with $R_A = R_B$ regardless of the individual values for r_1 and r_2. Alternatively, if the two strata, S_1 and S_2, were prognostically similar, with identical target rates of $r_1 = r_2$, the terms containing (r_1-r_2) would be zero, and the values for R_A and R_B would be equal, regardless of any disproportions in the values for k_A and k_B. But if the two strata have unequal target rates, so that $r_1 \neq r_2$, *and* if the strata are disproportionately distributed, so that $k_A \neq k_B$, the results for R_A and R_B will differ. By subtracting the entities noted in the preceding equations, we get

$$R_A - R_B = (k_A - k_B)(r_1 - r_2).$$

Thus, in the preceding example for cancer patients, $r_1 - r_2 = .70 - .20 = .50$ and $k_A - k_B = .85 - .40 = .45$. The difference $R_A - R_B = (.50)(.45) = .225 = 22.5\%$, which is the difference between the 62.5% and 40% noted earlier for the two cohorts.

The general principle here can be stated as follows. If $\Delta_k = |k_A - k_B|$ is the difference in proportional distribution of the two strata in two main cohorts, and if $\Delta_r = |r_1 - r_2|$ is the difference in the rates of the target event for those two strata, then the baseline difference in expected rates for the two main cohorts will be the product $\Delta_k \Delta_r$. The value of $\Delta_k \Delta_r$ is the bias introduced when two cohorts contain disproportionate amounts of patients from two distinctively different prognostic strata.*

A consideration of different prognostic strata is important not just for the issue of bias in compared cohorts, but also to avoid misleading conclusions about the results of maneuvers that have opposite effects on different prognostic strata within the same cohort.[15] For example, returning to the cancer population described earlier, suppose the surgery cohort and the radiotherapy cohort each contained 50% localized and 50% metastatic patients. Suppose, however, that surgery raises the survival rate by an increment of 15% in the localized patients and lowers survival by a decrement of 15% in the metastatic group; whereas radiotherapy has exactly the reverse effect. Thus, the survival rate after surgery would be 85% in patients with localized cancer and 5% for metastatic cancer; whereas radiotherapy would reduce survival to 55% in localized patients and raise survival to 35% in metastatic patients. The survival rate in the surgery cohort would then be

$$(.85)(.50) + (.05)(.50) =$$
$$(.425) + (.025) = 45\%$$

The survival rate in the radiotherapy cohort would be

$$(.55)(.50) + .(35)(.50) =$$
$$(.275) + (.175) = 45\%.$$

Consequently, if we looked only at the

---

*For two cohorts comprising people from three distinctively different prognostic strata, with target rates r_1, r_2, and r_3, the calculations would be as follows: Let k_A be the proportion of r_1-type patients and m_A be the proportion of r_2-type patients in Cohort A. The proportion of r_3-type patients will be $1-k_A-m_A$. For Cohort B, the corresponding values will be k_B, m_B, and $1-k_B-m_B$.

The expected target rates would be

For Cohort A, $R_A = k_A r_1 + m_A r_2 + (1-k_A-m_A)r_3$.

For Cohort B, $R_B = k_B r_1 + m_B r_2 + (1-k_B-m_B)r_3$.

By subtraction, the difference in cohort rates is

$R_A - R_B = (k_A-k_B)(r_1-r_3) + (m_A-m_B)(r_2-r_3)$.

Thus, if Δ_k and Δ_m, respectively, represent $|k_A-k_B|$ and $|m_A-m_B|$, and if Δ_{r_1} and Δ_{r_2}, respectively, represent $|r_1-r_3|$ and $|r_2-r_3|$, the bias can be specified as $\Delta_k \Delta_{r_1} + \Delta_m \Delta_{r_2}$. If only two prognostic strata are under consideration, the bias reduces to the $\Delta_k \Delta_r$ noted previously.

total survival rates, ignoring a prognostic stratification, we would conclude erroneously that surgery and radiotherapy had similar effects in the treatment of cancer, although the actual effects were completely opposite in the two prognostically different strata.

These problems in prognostic stratification can affect any type of cohort research, regardless of whether the study deals with intervention, cause, or course. In surveys of intervention, a prognostic stratification of cohorts is needed to avoid the bias that can arise when physicians assign treatment selectively. For example, if surgery is preferentially chosen for "operable" patients with localized cancer and is seldom offered when the cancer is metastatic, a surgical cohort will inevitably be biased for comparison with a cohort that receives radiotherapy or any other mode of therapy in which patients are not preselected for their "operability."

In pathogenetic surveys of cause of disease, the issues of prognostic stratification are more difficult to discern and to identify —mainly because epidemiologists have generally obtained so little information on the subject. The bias to beware is produced by patients' self-selection of the "causal" maneuver. Suppose that people who are "tense" have a lower life expectancy than people who are not. Suppose also that tense people are more likely to become cigarette smokers than people who are not "tense." Compared to a cohort of nonsmokers, a cohort of cigarette smokers may thus be disproportionately large in its quota of "tense" people. The subsequent comparative reduction in life expectancy of the smokers might then be due to the reduction caused by "tension" rather than by smoking.

In surveys of course of disease, a prognostic stratification is necessary to avoid misleading results in comparison of target rates from one era to the next. Thus, with better techniques of "early" cancer detection, a cohort of patients in 1970 might contain many more localized cancers than

a cohort found in 1940. The better survival rates in the 1970 cohort might then reflect earlier stages of detection rather than improved methods of treatment.

2. *Equal performance of maneuvers.* Another type of bias that is also commonly overlooked in cohort statistics is caused by inequalities in the performance of compared maneuvers. For example, in many surveys of treatment for acute myocardial infarction, the patients who received anticoagulants were also treated with elastic stockings, early ambulation, and chair rest; whereas the "control" group generally was treated with bed rest alone. Consequently, the differences in the physical therapy, rather than the presence or absence of anticoagulants, may have been responsible for differences in the outcome of the two cohorts. Another example of this type of bias would be the comparison of two different surgical operations, of which the first is performed by a highly skilled surgeon working with excellent anesthesiologic support, whereas the other operation is done by a less skillful surgeon working in a suboptimal anesthesiologic environment. In such circumstances, the better short-term outcome in patients who received the first operation might have little to do with the particular distinctions of the surgery itself.

A particularly important problem in treatment (such as diet or oral medication) that must be self-administered by a patient is caused by selectivity in the decisions of patients to maintain or reject the prescribed treatment. Suppose the natural rate of improvement for a particular condition is 30%, and suppose this rate is raised to 70% when patients receive either treatment A or treatment B. Suppose further, however, that treatment A is difficult to maintain (because of discomfort, poor taste, or some other feature) and is abandoned by 50% of the people who start it, whereas treatment B is more easily maintained and is continued faithfully by 90% of the patients. Suppose finally that we have not investigated the fidelity of maintenance for the two treatments, and that we are unaware of these distinctions. Our results would show the following rates of improvement:

For Cohort A, $R_A = (.70)(.50) + (.30)(.50) = .35 + .15 = 50\%$.
For Cohort B, $R_B = (.70)(.90) + (.30)(.10) = .63 + .03 = 66\%$.

If we considered only the total outcome in these two rates, we would falsely conclude that treatment B is inherently more effective than treatment A, when in fact the two treatments had equal potency. The difference in total outcome was due to differences in maintenance of the treatment, not in the inherent efficacy. If treatment A were reorganized in a more convenient manner that made its maintenance easier, the results might become just as good as those obtained with treatment B.

A practical example of this problem occurred during studies of antibiotic prophylaxis to prevent streptococcal infections and recurrences of rheumatic fever in patients with previous attacks of rheumatic fever.[26] For patients receiving monthly injections of long-acting benzathine penicillin, the attack rates of both infections and recurrences were substantially lower than those for patients who received daily doses of oral penicillin. Since the injection of penicillin ensured its receipt, and was almost always accomplished in the research clinic or in the patient's home, the fidelity of prophylaxis could be assured in the "injection" cohort. For the "oral" cohort, however, the daily ingestion of medication could not be supervised. Accordingly, in order to determine whether the superior results obtained with the injections were due to pharmacology or to maintenance, special procedures were established[13] to classify the fidelity of maintenance for the oral regimen as *excellent* and *not excellent*. When the injection group was found to have better results than the excellent oral group, the distinction could be attributed to pharmacology.

Even when the maneuver is assigned randomly by the investigator, rather than self-selected by the cohort, the patients who choose to maintain the maneuver (or who are able to maintain it) are a self-selected group, and the results may be biased by unrecognized distinctions that were involved in the selection process. For example, let us again assume that people who are "tense" are likely to die earlier than people who are "relaxed." Let us further assume that "relaxed" people will be much more likely to maintain a special dietary program than people who are "tense." Now suppose we perform a clinical trial of a special dietary program intended to reduce atherosclerosis. Having learned about the bias involved in failing to assess fidelity of a maneuver's maintenance, we carefully perform such assessments, and we then exclude from consideration the people who did not maintain the diet faithfully. Our group of faithful dieters will now be composed mainly of "relaxed" people, because the "tense" people will not have adhered to the dietary program. Our "control" group, which did not have to adhere to a diet, will be composed of a mixture of "tense" and "relaxed" people. Even if the diet has no effects on mortality, the resultant death rate will nevertheless be lower in the faithful dieters than in the "control" group, because the dieting cohort will contain a predominance of "relaxed" people, with low death rates.

3. Equal detection of target. Another type of transition bias, discussed earlier in this series of papers,[20] has been almost totally ignored in epidemiologic research, and acts as a major flaw in the validity of cohort statistics dealing with causes of disease.

Many acute ailments, such as streptococcal infections and thrombophlebitis, and many chronic diseases, such as lung cancer and coronary artery disease, are not detected unless the patient receives regular medical surveillance and/or special diagnostic testing. For example, as noted in necropsy examinations, about 20% of patients with lung cancer[25] and about 50% of patients with coronary artery disease[2] had not received the appropriate diagnosis during life.

Because so many major ailments can escape diagnostic identification, an important source of bias in compared cohorts is an unequal opportunity to have the target event detected. To avoid such bias, the two cohorts should be relatively similar in the frequency, intensity, and scope of medical examinations—particularly those techniques by which the target event is detected. For example, if lung cancer is the target event sought in a comparison of smokers and nonsmokers, the results may be biased if chest x-ray examinations were routinely performed more frequently in the smokers. If coronary artery disease is the target sought in a comparison of laborers and executives, the results may be biased if electrocardiograms were routinely performed more frequently in the executives.

To illustrate the quantitative aspects of this type of bias, let us assume that thrombophlebitis is detected when it occurs in 80% of a stratum that consists of women who have frequent medical examinations, but is detected in only 40% of a stratum of women examined infrequently. Let us assume further that a cohort of women taking the "pill" contains 75% of women from the first stratum and only 25% from the second, whereas a cohort of women using other forms of contraception contains 45% of women from the first stratum and 55% from the second. Finally, let us assume that r, the rate of development of thrombophlebitis, is the same for the "pill" as for other contraceptive agents. The reported rates of thrombophlebitis in the two cohorts would be as follows:
In the "Pill" cohort, $(.75)(.80)r - (.25)(.40)r = (.60)r + (.10)r = 70\% \ r.$
In the "Non-pill" cohort, $(.45)(.80)r + (.55)(.40)r = (.36)r + (.22)r = 58\% \ r.$
Thus, the reported rate of thrombophlebitis in the "pill" cohort would be substantially higher than the rate in the "non-pill" cohort, even though the "pill" had no differential effect on thrombophlebitis.

The algebra of this "tilted target" situation can be shown as follows: Let d_1 and d_2 be the different rates of detection for the target in strata 1 and 2. Let k_A and k_B be the proportions with which strata 1 and 2 occur in Cohorts A and B. Let r be the true rate of the target event, which is the same in strata 1 and 2. We would then find the following.

For Cohort A,
$$R_A = k_A d_1 r + (1-k_A)d_2 r$$
$$= k_A r \ (d_1-d_2) + d_2 r$$
and for Cohort B,
$$R_B = k_B d_1 r + (1-k_B)d_2 r$$
$$= k_B r (d_1-d_2) + d_2 r.$$
By subtraction,
$$R_A-R_B = r \ [(k_A-k_B)(d_1-d_2)].$$
If $\Delta_k = |k_A-k_B|$ and $\Delta_d = |d_1-d_2|$, this difference can be expressed as $r\Delta_k\Delta_d$, a value which indicates the bias produced by disparate detection of the target event in two strata distributed disproportionately in two cohorts. Thus, in the immediately preceding example, $\Delta_k = .75-.45 = .30$; $\Delta_d = .80-.40 = .40$; and $\Delta_k\Delta_d = (.30)(.40) = 12\%$, which was the difference between 70% and 58%.

These problems are an "incidence" counterpart of the fallacies discussed in the "prevalence" bias noted many years ago by Berkson.[4] Berkson pointed out that when the prevalence of certain manifestations was compared in patients hospitalized with different diseases, the results could be biased by disparities in the rates at which people with the compared diseases had been admitted to the hospital. In the fallacy under discussion here, the incidence of target events in cohort groups can be biased by disparate rates of examination procedures for detecting the occurrence of the target. Although both Berkson's point and the one cited here have generally been neglected in epidemiologic research, the lack of attention to such bias does not make it disappear and cannot provide scientific assurance that it is absent.

Such attention to bias in target detection is generally not a major necessity in therapeutic trials, because the investigator can usually make advance plans for the target event to be assessed equally in the different cohorts subjected to treatment. When the research is performed as a survey, however, the investigator cannot arrange for the target event to have been equally detected, and must beware that bias has occurred in the rates of detection for different cohorts. In intervention-cohorts, the therapeutic circumstances may have made the target event more likely to be detected with one form of treatment than with another. Thus, in an example cited elsewhere[18] for a clinical trial of antistreptococcal prophylaxis, streptococcal infections were more likely to be detected in patients receiving injected penicillin than in those receiving oral penicillin.

In cause-cohorts, phenomena associated with a "causal agent" may also have led to biased detection of the target disease. Thus, the frequent examination of "pill"-takers may produce a spuriously higher rate of thrombophlebitis than in the less frequently examined women who use other means of contraception. In course-cohorts, the different rates of disease[14] noted from one era to the next or in different geographic regions may be a reflection merely of the detection bias due to differences in diagnostic criteria and methods of case finding.

D. The reduction of transition bias

In certain research circumstances (as described later), some of the hazards just cited can be eliminated or minimized. In most forms of cohort statistics, however, various forms of bias are inevitable, and an investigator's main hope for scientific validity is to attempt to reduce or "adjust" the bias.

1. Allocation of maneuver. In the experimental circumstances of an interventional trial, the investigator begins with a defined candidate population. He creates the "treated" and "control" groups as he assigns the successive patients to be exposed or nonexposed to the maneuver under study. By allocating the maneuver according to principles of randomization, the investigator can attain three important goals: he can eliminate systematic bias in the allocation of maneuvers; and he can ensure that the compared cohorts will be concurrent in both populational source and calendrical time. The randomization procedure serves to remove systematic bias in allocation while assigning the compared maneuvers to cohorts derived from the same candidate population, during the same calendar interval.

The main systematic bias to be feared in these circumstances is the effect of previous transfer decisions that may render the candidate population unrepresentative of the patients to whom the results will be extrapolated. For example, when a parent population at a hospital is "screened" for admission to a therapeutic trial for a particular disease, certain patients may be excluded because they are "uncooperative," too ill to participate, or afflicted with major co-morbid ailments. As a result of these exclusions from the parent population, the candidate population will become disproportionately altered in a manner that impairs the validity of extrapolation to other patients with the "same" disease, despite the random allocation of treatment that formed cohorts from the candidate population.

The magnitude of this problem can be reduced if the candidate population is carefully identified, so that the extrapolation can be suitably cautious, and if a "screening log"[24] is kept to record the characteristics and outcome of the members of the parent population who were excluded from the trial. Thus, in a trial[22] of porta-caval shunt for patients with esophageal varices, perhaps the most striking result was that the candidate population, regardless of therapy, had a much better outcome than the members of the parent population who were not admitted to the trial.

In contrast to a therapeutic trial, the maneuver in a survey is chosen not by the investigator, but by nature, patients, or the patients' doctors. The investigator's inability to assign the maneuver is, in fact, the main feature that differentiates an *experiment* from a *survey*. In both types of research, the investigator can establish "control" groups for comparative purposes, but in a survey the investigator cannot *control* (i.e., govern, assign, allocate) the maneuver.

Because the exposure or nonexposure to the maneuver is not determined by the investigator, the cohorts of surveys are chosen quite differently from those of experiments. In an experiment, a candidate population is assembled and then divided into cohorts to be exposed or nonexposed to the maneuver. In a survey, the cohorts are determined, before the research begins, by their members having already been previously "assigned" to whatever maneuver they received. Since this assignment was not carried out by random allocation to a candidate population, the investigator must beware that the cohorts were rendered unequal in target susceptibility because of the decisions made when the maneuver was selected. In situations where the maneuver is chosen by doctors, a bias may arise because of pretherapeutic criteria that create prognostic disproportions among patients assigned to different modes of therapy. Thus, in cancer therapy, the criteria for "operability" usually provide a surgeon with patients who have better prognoses than those who are deemed "inoperable." Consequently, even when the cancer is left unresected, the "operable" patients have better outcomes than those who were "inoperable."[19] In situations where the maneuver is chosen by patients, prognostic differences may exist in people who select one type of maneuver in preference to another. Thus, people who choose to smoke cigarettes, to eat low-fat diets, or to use the "pill" may have distinctly different prognostic characteristics from people who do not choose these maneuvers.

Although such bias cannot be avoided in surveys, a scientific investigator will try to reduce its effects by "adjusting" the data. These adjustments consist of performing a prognostic stratification, and then comparing results of different maneuvers in the same prognostic strata. Thus, in a survey of treatment of cancer, the results

might be examined in patients who are in "good" or "bad" stages of disease. In a survey designed to determine whether the "pill" predisposes to cervical cancer, the initial gynecologic condition of the cohort groups can be determined. In one recent study,[39] for example, the women who chose to use the "pill" were found to have substantially more cervical dysplasia than non–pill users *before* contraceptive agents were begun. For surveys of cigarette smoking or high-fat diets, the personality, familial, and ethnic features of the cohorts can be assessed, and the populations can be divided into strata according to such possibly prognostic features as psychic status, ethnic background, and longevity of parents. The effects of the maneuvers can then be compared within similar strata of the cohorts.

The crucial issue in this type of adjustment is a *prognostic* stratification for the members of a cohort. The creation of the strata depends on the investigator's ability to recognize the particular initial-state properties or "risk factors" that affect prognosis for the target event. These properties cannot be chosen arbitrarily, and must be shown to correlate predictively with the target event.[15] Although certain demographic distinctions—such as age, race, and sex—are often used to establish strata in cohorts, these strata are not necessarily *prognostic* unless the demographic differences have been shown to affect susceptibility to the target event. Thus, if the prognosis for survival in cancer depended mainly on whether the cancer was localized or metastatic, and if the prognosis was otherwise the same for patients who were old or young, black or white, men or women, our search for bias would be concerned mainly with a possible disproportion between localized and metastatic strata. We would not be particularly concerned about demographic disproportions.

2. Ascertainment of maneuver. In an experimental trial or in a preplanned longitudinal survey, the investigator can make specific advance arrangements to ascertain the fidelity with which patients adhered to the assigned maneuver. He can then divide the patients according to *good* or *not good* compliance, and determine the outcomes in the different strata of "fidelity." These procedures can also be attempted when the survey is based on existing records compiled by other people, although the investigator is less likely to find that the necessary information was obtained and recorded.

In many modern trials or preplanned surveys of cohorts where such ascertainment could readily be achieved, however, the investigators have seldom made the required efforts. Adherence to maneuvers has been either omitted from assessment, or assessed only via questionnaires that were not rechecked or evaluated for reliability of answers. Thus, reports of success in the pharmaceutical treatment of angina pectoris, or in diet-plus-drugs treatment of obesity are seldom accompanied by data indicating the results according to the fidelity with which the prescribed regimen was maintained. In epidemiologic studies of the outcome of cigarette smoking or different types of dietary or exercise patterns, the investigators have seldom employed repeat questionnaires or other appraisals to check the accuracy of the history of the smoking, dietary, or exercise maneuvers in which the cohorts had engaged.[20] In the absence of such ascertainments and subsequent stratifications, the investigators have failed to "control" their cohorts for the hazard of an important source of transition bias.

3. Ascertainment of target detection. A preplanned longitudinal survey also allows the investigator to check the intensity of procedures for target detection in compared cohorts. Although such assessments are often incorporated into the protocol of therapeutic trials, the attempt to discern or exclude bias in equality of opportunity for target detection has been almost wholly absent in epidemiologic research. In almost all of the modern epidemiologic surveys of etiology of disease in cause-cohorts, no effort has been made to search for possible bias in target detection.

The investigators in many of these surveys have usually determined the occurrence of the target event not by an active research procedure, but by the passive "poll-bearing" analysis of death certificates.[20] This type of analysis cannot remove two types of bias that creates "tilted targets." The first is that the target event may occur without being recorded on the death certificate. Thus, such ailments as coronary artery disease or lung cancer are target events that can often occur without being detected during life.[2, 14, 25] Unless the disease has been diagnosed and unless the patient has been specifically noted to have died because of that disease, the death certificate will contain a "false negative" report of the target event. Although the investigators of etiologic cohorts have sometimes checked death certificates for "false positive" diagnoses, no reports have been published of efforts to detect and adjust the bias introduced by "false negative" reports.[14]

A second source of bias, even when attempts are made to check "false negative" diagnoses, is an unequal intensity of diagnostic procedures in compared cohorts. The data from death certificates do not indicate whether the compared cohorts were examined in equally assiduous manners. Since most etiologic cohorts engaged in self-selected maneuvers and received diverse forms of medical attention thereafter, the death certificate provides no scientific assurance that these unplanned, nonrandom activities were performed without bias. The assurance can be provided only with specific investigations of the intensity of target detection procedures. Such investigations, unfortunately, have not been performed or considered in contemporary epidemiologic strategies.

Although a scientific investigator establishes various types of "control" techniques

to eliminate bias in experimental procedures, epidemiologists have given almost no
attention to analogous forms of "control"
for *any* of the major sources of transition
bias in the cause-cohorts of etiologic research. A scientific effort to investigate
possible inequalities in susceptibility to
targets, performance of maneuvers, and
detection of targets has been strikingly
absent from modern epidemiologic statistics.

*4. Representation of antecedent popula-
tions.* If the compared maneuvers have
been randomly allocated, the cohorts will
usually be representative of the candidate
populations. If the maneuvers were not
randomly assigned, the investigator can
use prognostic stratification (as described
earlier) to help adjust for possible bias in
the assignment. Even when the maneuvers
were randomly allocated, however, a prognostic stratification is important to discern
the bias that may occur as a chance event
during randomization, and also to avoid
the problems cited earlier when maneuvers
have opposing effects in different prognostic strata.

In addition to these comparisons, however, an investigator would like to extrapolate his results beyond the candidate
populations from which the cohorts were
derived. As soon as he contemplates this
extrapolation, however, the investigator is
confronted by all of the populational transfers that occurred between the general
population and the candidate population.
In ideal circumstances, each of these transfers—from general to base to parent to
candidate population—should have been
performed via random sampling from the
antecedent population. In practical reality,
however, these goals are so difficult to
achieve that random samples are almost
never used in epidemiologic or clinical
research.[20] For example, none of the cohorts investigated in research on cigarette
smoking or the "pill" was obtained by random sampling from a base population of
smokers and nonsmokers, or pill users and
non–pill users. In the statistically designed

therapeutic trials of the past few decades,
none of the cohorts represented a random
sample of people with the particular disease or clinical condition under treatment.

In the absence of random sampling,
many types of bias can enter these populational transfers. For diseased cohorts, the
transfer from general population to base
population will be affected by medical
standards of practice with regard to "early"
detection of lanthanic disease in patients
who are asymptomatic or who have no
complaints related to the disease. The
transfer from base population to the parent
population found at a particular medical
setting will be affected by patients' iatrotropic stimuli,[12] by inter-iatric referral patterns, and by diverse personal, ethnic, social, or economic influences. The transfer
from parent population to candidate population will be affected by the stage of
severity of the disease, by the severity of
co-morbid ailments, and by the patients'
willingness to accept the proposed diagnostic and therapeutic procedures. All of
these features can alter the way in which a
cohort represents its antecedent populations
in proportions of people from different
strata within the disease.

For healthy cohorts, these transfers can
also be associated with various forms of
bias. For example, the "healthy people"
who form a candidate population by responding to a questionnaire may not all
be healthy. Consequently, unless the initial
state of each member of the candidate
population is checked appropriately, the
compared cohorts may contain disproportionate amounts of people who are
already ill, and who may even have developed the disease or target event that
was to be sought later on. Berkson[5] has
described the fallacy that can occur when
cohorts are created from disproportionate
numbers of sick and healthy people who
have returned questionnaires submitted to
a general population. After a "healthy"
candidate population has been assembled
by interviews or questionnaires, some of
the people may be rejected because of im-

proper or inadequate replies, and if the rejectees form a distinctive stratum, the cohort populations may be proportionately altered by the absence of members from that stratum.

In all of these transfers of diseased or healthy people, the main hazard of bias is an unequal susceptibility to the target event when the transferred people enter the candidate population that forms the compared cohorts. Consequently, an "adjustment" based on prognostic stratification is the investigator's best hope for reducing the bias that may arise during the "intake" of cohorts, and for increasing the validity of subsequent extrapolations. In order to perform the stratifications, however, the investigator must be aware of the possible sources of bias and must have suitable data for testing the outcome in different strata. Unfortunately, because prognostic distinctions have generally received so little quantification in modern clinical biology, the necessary data are seldom available, and the necessary stratifications are seldom performed.

Such stratifications are particularly important for the epidemiologic cohorts investigated for causes of disease. In clinical cohorts studied for the course or treatment of disease, an investigator can usually state the diagnostic or pretherapeutic criteria that differentiate his cohorts from other people who have the same disease. In therapeutic trials, he can often use previous clinical experiences to arrive at a suitable prognostic stratification even when specific survey data are not available to denote the strata. With these criteria for identification and stratification, the investigator can often clearly define the type of populations to which his results would apply.

In the cause-cohorts of epidemiologic research, however, an investigator begins with a generally healthy group of people and cannot classify them on the basis of an existing disease or previous experience with the course of that disease. Consequently, an epidemiologist must be particularly alert for the possibility that such "psychogenetic" features as psychic state, ethnic background, and parental longevity may be predisposing factors to such target events as disease and death. Nevertheless, the most common form of prognostic "adjustment" in epidemiologic cohorts is to stratify on the purely demographic basis of age, race, or sex. (The frequency of stratifications according to age is responsible for one of the uses of the word *cohort* in reference to a particular age group.) With such procedures, the results of a cohort may be inspected separately in such demographic strata as old people and young, whites and blacks, men and women, but the psychogenetic risk factors are seldom analyzed—probably because the necessary data are not readily available and would require rigorous investigative efforts to be obtained. An alternative type of demographic "stratification" consists of performing the same investigation in an additional cohort that has occupational or geographic properties different from those of a group that was studied previously. Thus, the results of a cohort containing people with the same occupation or in the same geographic region may seem more extrapolatable if similar results are found in other cohorts with different occupations or geographic regions.

These demographic stratifications, however, are based on arbitrarily chosen, conveniently available data. The stratifications are not necessarily *prognostic* unless the demographic factors have been shown to affect susceptibility to the target event. Even when age, race, sex, occupation, or geographic region have prognostic correlations, the role of psychic, ethnic, and familial factors cannot be ignored as even greater sources of prognostic bias. Thus, in a correlated prognostic stratification for mortality of healthy people, the longevity of parents, ethnic background, or psychic anxiety may be much more important as "risk factors" than the demographic aspects of sex, race, and occupation. The persistent neglect of these psychic and genetic features is an additional impairment to valid extrapolation for the cause-cohorts reported in modern epidemiologic statistics.

In the clinical populations studied as intervention-cohorts, many important phenomena are also regularly neglected during "staging" procedures or other attempts at prognostic stratification. Among the omitted clinical features that may delineate prognosis are the cluster and sequence of symptoms, the chronometry of clinical events, and the co-morbidity of associated ailments. Among the "decisional data" that may affect prognosis but that are usually ignored in statistical assessments are the iatrotropic stimuli, inter-iatric referral patterns, diagnostic criteria, pretherapeutic criteria, and patient acquiescence that have been discussed previously.

Since prognostic stratification is necessary to adjust for bias in the sampling procedure, in allocation of maneuver, and in differential effects of maneuvers, the existing defects in techniques of prognostic stratification constitute a major impediment to scientific progress in both epidemiologic and clinical forms of cohort research.

E. "Migration bias" and the unstable cohort

In all of the cohort problems just described, the members of the cohorts may have been unrepresentative of their antecedent populations and may have been compared unfairly, but each cohort was stable. Once its members had been noted, they persisted in their role as the denominator of any subsequent statistics. In one particular form of epidemiologic statistics, however, the data are presented as though they were obtained from a cohort, but the basic principle of cohort stability has been violated because of migration to and from the cohort.

This type of "migration bias" can occur when the rates of death are cited in "vital statistics" for a particular geographic region. For example, the death rate in Connecticut in 1967 for people aged 45 to 64 years was about 1%, according to tabulations of national vital statistics.[40] (In those listings, the death rate per 100,000 population in this age-regional group is cited as 1003.9. This rate is based on 6,405 counted deaths having occurred in an estimated 638,000 people.) Although this manner of citation suggests that the death rate was obtained in a stable cohort, neither the numerator nor the denominator of the rate came from a stable cohort. At the beginning of 1967, no attempt was made to count the number of people in Connecticut who were 45 to 64 years old; and at the end of 1967, no attempt was made to determine how many of those same people had died.

Instead, since the last census count was taken in 1960, the denominator of 638,000 people in 1967 represents an intercensal estimation, obtained with diverse "adjustments,"[3, 38] from people who had been counted seven years earlier in the age group 38 to 57. The numerator represents the counted number of deaths reported in Connecticut in 1967 at ages 45 to 64. Regardless of the accuracy with which the denominator was estimated, the cited death rate does not refer to a stable cohort. During the seven years since the 1960 census, many people who were originally in the 38 to 57 age group had moved away, and other people, who were 45 to 64 years old during 1967, had entered Connecticut from other geographic regions. If the death rate among the emigrants was the same as among the immigrants, the total rate for the apparent cohort would be unaffected. But if the emigrants were substantially healthier than the immigrants, or vice versa, the result for the apparent cohort would be distorted.

This type of bias must be considered when death rates are compared for different geographic regions at different eras. For example, if elderly people with a high death rate move to a region that is regarded as "good" for "old age," the death rate may soar for elderly people in that region. Instead of being regarded as a healthy locality, the region may then become regarded as unhealthy.

There is no readily available method of adjusting for this type of "migration bias." Even if the decennial census of geographic regions could be performed annually, the problem of intra-annual migration would still create difficulties. The migratory shifts in the denominators can be approximated by various methods,[3, 38] but migration is not accounted for in the numerators. One approach would be to arrange for standard death certificates to include data for not only the location of death and the "usual residence" of the deceased, but also an indication of how long the person had lived at the "usual residence" and the duration of time at the place where the person had lived previously. With appropriate analysis of such data, the numerator events could be more accurately demarcated for the denominator cohorts in whom the events presumably occurred.

• • •

Almost all of the problems just described in the "transition" bias of cohort research are caused by an investigator's inability to govern and regulate the lives of free-living people. The additional data that the investigator obtains for a human cohort and the additional stratifications that he performs are intended to compensate for the bias introduced by his lack of "control" over the procedures of sampling, allocation, maintenance, and target detection in human populations. Another activity performed in cohort research, however, is purely intellectual and is completely "controlled" by the investigator.

As the investigator reviews the assembled data for each potential member of the cohort, he must make certain critical decisions about the timing and chronologic sequence of events in that person's life. If the investigator makes these chronologic decisions improperly, he can create a type of bias quite different from the kinds just cited. The problems of "transition bias" are the result of selections made by nature, patients, and other doctors. The problems can be reduced or minimized by suitable identifications and stratifications, and, when

possible, by appropriate randomization and advance planning. The problems of "chronology bias," however, are created by the investigator himself; and the problems cannot be resolved by any of the tactics just noted. There is no way, in fact, to get rid of "chronology bias" because it is irremediable. When it occurs, the investigator has chosen the wrong cohort.

The problems of these distorted cohorts and the difficulties created by several other logical errors in statistical procedures for cohort analysis will be the topic of our next discussion two months from now.

References

1. Bailey, N. T.: Statistical methods for biologists, New York, 1959, John Wiley & Sons, Inc.
2. Beadenkopf, W. G., Abrams M., Daoud, A., and Marks, R. V.: An assessment of certain medical aspects of death certificate data for epidemiologic study of arteriosclerotic heart disease, J. Chron. Dis. **16**:249, 1963.
3. Benjamin, B.: Health and vital statistics, London, 1968, George Allen & Unwin, Ltd.
4. Berkson, J.: Limitations of the application of fourfold table analysis to hospital data, Biomet. Bull. **2**:47-53, 1946.
5. Berkson, J.: The statistical study of association between smoking and lung cancer, Mayo Clin. Proc. **30**:319-348, 1955.
6. Bradford Hill, A.: Statistical methods in clinical and preventive medicine, Edinburgh, 1962, E. & S. Livingstone, Ltd.
7. Bradford Hill, A.: Principles of medical statistics, ed. 8, New York, 1966, Oxford University Press.
8. Campbell, R. C.: Statistics for biologists, Cambridge, 1967, Cambridge University Press.
9. Cochran, W. G., and Cox, G. M.: Experimental designs, New York, 1950, John Wiley & Sons, Inc.
10. Dixon, W. J., and Massey, F. J.: Introduction to statistical analysis, ed. 3, New York, 1969, McGraw-Hill Book Co., Inc.
11. Doll, R.: Retrospective and prospective studies, chap. 4, *in* Witts, L. J., editor: Medical surveys and clinical trials, ed. 2, London, 1964, Oxford University Press.
12. Feinstein, A. R.: Clinical judgment, Baltimore, 1967, The Williams & Wilkins Company.
13. Feinstein, A. R., Spagnuolo, M., Jonas, S., Kloth, H., Tursky, E., and Levitt, M.: Prophylaxis of recurrent rheumatic fever. Therapeutic-continuous oral penicillin vs. monthly injections, J. A. M. A. **206**:565-568, 1968.
14. Feinstein, A. R.: Clinical epidemiology. II.

The identification rates of disease, Ann. Intern. Med. **69**:1037-1061, 1968.

15. Feinstein, A. R.: Clinical epidemiology. III. The clinical design of statistics in therapy, Ann. Intern. Med. **69**:1287-1312, 1968.

16. Feinstein, A. R., Pritchett, J. A., and Schimpff, C. R.: The epidemiology of cancer therapy. II. The clinical course: Data, decisions, and temporal demarcations, Arch. Intern. Med. **123**:323-344, 1969.

17. Feinstein, A. .R.: Clinical biostatistics. II. Statistics versus science in the design of experiments, CLIN. PHARMACOL. THER. **11**:282-292, 1970.

18. Feinstein, A. R.: Clinical biostatistics. V. The architecture of clinical research (concluded), CLIN. PHARMACOL. THER. **11**:755-771, 1970.

19. Feinstein, A. R.: Scientific defects in the staging of lung cancer, pp. 1005-1011, *in* Carbone, P. P., mod.: Transcription of NCI Combined Clinical Staff Conference. Lung cancer: Perspectives and prospects, Ann. Intern. Med. **73**:1003-1024, 1970.

20. Feinstein, A. R.: Clinical biostatistics. VII. The rancid sample, the tilted target, and the medical poll-bearer, CLIN. PHARMACOL. THER. **12**:134-150, 1971.

21. Fox, J. P., Hall, C. E., and Elveback, L. R.: Epidemiology. Man and disease, Toronto, 1970, The Macmillan Company.

22. Garceau, A. J., Donaldson, R. M., O'Hara, E. T., Callow, A. D., Muench, H., Chalmers, T. C., and the Boston Inter-Hospital Liver group: A controlled trial of prophylactic porta-caval shunt surgery, New Eng. J. Med. **270**:496-500, 1964.

23. Goldstein, A.: Biostatistics, New York, 1964, The Macmillan Company.

24. Greenberg, B. G.: Conduct of cooperative field and clinical trials, Amer. Statist. **13**:13-17, 28, June, 1959.

25. Heasman, M. A.: Accuracy of death certification, Proc. Roy. Soc. Med. **55**:733, 1962.

26. Irvington House Group: Rheumatic fever in children and adolescents. A long-term epidemiologic study of subsequent prophylaxis, streptococcal infections, and clinical sequelae, Ann. Intern. Med. **60**:(Suppl. 5) 1-129, 1964.

27. Kendall, M. G., and Stuart, A.: The advanced theory of statistics, New York, 1963, Hafner Publishing Co.

28. Lewis, A. E.: Biostatistics, New York, 1966, Reinhold Publishing Corporation.

29. MacMahon, B., Pugh, T. F., and Ipsen, J.: Epidemiologic methods, Boston, 1960, Little, Brown & Company.

30. MacMahon, B., and Pugh, T. F.: Epidemiology. Principles and methods, Boston, 1970, Little, Brown & Company.

31. Mainland, D.: Elementary medical statistics, ed. 2, Philadelphia, 1963, W. B. Saunders Company.

32. Mendenhall, W.: Introduction to probability and statistics, ed. 2, Belmont, Calif., 1967, Wadsworth Publishing Co., Inc.

33. Morris, J. N.: Uses of epidemiology, Baltimore, 1964, The Williams & Wilkins Company.

34. Remington, R. D., and Schork, M. A.: Statistics with applications to the biological and health sciences, Englewood Cliffs, N. J., 1970, Prentice-Hall, Inc., pp. 340-341.

35. Schor, S.: Fundamentals of biostatistics, New York, 1968, G. P. Putnam's Sons, Inc., p. 222.

36. Snedecor, G. W., and Cochran, W. G.: Statistical methods, ed. 6, Ames, Iowa, 1967, Iowa State University Press.

37. Sokal, R. R., and Rohlf, F. J.: Biometry, San Francisco, 1969, W. H. Freeman & Co.

38. Spiegelman, M.: Introduction to demography, revised ed., Cambridge, 1968, Harvard University Press.

39. Stern, E., Clark, V. A., and Coffelt, C. F.: Contraceptive methods: Selective factors in a study of dysplasia of the cervix, Amer. J. Public Health **61**:553-558, 1971.

40. Vital Statistics of the United States, volume II. Mortality. Part A. Tables 1-12 and 6-4, Washington, D. C., 1969, United States Department of Health, Education and Welfare.

CHAPTER 7

Sources of 'chronology bias'

In the previous paper of this series,[13] a cohort was defined as a group of people who are followed forward in time to observe the effects of a maneuver to which they have been exposed. The results are usually expressed statistically as a ratio, or rate, in which the denominator of the cohort contains the number of people exposed to the maneuver, and the numerator contains the number of those people who later developed a particular target event.

The type of target event that is sought in the "subsequent state" and counted in the numerator depends on the maneuver under investigation. In a cause-cohort, the maneuver is exposure to an alleged cause of disease, and the target event is the development of that disease. In an intervention-cohort, when the maneuver is an agent of prophylactic therapy, the target event is a condition to be prevented (such as a disease or death); and when the maneuver consists of remedial therapy, the target is a change in an existing condition. In a course-cohort, the maneuver is exposure to time or to the course of an established disease, and the target event may be a change in an existing condition or the development of a new one.

The "initial state" of the people contained in the denominator of a cohort also depends on the investigated maneuver. In studies of cause of disease or of certain types of prophylactic intervention, the cohort is deliberately chosen to be initially healthy, or at least free from the disease that is the target event. In studies of course of a disease or of interventional maneuvers that may alter the course, the cohort members must all be shown to have that disease. In certain studies of ontogenetic development, the cohort members must be initially healthy, whereas in other studies of effects associated with the passage of time, the cohort is taken from the members of a general population in a particular geographic region.

For scientific conclusions about the results, cohorts are regularly compared both "internally" to assess effects of the different maneuvers to which they were exposed, and "externally" to extrapolate the results to the antecedent populations from which the cohorts were derived. As discussed previously,[13] these comparisons are often made defective by "transition bias" in the formation and subsequent observation of the cohorts. The validity of external extrapolations may be impaired if the compared cohorts received disproportionate quantities of members from different prognostic strata during the transfer of each member from general population to base population to parent population to the candidate population from which the cohorts were selected. After the candidate populations are associated with the maneuvers that determine the cohorts, the validity of internal comparisons may be impaired if the contrasted cohorts are unequal in their initial prognostic susceptibility to the target event, in

This chapter originally appeared as "Clinical biostatistics—XI. Sources of 'chronology bias' in cohort statistics." In Clin. Pharmacol. Ther. 12:864, 1971.

performance of the compared maneuvers, or in opportunity for detection of the target event.

These diverse sources of transition bias can be adjusted or avoided if suitable data are obtained to permit analysis of the cohorts within different strata of people who are similar in prognosis, in performance of maneuvers, and in detection of targets. For prognostic analysis, the stratifications should be chosen according to clinical, psychic, genetic, or other factors that have been found to be distinctly predictive for the target event. The strata may be ineffectual if selected arbitrarily according to demographic data that are conveniently available but that have no cogent prognostic correlations.

Another type of transition problem is the "migration bias" that can occur in rates of target events for the general population of a particular geographic region. The effects of immigration and emigration make the population an unstable cohort, and the subsequent total rates may be biased unless they can be suitably adjusted for the exchanges of migration, or unless the rates in the two migrant strata are shown to be similar to those of the stable stratum.

These different problems in transition bias are an inevitable concomitant of the effort to study human populations whose free patterns of movement and personal decisions cannot be governed by the investigator. The investigator's best hope in these circumstances is to be aware of the potential for bias, to assemble appropriate data for checking the bias, and to analyze the results with suitable adjustments.

A quite different type of bias in cohort research, however, is not an inevitable feature of human life, and is entirely an intellectual creation of the investigator. This type of bias can be produced as the investigator deals with the complex subtleties of the diverse chronologic features that must be considered when cohorts are assembled and analyzed.

A. Chronologic issues in cohort research

At least four different aspects of time are involved in cohort research. One of these, which depends on the investigator, is the chronologic relationship between the events that transpire in the cohort and the time when the investigator collects the data used for research. The other three features of time depend on the members of the cohort. These features refer to a person's chronologic position in relation to the calendar, to his own life, and to his exposure to whatever maneuver is under investigation.

1. Investigative time. In studying a cohort, an investigator can begin his research before or after the members of the cohort undergo their exposure to the maneuver and its consequences. With either type of temporal approach, the cohort is followed forward from its initial state to its subsequent state, but if the investigator begins the research beforehand, he can collect the research data according to an advance plan, whereas if he begins the research afterward, he must collect his data from information observed and recorded by other people. Thus, if an investigator in 1950 decides to follow a cohort assembled in 1951-1952, he can try to devise special techniques for examining the members of the cohort and for obtaining the data. On the other hand, if an investigator in 1970 decides to follow that same 1951-1952 cohort, he must get his research data from existing records or from whatever other information had been noted during 1951-1952 and thereafter.

The temporal distinction refers to the time when the phenomena observed in the cohort are converted from their original descriptive data into the data collected for the research. This conversion can be planned before or after those phenomena take place. In both instances, the same cohort is followed in the same forward direction, and if the original data have been well observed and recorded, the investigator who does the research afterward should find the same results as the one who plans beforehand. For example, if an investigator wants to know the one-month mortality rate for premature babies at a particular hospital during 1951-1952, and if the hospital records are satisfactory, the investigator should presumably get the same results regardless of whether he planned his survey during 1950 or 1970.

The words *prospective* and *retrospective*

are sometimes applied to this temporal distinction in data collection, but these same words have also been applied, with quite different scientific connotations, to the forward or backward direction in which a population is followed. The distinctions are particularly important in statistical studies of etiology of disease. Such investigations are often called "prospective" if the investigator performs the type of forward longitudinal research described here, by following cohorts who are exposed or not exposed to a cause of disease, and by determining the rate at which the disease develops in the two cohorts. The etiologic research is often called "retrospective" if the investigator does not study cohorts. Instead, he begins with a group of diseased people and a contrived "control group" and he then looks backward to ascertain the rate at which the two groups had been exposed to the alleged cause.

The words *prospective* and *retrospective* thus have two distinctly different connotations according to the way in which they are used for investigative time or for investigative direction. In reference to collection of data, the *-spective* words deal with the order of timing for two different sets of events: whether the plan for assembling the research data precedes or follows the occurrence of the phenomena studied in the research. In reference to the direction of a temporal sequence, the *-spective* words deal with the forward investigation of members of a cohort toward the subsequent target event, or the backward investigation of a group of people in whom the target event has already occurred.

In the first usage of *-spective*, the main investigative hazard of "retrospection" is in scientific quality of data. Because the investigator could not "control" the original methods by which the population was observed and described, he may find that the recorded data contain diverse omissions, imprecisions, or other inadequacies. In the second usage of *-spective,* the main investigative hazard of "retrospection" is in

scientific logic. The sequential direction of phenomena has been completely reversed, so that the investigator looks not from cause toward effect, but vice versa.[8] The problem of scientific quality in data is always present in human research, regardless of the direction in which a population is followed, but when the population is followed backward the investigator inverts the logic of science and creates new problems in bias that transcend any of the "transitional" difficulties discussed previously, or the "chronologic" issues to be discussed here.

These additional types of "inversion bias" are too complex for further consideration now, and will be reserved for a later paper in this series. The main point to be noted here is that something must be done about the incompatible disparities in the two different uses of the words *prospective* and *retrospective*. The ambiguities created by the disparate connotations are confusing and destructive to clear thought. To eliminate these ambiguities, I propose that the *-spective* terms be eliminated from both types of usage.

We will then need two new sets of words to denote the timing of data collection and the directional pursuit of a population. Several alternate terms have already been suggested[1] for differentiating prior versus later plans for collection of research data. My own preference is to base this distinction on the Latin *legere* (to gather, collect, assemble) with its past participle *lectus*. If the research data are collected with advance planning before the observed events take place, the project can be called *prolective;* if the research data are collected from information that was recorded before the project began, the project can be called *retrolective*. As for the directional pursuit of a population, the name *cohort* already exists and seems satisfactory for describing a group of people who are followed forward. An appropriate name for a group of people who are followed backward will be considered later in this series of papers, during a more extended essay on the hazards of this type of inverted logic. The remainder of the current discussion is reserved for problems in the chronology of cohorts, regardless of whether the research is prolective or retrolective.

2. Secular time. Secular time, or *calendrical time*, refers to a particular date on a calendar, or to the interval between such dates. In some usages, the term *epoch* refers to an individual calendrical date, such as a particular day or year; and the term *era* is used to refer to the calendrical interval that spans two epochs. Thus, the decade between the epochs of 1920 and 1929 could be called the era of the 1920's.

A change that is noted between epochs or between eras is called a *secular change*, and, if the change shows a monotonic direction, a *secular trend*. Thus, the annual mortality rate for tuberculosis has shown[9] a downward secular trend during the 20th century. The survival rate for patients with Hodgkin's disease[6, 19] allegedly shows a rising secular trend during the past few decades, but the survival trend during the same era for breast cancer[6, 14, 18] has allegedly shown little or no rise.

A single cohort is usually uni-secular in that the pre-maneuver initial state of all of its members (as counted in the denominator of the statistics) occurred during a limited calendrical interval. To search for secular change in the effects of the same maneuver, results are often compared in uni-secular cohorts from different epochs or eras. Such comparisons are particularly common for course-cohorts and intervention cohorts. Thus, a uni-secular cohort from 1940-1949 might be compared with a uni-secular cohort from 1960-1969 to determine whether mortality rate has risen for coronary artery disease in the general population of a geographic region, or whether survival rate has improved for treatment of a particular cancer.

The main hazard of such comparisons arises from the different forms of transition bias described previously.[13] Although the investigator may believe that time itself is the only feature that has changed, other secular changes may have affected the proportions of different prognostic strata assembled in the denominator, the detection of target events in the numerator, and many important aspects of ancillary performance in whatever maneuver is under investigation.

Thus, the mortality rate for a particular disease at a particular region might be altered not by the progress of secular time but by different aspects of migration in the regional cohorts and by different techniques of detecting the disease. The survival rate for the treatment of cancer may also have changed not because of secular improvements in anti-neoplastic therapy, but because newer techniques of diagnosis have altered the prognostic strata exposed to treatment, and because newer methods of treating co-morbid ailments have prevented the deaths caused by diseases other than cancer. When the "same" maneuver is compared in cohorts of different secularity, therefore, the comparison may seem overtly "fair" in its chronologic aspects, but subtle sources of bias may arise from the transition problems cited earlier in transmigration, in prognostic strata, and in detection of target.

When cohorts of different secularity are used to compare different maneuvers, rather than the same maneuver, the comparison is usually promptly recognized as unfair because a change associated with secular transitions might be attributed erroneously to a change in the corresponding maneuvers. For example, because of temporal improvements in diagnosis and in ancillary therapy, patients with acute myocardial infarction today generally have better survival rates than such patients treated before the introduction of anticoagulants in the early 1950's. Consequently, when the outcome of a non-anticoagulant–treated pre-1950 cohort is compared with that of an anticoagulant-treated post-1950 cohort, the more recent cohort will usually show better results, but the difference might have little or nothing to do with the anticoagulants.[16] For this reason, compared cohorts should always be uni-secular unless the maneuver under consideration is secularity itself.

3. Life time. The age of each member of

a cohort may be regarded as *life time* or *generational time*. A group of people who were born in the same year, or within a few years of each other, may be called a *generation cohort* or an *age-specific cohort*.

When an ontogenetic occurrence, such as weight gain in newborn infants, is measured from the date of birth, the cohort obviously contains members whose initial-state age is similar. In many other circumstances, however, a cohort containing people of different ages may be divided into strata (or sub-cohorts) that are "age-specific." This type of age-stratification can be performed for at least three different purposes.

One type of age-stratification is used mainly for descriptive separation, as a way of "matching" the age of cohorts that are being compared for a maneuver other than age. For example, if we want to know whether people who lived in Connecticut in 1967 had better survival rates than those who lived in Florida, the maneuver under comparison is living in Florida versus living in Connecticut. To help get a fair comparison and to reduce the effects of transmigration, we might then contrast the results in different age groups—such as strata of people below age 45, 45-64, and above 64—in those two regions during 1967.

These are two main hazards of bias in such comparisons. The first is that the size of each cohort (or stratified sub-cohort) in the denominator is estimated rather than counted from decennial census data. The estimate for an intercensal year might be quite inaccurate if a substantial imbalance existed between immigration and emigration. A second hazard is not the numerical accuracy of the denominator, but the bias caused by disparate death rates in the two migrant populations.[13] Thus, if many healthy people in the age group from 45-64 moved to Connecticut from Florida, and if the same number of sick people in that age group moved to Florida from Connecticut, the denominators of the age-cohorts would be unaltered, but a major change could take place in the numerator data for deaths. Connecticut might then appear "healthier" than Florida, but only because of "migration" bias in the rates of death for the migrant members of the cohorts.

Another type of age-stratification is deliberately prognostic, to separate distinctions of target susceptibility among people of different ages. Thus, if elderly and young adults with maturity-onset diabetes mellitus have disparate survival rates, an age-stratification would be needed to evaluate the mortality effects of different forms of treatment. The main problem in this type of age-stratification is that it may not be cogently prognostic.[10] As discussed previously,[13] age is often a favorite variable for statistical stratifications because the data about age are usually reliable and easily available, but age is often not as prognostically important as certain clinical and co-morbid features of a diseased cohort, or psychic and genetic features of a healthy cohort. In such circumstances, a stratification based on age alone may be statistically impressive but biologically trivial. Unless the rate of the target event shows cogent changes with the different age strata, the "age-specific" rates may produce statistical fertilization without scientific fruit.

A particularly common type of age-stratification is performed for circumstances, such as the determination of general mortality rates, in which the cohort is a general population rather than a selected group of people who are either healthy or diseased. Since age is an important prognostic factor for mortality in a general population, the *crude death rate* (i.e. the number of observed deaths per number of people in that population) may be misleading because it contains no provision for the proportionate age distribution of the population. Consequently, although populations A and B have the same age-specific death rates in young and old people, population A, which contains a large proportion of elderly people, might have a substantially higher crude death rate than population B, which contains predominantly younger people. To avoid the bias contained in the crude death rates, we would therefore want to compare the rates for A and B within younger and older strata of the population.

Despite scientific clarity, these comparisons within strata do not have the statistical virtue of assessments based on a *single* index. Accordingly, in quest of such an index, epidemiologic statisticians regularly "correct" the age-specific rates with an "adjustment" that will allow the individual rates to be added together to form a single value. This type of "correction" is responsible for the "age-adjusted standard rates" that are a mainstay of epidemiologic statistics.

The adjustment depends on the distribution of ages and deaths in a selected "standard" population, and the method of "correction" is either *direct* or *indirect* according to the data available for the observed population that is to be "corrected." The details of the two methods are beyond the scope of this discussion, but they can be outlined as follows: In the direct method, the rates of death are known for the age-strata of the observed population; these rates are then multiplied by the proportionate distribution for each corresponding age-stratum of the standard population; and the sum of these products is the corrected death rate. In the indirect method, only the crude death rate and proportionate distribution of ages are known for the observed population; the observed age-proportions are then multiplied by the death rates for each corresponding age stratum of the standard population; the sum of these products is divided into the crude death rate of the standard population; and the result is used as a multiplicative factor that "corrects" the crude death rate of the observed population. Bradford Hill[4] has provided a particularly clear description of the rationale for these procedures and good numerical illustrations of the calculations.

The main problem to be noted here is the bias that is inevitable in both the direct and indirect corrections. In our previous consideration of "transition bias," we noted the difficulties that can arise when disproportions occur in the multiplication of ratios whose products yield the individual values added together to produce a final "rate." The same type of sum of products of ratios occurs in these death-rate "corrections." Since the "corrective" ratios depend entirely on the particular population that is chosen to be the "standard," the final results may vary dramatically according to the contents of that population.

As Fox, Hall, and Elveback[15] have pointed out, "One of the major weaknesses of the adjustment procedure lies in its lack of uniqueness, or in the influence which the choice of a standard population exerts on the outcome of the desired comparison." These authors suggest that "we do not want to compare summary rates at all" and that "no adjustment for age or other characteristic should be undertaken until the age- or other subgroup-specific rates have been studied carefully."

Despite these caveats, the adjustment procedure has not only maintained its current popularity in epidemiologic reports, but seems so well accepted that the authors often do not cite, and are not asked to indicate, which population was used for standardization and whether the method of standardization was "direct" or "indirect." In these circumstances, a reader who searches for scientific documentation of observations is unable to determine what was actually found in the observed age strata. Despite the unskeptical enthusiasm of the investigators who present such transmuted data and the remarkable credulity of the editors who accept the material for publication, the absence of suitable descriptions makes the published results neither interpretable nor reproducible.

4. Serial time. The fourth type of time to be considered in cohort research can be called *serial time* or *post-exposure time.* It is the length of time that has elapsed serially since "zero time," which is the inception of each member's exposure to the maneuver under surveillance. Unlike secular and generational time, which can be readily identified and classified, serial time is often difficult to ascertain.

The ascertainment presents no major problems in an experiment, since the investigator assigns the maneuver to the members of the cohort and can readily determine when the maneuver was applied, what was the initial state of each member before the exposure, and how much time elapsed until the occurrence of subsequent events. When the experimental data are assembled to form the statistical rates of the target event, the investigator can be sure that the virgule (or "fraction line") between numerator and denominator signifies the inception and subsequent performance of the maneuver for each member of the population.

In surveys, however, the investigator does not assign the maneuver, and may have many problems in deciding either what event to regard as the initiation of exposure to the maneuver, or when that event took place. In cause-cohorts, zero time may be the onset of a maneuver such as cigarette smoking whose exact date of initiation can seldom be accurately recalled. In course-cohorts, zero time may be the date of development of a disease whose specific date of onset can seldom be discerned. In intervention-cohorts, a particular mode of treatment may or may not be the first course of therapy for the selected disease.

The problems of defining and recognizing serial time, and the absence of suitable methods for analyzing this crucial chronologic feature of cohort research are responsible for many major scientific defects in the validity of contemporary cohort statistics. These problems will occupy the remainder of this discussion.

B. Zero time and the inception cohort

Since cohort statistics depend on the transition from an initial state to a subsequent state, each member of a cohort must have a chronologic reference point at which the "initial state" is identified, and from which the subsequent follow-up period begins. The characteristics of the initial state at that reference point are used to demarcate the people who are counted in the denominators of the cohort, or in the denominators of any stratifications of the cohort. The chronologic reference point is also used to measure the duration of time elapsed before occurrence of any target events cited in the numerators. Since the reference point has so central a role in the statistical data, its improper choice for the members of a cohort can create major, irremediable sources of bias.

1. The choice of zero time. Because the purpose of cohort research is to observe the effects of a maneuver, the logical choice of a reference date is zero time: the inception of the maneuver. Such a date, which is oriented neither to calendar nor birthday, would depend on the particular time in a person's life span or clinical course at which he became exposed to the maneuver under surveillance. Because of the problems noted earlier, the choice of zero time will differ with different types of maneuver.

If the survey is an ontogenetic examination of natural events that occur in postnatal life, the choice of zero time is obvious. It is the date of birth for the members of a generation cohort. For surveys in which the maneuver is exposure to a cause of disease, a suitable zero time would be the beginning of exposure to the alleged causal agent. For surveys or trials in which the maneuver is an intervention with prophylactic or remedial therapy, zero time would be the date of that intervention.

For pathogressive surveys of "clinical course,"[11] the choice of zero time is complicated by the examination of "natural history" in a group of diseased patients whose results are combined, regardless of therapy. Since some patients will have been "untreated" and since others will have received several courses of therapy, the choice of zero time should enable the patients to be mutually comparable at a date when therapy is first allowed an opportunity to affect "natural history." Accordingly, an appropriate zero time for each patient in such surveys would be either the date of the first treatment directed at the disease, or the date of the decision to give no specific therapy.

Thus, in a study of therapeutic intervention for a particular condition, zero time could be the date at which the intervention began, but in a study of "clinical course" for the same condition, zero time might be either the date of the *first* therapeutic intervention or of the therapeutic decision against specific intervention. For example, if we wanted to study the effects of radiotherapy in lung cancer, zero time would be the onset of the radiotherapy for each patient. To evaluate the results properly, we might then have to stratify the initial state of the patients according to surgical or other previous therapy, and also according to the "stage" of prognostic anticipations before radiotherapy began. On the other hand, if we wanted to study the clinical course of lung cancer,[11] zero time would be the first mode of treatment (selected among surgical exploration, radiotherapy, chemotherapy, or *no* anti-neoplastic therapy). We would then need to stratify the initial state mainly according to prognostic stages, since therapy had not yet occurred.

For the clinical course of certain ailments, the date of diagnosis is often the same as the date of the first therapeutic decision, since the two events may occur concomitantly. Thus, a diagnosis of rheumatoid arthritis is usually associated with a simultaneous decision about its therapeutic management, and so the date of diagnosis might be an appropriate zero time. In other circumstances, however, the choice of treatment may be delayed after diagnosis until specific pre-therapeutic requirements are evaluated. Thus, the treatment of chronic infections may await the results of tests for the infecting organism's sensitivity to antibiotics, and the treatment of a cancer may be delayed until the possibility and extensiveness of metastasis are determined. In the case of the infection and the cancer, the date of first therapeutic decision is often the best choice of zero time for pathogressive surveys of "clinical course." For certain chronic diseases, the study of "chronicity" may not begin until after an acute ailment has led to the detection of the disease. For example, in diabetes mellitus, the patient's initial diagnosis and treatment may occur in the hospital during an episode of acidosis, and the conventional plans of daily regulation at home may not be established until afterward. Consequently, for a survey of the clinical course of diabetic patients first diagnosed in a hospital,[17] a good choice of zero time might be the date of discharge after that hospital admission.

In all of the situations just described, the choices of zero time to begin serial time were oriented to the inception of each person's exposure to the maneuver under study. The choices did not depend on age or on secular aspects of the calendrical interval in which the cohort was chosen. These secular boundaries, however, determine the initial "parent population" from which the investigator selects the "candidate population" for his cohorts. In any type of cohort research, the members are assembled because they appeared at an appropriate site during a particular calendrical interval in which the investigator is interested. If the research deals with the course of disease D found during 1955-1959 at Hospital H, the cohort will be assembled from people noted to have the disease during that secular interval at the cited hospital. If the research deals with the effects of cigarette smoking in people who were healthy adults during 1950-1954, the cohort will be assembled from the healthy adult cigarette smokers who answered appropriate questionnaires during 1950-1954. Despite this common calendrical secularity in their manner of assembly, however, the members of the cohorts may have had major calendrical disparities in the date at which the individual zero times occurred.

The people who are uni-secular for a particular maneuver are not necessarily uni-serial for that maneuver. Thus, in a cause-cohort, the adults who were cigarette smokers during 1950-1954 had not all begun smoking during that time. Some people had started smoking many years before 1950-1954, whereas other people had begun more recently. Similarly, in a course-cohort, the people who are admitted to the same hospital with the same disease during the same calendar interval have nevertheless had the disease for varying lengths of time. For some patients, the therapeutic maneuver assigned during that admission was the first course of treatment for the disease, but for other patients, the treatment may have been a second, third, or later episode of therapy.

In addition to this problem of uni-seriality for the maneuver, a problem of unizonality exists for a group of patients assembled at a hospital or other medical center. The bias of multi-zonality was considered previously in reference to transmigration for a general population in a particular region. The rate of subsequent deaths or other events in the apparent cohort could be distorted by disproportions in the rates with which healthy and sick people enter or leave the region. Analogously, the rates of post-therapeutic events for the diseased population at a particular hospital may be biased by the patterns of admission and referral to that hospital.

For example, a large medical center that provides special types of radiotherapy or chemotherapy for cancer may receive many pre-moribund patients who are referred after having had "unsuccessful" surgical treatment at a neighboring "satellite" hospital. If data for these referred post-surgical patients are added to the data for patients whose surgery was first performed at the medical center, the combined post-surgical results may seem worse at the medical center than at the "satellite."

2. The inception cohort. The diverse forms of bias that can result from these different patterns of serial exposure and zonal migration after zero time can be avoided if the group under study is an *inception cohort*. An inception cohort consists of a group of people in whom "zero time" for the investigated maneuver occurred at the same investigative locale and during the same secular interval.

Thus, if the maneuver is the ontogenetic risk of death during 1967 for the general population of people in Connecticut who were 45-64 years of age on their preceding birthday, an inception cohort would consist of the people with that age and in that region on January 1, 1967, regardless of whether any members of the cohort subsequently moved away or became older than 64. The inception cohort would exclude any appropriately aged "immigrants" who moved to Connecticut during the year, or people already living in Connecticut who became 45 years old after January 1, 1967. If the maneuver is the first course of treatment during 1953-1959 for patients with lung cancer at either of two "index" hospitals,[11] an inception cohort would consist of all those people whose first course of treatment took place at either one of those two hospitals

during the cited secular interval. The inception cohort would exclude people with lung cancer who were in one or both of the two "index" hospitals during the cited interval, but whose first treatment had taken place at some other hospital or at a date before 1953 or after 1959.

According to these specifications, an inception cohort is uni-serial, uni-zonal, and uni-secular. The members of the cohort are uni-serial in that the initial state cited for each member in the denominator refers to his condition at zero time, when the studied maneuver began; the cohort is uni-zonal in that the maneuver for each member was initiated in the particular zone (city, state, hospital, or other medical setting) at which the cohort was assembled; and the cohort is uni-secular in that the uni-serial, uni-zonal zero time took place within the secular interval of the assembly.

The bias that can occur when cohorts are multi-zonal or multi-secular has already been discussed. Such bias is caused by the "transition" problems described earlier, and the bias can be reduced or eliminated with appropriate attention to stratifications and other suitable procedures that can separate zonal or secular prognostic distinctions within the observed cohort. The remainder of this discussion is devoted to the bias that can occur when a cohort is multi-serial rather than uni-serial, or when a uni-serial cohort is "aborted" by subsequent elimination of some of its starting members. Such bias cannot be removed by stratification or by any other procedure of taxonomy or mathematics. The bias is irremediable if the observed cohort has been permanently distorted by the omission of unknown numbers of people whose data are disparate from the reported results.

C. The bias of "survival" cohorts

Unless a uni-secular cohort is restricted to members whose zero time occurred during that secular interval, many of the members will actually be survivors of other cohorts with zero times that occurred secularly at an earlier date. For example, if we decide to study the subsequent clinical course of a group of patients noted to have lung cancer at a particular hospital during 1953-1958, any such patients whose first treatment occurred during 1949-1952 are survivors of the earlier cohort. If the survival rate for newly treated patients is the same as that for those who have already survived several years after first treatment, then we need not attempt to distinguish the "old" and the "new" groups. But if survival rates are different for patients alive at different serial times after zero time, our failure to make the distinctions can be scientifically disastrous.

Consider a group of n people with a disease D, for which the short-term survival rate is q and the long-term survival rate is r. The number of people who die early is $(1-q)n$; the number of people who are dead after the long-term interval is $(1-r)n$; and the number of people who die between the short-term and long-term dates is $(1-r)n - (1-q)n = (q-r)n$.

Now suppose an investigator decides to study this disease but does not specifically obtain a uni-serial zero-time cohort. Instead, he happens to assemble a group of people who were available after the "short-term" period had concluded. Since the short-term deaths have already occurred in people with disease D, the assembled cohort will be drawn from qn people, rather than n people in whom the disease began. Of those qn people, $(q-r)n$ will die during the long-term observation, leaving rn survivors. When the investigator calculates the survival rate for his observed cohort, he divides the survivors by the number of people with which he began, and he obtains $rn/qn = r/q$. If he had started with a true inception cohort, however, the correct survival rate would have been r, not r/q. By using a "survival cohort," he has biased the true survival rate by a factor of $1/q$.

To illustrate this phenomenon with specific numbers, let us consider a disease in which 50% of the victims die over a long-term period, but most of the deaths occur quickly, so that 40% of the population dies during the first few months. Thus, if we studied 100 people from the inception of the disease, 40 would die in a short-term period and 10 more would die during the long-term period, so that 50 people survive at the end of the long term. If an investigator assembles a cohort of 60 people in whom the disease had begun a short period previously, those people will represent 60 survivors from an original cohort of 100 people, and 10 of the 60 people will die

thereafter. The investigator may then fallaciously conclude that the long-term survival rate for the disease is 50/60 = 83%, instead of the correct long-term rate, which is 50%. The bias in survival was a factor of 1/.60, where .60 was the short-term survival rate.

If an investigator compares two cohorts that have the same long-term survival rate of r, but different short-term survival rates of q_1 and q_2, and if he selects his cohorts after the short-term period, the spurious long-term rates that he will get for the two cohorts will be r/q_1 and r/q_2. The ratio of these spurious long-term rates will be $r/q_1 \div r/q_2 = q_2/q_1$. Thus, if both cohorts have a long-term survival of 20%, but if the short-term survival rate is 40% for one cohort and 80% for the other cohort, the spurious long-term rates that will be calculated for the two cohorts are

$$\frac{.20}{.40} = 50\% \text{ for the first cohort and } \frac{.20}{.80} = 25\%$$

for the second. The observed long-term rate for the first cohort will therefore seem twice as high as that for the second cohort, even though the rates for the two cohorts are actually the same.

Now suppose two cohorts contain a mixture of two subgroups with different short-term survival rates, q_1 and q_2, and the same long-term rate, r. Suppose the proportion of people from the first subgroup is k_A in Cohort A; the proportion of people from the second subgroup in Cohort A will be $1-k_A$. Suppose the corresponding proportions in Cohort B are k_B and $1-k_B$. Because the long-term rates in the two subgroups are the same, the long-term results in Cohorts A and B should be the same if they were selected as inception cohorts, regardless of the proportions k_A and k_B. If the cohorts were selected after a short-term post-inception interval, however, the observed survival rates will be as follows:

$$\text{For Cohort A, } R_A = k_A \left(\frac{r}{q_1} \right)$$

$$+ (1-k_A) \left(\frac{r}{q_2} \right) = k_A r \left(\frac{1}{q_1} - \frac{1}{q_2} \right) + \frac{r}{q_2}$$

$$\text{For Cohort B, } R_B = k_B \left(\frac{r}{q_1} \right) +$$

$$(1-k_B) \left(\frac{r}{q_2} \right) = k_B r \left(\frac{1}{q_1} - \frac{1}{q_2} \right) + \frac{r}{q_2}$$

The difference in the observed rates will be

$$R_A - R_B = r(k_A - k_B) \left(\frac{1}{q_1} - \frac{1}{q_2} \right)$$

If $\Delta_k = |k_A - k_B|$ is the disproportion in the subgroups, and if $\Delta q = \left| \dfrac{1}{q_1} - \dfrac{1}{q_2} \right|$ is the difference in the reciprocals of the short-term survival rates, the bias introduced by disproportionate subgroups in two survivor cohorts will be $r\Delta_k\Delta_q$.

For numerical example, let us consider the two subgroups described in the previous paragraph. Both subgroups have a long-term survival of 20%, but the short-term survivals are 40% and 80%, respectively. Now let us form two disproportionate cohorts. Cohort A contains 75% of its patients from the first subgroup and 25% from the second. Cohort B contains 30% of its patients from the first subgroup and 70% from the second. If these cohorts are formed as "survivor cohorts" after the short-term post-inception period has ended, the observed survival rates will be as follows:

$$\text{For Cohort A, } R_A = (.75)\left(\frac{.20}{.40}\right)$$

$$+ (.25)\left(\frac{.20}{.80}\right) = .375 + .0625 = 43.57\%$$

$$\text{For Cohort B, } R_B = (.30)\left(\frac{.20}{.40}\right)$$

$$+ (.70)\left(\frac{.20}{.80}\right) = .15 = .175 = 32.5\%$$

According to the formula stated earlier, $\Delta_k =$

$$|.75 - .30| = .45; \Delta_q = \left|\frac{1}{.40} - \frac{1}{.80}\right| = |2.5 - 1.25|$$

$= 1.25$; and $r = .20$. The value of $r\Delta_k\Delta_q = (.20)(.45)(1.25) = (.09)(1.25) = 11.25\%$, which is the same result found by subtracting 32.5% from 43.75%. Thus, as the result of the bias introduced into "survival cohorts" composed of disproportionate subgroups with disparate short-term survival rates, we would have found a long-term survival rate in one cohort that was 11.25% higher than in the other. In reality, however, the two survival rates were the same.

The use of "survival cohorts" can thus create major distortions in cohort statistics unless the investigator ascertains that the inception cohorts would have been similar in their short-term (and intermediate) survival rates. Recognizing these distinctions, an investigator may try to stratify his survival cohorts for the duration of time elapsed since the inception of the maneuver. But this type of stratification does not eliminate the bias, since the members of the compared uni-serial strata will represent the survivors of a series of unspecified inception cohorts, each of which began at the onset of each of the different serial durations. The comparisons within uni-serial strata may be satisfactory, but the actual rates of the cohorts will not be accurate or extrapolatable.

1. The multi-serial cross-section. An investigator obtains a "multi-serial cross-section" when he assembles, from some conveniently available source, a group of people in whom the maneuver to be studied was initiated at diverse times before the group was assembled. Since the forward investigation of the effects of the maneuver begins secularly at different serial times rather than at "zero time" for each person, the group is multi-serial. Furthermore, because of this multi-seriality, the group is not an inception cohort; it is a "cross-section", comprising survivors from the inception cohorts that previously began the maneuvers at a "zero time" denoted by each of the diverse serial times. The use of multi-serial cross-sections, rather than inception cohorts, constantly occurs in statistical studies of the causes and courses of disease.

a. Epidemiologic studies of cause. A favorite tactic of epidemiologists is to assemble an apparent cause-cohort by a "rancid-sampling" technique.[12] The group under study is obtained from responses to mailed questionnaires or from the data of a "chunk" population that is conveniently accessible to the investigator.

The "transition bias" inherent in such procedures has already been discussed previously.[13] The parent population may not be representative of the base population because of selectivity in choice of the "chunk" of people to whom the questionnaires were sent, or for whom "baseline" data were readily available. The candidate population that emerges from this parent population may not properly represent the parent group because of bias in the willingness of the solicited people to return questionnaires or participate in research. Since the initial state of the cohort members is not carefully examined, the cohorts may contain a disproportionate mixture of sick and healthy people from the candidate population. Since the performance of the maneuver is seldom checked for reliability of description, bias can result from misclassification of the maneuvers as the "cohorts" are identified. Since the opportunities for detection of the target are not ascertained, bias can occur from the inequalities that produce "tilted targets."[12]

Beyond all of these forms of transition bias, however, such investigations contain the chronologic bias, arising from multiserial cross-section, that confounds any of the interpretations of results. Thus, if the research deals with the effects of cigarette smoking in a cross-section of people obtained during 1950-1954, the people in that cross-section who have been smoking for more than 20 years are the survivors of an inception cohort that began smoking at least 20 years previously. The people who have been smoking for 15-20 years are the survivors of an analogous inception cohort from 15-20 years before. The same problem of selective survivorship applies to all members of the cross-section except the people who began smoking during 1950-1954. The latter group of people constitute the only component of the "cross-section" that can be regarded as an inception cohort.

b. Epidemiologic studies of course. This same problem in multi-seriality occurs when an investigator attempts to study the effects of aging not by observing a cohort, but by taking a series of "longitudinal cross-sections" of people at different ages.

For example, if we wanted to know the way that serum cholesterol normally changes at 5-year intervals from age 40 to age 60, the scientific procedure would be to obtain a cohort of healthy 40-year-old people, determine their cholesterol values, and repeat the determination in each member of that cohort at 5-year intervals for the next 20 years. An alternative to this prolective approach would be to perform the study retrolectively through diverse records inscribed more than 20 years ago. We would try to find an appropriate cohort of people who were 40 years old at that time and in whom suitable data would later be available. We could then follow that cohort retrolectively by examining their subsequent records, checking the cholesterol results obtained at quinquennial tests, and noting the changes during the next 20 years.

Both of these cohort approaches would use valid scientific logic but might be difficult for the investigator. The prolective approach would require that he be willing to wait 20 years before he gets the answer to his question. The retrolective approach would require his tolerance (and adjustment) of the many situations in which cholesterol values were not obtained at the proper quinquennial intervals. And both approaches would require vigorous efforts to get suitable follow-up information for people who might become or had been "lost" from the cohort.

Since the scientific procedure is so difficult, many epidemiologic investigators prefer a different tactic, which provides suitable data for each person, which eliminates a period of waiting for results, which requires no effort in follow-up activities—and which destroys the scientific logic of cohort research. The investigator assembles a group of "healthy" people who are 40 years old, another group who are 45, another group who are 50, and so on through to a group who are 80 years old. In each group, the investigator determines the cholesterol values. From the distribution of the cholesterol values at these different ages, the investigator then draws conclusions about the change in cholesterol with aging.

Since each of these age groups represents the survivors of a cohort of people from the previous age group, this type of "longitudinal cross-section" permits no valid scientific conclusions. For example, suppose people with elevated cholesterol values at any age have an increased fatality rate. Each surviving cohort may then have a lower average cholesterol value than its predecessor, leading to false decisions about the way that serum cholesterol is altered by "normal" aging.

c. Clinical studies of course. In clinical surveys of the course of a chronic disease, an investigator may select his "cohort" from a group of people who were attending a special clinic for that disease. For example, to assess the future rate of vascular complications in patients with diabetes mellitus, an investigator may follow all the people who appeared in a Diabetes Clinic during 1950-1952. After determining the state of those same people in 1965-1967, the investigator may prepare statistics about the 15-year rates of survival and vascular complications in diabetes. He may even divide those rates according to the "good" or "bad" way in which glucose regulation was "controlled" by different groups of patients.

The bias in such studies should already be apparent to the reader. The initial population is a multi-serial cross-section of survivors from diabetic cohorts whose disease was first diagnosed at diverse "zero times" before the investigator began his research. Without knowing the results of those previous inception cohorts, the investigator has no way of determining how badly he has biased the results that will later be found in his multi-serial "survival cohort."

2. *The aborted cohort*. In all of the instances just cited, an investigator was studying a multi-serial cross-section rather than an inception cohort. In the last type of bias to be cited here, the investigator begins with an inception cohort, but alters its results by an improper removal of certain members of the cohort from the statistical data. This type of "aborted cohort" is created when the denominator of people who were exposed to the maneuver under study is reduced by an event that occurred *after* the maneuver was initiated. Such "abortions" can take several forms.

a. The "follow-up cohort." When certain members of a cohort become "lost" to follow-up, an investigator may confine the statistical results to those members for whom follow-up data are available. The conclusion will be biased unless the "lost" members and the "maintained" members have the same rates of the target event. For example, suppose an investigator has satisfactory follow-up data for 60 members of a cohort of 100 people, and finds that 30 of those 60 people survived. If

he ignores the 40 people who are "lost," he concludes that the survival rate is 50% (= 30/60). Suppose he tracked down those 40 missing people, however, and found that only 5 of them had survived. The true survival rate would now be 35% (= 35/100).

In the hope of eliminating this type of bias, many investigators resort to a "life-table" method[3, 5] of analysis for dealing with lost members of a cohort. The belief that a life-table analysis will remove such bias is one of the many fallacious delusions that permeate the strategies of contemporary biostatistics. The life-table procedure is useful only for "adjusting" the discrepancies that occur if the members of a cohort have been followed for unequal lengths of time. The procedure does not "adjust" for unequal rates of outcome among "maintained" and "lost" members of the cohort. In fact, the life-table adjustments are based on the assumption that the "maintained" and "lost" members have had the *same* rates of the target event. If these rates are substantially different, the difference is incorporated as a significant bias in the life-table calculations.

The only way to eliminate such bias is for the investigator to perform scientific research rather than statistical adjustments, and to make vigorous efforts to ascertain the fate of the "lost" members. With suitable ingenuity in the activities of tolpery,* an investigator should be able to learn what has happened to almost all members of the cohort, particularly if the "target event" is life or death. The failure to perform adequate tolpery in cohort research is scientifically inexcusable, but is often condoned in the belief that adequate follow-up is unnecessary, since a life-table analysis will presumably compensate for the investigator's delinquency.

Despite heroic efforts in tolpery, an investigator may still occasionally be unable to obtain suitable follow-up data for everyone. In such circumstances, his best method of "compensation" for bias is not recourse to a life-table analysis but the performance of a prognostic stratification for the lost members of the cohort. If the prognostic distribution of the lost group is essentially similar to that of the maintained group, the investigator can be justified in assuming that the outcome rates of the

---

*This word was coined[10] several years ago to refer to the process of tracing lost persons.

two groups would have been similar. He can then analyze his data in the maintained group via direct numerical rates for the target event or, if appropriate, via a life-table procedure.

If the number of lost members is quite small relative to the size of the maintained group, the investigator may even be justified in ignoring the lost members. Thus, if k_M is the proportion of maintained members, with target rate r_M; and if $(1-k_M)$ is the proportion of lost members, with target rate r_L, the true target rate for the cohort is $k_M r_M + (1-k_M)r_L$. If k_M is very close to 1 (i.e., almost all the cohort has been maintained), the value for $(1-k_M)$ will be quite small and the term, $(1-k_M)r_L$, will be small regardless of the value of r_L. The true result will then be closely approximated by the value of r_M found only in the maintained members.

This principle can be illustrated with data from the example cited earlier, where the investigator had lost 40 members of a cohort of 100 people, and where the numerical values were k_M = .60, $(1-k_M)$ = .40, r_M = .50, and r_L = .125. The true survival rate would have been $(.60)$ $(.50) + (.40) (.125) = .30 + .05 = 35\%$, whereas the survival rate in the maintained patients was .50, or 50%. If this investigator had started with 1,000 people, however, and had lost only 40, the values for k_M and $1-k_M$ would now be .96 and .04, respectively. If r_M and r_L had the same values as before, the true survival rate would be $(.96)$ $(.50) + (.04) (.125) = .48 + .005 = 48.5\%$, which is reasonably close to the 50% that would be found exclusively in the maintained members.[*]

b. The "post-operative" cohort. Another type of "aborted" cohort occurs in many reports of surgical treatment for diverse diseases. The results are often based not on all the patients who received the operation, but on those who survived beyond the post-operative period. Such calcula-

tions obviously distort the outcome for the operation itself.

c. The "adherence" cohort. A pharmaceutical counterpart of the surgical fallacy just noted occurs when the results of a cohort are reported only for those members who faithfully adhered to the prescribed regimen. People who abandoned the treatment or who complied poorly are omitted from the results. This type of "adherence cohort" has been especially common in reports of treatment for obesity,[7] but has been used in various other appraisals of pharmaceutical agents.

d. The "retrolectomy" cohort. In all of the circumstances just cited, the investigator knew the full size of his cohort's denominator, but curtailed its magnitude deliberately. In the last type of "aborted" cohort to be noted here, the size of the denominator is curtailed inadvertently.

When a cohort is obtained retrolectively from a survey of data available at a particular zonal site (such as a hospital), the full magnitude of the appropriate cohort may be reduced by various factors that create a bias of which the investigator is unaware. For example, the incidence rates of myocardial infarction at a hospital will be falsely low if the investigator gets his cases exclusively from the records of patients formally discharged from the hospital, and fails to check both the emergency room data (to learn about people who died before an "admission record" was created) and the necropsy protocols (to learn about people whose diagnosis was discovered as a "necropsy surprise").

The detection of cases of diseases listed in the files of the Medical Record Room will be affected by the ability of the record-room staff to maintain accurate diagnostic files, to retrieve the appropriate medical records, and to recall records that have been sequestered in other locations. The ultimate results will also be affected by the criteria the investigator uses for allowing patients into the cohort. For example, the survival rates for lung cancer will be falsely elevated[11] if an investigator insists on histologic proof of diagnosis, and refuses to accept patients with cytologic evidence alone.

These and other sources of bias in collecting a cohort during retrolective research must be carefully checked to avoid the "abortions" caused by inadvertent "retrolectomy."

---

[*]In a laudable attempt to test the validity of life-table techniques, Bailar, Lowry, and Goldenberg[2] examined the survival results in a cohort of breast cancer patients for whom "lost" cases were later "found." The authors noted "that the true experience of the patients originally classified as lost was definitely better than that of the (maintained) patients," but the life-table results based on the usual assumptions about missing patients seemed quite similar to the actual result after the originally lost cases were included. One probable reason for the similarity is that the "lost" cases occupied so small a proportion of the original cohort, which consisted of 1,576 "maintained" and 83 "lost" patients. Since k_M was .95 (i.e., 1576/1659), the results should have been similar no matter how the lost cases were managed statistically.

• • •

The many scientific violations caused by transition bias and chronology bias are unfortunately the rule, rather than the exception, in contemporary biostatistical data. The fallacies have been overlooked in the educational upbringing of statisticians and clinicians, and are seldom considered when clinical investigators receive statistical advice. The subject of cohort research is regularly discussed in the training of epidemiologists, but its scientific requirements are often disregarded or glossed over. Many egregiously defective epidemiologic projects are presented to students not as "exercises" for critical review to detect major scientific flaws, but as "classics" for apathetic emulation to learn "standards" of research methodology.

Because the problems have been so ignored by statisticians, clinicians, and epidemiologists, the collection of statistics for cohorts or pseudo-cohorts has proceeded essentially as an act of body counting, without development of the fundamental scientific principles and logical guidelines that have been created for other forms of modern research. The basic scientific demands that might be made for demonstrating validity in laboratory investigations or in any other type of disciplined research have been singularly absent from the methods of cohort statistics. Some of the defects are now being remedied as epidemiologists abandon their passive collection of mailed questionnaires and death certificate data and begin to perform active "field studies"; as clinicians recognize that "clinical experience" must be carefully specified and quantified to be accepted in modern science; and as statisticians increasingly discover that human populations cannot be properly analyzed with theories developed exclusively from imaginary abstractions, agricultural plots, brewery vats, and fruit flies. In the meantime, however, great heaps of existing data and interpretive concepts have been produced by methods that have no more validity in modern science than the tactics of alchemy would have in modern chemistry. These enormous methodologic deficiencies would inevitably lead to the massive controversies that now exist about the conclusions drawn from statistical studies of cause, course, and treatment, particularly for chronic diseases.

No single, prompt or easy cure can be proposed for these intellectual maladies. A first step, however, is to recognize that the maladies exist, that they are serious, that they require active "therapy," and that they cannot be remedied by preserving either the ignorance with which they are neglected or the self-delusions with which they are minimized. Because biostatistical clinical epidemiology is a relatively new scientific domain, it can be expected to create and to shelter many major blunders before its scientific methods become well developed. For that development to occur, scientific investigators must regain the skepticism, curiosity, and intellectual discipline that are the *sine qua non* of science, but that have often been obliterated during the collection of statistical numbers. By recalling and renewing the principles of scientific research, the investigators can begin to advance beyond the entrenched complacency of "established" doctrines that would promulgate, as models for the future, the failures of the past.

References

1. Apley, J.: A word wanted, Lancet **1**:784, 1954. (Letter to Editor.)
2. Bailar, J. C., Lowry, R., and Goldenberg, I. S.: A note on the follow-up of lost patients, *in* National Cancer Institute Monograph No. 6: End results and mortality trends in cancer, September, 1961, United States Department of Health, Education and Welfare, pp. 123-127.
3. Berkson, J., and Gage, R. P.: Calculation of survival rates for cancer, Mayo Clin. Proc. **25**:270-286, 1950.
4. Bradford Hill, A.: Principles of medical statistics, ed. 8, New York, 1966, Oxford University Press.
5. Cutler, S. J., and Ederer, F.: Maximum utilization of the life table method in analyzing survival, J. Chron. Dis. **8**:699-712, 1958.

6. End Results Section, Biometry Branch, National Cancer Institute: End results in cancer, Report No. 3, 1968, United States Department of Health, Education and Welfare, National Cancer Institute, Bethesda, Md.

7. Feinstein, A. R.: The treatment of obesity: An analysis of methods, results, and factors which influence success, J. Chron. Dis. **11**:349-393, 1960.

8. Feinstein, A. R.: Clinical judgment, Baltimore, 1967, The Williams & Wilkins Company.

9. Feinstein, A. R.: Clinical epidemiology. II. The identification rates of disease, Ann. Intern. Med. **69**:1037-1061, 1968.

10. Feinstein, A. R.: Clinical epidemiology. III. The clinical design of statistics in therapy, Ann. Intern. Med. **69**:1287-1312, 1968.

11. Feinstein, A. R., Pritchett, J. A., and Schimpff, C. R.: The epidemiology of cancer therapy. II. The clinical course: data, decisions, and temporal demarcations, Arch. Intern. Med. **123**:323-344, 1969.

12. Feinstein, A. R.: Clinical biostatistics. VII. The rancid sample, the tilted target, and the medical poll-bearer, CLIN. PHARMACOL. THER. **12**:134-150, 1971.

13. Feinstein, A. R.: Clinical biostatistics. X. Sources of 'transition' bias in cohort statistics, CLIN. PHARMACOL. THER. **12**:704-721, 1971.

14. Forrest, A. P. M., and Kunkler, P. B.: Prognostic factors in breast cancer, Baltimore, 1968, The Williams & Wilkins Company.

15. Fox, J. P., Hall, C. E., and Elveback, L. R.: Epidemiology. Man and disease, Toronto, 1970, The Macmillan Company.

16. Gifford, R. H., and Feinstein, A. R.: A critique of methodology in studies of anticoagulant therapy for acute myocardial infarction, N. Engl. J. Med. **280**:351-357, 1969.

17. Kaplan, M. H., and Feinstein, A. R.: The importance of co-morbidity in the outcome of diabetes mellitus, J. Clin. Invest. **50**:52A, 1971.

18. MacDonald, I.: The natural history of mammary carcinoma, Am. J. Surg. **111**:435-441, 1966.

19. Ultmann, J. E., Cunningham, J. K., and Gellhorn, A.: The clinical picture of Hodgkin's disease, Cancer Res. **26**:1047-1060, 1966.

CHAPTER 8

Credulous idolatry and randomized allocation

The process of randomization can be used statistically in at least three different ways in scientific research. In the first way, randomization is employed to select a sample of people who will represent a larger parent population. As discussed in the first paper[16] of this "trio" on randomization, random samples are regularly chosen for research in social or political science, but seldom in clinical or epidemiologic investigation. In the second use of randomization, an inferential test of "statistical significance" is performed through random rearrangements that show the relative frequency with which "exceptional" results would occur among all the distinctive permutations of data for the investigated people. As discussed at our last meeting,[17] this type of "permutation" or "randomization" test for the observed data has major advantages over its conventional counterparts in t-tests or χ^2 tests, but is also seldom employed in current biostatistical activities.

The third use of randomization is for allocating the therapeutic (or other) maneuvers under investigation in a research project. This procedure is the topic of the current paper, which concludes this subseries on randomization.

A. Problems in the investigation of maneuvers

In most clinical or epidemiologic research, the main purpose is to observe the effects of a principal maneuver. In therapeutic research, this maneuver is usually administration of a prophylactic or remedial agent. In etiologic research, the maneuver is exposure to an alleged cause of disease.

The investigator's ability to allocate the observed maneuver is what distinguishes an experiment from a survey. In an experiment, the investigator makes specific plans by which each person under study is assigned to receive either the principal maneuver or a comparison maneuver. In a survey, the investigator cannot govern or "control"[14] the maneuvers under scrutiny. They are (or have been) chosen in diverse ways that were not pre-arranged according to a specific plan of assignment. To discuss the strategy used for assigning maneuvers, we must therefore confine our attention to experiments, rather than surveys. This restriction will exclude almost all the contemporary epidemiologic studies of causes

This chapter originally appeared as "Clinical biostatistics—XXIV. The role of randomization in sampling, testing, allocation, and credulous idolatry (conclusion)." In Clin. Pharmacol. Ther. 14:1035, 1973.

of disease. The maneuvers investigated in those etiologic surveys were generally self-selected by the patients or encountered in nature, without experimental assignment.

Since the main form of clinical experiment performed in medicine today is a trial of therapy, our concern in the rest of this discussion will be with the allocation of treatment in therapeutic trials. Although a randomized allocation of treatment has sometimes been heralded as the most important scientific advance in the evaluation of therapy, the introduction of at least two other methodologic principles—concurrent comparison and objective observation—has been equally if not more important.

1. Concurrent comparison of maneuvers. For many centuries of medical research, therapeutic maneuvers were investigated without regard to one of the elemental requirements of science. There were no "controls." An investigator usually assembled his treated cases, reported their results, and ascribed the results to the treatment, while ignoring the possibility that the same effects (or even better ones) might have occurred without treatment. Only in the past two centuries have medical investigators begun to recognize these errors of *post hoc* reasoning and to try to avoid them by concurrently observing a "control" group of people who receive no treatment or an alternative form of treatment.

The idea of using a "control" or comparison treatment in therapeutic research has become generally accepted only in the past few decades, and is still not accepted unanimously. The problem has been ascribed to ethics, rather than science. Wanting to choose the best available therapy for each patient, a physician may be ethically reluctant to employ a possibly "inferior" treatment. Although physicians throughout the centuries have deluded themselves about the superiority or inferiority of different modes of therapy, at any point in time a physician will usually establish a ranking of preferences for the available agents, and will want to reject anything other than the one that seems best.

This problem arises whenever a new pharmaceutical substance, whose potential benefit has been shown in preliminary investigation, is to receive formal comparison against a placebo. A particularly dramatic example of the problem occurred when a vaccine was created to prevent poliomyelitis. Although controlled clinical trials were scientifically necessary to demonstrate the value of the vaccine, many physicians had major moral qualms about the otherwise preventable paralysis that might occur in the untreated control group. A simple example of clinical delusions about therapeutic preferences occurred when the administration of oxygen to premature babies was suspected of causing the epidemic of retrolental fibroplasia that took place about 20 to 25 years ago. At first, when the oxygen was regarded as desirable, a controlled trial was opposed because the "control" babies would be denied a beneficial treatment. Later, when the oxygen was regarded as hazardous, a controlled trial was opposed because the treated babies would be needlessly exposed to danger.[23]

To make comparative therapeutic decisions, the doctors who object to concurrent comparison with a differently treated group will often rely on the results obtained in the past with "historical controls"—the patients treated before the new agent became available. These comparisons may not always be valid because of the bias introduced by unrecognized secular changes in the characteristics of the treated patients and in ancillary modes of therapy. This hazard, however, has not prevented the recognition of certain particularly powerful and effective agents. Many of the most thoroughly accepted current drugs—including morphine, digitalis, aspirin, insulin, penicillin, and corticosteroids—were established on the basis of "historical controls," without concurrent comparisons.

In modern biostatistical practice, a concurrent comparison maneuver has become regarded as essential to proper design of research, although many problems of choosing these maneuvers remain scientifically unresolved.[8, 14] Among the prominent problems are whether to test the active agent against a placebo, a comparison treatment, or no treatment; and decisions about the number of concurrent maneuvers to be compared in a single study, the choice of parallel vs. successive (or "cross-over") comparisons, and the standardization of ancillary treatment.

Although the scientific need for concurrent comparison is now generally accepted, the main medical difficulty is in the "ethics" of satisfying that need. This difficulty involves ideas and concepts that are quite different from those entailed in choosing a method for allocating the maneuvers to be compared.

2. *Objective observation of results.* As physicians increasingly appreciated the requirement for concurrent comparisons of treatment, the idea of *controlled clinical trials* became well established. It soon became regarded as so important a methodologic advance that it was cited in the titles of publications. A report of therapy that formerly might have been called "The use of Excellitol in the treatment of headache" would now be entitled "A controlled clinical trial of Excellitol in the treatment of headache."

Despite the scientific improvements produced by concurrent comparisons, a major defect still remained: the results were not being observed objectively. As long as a patient knew whether or not he was receiving treatment, his responses might be affected by that knowledge. Accordingly, in controlled studies of pharmaceutical agents, the patients who might have received no treatment were instead given a placebo and were kept ignorant of whether their therapy was the "active" agent or the placebo.

This "single-blind" technique could remove the patient's subjective bias, but would not alter the subjectivity of the physician who observed and recorded the results. As long as he knew what treatment the patient was getting, the doctor's prejudices might influence the patient's perception of his own responses or the way that the doctor interpreted and reported the responses. Consequently, the "double-blind" technique[24] was developed for controlled clinical trials. The physical appearance of the placebo was made similar to that of the "active" agent, and both the patient and the doctor were kept unaware of the treatment being given in a particular case. The double-blind technique soon became so well regarded that its application was often added to the methodologic ingredients noted in the titles of research reports. Thus, the paper cited earlier might now be labelled as, "A double-blind controlled clinical trial of Excellitol in the treatment of headache."

Despite valuable contributions, the double-blind administration of treatment has not totally solved the problem of getting objective observations. The double-blind technique has some distinct limitations. It solves only one part of the problem; the solutions it offers are sometimes more apparent than real; and it creates some new problems of its own.

A double-blind technique can best be applied when the treatment is either an oral medication or an injection. (To compare an oral medication against an injection requires two sets of placebos—one given by injection and the other orally. Each patient then must receive both an injection and an oral medication, one of which is a placebo.) The double-blind technique is difficult or impossible to apply when the investigated treatment is non-pharmaceutical, such as verbal psychotherapy, surgery, renal dialysis, or the application of such prosthetic devices as braces and artificial limbs. Although a sham surgical procedure was performed about 15 years ago[2] by a type of double-blind technique, the ethical aspects of such operations would be difficult to defend today even if the operations were clinically feasible.

For pharmaceutical investigations, the double-blind technique is sometimes "double-blind" in name only, because the identity of the injected or oral active agents may be difficult or impossible to conceal. The active agent may be recognizable from a property that is present on administration (the "sting" of the injection; or the taste or odor of the oral medicine) or from an associated side effect (such as bradycardia or change in sedimentation rate) that occurs afterward. Because of these clues to the identity of the agents, many clinical trials have been "double-blind" *de jure* but not *de facto*.

A greater disadvantage of the double-blind technique is the problems it creates in the design and conduct of trials for certain forms of treatment. The double-blind technique is difficult to maintain when the therapeutic agent must be "titrated" to an optimum individual dose for each patient. This problem can be managed by allowing both the placebo and the active agent to be given in escalating dosage—but the identity of the agents is often recognized during the adjustment process and besides, the process is logistically cumbersome to carry out. To avoid using such adjustments, the therapeutic agents may be prescribed throughout the trial in an invariant dosage rather than in flexible amounts. The results are then acceptable as a successful exercise in double-blind design, but are often useless as an act of clinical science because they are not based on the realities of clinical practice.

A different type of problem occurs when the dosage of a treatment, such as anticoagulants, must be regulated according to the values of an associated laboratory test, such as prothrombin time. In this circumstance, the physician who regulates the dosage must be aware of the identity of the therapeutic agent. This problem can be solved by using two sets of clinical examiners in the trial. One set of examiners, aware of the treatment, act to regulate the dosage. The other set, who are kept "double-blind," make the necessary observations of the key clinical variables under investigation. This two-examiner technique, which can also be applied to solve the first type of problem in dosage regulation, has been used with reasonable success,[27] but it increases the expenses and logistic complexity of a clinical trial, and it carries the risk that the "unblinded" examiner may inadvertently reveal the identity of the treatment to either the patient or to the "blinded" examiner.

Despite these difficulties, the double-blind technique has made obvious major contributions to the scientific quality of clinical trials. The prime objections that are still often raised against the technique are based not on any of the foregoing problems, but on ethical and intellectual issues.

Ethically, a doctor who has vowed to give his patients the best possible care may believe he cannot fulfill that vow if he is unaware of the treatment each patient is getting. This belief was more justified in the past than it is today, when stringent criteria are often used to restrict a trial to patients with minimum likelihood of adverse reactions to treatment, and when diverse "fail-safe" procedures are employed to deal with any adverse reactions that may occur during the trial. Nevertheless, certain doctors remain dissatisfied with these safeguards, and will refuse to allow themselves or their patients to participate in studies where the doctor does not know the identity of the treatment.

Intellectually, the major objection to double-blind trials is that they may create a false sense of security that allows neglect of important scientific challenges in the construction of indexes, scales, and criteria for assessing the outcome of therapy.[11, 13] The most important responses to treatment are often expressed in "soft data" that contain verbal comments such as *better* or *worse*, or rating scales such as *excellent, good, fair*, and *poor*. These indexes of expression are "soft" because their ingredients are often unspecified; the elements of the scale are seldom clearly demarcated; and no criteria are provided for using the indexes and scales.

The double-blind technique can prevent bias when these expressions are employed, but they are often undefined and non-reproducible because they lack detailed specifications and criteria. With adequate scientific attention to those details, the data would become much more objective, "hard," and precise—but the necessary attention is usually diverted or distracted into other channels. Thus, the poor scientific quality of these non-reproducible expressions may fail to arouse concern because they are used in a double-blind manner, so that none of the compared therapeutic agents will be subjectively favored when the criteria-free rating scales are applied. An analogous complacency would lead to the belief that a scientific investigator need not be able to reproduce what he does as long as he does it without bias.

The *clinimetrics* needed to construct suitable indexes, scales, and criteria for therapeutic accomplishment will be discussed in future papers of this series. For the moment, we can consider some of the major defects that arise when the absence of clinimetric science is condoned by the usage of double-blind techniques. Perhaps the worst defect produced by this line of reasoning is the current lack, as noted previously,[10] of any operational algorithms or criteria for identifying, i.e., diagnosing, an "adverse drug reaction." Despite the reams of literature issued by investigators and federal regulators on the subject of "safety," there currently exist no citations of reproducible clinical methods for arriving at the operational decision that a particular post-therapeutic effect noted in a patient is an "adverse drug reaction." To decide about "safety," investigators often rely on listing a series of "effects" whose cause has not been rigorously identified, and on counting whether the "effects" are more frequent in the treated or control members of the "double-blind" groups. Thus, if an epidemic of influenza passes through the community, there is no specified intellectual mechanism for deciding that the acute fevers, coughs, malaise, etc.

should be ascribed to the influenza. Instead, these symptoms may become listed as "effects" of therapy, and if they happen to appear more commonly in the active treatment group than in the controls, they will then be cited as "adverse side effects" of the treatment. Perhaps the silliest known extreme of this unscientific method for collecting statistics occurred in a survey where gonorrhea was "discovered" to be a frequent "adverse side effect" of therapy with oral contraceptive pills.

B. Problems in the allocation of maneuvers

The main reason for devoting so much discussion to the two foregoing issues (concurrent comparison and objective observation) is that the advantages and disadvantages of these procedures are sometimes mistakenly attributed to the use of randomized allocation in clinical trials. Physicians who argue against the merits of "randomized trials" are often concerned with defects that really arise not from the process of randomization, but from either inappropriate arrangements of treatment or unsatisfactory aspects of the double-blind technique. Conversely, some of the strongest advocates of randomized trials may ascribe to randomization certain virtues that really belong to control groups and double-blind observations. For example, in one recent indictment[1] of unsatisfactory designs in investigations of cancer therapy, the authors urged the more frequent application of randomization—but the major faults cited in the reported studies were the absence of concurrent control groups.

Assuming that we have properly chosen the comparison treatment(s) and a suitable method for making objective observations, we can now turn to the method of allocating the therapeutic regimens to the patients who enter the trial. In rare situations, the patients may already be assembled and available all at once for their therapeutic assignment. More commonly, the individual patients will enter the trial sequentially over a period of time. The method of allocation is used to determine the treatment assigned to each member of this sequence. When the sequential allocations are completed, each patient has been assigned to a regimen, thus defining the treatment groups.

The goal of this allocation process is for each treatment group to achieve equality in composition. The groups also are usually made equal in size, because numerical equality offers the greatest chance of attaining "significance" in the subsequent statistical tests to be performed when the results of the groups are compared. (Occasionally, however, for reasons discussed previously,[8, 14] we may deliberately want the numbers of patients to be distributed unequally among the treatments in ratios such as 1:2 or 1:1:2.) If an equal size of each group were the main goal, no problem would exist in the method of allocating treatment. The regimens could simply be assigned to patients in an alternating manner that preserved equal numbers in the therapeutic groups, and there would be no need to discuss randomization or any other procedure for arriving at an "unbiased" assignment. The demands of science are much greater, however, than the mere statistical convenience of equal numbers in the compared groups. For scientific comparison, the groups must be equal in composition, not just in numbers.

To decide that groups of people are equal in composition is a subtle, complex problem that will be outlined here only briefly because it received extensive discussion earlier[12] in this series. In studies of therapy, the key issue in "composition" is prognostic similarity for the target event that is to be altered or prevented by the treatment. We might therefore try to give the groups an exactly homogeneous composition by selecting only patients with identical prognoses. Such an attempt would be clinically unrealistic, since the use of therapeutic agents is seldom confined to patients with identical prognoses. The attempt would also be intellectually unfeasible, since different patients have different prognoses and we seldom can predict individual outcomes well enough to be assured that any two patients are prognostically identical.

Instead, we classify the patients into distinctive subgroups, or strata, with different prognostic expectations that are expressed in such titles as *good risk, fair risk,* and *poor risk.* We then determine equality of composition in the therapeutic groups according to the proportionate distribution of these prognostic strata. Thus, if a group assigned to Treatment A contains 19% good risks, 40% fair risks, and 41% poor risks, it is essentially similar in composition to a Treatment B group that contains 17% good risks, 41% fair risks, and 42% poor risks. It would not be similar to a group containing 30% good risks, 12% fair risks, and 58% poor risks.

Equal prognostic composition of the compared groups is a dominant scientific necessity in the evaluation of therapy, and is the major reason for insisting that treatment be allocated in an unbiased manner. If the clinician who assigns the treatment is aware of both the patient's condition and the proposed treatment, there is always a chance that the clinician's prejudices may act consciously or subconsciously to alter the proposed allocation by changing the treatment or the patient's position in the allocation sequence. The clinician may prefer to assign the better risk patients to Treatment A and the poorer risk patients to Treatment B, or vice versa, thus altering the proportionate composition of the treatment groups.

The annals of therapeutic allocation contain diverse instances of situations in which an arrangement (such as alternative days of the month or odd-and-even unit numbers) that allowed the physician to anticipate the proposed treatment was followed by acts of clinical prejudice that distorted the pre-determined plans. (Mainland's textbook[23] provides an excellent discussion of these difficulties.) Consequently, to allow the therapeutic groups to have equal composition, we would want the treatments to be allocated without the clinician being able to know in advance what will be assigned to each patient.

The method of achieving this goal is to remove the clinician from the assignment of treatment. His prejudices can be avoided* if he is unable to anticipate the schedule of the assignments made by some other human or inanimate mechanism. This decision—to assign treatment by a mechanism other than the option of individual clinicians—is the last major step in the reasoning. The only remaining step is to select the mechanism that will arrange the sequence of the assignments.

C. The merits and problems of randomization

The assignment mechanism proposed by R. A. Fisher[18, 19] has now become almost universally accepted. The decisions are left to chance alone. The sequence of therapeutic agents is allocated according to a randomization process that uses the random numbers provided by suitable tables or generated by an appropriate computer program.[21]

1. Advantages of randomization. The random allocation of treatment is believed to have four principal advantages:

a. It removes any bias that might occur if clinicians made selective choices of treatment.

b. If the patients were not previously divided into distinctive prognostic strata, the randomization procedure could be expected (within the limitations of chance) to distribute the strata in equal proportions among the groups under comparison.

c. If randomization were performed within previously defined prognostic strata, the randomization procedure could be expected (within the limitations of chance) to provide equal distribution of any important prognostic factors that had been overlooked during formation of the strata.

d. For later analysis of data, the procedure would allow the results to be appraised statistically with tests whose interpretation requires, as a basic assumption, the random assignment of treatment.

As we shall see later on, these advantages have sometimes turned out to be illusory, delusive, or unnecessary in clinical investigation. Nevertheless, after the apparent success of randomization in the agricultural research where it was first employed, the idea was soon accepted by the statisticians who have become authoritative figures in the planning of clinical research. Randomization has now become regarded as a paramount principle and even as a *sine qua non* of scientific design in the human experiments that are called "clinical trials."

2. Clinical objections. After the idea of randomization was accepted by statisticians, it encountered considerable difficulty in being accepted by clinicians. Some of the clinicians' objections, as noted earlier, were misdirected. Other objections, however, were more appropriately aimed at the act of randomization itself.

a. For some clinicians, the formal mechanics of randomization seemed needlessly complex. Why go through all the trouble of using random number tables or other statistical paraphernalia? Why not simplify matters by allocating treatment alternatively to successive patients, or according to odd-or-even unit numbers or days of the week?

b. For other clinicians, the main objection to randomization was its logistics. If the randomization were planned within different prognostic strata, a separate randomization schedule had to be maintained for each stratum, and each patient's location among the strata had to be clearly established before the schedule could be used. If the randomization schedule in a multi-center collaborative trial were maintained at a central headquarters, the investigators at each center would have to telephone or write to the coordinating unit for each therapeutic assignment.

---

*The potential for prejudice is not totally removed, of course. After noting the assigned treatment, the clinician could always persuade the patient to refuse it—but we would then be dealing with a different type of prejudice. The original treatment would still have been allocated without the clinician's bias.

c. For yet other clinicians, the major problem was in ethics. Even if a doctor could accept the ideas that he might be using a possibly "inferior" treatment and that he might not know whether he was using it, the notion of choosing each patient's therapy entirely by chance was still anathema. Besides, in soliciting informed consent from a patient, a physician might fear that he would seem foolish if he confessed that his profound exercise of clinical judgment had been abandoned, and that the choice of treatment had been relegated to something as apparently frivolous as the equivalent of a tossed coin.

The current widespread acceptance of randomization is attributable to the success with which these objections have been countered:

a. The difficulty in using systematic "alternation," rather than randomization, is that it does not prevent (and may even abet) the hazard of potential bias, as noted earlier.

b. The difficult logistics of a complicated allocation schedule would occur for any trial involving multiple strata or multiple centers, no matter what scheme was used for the mechanism of allocation.

c. A doctor's ethical objections about an "inferior" therapy could be answered by noting that controlled trials are usually proposed when a true dilemma exists, so that none of the compared treatments can be definitively regarded as superior or inferior. And the doctor's ethical objections about the "frivolity" of a randomized assignment of treatment could also be readily countered. If all the work of a clinical trial is required to get a scientific answer to the question of therapeutic superiority, and if the scientific validity of the trial requires the elimination of the doctor's possible bias in assigning treatment, it would be "frivolous" to use any method of allocation that might allow such bias to occur.

The counter-arguments just cited provided a successful rebuttal to the outstanding objections rated against the use

of randomization in clinical trials, and it has now won the day. Randomization is not only generally established in the design of the trials; it has also become widely regarded as the *only* valid method of allocating treatment.

3. Disadvantages of randomization. Despite these obvious merits, the process of randomization has serious disadvantages that arise not from its scientific accomplishments, but from its intellectual distractions. Many challenging problems in the design, pertinence, and value of therapeutic trials have not yet been solved. These problems, which have nothing to do with randomization itself, have a much greater scientific, clinical, and human importance than the issue of whether or not therapy was randomly allocated. But the problems have been generally ignored, neglected, or disdained. The statistical consultants who might have convinced clinicians that the problems warranted attention have been preoccupied with efforts mainly to "sell" the idea of randomization. And the clinicians, having been "sold" on the idea, began to use it as an excuse to avoid any further concern with the problems, because randomization had been promulgated as a panacea that cured or prevented any intellectual maladies in planning therapeutic research.

As randomization continues to receive this credulous reverence from both statisticians and clinicians, the scientific, clinical, and human problems continue to fester. The adverse consequences of these unsolved problems are relatively minor in the small-scale trials conducted to test the short-term pharmaceutical effects of individual new drugs. The consequences have been much greater and more strikingly evident, however, in the massive, multi-center clinical trials that are concerned with "natural history" and the long-term effects of therapy.

a. The choice of the compared treatments. Randomization has nothing to do with the choice of the treatments or dosage schedules that are compared in a therapeutic trial. Because this choice may not be given adequate consideration, however, many randomized clinical trials have been poorly designed. A mode of treatment that should have been compared is omitted; or an included treatment is given at a dosage schedule that is clinically improper or inapplicable.

The total therapeutic efficacy of many regimens has been inadequately measured, because the active agent given to one group of patients was compared only against the results of placebo in a second group. To quantify the total efficacy would have required comparison with a third group of patients, receiving no treatment.[13] As a result of these omissions, statistical measurements of therapy have often dealt with pharmaceutical but not therapeutic effectiveness. The total therapeutic effect arises as a combination of pharmaceutical action together with the doctor's behavior and the patient's anticipation. In the absence of a wholly untreated group, no quantitative attention is given to the important effects, on doctor and patient, of knowledge that a potentially useful pharmaceutical agent is available.

Many illustrations of unsatisfactory dosage schedules can be found in the published medical literature. Perhaps the best known recent examples* occurred in the celebrated UGDP study,[29] where oral agents that are often given in flexible amounts were prescribed in fixed dosages, and where one group of patients received insulin in a permanent, invariant dosage for the entire duration of the trial. The use of insulin in this inflexible manner is contrary to the recommendations stated in all textbooks dealing with pharmacology, internal medicine, or diabetes mellitus.

b. The elimination of pre-therapeutic bias. The act of randomization provides

protection only against the bias introduced by human selectivity in the assignment of treatment. Randomization does not protect against its own introduction of bias, through distortions that may occur as an act of chance when the treatment groups are formed during the "luck of the draw."[16]

The devout belief that randomization completely prevents pre-therapeutic bias has sometimes diverted clinical investigators from appreciating obvious inequities in the composition of the compared groups. For example, after the randomization performed in the UGDP study, 189 patients in one group with a total of 362 baseline "risk factors" were contrasted with 185 patients in another group that contained a total of 306 risk factors. The mean value for the first group, 1.92, was 16% higher than the mean value for the second group, 1.65, and this clinically significant difference was also "statistically significant" ($t = 2.17$, $P < 0.05$). Nevertheless, the baseline disparities were dismissed with the statement that "all in all, the luck of the draw was not too bad."[4]

The occurrence and consequences of randomization bias have been discussed previously in this series[12, 16] and elsewhere.[26] This type of bias, which can invalidate the results of a clinical trial, can be either prevented or compensated with appropriate precautions. The precautions involve the selection, formation, and application of cogent prognostic strata either before the random allocation of treatments or afterward during the analysis of subsequent results. Nevertheless, the problems of prognostic stratification have been frequently ignored during the apotheosis of randomization alone.

c. The analysis of prognostic strata. Even if the randomization has produced a perfectly equal distribution of prognostic distinctions, the results must still be analyzed within suitable prognostic strata. No sensible biologist would want to compare the results of treating a mouse with those of treating an elephant; and no thoughtful

---

*Because the UGDP study was intended to be a "model" of methodology in clinical trials and because it has received such extensive public discussion, the procedures used in that "model" will provide familiar examples of some of the problems cited here and in subsequent sections.

clinician would want to mix the results of a poor-risk group with those of the good risks. Nevertheless, when the data of a therapeutic trial are evaluated only in the randomized treatment groups, without regard to prognostic stratification, this type of unscientific mixture is perpetrated.

An excellent example of this phenomenon occurred in the UGDP trial. Three different types of tests of "statistical significance" were performed for the post-therapeutic results in the randomized groups, but no statistical tests were published for comparisons of what had happened after treatment *within* similar prognostic strata. When the treated groups were divided into the UGDP version of prognostic strata, the statistical tests dealt only with the baseline comparability of the strata, not with the post-therapeutic results in each stratum.

The reasons for analyzing results within prognostic strata have been previously[12] discussed in detail. The analyses are necessary to avoid false positive conclusions, if the active treatment is massively effective in one stratum but not in any others; and false negative conclusions, if the patients in different strata respond in opposite ways to different treatments. The stratification is also a fundamental scientific requirement, as noted later, for any attempt to extrapolate the results to patients beyond the immediate group who participated in the trial.

d. The formation of clinimetric indexes. The blind worship of double-blind techniques is not solely responsible for the current lack of attention, as noted earlier, to suitable "clinimetric" indexes for evaluating therapeutic accomplishment. A clinician who feels assured that his data will be valid if he uses randomization may then delude himself into the false belief that statistical validity confers scientific validity or clinical credibility. A concern with the creation of valid indexes of therapy will thus seem like an unnecessary procedure.

An example of this problem occurred for the "natural history" and clinical outcomes

that were analyzed in the UGDP trial. Certain crucial changes in patients' clinical conditions were defined according to statistically established indexes that were quite disparate from clinical reality.[9] (Perhaps the most bizarre of the indexes were the appraisal of peripheral neuropathy according to biothesiometric measurements of an index finger, and the identification of congestive heart failure only according to "use of digitalis".) Investigators who plan future studies of the long-term clinical course of maturity-onset diabetes mellitus will have to develop, *de novo*, the necessary clinimetric indexes that were omitted from the UGDP methodologic "model."

D. Intrinsic problems of randomized allocation

The four major scientific defects that have just been cited cannot be directly attributed to the use of randomization in allocating therapy. The defects are not caused by randomization and cannot be altered by it. The reason for associating these defects with randomization is that their continued neglect has been encouraged by devout faith in the panchrestic virtues of a random allocation.

Having been taught to believe that a clinical trial was well designed if the treatments were randomly allocated, clinical investigators have had no incentive to confront the massive scientific problems that remain despite the act of randomization. Having noted the success of randomization in allocating the treatments studied in agricultural research, biostatisticians have advocated the additional idea that sick people could be compared, like plots of inanimate soil, mainly as a mathematical exercise in "hypothesis testing." As both clinicians and statisticians have given homage to the avatar of randomization, the major scientific defects of clinical trials have been neglected and perpetuated.

Several other illusions of randomization, however, can be intrinsically associated with it. Some of these illusions represent claims for merits that are not possessed by randomized allocation, and others represent its inherent flaws.

1. Universal randomization. The suggestion is sometimes offered that many current problems in evaluating new treatment would be solved if randomization were universal—so that every new treatment were tested with a randomized trial, starting with the first patient on whom the treatment is tried. The suggestion has some obvious values, but it is incompatible with reality.

One prominent difficulty is that too many new treatments are constantly being proposed. The facilities for doing clinical research are not extensive enough to allow every new agent to be tested with all the detailed protocol and statistical organization of a randomized therapeutic trial. Another difficulty is that long-term evidence of safety and efficacy must generally be assembled from survey data, rather than trials, because all the patients (and the investigators) can seldom be maintained in a clinical trial for a period of observation long enough to be truly "long-term." Perhaps the most important difficulty, however, is that patients would not be suitably protected from harm if major trials were begun before any substantial "pilot" evidence had been assembled to show the benefit of potentially hazardous agents.

For example, the current disrepute of cardiac transplantation and thalidomide occurred without the use of randomized trials, and the flaws of both these treatments might have taken longer to detect and might have been even more disastrous if their initial tests had been performed in the conventional "controlled" manner. The defects of cardiac transplantation and thalidomide were both evident by comparison with "historical controls," and the thalidomide hazards could have been noted, prior to human usage, had suitable tests been conducted in animals.

Before a large-scale randomized trial is planned, sufficient preliminary evidence should be assembled to demonstrate that the agent is potentially safe enough and effective enough to warrant all the efforts of the trial. Some of this evidence can come from animal experiments, but most of it will usually come from surveys of early clinical applications in patients. Furthermore, in circumstances where a randomized trial will not or cannot be performed, such surveys, after brief or extensive clinical usage of a therapeutic agent, will often provide the only opportunity to evaluate its merits. For these reasons, much of the energy now expended in calling for universal randomization might be better used in demands for improving the quality of the surveys. These improvements will require attention to the same defects that continue to mar the design of randomized trials: the need for better methods of specifying comparative treatment, searching for bias, forming prognostic strata, and developing clinimetric indexes.

With such methods, the results found in the preliminary surveys may either eliminate the need for a randomized trial or allow the subsequent trial to be planned in a way that provides valid, useful results. Without such methods, clinical investigators may simply replace poorly designed universal non-randomized surveys with poorly designed universal randomized trials. The demand for more and earlier randomized trials is reasonable, particularly when an agent has been surveyed long enough to document its potential value. Neither science nor society will be well served, however, by an "improvement" that merely exchanges one form of unsatisfactory research for another.

2. Sophistic randomization. The randomized allocation of therapy is an act of sophistry when randomization is applied ritualistically to a situation in which a conventional clinical trial would subvert the basic objective of the research.

For example, suppose we wanted to evaluate a non-prescription (over-the-counter) pharmaceutical preparation. To perform such an evaluation properly, we must recognize a unique feature of usage for over-the-counter drugs: no doctor is involved. The "patient" is responsible for the decision to take the drug, for the anticipation of its effects, and for the observation of those effects. If we impose an outside physician-like prescriber or observer in a clinical trial intended to evaluate an over-the-counter drug, we have destroyed the setting in which the drug is ordinarily taken. Regardless of whatever conclusions are reached in such a trial, they may not be pertinent for the circumstances in which the drug is usually employed. This clinical form of the Heisenberg principle[20] in physics—that the act of observation alters the observed phenomenon—creates enormous problems in any attempt to evaluate the safety and efficacy of over-the-counter preparations. Such evaluations are possible, but their appropriate design requires much more thought and effort than the simplistic use of a conventional randomized clinical trial.

Another example of sophistry in the devotion to randomized trials occurs when a particular drug is effective in only 1 of 25 people who take it. For 24 of those people, the agent is worthless; but for the twenty-fifth, the result is highly desirable. If this drug is used to treat a common condition in a population containing 100,000,000 people, we might thus find 4,000,000 people who would be delighted with the drug's safety and efficacy. Now suppose, however, that the drug is tested in a conventional randomized clinical trial, performed on 50 people. A distinct improvement is found in none of the 25 people who received placebo and in only one of the 25 who received the active drug. Because the difference in the improvement rates appears clinically trivial and is not statistically significant, the drug is deemed ineffectual and is not allowed to be marketed. The benefits that might be accrued by 4,000,000 users are ignored in favor of the results found in the randomized trial.

(This problem could be managed with the use of randomization if an appropriate stratification were performed beforehand. Assemble a population of people who have tried the drug and believe that it is effective. In a double-blind manner, randomly assign the people to "cross-over" to a placebo substitute, and determine whether they can tell the difference.)

These two examples are but a few of the many that could be cited to illustrate circumstances in which the proper evaluation of therapy requires suitable plans for subtle distinctions that cannot be managed merely with faith in randomization alone.

3. Inappropriate statistical claims. An argument often presented in favor of the routine use of randomized allocation is that it is prerequisite to the subsequent application of tests of "statistical significance." According to this argument, such tests are valid only if the maneuvers were randomly assigned.

There are at least four reasons why this argument is either wrong or hypocritical:

a. Tests of "statistical significance" are regularly applied, often by major members of the statistical pantheon, to epidemiologic trohocs[15] and to other groups examined in clinical, epidemiologic, or psychologic surveys where neither the sampling nor the allocation was performed randomly.

b. The statistical ideas about randomization and the "validity" of a "significance" test are based on the idea of extrapolating the results to the parent population. This idea requires that the people under study be randomly selected from the parent population. Such a selection does not occur in most therapeutic trials. The patients may receive a randomized allocation of therapy, but they do not themselves represent a random sample of persons with the condition under treatment.

c. As noted in the previous paper,[17] a "permutation" or "randomization" test can be used to appraise the significance of numerical differences in data, regardless of whether the compared maneuvers were allocated randomly, and regardless of whether the groups under study were randomly chosen from the parent population.

d. The demand for randomized allocation of therapy was not accepted by all leading statisticians in the past, and has been revised or abandoned by some prominent statisticians today. Almost 40 years ago, W. S. Gosset[28] (the "student" who devised the t-test) strongly advocated the use of certain systematic arrangements that he called "balanced." In more recent literature, D. R. Cox[6] has noted "the limited usefulness of randomization in very small investigations" and has described other circumstances where it seems "undesirable." D. V. Lindley[22] has stated that "randomization is quite unnecessary either in the design or analysis of experiments." W. J. Youden,[30] in proposing the use of "constrained randomization," pointed out that randomization is "required only when the order or position of the experimental unit (in the therapeutic sequence) influences the performance of the units," and that an unconstrained randomization may produce an "obviously undesirable" arrangement "that may doom the particular experimental program."

In several newly proposed methods of therapeutic allocation, randomization is abandoned in favor of other techniques that include the sequential cost function procedure of Colton,[3] the "play-the-winner" methods described by Zelen[31] and by Nebenzahl and Sobel,[25] and the multi-stage adaptations of Cornfield, Halperin, and Greenhouse.[5] These new proposals, whose merits are beyond the scope of this discussion, serve to demonstrate that authoritative statisticians have begun to think about the previously unthinkable act of assigning therapy by methods other than randomization.

4. Uncertain statistical tactics. Clinical investigators who do their own statistical tests have discovered a peculiar quirk in the calculation of variance and its square root, the standard deviation. For this calculation, we find the group variance (i.e., the sum of the squared deviations from the mean), which is expressed as $\Sigma x_i^2 - n\bar{x}^2$, where each x_i represents the individual values for n people, with a mean of $\bar{x}$. To convert this group value to the "mean"

variance for individual members, we would expect to divide by n. In fact, however, the divisor used in modern statistical procedures is n-1.

The reason for this change is immersed in principles of "estimation theory" and is beyond the scope of this discussion. Basically, the idea is that we divide by n when the group variance is determined from data for the entire parent population. With the data of a random sample, however, the variance of the parent population is better "estimated" if the divisor is n-1. Consequently, in the current routine ritual for tests of "statistical significance," n-1 is used in the denominator when group variance is converted to variance and standard deviation.

This ritual may not be appropriate, however, when statistical significance is tested for the groups compared in a clinical trial. We deal with a collection of people who entered the trial. Not having been randomly selected, these people may not represent anything other than themselves, and they may not allow any generalization of results. Our statistical tests will apply only to this collection of people. In the clinical trial, the collected people form the "parent population" that is then randomly divided into the sub-collections or "samples" who constitute the treated groups. In this process we examine every member of the "parent population," because a randomized therapeutic trial contains all of the people who entered it. The appropriate number to use for calculating the pooled variance for that entire "parent population" would therefore seem to be n, rather than n-1.

The only justification for dividing by n-1 is if we want to use the trial not for a direct analytic comparison of two (or more) treatments, but for estimating parameters in an external population that was not observed. Such an estimation cannot be justified, however, because the external population was not randomly sampled. Consequently, the statistical tests used in many clinical trials may have been performed improperly, with the calculated values of t (or other statistical scores) being made too low because the pooled variances, based on a divisor of n-1 rather than n, were too high. Had the more appropriate computation been performed, many t values that were regarded as "not significant" might have become "significant," particularly in trials with small numbers of patients.

This point is worth noting for data analysts who use programmed desk calculators or computers in which variance is routinely determined with the n-1 formula. On the other hand, when the sample size is so small that differences between n and n-1 may create major changes in the results, the data should probably *not* be analyzed with t-tests or with any other procedures that depend on estimating variance. The preferable alternative is to use a permutation test,[17] which is not affected by variances or by disputes about n versus n-1.

E. The cardinal defect of randomized allocation

The statistical point that has just been discussed leads us to the clinical point that is the unalterable, cardinal flaw of all trials performed with randomized allocation of therapy. The results are highly limited. They may not pertain to anyone other than the group of people who participated in the trial. If these people are *not* a random sample of the disease or condition under treatment, the results cannot be validly extrapolated for statistical purposes, but a clinician may not care about this issue. The extrapolation that concerns him is clinical. If the treated population was not a random sample, whom did the patients represent? And to what kind of patients can the results apply?

Amid the many randomized therapeutic trials that have been performed in the past few decades, I do not know of a single investigation in which the patients under study were chosen randomly. The participating patients have been the "chunk samples" of people found in hospitals, out-patient clinics, doctors' offices, and other sites convenient to the investigators. The participants have never been chosen randomly from the parent population of patients who

might have been eligible for the trial. After the participants were assembled, their treatment may have been allocated randomly, but the participants themselves were not randomly selected.

These problems create major uncertainties about whether the results of a clinical trial will be applied to patients who are similar to those in whom the trial was performed. If the condition under treatment is a reasonably homogeneous entity, such as a Colles fracture in healthy adolescents, the results found in one group of patients might readily be extrapolated to another. If the treated condition has a heterogeneous clinical spectrum, however, the results cannot be easily generalized because of possible disparities in the types and proportions of the disease spectrum represented by the patients in the trial.

This difficulty regularly occurs for patients in the diverse clinical spectrums found during therapy for many acute medical ailments as well as for all chronic diseases—such as diabetes mellitus, cancer, pulmonary emphysema, and coronary artery disease. We cannot be sure that the clinical characteristics and spectral distribution of patients with such ailments as pneumonia, functional bowel distress, stroke, or inoperable cancer are the same for a private referral clinic as for a municipal ward service. We cannot be sure that the types of patient treated by Dr. A, who performed the trial, are the same as those of Dr. B, who plans to apply the results. In some circumstances, we cannot even be sure that the results found in one subset of patients are pertinent to what was noted in another subset of patients within the same trial. (The major contrast that can arise for patients in the same multi-center trial was demonstrated in the UGDP study, where the fatality rates, regardless of therapy, ranged from 1% (1/87) in one participating center to 26% (23/90) in another.)

To be able to apply the conclusions of a clinical trial reproducibly, clinicians must have satisfactory data to identify the post-therapeutic results found in the different kinds of patients under treatment. The patients cannot be suitably identified if they are described only according to a diagnostic label that does not denote important clinical distinctions of their condition before and after treatment. The crucial role of the cogent stratifications described earlier and previously[12] is to permit these distinctions to be designated. When such stratifications are absent, a clinical reader has no way of knowing whether and how the results of a trial can be extrapolated. Even when the stratifications are well performed, the results may still be difficult to apply if the trial was designed with overly rigid admission criteria that created a "pure-disease sample," a "compliance sample," or some other highly restricted group that differs greatly from the patients encountered in ordinary clinical practice.

For both these reasons—the clinically constricted spectrum of the admitted patients and the failure to perform suitable stratification of those who were admitted—many randomized trials have been performed as a type of *in vitro* experiment that must be followed by extensive *in vivo* tests. The trial may show the relative efficacy and safety of the therapy for the group of people under scrutiny, but the results may not be readily interpretable or applicable to patients elsewhere. Even when the data are suitably stratified, the number of patients in the strata may be too small for satisfactory generalization. Consequently, to make appropriate interpretations and applications, clinicians must rely either on additional clinical trials or, more commonly, on surveys of the results noted when the treatment was or becomes used in the diverse types of patients who may have been excluded from the trial or inadequately identified during it.

These intellectual and clinical problems are regularly ignored when sweeping conclusions are zealously drawn from either a single trial or a relatively small number of trials. The careful formation of scientific conclusions is particularly important for the regulatory agencies and other influential members of the medical community who make decisions about the efficacy, safety, and applicability of new (or old) forms of treatment.

1. Issues in efficacy. A single trial may demonstrate that an agent is efficacious, but cannot prove the absence of efficacy. As shown in the earlier example of an agent that worked well for 1 of every 25 people, the trial may not have included enough members of the strata of "responsive" patients. A trial may also give a falsely "negative" result because of the "cancellation" created by opposing effects in different strata, or because of other forms of insensitive design, as discussed by Cromie.[7] Even if efficacy was demonstrated, the results of the investigated group or of other patients must be carefully analyzed to determine whether the efficacy pertains to all the treated patients or only to certain strata.

2. Issues in safety. No clinical trial can prove that an agent is safe. The trial can show only that the agent brought no harm to the people who received it. The agent may not have been maintained long enough for toxic effects to develop, or the trial may not have included the particular kinds of patients for whom the agent is unsafe. For example, in a clinical trial confined to men and post-menopausal women, thalidomide might readily be shown to be an effective, harmless sedative. Conversely, when lack of safety is implied in a clinical trial, the data must be carefully examined to determine whether the "adverse reactions" were actually due to the indicated agent and whether the reactions occurred in all the treated patients or just in certain susceptible strata.

3. Issues in applicability. For all the foregoing reasons, the ultimate safety, efficacy, and applicability of therapeutic agents cannot be established only with randomized clinical trials and must be determined from supplementary data. The results of a single trial or of a few trials cannot possibly encompass the diverse types of patients and reactions that may be encountered when a therapeutic agent comes into general use. The trials can serve only to indicate that a new agent should be allowed into the clinical "market" or that an old agent should be reappraised— but the trials do not necessarily allow definitive conclusions. Only the additional information of general clinical experience (with or without randomized trials) can provide a satisfactory view of the broad scope of human illness that is merely glimpsed, and sometimes distorted, by the investigative artefacts imposed during the trials.

The ability to generalize the results of randomized trials would be greatly enhanced if better techniques were developed for identifying and stratifying clusters of patients with distinctive prognostic characteristics. Many current arguments about safety and efficacy could be readily resolved if the anecdotal opinions reported as clinical experience, the non-random evidence assembled in clinical surveys, and the imprecise mixtures tabulated in randomized trials were all improved to allow a specification of distinctive clinical strata and an analysis of results within those strata.

• • •

In the meantime, however, randomized trials will continue to be an essential ingredient in therapeutic progress. Assuming that all other plans for a trial have been made in a satisfactory manner, randomization (preferably within well-demarcated prognostic strata) offers the best current method for allocating the sequence of therapy. The idea of randomized allocation will retard therapeutic progress, however, if randomization continues to be regarded as the principal ingredient in that progress, and if all of the more important clinical and scientific components continue to be neglected.

References

1. Chalmers, T. C., Block, J. B., and Lee, S.: Controlled studies in clinical cancer research, N. Engl. J. Med. **287:**75-78, 1972.

2. Cobb, L. A., Thomas, G. I., Dillard, D. H., Merendino, K. A., and Bruce, R. A.: An evaluation of internal-mammary-artery ligation by a double-blind technic, N. Engl. J. Med. **260:** 1115-1118, 1959.

3. Colton, J.: A model for selecting one of two medical treatments, J. Amer. Stat. Assn. **58:** 388-400, 1963.

4. Cornfield, J.: The University Group Diabetes Program. A further statistical analysis of the mortality findings, J. A. M. A. **217:**1676-1687, 1971.

5. Cornfield, J., Halperin, M., and Greenhouse, S.: An adaptive procedure for sequential clinical trials, J. Am. Stat. Assn. **64:**759-770, 1969.

6. Cox, D. R.: Randomization, Biometrics **27:** 1114, 1971. (Abst.)

7. Cromie, B. W.: Errors in providing data for statistical analysis, Proc. Roy. Soc. Med. **59** (Suppl.):64-68, 1966.

8. Feinstein, A. R.: Clinical biostatistics. III-V. The architecture of clinical research, CLIN. PHARMACOL. THER. **11:**432-441, 595-610, and 755-771, 1970.

9. Feinstein, A. R.: Clinical biostatistics. VIII. An analytic appraisal of the University Group Diabetes Program (UGDP) study, CLIN. PHARMACOL. THER. **12:**167-191, 1971.

10. Feinstein, A. R.: Clinical biostatistics. IX. How do we measure "safety and efficacy"? CLIN. PHARMACOL. THER. **12:**544-558, 1971.

11. Feinstein, A. R.: Clinical biostatistics. XII. On exorcising the ghost of Gauss and the curse of Kelvin, CLIN. PHARMACOL. THER. **12:**1003-1016, 1971.

12. Feinstein, A. R.: Prognostic stratification series, CLIN. PHARMACOL. THER. **13:**285-297, 442-457, 609-624, and 755-768, 1972.

13. Feinstein, A. R.: The need for humanised science in evaluating medication, Lancet **2:** 421-423, 1972.

14. Feinstein, A. R.: Clinical biostatistics. XIX. Ambiguity and abuse in the twelve different concepts of 'control,' CLIN. PHARMACOL. THER. **14:**112-122, 1973.

15. Feinstein, A. R.: Clinical biostatistics. XX. The epidemiologic trohoc, the ablative risk ratio, and 'retrospective' research, CLIN. PHARMACOL. THER. **14:**291-307, 1973.

16. Feinstein, A. R.: Clinical biostatistics. XXII. The role of randomization in sampling, testing, allocation, and credulous idolatry (Part 1), CLIN. PHARMACOL. THER. **14:**601-615, 1973.

17. Feinstein, A. R.: Clinical biostatistics. XXIII. The role of randomization in sampling, testing, allocation, and credulous idolatry (Part 2), CLIN. PHARMACOL. THER. **14:**898-915, 1973.

18. Fisher, R. A.: The arrangement of field experiments, J. Ministry Agriculture **33:**503-513, 1926.

19. Fisher, R. A.: The design of experiments, ed. 8, New York, 1966, Hafner Publishing Co.
20. Heisenberg, W.: The physical principles of the quantum theory, Chicago, 1930, University of Chicago Press.
21. Landis, J. R., and Feinstein, A. R.: An empirical comparison of random numbers acquired by computer-generation and from the Rand tables, Comp. Biomed. Res. **6**:322-326, 1973.
22. Lindley, D. V.: Is randomization necessary? Biometrics **27**:1114, 1971. (Abst.)
23. Mainland, D.: Elementary medical statistics, ed. 2, Philadelphia, 1963, W. B. Saunders Co.
24. Modell, W., and Houde, R. W.: Factors influencing clinical evaluation of drugs. With special reference to the double-blind technique, J. A. M. A. **167**:2190-2199, 1958.
25. Nebenzahl, E., and Sobel, M.: Play-the-winner sampling for a fixed-sample-size binomial selection problem, Biometrika **59**:1-8, 1972.
26. Radhakrishna, S., and Sutherland, I.: The chance occurrence of substantial initial differences between groups in studies based on random allocation, Appl. Stat. **11**:47-54, 1962.
27. Seaman, A. J., Griswold, H. E., Reaume, R. B., and Ritzmann, L.: Long-term anticoagulant prophylaxis after myocardial infarction. Final report, N. Engl. J. Med. **281**:115-119, 1969.
28. Student (W. S. Gosset): Comparison between balanced and random arrangements of field plots, Biometrika **29**:363-379, 1937.
29. University Group Diabetes Program: A study of the effects of hypoglycemic agents on vascular complications in patients with adult-onset diabetes. I. Design, methods and baseline results; and II. Mortality results, Diabetes **19**:747-830 (suppl. 2), 1970.
30. Youden, W. J.: Randomization and experimentation, Technometrics **14**:13-22, 1972.
31. Zelen, M.: Play the winner rule and the controlled clinical trial, J. Amer. Stat. Assn. **64**:131-146, 1969.

CHAPTER 9

Consequences of 'compliance bias'

Most discussions of *compliance* are concerned with a patient's maintenance of an assigned therapeutic regimen. Since no drug, diet, or other agent of therapy can work unless it is taken, one of the main clinical reasons for studying compliance is to increase it. By finding out why patients fail to comply and how we can encourage compliance, we hope to develop better ways of enabling a presumably beneficial therapeutic regimen to accomplish its benefits. With these goals in mind, we may investigate the various clinico-socio-behavioral features that are determinants of compliance and the educational-communicational-packaging features that may enhance it.

A substantial literature has begun to develop on compliance with therapeutic regimens. The references cited here are only a few of the many studies[1, 2, 11, 12, 16-18, 21] specifically devoted to this topic, and a detailed compendium[13] of the literature was recently assembled for a major "Workshop/Symposium" conducted at the McMaster University Medical Center in Hamilton, Ontario, Canada. The organizers of that meeting, Drs. David L. Sackett and R. Brian Haynes, have also begun to issue

a newsletter that contains an ongoing account of new developments in the field.

In trying to achieve or increase compliance with a therapeutic regimen, we begin with the basic assumption that the therapy is desirable—that it is safe, effective, and worth using. Once these virtues have been established, the regimen will warrant the efforts by both medical personnel and patients to ensure that it is maintained as prescribed. On the other hand, the complex spectrum of compliance has effects that can alter the basic data analyzed to determine the virtues of a regimen. These ramifications of compliance are the focus of discussion in this essay. Unless suitable biostatistical attention is given to the diverse patterns and effects of compliance, it can act as a source of confusion and distortion in the original therapeutic data. If various forms of "compliance bias" are not properly recognized and adjusted, a valuable therapeutic regimen may be dismissed as worthless or an ineffectual treatment may be promulgated as good.

In this essay, I should like to discuss six features of compliance that can affect the biostatistical data and interpretations. These features relate to issues in regimen compliance, the evaluation of compliance, the non-compliance "control", protocol compliance, the "compliance sample", and the "compliance-confounded cohort".

This chapter originally appeared as "Clinical biostatistics—XXX. Biostatistical problems in 'compliance bias.'" In Clin. Pharmacol. Ther. 16:846, 1974.

A. Regimen compliance

The first point to be considered is the way that the results of a therapeutic regimen can be distorted by the compliance it receives. Let us assume that an index of success has been established in a randomized, double-blind therapeutic trial, comparing Drug A vs. Drug B. Let us further assume that the two drugs are equally effective. Despite this equivalence in efficacy, compliance bias can alter the results of the trial so that a major difference can falsely occur in the success rates of the two drugs. The observed success rate might be 50% for Drug A and 66% for Drug B.

A false difference of this magnitude could occur as follows: Suppose that the condition under treatment has a 70% success rate when either Drug A or B is faithfully maintained and a 30% success rate when either drug is abandoned. Now suppose that Drug A has an unappealing taste, appearance, or schedule of administration so that it is faithfully maintained by only 50% of the patients assigned to it, whereas Drug B receives excellent compliance by 90% of the patients. With these distinctions, if 200 patients were assigned to Drug A, 100 patients would maintain the drug faithfully and 70 of these 100 would have a successful outcome. Of the 100 patients who abandon the drug, 30 would be successful. The net result for Drug A would be 100 successes per 200 patients—an overall success rate of 50%. With Drug B, 180 of the 200 assigned patients would maintain excellent compliance and 126 (70%) of them would have a successful outcome. Of the 20 patients who abandon the drug, 6 (30%) would be successful. The total success rate for Drug B would thus be 132/200, or 66%.

The difference between the two success rates would be large enough (16%) to be clinically significant and the magnitude of the sample sizes cited here would also make the difference "statistically significant" at $P < .005$ ($\chi^2 = 10.5$). If we had not attempted to investigate and analyze compliance, however, we would be unaware of its role in causing the difference. We would then conclude erroneously that Drug B is pharmacologically more effective than Drug A, although the actual cause of the difference arose as a matter of compliance, rather than pharmacologic efficacy.

The mathematical calculations just cited can be simplified by the following algebraic procedure. Let p_D be the proportion of patients who maintain good compliance for Treatment D. Let q_D, which is $1-p_D$, be the proportion of patients who do not maintain good compliance. Let r_1 be the rate of an outcome event (such as "success" or a cardiovascular complication) in patients who maintain good compliance. Let r_2 be the rate of this outcome event in patients whose compliance was not good. With these conventions, the rate of the outcome event for the cohort of patients receiving Treatment D is $p_D r_1 + q_D r_2$. Thus, in the foregoing example, the success rate for Drug A is $(.50 \times .70) + (.50 \times .30) = .35 + .15 = .50 = 50\%$. The success rate for Drug B is $(.90 \times .70) + (.10 \times .30) = .63 + .03 = .66 = 66\%$.

The effect of compliance bias in the situation just described was to cause a false difference in the apparent efficacy of two drugs that actually had equal pharmacologic action. An analogous set of problems might work in the opposite direction to produce a false difference in the adverse-reaction rates of two drugs with equal toxicity.

B. Evaluation of compliance

Since distinctions in compliance can affect the appraisal of a therapeutic regimen's efficacy and safety, the evaluation of compliance is an important, although often neglected, aspect of clinical biostatistics. Probably the main reason for this neglect is that compliance is an entirely subjective and human phenomenon. Its data are extremely "soft". The degree of compliance is determined by the patient; the act of compliance usually occurs in circumstances where it cannot be directly observed by the investigator; and its appraisal depends on what the patient decides to do and report about it. In an era devoted to the analysis of "hard" data, compliance is a variable that lacks scientific appeal, no matter how important the phenomenon may be.

The prejudice against this type of information has been well summarized by the recent Nobel laureate, Konrad Lorenz[15]:

> If the subject of investigation happens to be human, he or she is being literally dehumanized by being prevented from showing any response which a guinea pig or a pigeon might not show as well (in fact, the same experimental set-up is often applicable to animal and human subjects). Worse, in that kind of experimentation, the experimenter himself is not permitted to be quite human, as he is strictly prevented from using most of the cognitive mechanisms with which nature endowed our species. ...The worst of this widespread contempt for description is that it discourages people from even trying to analyze really complicated systems.

1. Types of data. For investigators who are willing to cope with complicated human systems, three different methods can be used for getting data to describe and evaluate compliance. Perhaps the most objective technique is to measure the presence of the drug (or one of its metabolic products) in the urine. The main disadvantage of this method is that it pertains only to the one specimen for which the test was made. The result does not indicate the patient's compliance during all the other times for which no urine tests were performed. Furthermore, the single urine test may not be able to indicate whether the drug was correctly taken in the prescribed pattern even on the day of the test.

A second quantitative technique is based on dosage unit counts. At each visit, the patient is given a fixed number of doses in a container that is returned for its remaining doses to be counted at the next visit. This technique provides quantitative data, but it will fail if the patient forgets to bring the container, and the "pill count" cannot demonstrate whether the medication was taken in the desired pattern or disposed in various unprescribed manners.

The best way of finding out what a patient has done is to ask the patient directly. From the reply, an investigator

can learn the qualitative and quantitative information that is not provided by the other two techniques. For getting the totality of data needed to evaluate compliance, a well-constructed interview technique cannot be replaced by any of the available "objective" methods. Furthermore, a patient who deliberately wants to disguise the truth can subvert the "objective" procedures as well as the information provided in the interview.

The interview technique, however, is patently subjective. It depends completely on the patient's recall and reliability and also on the skill of the interviewer. An interviewer who is punitive or whose manner is otherwise unacceptable to the patient may not elicit accurate data. For these reasons, the interview technique is often used as the prime source of compliance data, but one of the "objective" techniques is added to verify the patient's reliability. A patient would be regarded as truly compliant only if the information stated in the interview is consistent with the results of the objective test.

2. Types of rating. Regardless of what method is used for assembling data about compliance, the results must be cited in a manner that allows the data to be analyzed. Since compliance cannot be expressed in dimensional terms (which might be used for such variables as *height* or *serum cholesterol*), the investigator must choose a scale that provides a rating. The scale that is chosen can be a dichotomous partition (such as **good** and **not good**) or a set of ordinal ranks, containing such categories as **poor, fair, good,** and **excellent.** For many analytic purposes, a dichotomous partition will suffice, since the investigator may want to engage only in a simple comparison in which the outcomes of the good group or not-good group are contrasted against all others.

The choice of criteria for these ratings will obviously be affected by the type of regimen under study and the purpose for which it has been prescribed. For example, the criteria for good compliance may differ if a daily antibiotic is being taken to prevent rather than to eradicate an infection. To illustrate this distinction, I shall list here two sets of criteria used during investigations[4-6] of daily oral antibiotics in the prevention of Group A streptococcal infections and rheumatic recurrences in a population of children and adolescents who had all had at least one previous episode of acute rheumatic fever:

Dose of drug	Oral Penicillin G 200,000 units daily	Oral Penicillin G 400,000 units 3 times daily for 10 days
Purpose of regimen	Continuous pro-phylaxis against streptococcal infection	Eradication of streptococcal infection
Criterion of "good" compliance	Reliable history *and* no more than 5 days missed per month *and* no 2 days missed consecutively	Reliable history *and* no more than 1 dose missed during the 10 days

Regardless of whether the reader agrees or disagrees with the details of these criteria, they demonstrate the fact that different types of therapeutic regimens will require different criteria for ratings of compliance.

C. The non-compliance "control"

Although the scientific prejudice against talking to patients is one of the main reasons that compliance has been so neglected as an important variable in statistical analyses, another type of prejudice has caused clinical investigators to lose other valuable data related to compliance. This prejudice is the tendency of doctors to dismiss patients who reject the doctors' recommendations.

In ordinary clinical practice, a patient who fails to carry out the doctor's recommendations is performing an important experiment that the doctor was unwilling to undertake. The patient has decided, in effect, to test a counter-hypothesis. If the experiment fails, the failure helps support the propriety of the doctor's original therapeutic decision. If the experiment succeeds, the doctor has learned that success does not always require the original plan of action. Consequently, a patient who refuses to comply with an offered treatment becomes a type of "control" whose results can be compared with those of patients who received the treatment.

Nevertheless, in ordinary clinical practice, a patient who appears to reject the doctor's recommendations is often rejected by the doctor. Because the patient may then be actively or passively urged to seek medical attention elsewhere, the doctor may miss the opportunity to learn the results of the counter-experiment. This type of loss may be a necessary event in circumstances where a busy practitioner wants to use his time "efficiently" and has no intention of ever tabulating his therapeutic results. The loss is highly undesirable, however, if the practitioner's data ever become items of biostatistics.

An illustration of the problem has regularly appeared in surveys reporting the outcome of therapy for cancer. In such surveys, the results of surgically treated patients have generally been compared against those of patients who received radiotherapy or chemotherapy. This comparison is unfair because the non-surgical patients were not an "operable" group; they were usually deemed "inoperable" and referred for other modes of treatment. For an unbiased comparison, the group of "operable" patients who received surgery should be contrasted with a group of "operable" patients who received some other treatment.

This type of contrast would be deliberately arranged in a randomized therapeutic trial, but very few such trials have been conducted for "operable" patients. Consequently, the only source of "operable" non-surgical patients in ordinary clinical practice is the people who were deemed "operable" and who refused the offered surgical treatment. These "non-compliant" patients would be a reasonable control group for the surgically treated patients;

but the non-compliant patients are usually rejected by their surgeons and seldom receive follow-up examinations for their outcomes to be noted, recorded, and analyzed.

Non-compliant patients can also serve as an important "control" group in circumstances where the results of placebo therapy are not available. For example, when several antibacterial agents were receiving randomized clinical trials to compare their value in preventing streptococcal infections, ethical considerations militated against the examination of results in groups treated with placebo. In the absence of a placebo-treated group, however, major problems arose when two of the "active" drugs were found to yield essentially similar results[5]. Was either drug really more effective than placebo? The issue was resolved when the streptococcal attack rate in compliant patients (who maintained "good prophylaxis") was found to be substantially lower than in patients who failed to comply.

Another opportunity to make analytic use of compliance distinctions occurred during an investigation of the role that tonsil size might play in predisposing rheumatic children and adolescents to streptococcal infections.[6] Among the patients who maintained good continuity of antibiotic prophylaxis, the attack rate of streptococcal infections was unaffected by tonsil size. Among patients who did not maintain good prophylaxis, the streptococcal attack rate increased with increasing size of the tonsils.

D. Protocol compliance

In all the issues discussed so far, the idea of *compliance* referred only to the patient's acceptance or maintenance of an assigned therapeutic regimen. Another important aspect of compliance refers to the maintenance of a research protocol. During the course of a therapeutic trial or other investigation, many planned procedures must be carried out by both investigator and patient. The compliance or non-compliance given to these protocol procedures can affect the results of the research.

1. Compliance by investigator. The likelihood of violating a research protocol is particularly high when multiple investigators are collaborating. The violations usually arise because of poor communication among the collaborators or inadequate attention by individual investigators. One frequent violation occurs in the criteria for admission to the trial. For example, in the UGDP cooperative study[19] of therapy for diabetes mellitus, 9% of the admitted patients did not fulfill the minimum standards of glucose intolerance that had been established as diagnostic criteria for diabetes mellitus. Aside from the ethical problems produced by this type of protocol violation, it can create a major statistical problem if the results in the "ineligible" and "eligible" patients are substantially different.

Another type of violation, which is often inadvertent, is the investigator's development of the ability to discern the identities of the drugs being studied in a double-blind trial. This "unmasking" is particularly likely to occur if the active drug can be recognized from a physiologic side effect—such as the bradycardia that often occurs with beta-blocking agents. The consequence of this type of protocol violation is the delusion that symptoms and other subjective data have been determined with the presumptive "objectivity" of an effectively maintained double-blind technique. If doctors (or patients) become successfully able to differentiate the active drug from the placebo, the clinical trial is converted into a pseudo-double-blind exercise, having all the logistic disadvantages of double-blind research and none of the scientific advantages.

A third protocol problem in therapeutic trials is the need to exclude supplementary drugs that might affect the results of the main drug under investigation. The violation of this specification of a protocol is often overlooked if the violations have occurred with equal frequency in each group of patients receiving the compared therapeutic regimens. Since the qualitative characteristics of the "ineligible" medications may not be equivalent for each group of patients, the differences may be responsible for distinctions that become erroneously attributed to the principal therapeutic agents.

Of the many other potential issues in investigator non-compliance, the only one to be cited here is the problem of preserving the "letter" of a research protocol while ignoring its "spirit". For example, suppose we are conducting a therapeutic trial to determine whether the maintenance of normoglycemia will prevent vascular complications in adults with diabetes mellitus. If we prescribe a fixed dosage of an oral hypoglycemic drug and determine whether the patient complies with the prescribed regimen, we have adhered to the specifications of the protocol. On the other hand, if we fail to check whether the patient's blood sugar is actually being maintained in a normal range or if we fail to adjust the dose of the drug so that it produces normoglycemia, we have not complied with the basic idea of the research.

There are many other ways in which an investigator's non-compliance with protocol can distort the research data. Nevertheless, the published reports of a research project often contain no indication of efforts made to check whether protocol compliance has occurred. An interesting aspect of the peculiar "double standard" used on the current research scene is that pharmaceutical companies are expected to monitor the compliance of clinical investigators who perform trials of new drugs, but an analogous monitoring may not be demanded when a federal agency sponsors a multi-center therapeutic trial involving investigators at academic institutions.

2. Compliance by patient. While complying with the prescribed medication, a patient may violate the prescribed protocol in several different ways. One violation consists of breaking the double-blind code.

A recent example of this problem was provided by Chalmers[3]. He described the way in which a sophisticated group of patients (employees of the National Institutes of Health), who were participating in a double-blind clinical trial, tasted the contents of the capsules to distinguish vitamin C from placebo. According to Chalmers, the rates of the outcome event in the trial were substantially different for patients who did or did not correctly identify their medication.

Another important form of patient non-compliance is improper attendance for repeated examinations after treatment is initiated. If a patient scheduled to have a particular test done at 4 weeks and at 8 weeks after treatment appears only at 6 weeks, where do the results of the 6-week test get counted? Suppose the patient does not appear often enough to have all the periodic tests that are needed to rule out episodic events, such as asymptomatic streptococcal infections or anicteric hepatitis. How are the incomplete data to be analyzed? There are no simple statistical answers to these questions. Each decision requires subtle judgments according to the particular circumstances that are involved.

The ultimate act of non-compliance, of course, is the patient's decision to drop out of a study altogether. Except for one issue to be cited later, the problems of analyzing data for drop-out patients are beyond the scope of this discussion, and will be reserved for a later installment in this series. The problems are difficult, complex, and not always well managed by the actuarial ("life-table") analyses that are usually proposed as a solution.

E. The "compliance sample"

A different type of biostatistical problem arises when a therapeutic trial is conducted with a "compliance sample" of patients. Such a sample arises in the following way: Before admission to the trial, the patients who are otherwise eligible are screened to determine their ability and willingness to comply with both the protocol and the therapeutic regimens under investigation. Patients whom the investigators regard as non-compliant are then excluded from admission, so that the trial is conducted with the group of seemingly cooperative patients who constitute the "compliance sample". A clue to the existence of such a sample can be noted from an account of the criteria used for excluding patients from a trial. These criteria customarily depend on various features of diagnosis, prognosis, co-morbidity, or co-medication. If the criteria also include a statement about "willingness to cooperate", the investigators have used a compliance sample.

To choose patients in this way seems perfectly reasonable. After all, in conducting a therapeutic trial, the investigators do not wish to expend major amounts of time and vigorous research efforts on patients who are not likely to maintain the proposed medication or appear for the proposed examination procedures. By screening out the non-compliant patients, the investigators would eliminate wasted energy and increase the efficiency of the research activities.

In attaining this efficiency, however, the investigators take a substantial risk. The risk is that the compliant patients may not properly represent the people who have the condition under treatment. The risk is tiny if the excluded non-compliant patients constituted only a small proportion of the total group of otherwise eligible patients. If the excluded group occupied a large fraction of the eligible cases, however, the results of the trial may be seriously compromised, particularly if compliance and therapeutic responsiveness are inter-related. The results of the trial may be pertinent for compliant but not for other patients with the same clinical condition.

An example of this type of problem occurred in the recent Veterans Administration Cooperative Study[20] of the treatment of hypertension. Because the results provided "hard" (randomized) evidence of the value of treating patients with asymptomatic hypertension, the trial has received many justified praises for the excellence with which it was designed and conducted. Nevertheless, the group under study contained a highly restricted compliance sample of hypertensive patients. The selection procedure was described as follows[9]:

> Since an appreciable number of dropouts would jeopardize the study, we wished to minimize their occurrence as much as possible. "Skid row" alcoholics, vagrants, psychopaths, antagonistic personalities, mentally incompetent persons who are not properly cared for at home, and all those who for one reason or another could not return to clinic regularly are therefore excluded from the trial. In addition, the pre-randomization trial period serves to eliminate other potential dropouts that are missed during the initial evaluation.

The VA investigators have not published data on the number of otherwise eligible patients whose anticipated (or demonstrated) non-compliance kept them from being admitted to the trial. It has been estimated[10] that between one half to two thirds of the patients with eligible blood pressures were excluded from entry. The exclusion of this large proportion of patients would not affect the results found in the compliant patients who were treated in the trial, but would impair the ability to draw general conclusions about the treatment of other patients with hypertension. Docile hypertensive patients who are willing to comply in such a trial may have their vascular systems benefitted by therapeutic agents that lower blood pressure; but these agents may not work as well on the many non-docile hypertensives who are non-compliant.

As public campaigns are mounted to deliver appropriate treatment to all patients with hypertension, the results (if noted and evaluated) may be somewhat disappointing. If the rate of vascular complications is not reduced as much as was expected, the disparity may arise from the unresponsiveness of the non-compliant patients whose therapeutic refractoriness had not previously been discovered.

F. The "compliance confounded cohort"

The last problem to be cited here is particularly subtle and complex. It can arise if the ability to comply with a therapeutic regimen is also related to the event that is to be noted as the main outcome of treatment. If compliance ability and outcome event are closely related, the results will be distorted by a confounding variable. Regardless of treatment, the cohort of people who can comply with treatment will be destined to have an outcome-event rate that differs substantially from the corresponding rate in the people who do not maintain compliance. Consequently, an ineffectual regimen may falsely appear to be distinctly beneficial (or detrimental) to the people who maintain it.

To illustrate this point, suppose that people who have a high degree of the particular kind of inner drive or stress that might be called psychic *tension* are more likely to develop cardiovascular disease than people who are not psychically tense. Let us now suppose that an unappealing and difficult-to-maintain new diet has been proposed as an agent that prevents cardiovascular disease. Let us further assume that the diet is actually ineffectual. Finally, let us assume that the tense people have great difficulty in complying with this new diet, whereas non-tense people are much more able to comply. Under these conditions, when the diet is prescribed for a large population, the rate of cardiovascular disease will be lower in people who maintain the diet than in people who do not. The false conclusion may then be that the diet effectively prevents cardiovascular disease.

Since this type of problem may arise in the multiple risk factor intervention trial (MRFIT) now being launched[14] throughout the United States, I shall cite some contrived numerical data to illustrate the possibilities.

Let us assume that we can identify a tense group of people who will also have a 30% rate of cardiovascular events during the interval under study. In non-tense people, the corresponding rate is 5%. Let us further assume that the population under study consists of 70% non-tense people and 30% tense people. If nothing were done to this population, we would expect the overall rate of cardiovascular events to be

$$(.70) (.05) + (.30) (.30) =$$
$$.035 + .09 = .125 = 12.5\%$$

Now suppose that the entire population enters a randomized clinical trial in which the action of a special new diet is being tested. Half the population is assigned this new diet and the other half continues to maintain its usual dietary pattern.

The compliance problem might now occur as follows. For the people who are not receiving a special diet, there is no difficult regimen acting as a provocation to drop out. The only drop-out incentive is the "nuisance" of participating in the clinical trial itself. Consequently, the drop-out rates in the no-diet patients would be the usual attrition to be expected in any trial, and the rates would be similar in the tense and non-tense patients. Let us assume that these drop-out rates are 5% in each group. The remaining population in the no-diet cohort will thus be composed of 95% of the starting members of each psychic group, and will be 95% of its original size. [This figure can be verified as $(.95) (.70) + (.95) (.30) = .665 + .285 = .950 = 95\%$.]

For the patients in the cohort assigned to receive the special diet, the difficulties of maintaining the diet will create a strong stimulus toward dropping out. Among non-tense patients, let us assume that the drop-out rate is 10%, twice as high as the rate in similar patients not receiving the diet. Among tense patients, the problems of maintaining the special diet are formidable, so that 80% of these patients drop out.

The total group of people who maintain the special diet will thus be reduced to 69% of the original cohort. [This figure can be verified as $(.70)$ $(.90)$ + $(.30)$ $(.20)$ = $.63$ + $.06$ = $.69$ = 69%.] This rate of compliance will not seem unusually low, because a relatively high drop-out rate would be anticipated for people assigned to the special diet.

Now let us consider what will be observed as the outcome rates for cardiovascular events in this study. For the cohort of people who continued to participate in the no-diet group, the event rate would be 5% in the 66.5% of non-tense people and 30% in the 28.5% of tense people. The total event rate would be $(.05)$ $(.665)$ + $(.30)$ $(.285)$ = $(.03325)$ + $(.0855)$ = $.11875$. When adjusted for the population of no-diet people who actually completed the trial, this rate would be $(.11875)$ / $(.95)$ = $.125$ = 12.5%. For the cohort of people who continued to maintain the special diet, the event rate would be 5% in the 63% of non-tense people and 30% in the 6% of tense people. The total event rate for the special diet group will therefore be $(.05)$ $(.63)$ + $(.30)$ $(.06)$ = $.0315$ + $.018$ = $.0495$ = 4.95%. When adjusted for the special-diet people who actually completed the trial, this rate would be $(.0495)$ / $(.69)$ = $.072$ = 7.2%.

If we knew nothing about the relationship of personality, compliance, and cardiovascular rates in tense vs. non-tense people, we would observe only the outcome rates. Without a stratification for psychic state, we would not be aware of the differential drop-out distinctions that had produced the differences in outcome, and we might draw conclusions based only on the gross outcomes. Thus, in a randomized clinical trial comparing a special diet vs. no diet, we would have noted that the people who maintained the special diet had a cardiovascular event rate of 7.2%; and that the people who maintained no special diet had a corresponding rate of 12.5%. The special diet would appear to

have reduced the cardiovascular event rate by $\frac{12.5 - 7.2}{12.5}$ = $\frac{5.3}{12.5}$ = 42.4%. This magnitude of reduction would obviously seem clinically significant; and furthermore, with the large numbers of patients entered into the trial, the difference would also be statistically significant[*].

The obvious conclusion would seem to be that the special diet had reduced the rate of cardiovascular disease by more than 40%—and yet the conclusion would be totally wrong. The apparent benefits of the diet, which we know was actually ineffectual, would have arisen only from the fact that it received compliance mainly from people destined to have a low rate of cardiovascular events.

At this point in the discussion, a student of clinical trials would immediately note that the analysis presented thus far is incomplete. We have not yet looked at the results of the drop-out patients. Under the conditions noted earlier, we should find a substantial difference in cardiovascular rates in the two groups of patients who dropped out. These rates would be 12.5% in the no-diet group and 24.4% in the special-diet group. The explanatory calculations are as follows. In the no-diet group, the non-tense drop-outs would contain $(.70)(.05)$ = $.035$ and the tense drop-outs would contain $(.30)$ $(.05)$ = $.015$ of the original population. The cardiovascular rate in this group of drop-outs would be $[(.035)$ $(.05)$ + $(.015)$ $(.30)]$ / $.050$ = $[.00175$ + $.00450]$ / $.050$ = $.00625/.05$ = $.125$ = 12.5%. In the special diet group, the non-tense drop-outs would contain $(.70)$ $(.10)$ = $.07$ and the tense drop-outs would contain $(.30)$ $(.80)$ = $.24$ of the original population. The cardiovascular rate in this group of drop-outs would be $[(.07)$ $(.05)$ + $(.24)$

---

[*]With calculations that are too extensive to be repeated here, it can be shown that this difference in the two groups of compliant patients will have a P value below .05 (by χ^2 test) if as few as 636 patients are initially enrolled in the trial.

$(.30)] / .31 = [.0035 + .072]/.31 = .0755/ .31 = .244 = 24.4\%$. The finding that one drop-out group had a cardiovascular rate twice as high as the other drop-out group should immediately alert our suspicions that something extremely peculiar has happened.

Furthermore, if we look at the results of all patients who were randomized, regardless of those who dropped out, we would find that the cardiovascular rates are the same. In the no-diet group, the rate would be $[(.11875) + (.00625)] / [(.95) + (.05)] = [.12500] / 1.00 = 12.5\%$. In the special diet group, the rate would be $[(.0495) + (.0755)] / [(.69) + (.31)] = [.1250] / [1.00] = 12.5\%$. This similarity in cardiovascular rates for the two randomized groups, regardless of drop-outs, would help confirm the existence of some strange phenomenon among the drop-out cases.

To get all this additional information, however, would require that the therapeutic trial be conducted with an extraordinary passion for getting complete, detailed follow-up data for all patients who have dropped out. This intensity of follow-up surveillance almost never occurs in a therapeutic trial. If the outcome event is death, the investigators can usually learn about its occurrence in drop-out patients who have otherwise been "lost to follow-up"; but if the outcome event is a non-fatal cardiovascular event (such as angina pectoris, myocardial infarction, intermittent claudication, or stroke), the occurrence or non-occurrence of this event is difficult to document in a standardized manner for living patients who have been lost to follow-up. Because of these difficulties in the follow-up of dropped patients, the investigators may be strongly tempted to confine their main analyses to the patients who, complying with the research protocol, continued under observation. If this temptation is accepted, the investigators will reach the erroneous conclusion described earlier.

The possibility of this type of error is a major hazard in the work of the MRFIT study. An abundance of evidence has now been assembled to suggest that a distinctive relationship exists between certain personality types (or psychic states) and subsequent cardiovascular disease. The main issue is no longer whether such a relationship exists, but how to identify it—by which particular psychologic test or other psychiatric examining instrument can we best discern the people who are especially susceptible to cardiovascular disease. Another reasonable belief is that the people who have this particular psychic constitution may be unwilling or unable to maintain the particular forms of special dieting or other interventions that are prescribed as "active therapy" in the MRFIT trial. Since the "control" group will receive no diet, rather than an equally unpalatable but standard diet, the MRFIT investigation thus possesses all the ingredients needed for a major scientific error in the interpretation of results.

The most cogent way of avoiding this error is for the patients' psychic condition to be examined with test procedures that are as thorough as those used for examining the condition of serum lipids. With such data, the investigators could identify the different degrees of psychic "risk", and could use the results for the analyses needed to demonstrate that compliance bias is absent. This approach may not be scientifically appealing, however, because the questionnaire and other written instruments used for examining psychic status have not received intensive attention from epidemiologists. The ideologic belief of most contemporary epidemiologists has been that "risk factors" arise from nurture but not from nature—from such environmental features as food, water, tobacco smoking, and exercise; but not from such constitutional features as heredity and psychic status. Because of this ideologic belief, both heredity and psyche have been generally ignored in epidemiologic research, and suitable scientific instruments have not been developed or applied for obtaining the necessary data in large cohort studies.

In the absence of suitable psychic examinations and correlated data analyses, another way of trying to avoid the cited error is for all the MRFIT patients to continue to receive intensive medical surveillance, even if they drop out, so that the detection of cardiovascular events is equally performed for everyone, regardless of regimen compliance. If the cardiovascular rates are different for *non-compliant* patients in the several therapeutic regimens, the investigators will have received a major signal that their basic data may be distorted by a compliance-confounded cohort. Equality of diagnostic surveillance may not be achievable, however, because the drop-out patients may be unwilling to continue to return to the MRFIT clinics for the necessary examinations. To cope with this problem, the investigators may need to arrange night clinics, home visits, or other special procedures that will allow drop-out patients to receive suitable follow-up examinations for detecting cardiovascular events.

• • •

These six features of compliance should suffice to indicate its intricacies and its potential for creating major biostatistical delusions. Compliance bias can be added to selection bias,[7] detection bias,[7] and chronology bias[8] as another prime source of the confounding variables that produce fundamental errors in biostatistical analysis. Confounding variables in biostatistics are like counter-hypotheses in any other form of scientific research. If the investigator does not contemplate and rule out the counter-hypotheses, they may vitiate his chosen hypothesis and invalidate his research. Like the biases due to inequities in selection, detection, and chronology, compliance bias will not disappear merely because an investigator hopes or wishes that it does not exist. It also will not disappear if the data analyst tries to "adjust for bias" by using age, race, sex or other variables that are conveniently available, instead of concentrating on the "inconvenient" variables that create the confounding.

To acquire the data needed for analyzing compliance and ruling out the existence of compliance bias, investigators will have to restore attention to a traditional activity of clinical medicine: talking to the patient. The investigators who have neglected or abandoned this information because it is scientifically "soft" have created the hazard of a clinical science that is "hard" but often irrelevant or erroneous. By perpetuating a restricted focus on "hard" data while ignoring important "soft" data that are obtained by direct conversation with patients, biostatisticians have abetted the malefaction. In addition to the cited scientific defects, however, therapeutic investigations that depend only on "hard data" create an important humanistic hazard. The idea may be established that biostatistical analyses are unable to distinguish between an act of patient care and an exercise in veterinary medicine.

References

1. Boyd, J. R., Covington, T. R., Stanaszek, W. F., and Coussons, R. T.: Drug defaulting. I. Determinants of compliance; II. Analysis of noncompliance patterns, Am. J. Hosp. Pharm. **31**:362-367; 485-491, 1974.
2. Blackwell, B.: The drug defaulter, CLIN. PHARMACOL. THER. **13**:841-848, 1972.
3. Chalmers, T. C.: Quoted in Internal Medicine News, p. 4, Oct. 11, 1973.
4. Feinstein, A. R., Wood, H. F., Epstein, J. A., Taranta, A., Simpson, R., and Tursky, E.: A controlled study of three methods of prophylaxis against streptococcal infection in a population of rheumatic children. II. Results of the first three years of the study, including methods for evaluating the maintenance of oral prophylaxis, N. Engl. J. Med. **260**:697-702, 1959.
5. Feinstein, A. R., Spagnuolo, M., Jonas, S., Kloth, H., Tursky, E., and Levitt, M.: Prophylaxis of recurrent rheumatic fever. Therapeutic-continuous oral penicillin vs. monthly injections, J. A. M. A. **206**:565-568, 1968.
6. Feinstein, A. R., and Levitt, M.: The role of tonsils in predisposing to streptococcal in-

fections and recurrences of rheumatic fever, N. Engl. J. Med. **282**:285-291, 1970.

7. Feinstein, A. R.: Clinical biostatistics. X. Sources of 'transition bias' in cohort statistics, CLIN. PHARMACOL. THER. **12**:704-721, 1971.

8. Feinstein, A. R.: Clinical biostatistics. XI. Sources of 'chronology bias' in cohort statistics, CLIN. PHARMACOL. THER. **12**:864-879, 1971.

9. Freis, E. D.: Organization of a long-term multiclinic therapeutic trial in hypertension, *in* Gross, F., editor, with the assistance of Naegeli, S. R., and Kirkwood, A. H.: Antihypertensive therapy. Principles and practice. An international symposium, New York, 1966, Springer-Verlag, pp. 345-354.

10. Freis, E. D.: Personal communication.

11. Gillum, R. F., and Barsky, A. J.: Diagnosis and management of patient noncompliance, J. A. M. A. **228**:1563-1567, 1974.

12. Gordis, L., Markowitz, M., and Lilienfeld, A. M.: Why patients don't follow medical advice: A study of children on long-term antistreptococcal prophylaxis, J. Pediatr. **75**:957-968, 1969.

13. Haynes, R. B., and Sackett, D. L.: An annotated bibliography on the compliance of patients with therapeutic regimens, Department of Clinical Epidemiology and Biostatistics, McMaster University Health Sciences Centre, Hamilton, Ontario, Canada, 1974. (Mimeographed pamphlet.)

14. Kaelber, C. T.: Quoted in Medical News, J. A. M. A. **227**:1243-1244, 1974.

15. Lorenz, K. Z.: The fashionable fallacy of dispensing with description, Naturwissenschaften **60**:1-9, 1973.

16. Mazzullo, J. M., Lasagna, L., and Griner, P. F.: Variations in interpretation of prescription instructions. The need for improved prescribing habits, J. A. M. A. **227**:929-931, 1974.

17. Roth, H. P., Caron, H. S., and Hsi, B. P.: Measuring intake of a prescribed medication. A bottle count and a tracer technique compared, CLIN. PHARMACOL. THER. **11**:228-237, 1970.

18. Stewart, R. B., and Cluff, L. E.: A review of medication errors and compliance in ambulant patients, CLIN. PHARMACOL. THER. **13**:463-468, 1972.

19. University Group Diabetes Program. A study of the effects of hypoglycemic agents on vascular complications in patients with adult-onset diabetes. Part I: Design, methods, and baseline characteristics. Part II: Mortality results, Diabetes **19**(Suppl. 2): 747-830, 1970.

20. Veterans Administration Cooperative Study Group on Antihypertensive Agents. Effects of treatment on morbidity in hypertension. II. Results in patients with diastolic blood pressure averaging 90 through 114 mm Hg, J. A. M. A. **213**:1143-1152, 1970.

21. Wilson, J. T.: Compliance with instructions in the evaluation of therapeutic efficacy. A common but frequently unrecognized major variable, Clin. Pediatr. (Phila.) **12**:333-340, 1973.

SECTION TWO

OTHER ARCHITECTURAL PROBLEMS

The difficulties noted in the preceding section can be magnified or embellished in the several ways that are discussed in the next few chapters. The first problem arises from a misplaced confidence in the prophylactic or remedial powers of statistical consultation. The statistician usually has many valuable tricks up his sleeve, but the sleeve may sometimes be empty or the trick may be a delusion. The second problem arises as another misplaced confidence, caused by the disparity between mathematical ideas based on random sampling and the medical reality of "samples" that are never selected randomly. Beyond the potential bias of a "rancid" sample, an investigator can add further distortion to the data by using the unequal examination procedures that create "tilted targets."

A prominent source of confusion is the ambiguity with which the concept of "control" is used and abused in the design of research. In most scientific plans and in statistical courses on "experimental design," the control is the comparative maneuver, but neither scientific nor statistical instruction contains specific attention to important issues in choosing either the comparative maneuver or the control group of people who receive it. To confound the confusion, the idea of control also has been applied to at least ten additional ideas in medical research.

A "case-control" study is the most frequent situation in which the idea of control is diverted from its customary scientific connotation and is applied to an effect rather than a cause. In case-control research, a group of diseased people is compared against a group of controls who do not have the disease. The comparison can be used in a "cross-sectional" study to examine the diagnostic utility of a particular marker (or test) in discriminating between diseased and nondiseased people. Alternatively, the case-control study can be "retrospective," aimed at examining an etiologic suspicion. In both types of case-control arrangement, the standard forward architecture of scientific research is drastically altered and the choice of a suitable control group becomes the crucial feature that determines the value of the results. Since mathematical principles again offer no help in making this choice, the decision requires careful scientific strategies.

Although diverse mathematical tactics have been developing for manipulating the quantitative results of both types of case-control study, rigorous standards have not yet been established for the scientific principles of a satisfactory research architecture. In diagnostic case-control studies, the key issue is the degree of discrimination that is sought within the diverse spectrum of diseased and non-diseased people. In etiologic case-control studies, the key issue is the development of suitable procedures to avoid the many biases that are inevitable when cause-effect reasoning is conducted in a logically backward temporal direction.

CHAPTER 10

Statistical malpractice—and the responsibility of a consultant

A pathologist has often been called a "doctor's doctor." In situations in which necropsy, biopsy, or cytology can provide confirmation for diagnostic reasoning, the pathologist is the consultant to whom clinicians have traditionally turned for verification or occasional refutation of the decisions reached during the preceding diagnostic activities. A statistician has now become the "researcher's doctor." He is the consultant to whom investigators regularly turn for advice about decisions made during research. The statistician is the consultant who is often asked to check the design of a research project, to plan the analysis of the data, and to help interpret the results.

Statisticians have not always held this crucial role in the world of medical research. Until the past few decades, clinical investigators were strongly distrustful and sometimes actively antagonistic about the scientific value of statistics. A century ago, when Claude Bernard was establishing experimental discipline in medical research, he denounced "mathematicians (who) . . . simplify too much and reason about phenomena as they construct them in their minds, but not as they exist in nature." Saying that ". . . statistics can never yield scientific truth (or) . . . establish any final scientific method," Bernard urged clinical investigators to "reject statistics as a foundation for experimental therapeutic and pathological science."[1]

When Pierre Louis, more than a century ago, was developing and advocating his "numerical method" for the appraisal of therapy,[19] his clinical espousal of statistics was opposed by most of the leading clinicians of the day.[11, 21, 32] The sentiment was summarized in the remarks of the renowned Armand Trousseau:[34]

> If the application of statistics to medicine were not rated too high, if it were not considered as the very keystone of the arch of all science . . . I should only praise it, because I really believe it to be useful; but there is so much noise made about such poor results. . . . I reproach (the statisticians) . . . for counting too much . . . and for declining to put any mind into the facts. . . . This mathematical exactitude . . . is only a relative precision, for it changes under the observation of the same man, according to the year, the season, and the reigning medical constitution.

From beyond the clinical world, the fortune of statistics has borne such recent taunts as Darrell Huff's[26] provocative book, *How to lie with statistics*, and Arthur Koestler's remark that "Statistics are like a bikini bathing suit: what they reveal is interesting; what they conceal is vital." From within the statistical fraternity, an "anthology" of diverse misuses and abuses

With the same name, this chapter originally appeared as "Clinical biostatistics—VI." In Clin. Pharmacol. Ther. 11:898, 1970.

of statistics has been provided in the text by Wallis and Roberts.[37]

Despite these caveats, statisticians have managed not only to endure in the world of clinical research, but more recently to prevail. The editors of good medical journals now insist on appropriate statistical reviews before manuscripts are accepted for publication, and at one leading journal[9] the word "significance" has been removed from general circulation and reserved for use only in a statistical context. At the extremes of mathematical obeisance, the editor of a psychologic journal[30] has decided to accept only manuscripts that have the "super-significance" demonstrated by P values of less than 0.01.* In concepts about etiology of disease, statistical "proofs" for the causes of chronic diseases are now generally accorded the respect that was once reserved for Koch's experimental postulates about acute infectious disease. Statistical validation has been emphasized by the FDA in a recently issued series of guidelines for sanctioning claims about new drugs. Advance approval and concomitant participation by statisticians have become a prerequisite demand before large-scale clinical trials will be funded by suitable agencies. And courses in statistics have become standard parts of the curriculum leading to doctoral degrees in either medicine or biology.

To achieve this status, the statistician may have had to fight an uphill battle and may still bear many scars of the conflict, but he has now clearly arrived. Furthermore, his consultative authority has been expanded in recent years to include prevention, and not just diagnosis and treatment, for the "ailments" of clinical research projects. His assistance, which was formerly sought remedially after a project was completed, is now often solicited prophylactically before the project begins. His ideas, which were formerly applied mainly to the choice and application of statistical tests after the investigator had planned the research, are now often solicited early enough to affect and sometimes to govern the basic design of the project.

Statisticians have welcomed the new challenges and have recommended this expansion of their roles. After a generation of exposure to books and courses on statistical concepts of "experimental design," the statistician has begun to feel relatively confident about his skill in planning research, and, for several decades, statisticians have urged that they be consulted "before you begin the project, not afterward." In receiving the constantly increasing flow of investigators who come as "patients," the statistical consultant has willingly accepted the authority, prestige, and other rewards that go along with his role as the researcher's doctor.

As every practicing medical doctor knows, of course, a patient's consultant cannot accept authority without also accepting responsibility. A physician who takes on the problems brought to him by a patient also becomes responsible for what he does in their management. He must be fully attentive to the subtleties as well as the grossly overt aspects of the problems; he must not perform procedures for which he is untrained or unqualified; he must guard against breaches of accepted ethical standards; and he must be ready, when necessary, to defend his actions if they are questioned by a jury of his peers or in a court of law.

In accepting authority as a consultant in clinical research, how well has the statistician accepted the responsibility? What sort of "licensure" or "boards" are used to test his qualifications, and what kind of "pathologist" or "review panel" serves to detect his failings? When he performs experiments by applying untested theories or unproved models to a research project, does he obtain informed consent from the investigator who is his "patient"?

---

*The hegemony of statistical doctrines has not been confined to biomedical publications. In the literature of social science, the traditional deference to a statistician's *imprimatur* has recently been subjected to the "radical" proposal that primary attention be given to the concepts and methods of the research, rather than to the data and the statistical analysis.[38]

By what kind of Pythagorean or other oath does he pledge the quality and ethics of his practice? How often does he commit malpractice? How are his instances of malpractice detected, guarded against, or compensated for?

These issues have rarely been discussed in the literature of statistics and are seldom considered during a statistician's education. Sporadic papers have appeared about the errors committed during consultative activities,[29, 36] and the retiring president of a statistical society may occasionally use his farewell address to warn his colleagues about certain intellectual or practical blunders.[33, 39] In such an address two years ago, Frank Yates[39] complained that "the standard of much day-to-day statistical work is regrettably low. These matters . . . are primarily the responsibility of the university statistical departments and are a direct consequence of the present-day obsession with advanced theory, largely divorced from practice." Yates also quoted an earlier concern of Sir Ronald Fisher: "We are quite in danger of sending highly trained and highly intelligent young men out into the world . . . with a dense fog in the place where their brains ought to be."

These random censures by leaders of the profession have not brought a tradition of introspective review and constant self-criticism to statistical consultants. In the educational processes and literature of statistics, there is no counterpart of a clinicopathologic conference, in which a consultant's errors are regularly sought, identified, and revealed for public discussion. In the meetings and publications of biostatistical societies, the parochial contents may prevent statisticians who work with clinical topics from receiving regular exposure to comments or suggestions from connoisseurs of the topics. Although statisticians are constantly asked to speak at clinical meetings, to referee papers submitted to clinical journals, and even to write instructive papers for the clinical readers of those journals, the converse

phenomenon does not occur in the world of biometry. The editors of biostatistical journals do not invite clinicians either to review or to write appropriate papers, and the people who plan statistical seminars on topics in clinical research almost never solicit the attendance of expert clinicians who might contribute occasional insights and touches of reality to the proceedings.

The need for vigilant critical self-appraisal by biometricians has been accentuated in recent years because of the increased opportunity both for statistical consultants to commit malpractice and for the malpractice to have catastrophic effects. In the days when a statistician worked mainly *post hoc* to perform statistical analysis for a completed research project, his choice of the wrong analytic procedures might create an intellectual nuisance, but would not affect either the basic design or the primary data of the project. After the statistical errors were discovered, they could always be rectified later with a better set of analyses. If the statistician gives improper advice before a project begins, however, he can distort both the design and the data, so that the project may not be salvageable later. After the statistician's misdeeds in planning are recognized and corrected, the entire project would have to be repeated. The repetition is not too difficult for relatively small projects, but such projects are seldom the ones for which statisticians are asked to provide advance consultation. The type of research that is most difficult to repeat is a massive project in which many observations are performed during many years. This type of project, as exemplified by a large-scale cooperative clinical trial, is the type of research that has been increasingly delegated to the design of statistical authorities and that offers them the greatest opportunity for transgressions that cannot be remedied easily, if at all.

The complex logistics of a large-scale clinical trial create major difficulties for every aspect of the review, appraisal, and verification that research must receive to be accepted in the scientific community. For purposes of review, the primary data of a modest-sized project are readily available for inspection, but the raw data of a mammoth clinical trial may be diffused among a vast array of coded pages or transformed into a dense bulk of computerized conversions. For purposes of analysis, the numerical summaries of a relatively small project can generally be shown entirely in simple tabulations; but in a large clinical trial, even the summaries may be too abundant for complete citation. In the material selected for publication, crucial information may be omitted, dispersed among a plethora of tables, or obscured by conversion into percentages, regressions, and other statistical "adjustments." And the clinical trial can seldom be repeated. The repetition would require assembly of another group of investigators who are willing to devote many years of labor in the new effort and who are able to acquire the necessary funds for its support. Even if new investigators and funds can be obtained, however, the new data may still not settle an existing argument, because the previous workers may claim that the populations under investigation were different.

For all these reasons, the basic strategies of design and analysis in a clinical trial must be particularly circumspect and above suspicion. When disputes arise about the conclusions, statistical deficiencies in planning the basic strategies can have devastating consequences. The investigators will have worked prodigiously for results that cannot be either reliably analyzed or confidently utilized. In addition to the effort already invested in the project, large amounts of energy may be consumed in the controversies that follow as the participating investigators and statisticians, committed emotionally to their years of devoted but possibly misdirected labor, become even more fervently committed to defending their results against the inevitable criticism. The sponsoring agency, re-

luctant to recognize or admit that it has expended large sums of money for a badly flawed product, may leave its position "above the battle" and become actively embroiled as a partisan in the disputes. The patients whose future therapy should have been enlightened by the results are left instead to the uncertainties of medical dissension about whatever treatment has emerged as extolled or condemned.

Although misdesigned clinical trials have not yet been given specific attention, some of the problems in meeting the general challenges of statistical consultation have recently begun to receive public comment among biometricians. Within the past few years, these problems have been contemplated[3-7, 23, 27, 41] in major papers, abstracts, and letters to the editors of such journals as *Biometrics, Technometrics,* and *The American Statistician.* A particularly extensive presentation and discussion of the issues recently appeared in the *Journal of the Royal Statistical Society.*[33A] My object in the remainder of this discussion is to augment this established foundation of constructive criticism.

Having worked both as a clinical investigator and biostatistical consultant for many years, I have had an unusual opportunity to observe defects in activities that occur bilaterally on the clinical biostatistical street. In several recent publications, I have described what seem to be some of the main failings of my fellow clinicians.[10-12] I would be less than fair to my statistical colleagues if I neglected to note some of the apparent imperfections on their side of the street.

To illustrate the problems, I shall contrast the way that statisticians and clinicians are prepared for and perform their activities as consultants. The clinical analogies seem appropriate for these illustrations, because clinical consultants have a tradition and heritage that is more than 2,500 years old. Statisticians may not always admire the way that clinicians recite experiential anecdotes, make unquantified judgments, and deliver personal care, but we cannot deny that clinicians have been deliberately prepared for their role as consultants, and that they have had enormous experience and frequent success. As statisticians, we might be able to profit by studying their methods.

1. Formulating a problem

In consulting a medical doctor, a patient is not expected to express his problem in a clear, articulate, well-organized manner. The patient believes that the doctor will know what questions to ask and will know how to organize the information in a manner suitable for characterizing the problems and planning their management. Consequently, one of the first things that a clinical consultant learns is an intellectual structure for getting and arranging the information used to formulate patients' problems. The structure, reflected in the contents of the history and physical examination, contains such components as the *chief complaint, present illness,* and *review of systems,* and the formulation is expressed in such terms as *diagnosis, pathogenesis, prognosis,* and *therapy.*

A statistical consultant, however, has not been specifically trained in an intellectual discipline suitable for acquiring the necessary data and formulating the logical problems of a research project. As noted earlier in this series, statistical courses in "experimental design" are inadequate both for the "experiments" and for the "design" of the work done in clinical research. Many clinical projects are conducted as surveys or methodologic explorations, not as experiments, and even for projects that are truly experiments, statistical principles do not distinguish the critical differences between interventional and explanatory experiments.[14] In "design," statistical principles do not contain details of the fundamental scientific concepts needed to plan the basic architecture of clinical research, and a specialized knowledge of statistics does not become cogent until the major parts of the architectural design have been completed.[15] An excellent statistical consultant, of course, becomes a connoisseur of the necessary scientific concepts and constantly recognizes their intellectual priority in the design of research. But he must depend on his willingness and ability to make these perceptions after he begins his consultative activities. The details and importance of the scientific principles are not usually transmitted as part of his undergraduate or postgraduate instruction.

The preparation for work as a consultant thus contains antipodal contrasts in the education of clinicians and statisticians. A clinician is taught to identify and formulate patients' problems in a carefully structured manner; but he is then left to develop diverse tactics of "judgment" for managing the outlined problems. A statistician is taught a carefully organized set of mathematical structures for managing an outlined problem; but he is left to develop diverse judgmental methods for identifying and formulating the problem. The clinician may emerge able to express the right questions but unable to find the answers; the statistician may emerge with the right answers but unable to select the questions.

The difficulty in outlining details of scientific architecture in clinical research would not be a major occupational hazard for a statistician if he could rely on his "patients" to provide the outline. Unfortunately, however, in appearing as a "patient" for the statistician, the clinician is often unable to provide a well-organized account of the "chief complaint" or other intellectual maladies of his problems in research. The clinician may have learned how to be a medical consultant for patients, but not how to be a "patient" for statistical consultants. Like the statistician, the clinician has also had no rigorous instruction in the methodology of scientific investigation. The clinician's "basic science" courses in medical school taught him an array of facts and laboratory procedures that are not readily applicable in clinical investigation[17]; his courses in statistics, if any, were not concerned with scientific architecture in research and usually dwelt mainly on theories of probability and on techniques of performing statistical tests; his clinical training exposed him to the unquantified anecdotage and logical imprecision that he often seeks to escape by getting consultative help; and nowhere did he receive any formal instructions about how to express a clear, succinct objective in his research and how to formulate a sequence of scientific procedures for attaining the objective.

The biostatistical consultation may thus become a peculiar paradox. A "patient" who has ideas about research but who may not know how to express them precisely or quantitatively comes to seek help from a statistical "doctor" who knows about precision and quantification, but who may not know how to express ideas about research.

2. Taking a history

In taking a history, any good clinician knows how to deal with a patient who is excessively garrulous, reticently uncommunicative, or flagrantly imprecise. The clinical consultant will usually interrupt garrulosity, probe reticence, and delineate imprecision. Moreover, if the patient is unable to provide a satisfactory history, the clinician knows how to improve it by enlisting the aid of family, friends, or interpreters. The clinician becomes adept at developing these interrogational skills not only because he has learned a basic intellectual architecture to indicate what information is necessary, but also because he knows that he is obligated to get the information. The standards and traditions of his consultational craft demand that he do so.

As a statistical "patient," however, the clinician may, for the reasons cited previously, give a poor history. Aside from knowing that he ought to have *controls* and that *randomization* and *double-blind* are good things, the clinician "patient" may be garrulous, reticent, or imprecise in trying to describe the "ailment" of his re-

search. He may talk interminably about the work he has done for the past 10 years and may discuss a variety of conjectures about the mechanism of the phenomenon he is studying, without ever stating the objective of the current project. He may become reticent about expressing a specific objective when he arrives with a pile of data and wants to know "If I've got anything significant here," or when he says "I'm interested in studying phenomenon X," without indicating what aspect of X is to be assessed for what purpose. He may become imprecise and refer only to a nebulous "judgment" and "experience" when he is asked to provide statements of criteria, evidence of validation, or tests of reproducibility for the phenomena under investigation.

A clinical consultant who was confronted with such a poor history-giver would know what to do about the situation. The clinician's knowledge of the necessary medical outline would help him determine what information to get, and his traditional obligation to get the information would evoke the necessary effort to do so. The statistician, however, may have neither the knowledge nor the obligation appropriate for his task. Having no specific scientific outline as a guide that might ease the history-taking and having no professional traditions that create a responsibility for extracting the crucial information, the statistical consultant may meet the challenge with several varieties of evasion.

One type of evasion is used for an investigator who comes with a collection of assembled data but who has difficulty describing what the research was about and what the data are supposed to show. The statistician gets rid of the "patient" by saying, "Let me have your data." In isolated comfort, the statistician can then process the data with a series of analytic statistical tests. A somewhat different evasion is used for an investigator who comes with an imprecise proposal for a clinical research project. After a few questions about confounding variables and hard endpoints, the consultant says, "Let me have your protocol," which can then be contemplated and manipulated in the privacy of the statistician's theories about "experimental design."

In both types of evasion, the statistician deprives himself of an adequate history and scientific formulation of the problems. Working in a Procrustean manner, he may take his knowledge of statistical tactics and adapt the research problems to fit those tactics, instead of choosing or adapting his tactics to fit the problems.

3. The management of therapy

With advances in technology, clinicians may sometimes order myriads of laboratory tests rather than take a history or think. The availability of digital computers has had similar effects on statistical consultants. In the "ancient" days when all the statistical computations had to be done with a desk calculator, a statistician had the incentive to be selective in choosing analytic tests, if for no other reason than to spare himself the labor of the calculations. If data were available for 14 variables, only two of which were deemed important, the statistician would analyze those two variables. Today, with almost no effort, a statistician can get a computer to massage all 14 variables in diverse ways, to perform "factor analyses" on the lot, and to prepare a matrix of correlations for each variable with every other variable. Receiving the enormous pile of print-out, the investigator may have to spend days or weeks searching for what he wanted. He may not find it at all, but the magnitude of the computations will usually convince him that the consultant has done a "thorough" job.

A different statistical counterpart of defective clinical practice occurs when the statistician "treats" the protocol of a clinical trial without having established a careful "diagnosis" of what is wrong or what needs to be done. Clinicians may sometimes, in "shotgun" manner, dispense

antibiotics for fever or tranquilizers for anxiety, without probing deeply into the sources of the fever or the anxiety. But statistical consultants may also, in an *ex cathedra* pronouncement, prescribe fixed dosages, "pure" populations, randomization, double-blind procedures, dimensional measurements, and hard endpoints, without determining whether these standard agents of the statistician's "therapeutic armamentarium" will distort the objective of the research or invalidate the results.

The practitioner of this type of statistical shotgun therapy may be as difficult to convince of his malefactions as is the clinician who uses antibiotics and tranquilizers indiscriminately. As justification for the treatment, the clinician can usually point to the patient's subsequent improvement, and the clinician may become incensed if his judgment is later questioned for having caused possibly needless expense and risk to a patient who might have either improved without the chosen drugs or improved more rapidly with others. As justification for shotgun statistical treatment, the statistician can usually offer certain obvious improvements of a faulty protocol, and he may become incensed if his efforts in bringing well-established statistical principles to the project are decried as being so consummately statistical that the results are not meaningful in clinical science.

A shotgun statistical design of a clinical trial can create many problems that have been discussed in detail elsewhere.[11-15] The basic difficulty is that the results of the trial become useless for scientific clinical reality, because crucial clinical activities were either omitted or distorted in order to fit the demands of statistical approbation. A drug that ordinarily requires flexible dosage has not been tested properly if given in fixed dosage. If patients with comorbid diseases are excluded from a trial in order to test a "pure" population with the "main" disease, the results may be free of confounding variables but also free of any realistic significance for the "impurities" constantly encountered in patients. The results of a trial cannot be related to clinical practice if prognostically heterogeneous patients are combined, randomized, and analyzed as a single group without previous or subsequent division into homogeneous prognostic strata. The investigator's time is wasted when double-blind procedures are used unnecessarily, and everyone's time is wasted when double-blind tactics are needed but omitted in circumstances in which their application might have been difficult, requiring a second set of participating observers. The objective of the research becomes distorted when the quest for dimensional measurements creates the "substitution game,"[40] in which the index variables are transferred from the qualitative facts that the clinician really needed to know into unimportant data that he can measure. The conduct of the trial becomes an "ordeal"[18] when the desired clinical targets that are abundant in "soft data" are displaced into uncommon "hard data" endpoints that may require needlessly prolonged observation of needlessly huge numbers of patients.

Aside from the practical difficulties created by shotgun designs, the continued acceptance of such procedures is detrimental to the progress of clinical science. One of the main reasons for the neglected prognostic heterogeneity, displacement of targets, and other defective tactics just cited is that the statistician wants to avoid using imprecise concepts and unreliable data. He eliminates patients with comorbid diseases because the clinician has not adequately classified the diseases or their consequences; prognostic strata are not analyzed because clinicians have not delineated the specifications of the strata; and "soft data" variables are displaced because the data are neither observed nor interpreted in a reproducible manner. Rather than accept information that has little or no scientific validity, the statistician may prefer to do what seem scientifically and statistically valid—even at

the risk of producing meaningless science.

This type of consultative advice is tantamount to giving only pills and injections to a patient who really needs vigorous physical exercise or intensive psychotherapy. A good clinical consultant will not allow pharmaceutical substitutes to replace a patient's need to work out his own problems, and a good statistical consultant should not allow clinicians to escape the scientific defects of their own intellectual inertia. If comorbid diseases and prognostic strata have not been properly classified, the statistician should insist that clinicians make suitable efforts to do so. If subjective variables and "soft" data are critically important, they should not be replaced by what is objectively measured, "hard," and irrelevant. The statistician should demand, instead, that the clinician develop the observational procedures, indexes, and criteria[16] that will "harden" the important "soft" data while preserving them for analysis. A clinician who has not yet developed the intellectual "muscles" that will enable him to "walk" scientifically will never develop this skill if he constantly avoids the necessary effort by being pushed in a statistical "wheelchair."

By absolving the clinician of the need to improve his own important data and judgmental activities, statistical consultants perpetuate the atmosphere that evoked such scientific and clinical distress about statistics more than a century ago. Said Armand Trousseau,[35] "This (statistical) method is the scourge of the intellect: it transforms the physician into a calculating machine, making him the passive slave of the figures which he has massed up. . . . You wish the pupil to see only crude facts and to stifle his intellect: and when, by means of this dismal labor, his mind has been to some extent mutilated, you will ask him to show mental vigour . . . and prolific thought." Said Claude Bernard,[2] "Against these antiscientific ideas we must protest with all our power, because they help to hold medicine back in the lowly state in which it has been held so long."

4. The arrogance of power

Because so many human illnesses are self-limited and will subside no matter what is done clinically, every medical doctor will usually have a high "success" rate in his therapeutic activities. This natural rate is augmented by the dramatic cures achieved with antibiotics, surgery, and other modern therapeutic agents, and even when the doctor's therapy fails to cure, his personal concern and compassion can provide comfort. The freqency of these successes make most patients devoted to their doctors, and the emotional overtones associated with human sickness may make many patients devoutly worshipful of the consultant whose work seemed to provide relief or remedy.

This type of deification is one of the main intellectual hazards of a clinician's occupation. A thoughtful clinician, recognizing the deifying propensity of his patients, may often use it therapeutically, but he must constantly beware that he does not begin, consciously or unconsciously, to believe in all the power, glory, and omniscience that have been attributed to him. Not all clinicians, however, are able to resist this belief, which may lead to various forms of arrogance in the way a clinician thinks about his activities, receives critical appraisal, and interacts with other people.

Although a clinician's basic personality and character are his main prophylaxis against this behavioral malady, certain professional safeguards can help protect him and the public. He must pass standard examinations to be licensed as a practitioner and additional "boards" to be certified as a specialist. An internist receives frequent diagnostic "exposure" at clinicopathologic conferences, and a surgeon's removal of tissue is constantly reviewed by special committees. The procedures for accreditation of hospitals provide a means of reviewing medical record-keeping and

for ascertaining that all deaths are checked either at necropsy or with other types of evaluation. A clinician who participates in the activities of a teaching hospital will receive frequent interrogation and intellectual provocation during his "rounds" with house staff and students. The various recent demands for suitable instruction and "disclosure" to patients have improved the ethical tactics of clinical investigators, and the spreading epidemic of legal suits for malpractice has made all practitioners more careful of their decisions and explanations. These activities alone are obviously not adequate to thwart the development of unrestrained arrogance in a clinician's exercise of the power delegated to him, but they can help. And although a clinician may be able to "bury his mistakes," he is seldom able to hide them from himself or his colleagues.

A statistical consultant, by contrast, has no such restraints in his professional activities. There are no types of licensure or accreditation procedures after he receives his academic degree; there are no *routine* reviews by outside critics of his professional performance; there are no younger minds regularly available or assigned to probe and question his consultative judgments in each of his tasks; there is no code of ethics to keep him from "experimenting" without adequate explanation to his "patients"; there is no threat of legal action to make him worry about engaging in malpractice. The statistician need not even bury his mistakes. If adequately glorified, they can be published.

Moreover, although patients have become increasingly wary of their clinical consultants and are less likely to engage in abject, mute worship, the statistician's clientele now seems more credulous, taciturn, and reverent than ever before. In 1932, Major Greenwood[20] identified the early stages of this trend:

> Even as recently as 20 years ago, medical writers would still challenge peremptorily the demand that their data should be treated

statistically at all . . . (but) the writer . . . now seeks for some technical "formula" by the application of which he can produce "significant" results. . . . The change has been from thinking badly to not thinking at all, from thinking that statisticians were triflers to believing that statisticians are patentees of more or less powerful magic.

This trend has now advanced to the current state described by Remington and Schork[31]:

> Certainly the statistician holds no special qualifications in the area of careful consideration and reflection into experimental inference, but all too frequently today the investigator abdicates his responsibility in these areas to the statistician. . . .

The clinician has many reasons for this willingness to delegate authority and responsibility to his statistical consultant. Some of the reasons are the external demands imposed by the contemporary fashions of editors and granting agencies, but many of the reasons are internal, representing the insecurities caused by the clinician's absence of training in scientific methodology and by misdirected training in statistics.

The likelihood of gullible homage to a statistical consultant is particularly high in populational research such as clinical trials. A clinical investigator who does laboratory research usually has definite ideas about experimental design and analysis, and usually asks the statistician afterwards only for technical assistance in performing the analytic tests. The clinician who does populational research, however, may have had little or no exposure to scientific principles of clinical epidemiology. His previous research experience may have been obtained in laboratory activities, in which precise objective data can be obtained with equipment constructed by an engineer, requiring no demands on the clinician's ability in clinical observation and interpretation. Knowing that controlled clinical trials are needed to remedy the defects of earlier therapeutic studies, but not knowing how to plan the details of new trials, the clinician relies on the statistician's

knowledge of "experimental design." Because laboratory investigation brought no improvement to the clinician's defective methodology, he may readily accede, for the sake of science, to the statistician's removal or denigration of "soft" clinical data and judgment. Furthermore, since the clinician has had almost no training in how to maintain or process large amounts of data, he may also be delighted to delegate the entire planning of these chores to the statistician or to the statistical-computer group.

Thus, aware of his own ignorance about scientific methodology and data processing, impressed by the statistician's credentials in "experimental design," and obsessed by the hope that the statistical procedures will offer panaceas for all ailments in research, the clinician "patient" is often deeply grateful merely to be admitted to the office of a statistical "doctor." Anything given as help thereafter is received humbly and reverently, particularly if it leads to the acceptance of a paper for publication or of a research proposal for funding. Since the clinician seldom understands what has been done statistically, he is seldom critical of it, and, when asked to be critical, his only lament may be about the statistician's occasional delays in giving help. This reluctance to appraise the quality of the help may be due to the clinician's insecurity about statistics, but he may also fear any comments that might make him seem an "ungrateful patient."

Receiving this awed idolatry from clinicians who are themselves regularly idolized, the consultant's consultant is particularly susceptible to the risk of developing the same forms of intellectual arrogance that may occur in any authority whose pronouncements are regularly accorded an unquestioned omniscience.

5. The threat of clarity

A complaint that patients sometimes lodge against clinical consultants is that intricate concepts are not explained or that simple concepts are obfuscated into oro-tund Latin phrases and professional jargon. The threat of clarity, as Hardin[22] has noted, often perpetuates a verbal mumbo-jumbo that can mask the absence of knowledge or understanding. A good clinician feels no such threat, however, and is usually prepared to explain what he knows or to say "I don't know" when he does not. One of the hallmarks of a good clinician, in fact, is the ability to express complex information, without con-descension, in terms that are clear, simple, and comprehensible to a patient. A major advantage of preceptorial training for young clinicians is the opportunity to learn this type of communicative skill by ob-serving its performance.

The training of a statistical consultant, however, does not usually include this type of preceptorial exposure, and he may not have received many challenges to his skill in explanation. As Hotelling[25] has pointed out, statisticians are not even regularly asked to be able to supply proofs for the *mathematical* validity of their tests and procedures. Added to these problems is the statistician's protracted exposure to the convoluted writing and murky prose that sometimes appear in the highest echelons of statistical literature. In view of these many handicaps to communica-tion, a statistician's "patient" should not be surprised if the consultant seems either unconcerned about providing explanations or unable to provide good ones when he tries.

This problem in communication would not be particularly important if the con-sultant could rely on his "patients" to badger him into giving satisfactory expla-nations for statistical tactics. A patient who keeps saying "I don't understand" will often inspire or goad his clinical con-sultant into new expression of old ideas, old expression of new ideas, or other intellectual shufflings that will, in pro-viding better explanation to the patient, often enlighten the clinician as well. Un-fortunately, however, in consulting a statis-tician, the clinician "patient" is usually reluctant to confess his initial ignorance or to repeat the confession after receiving an improvised but unsatisfactory explana-tion. Accustomed to playing the role of omniscient savant for his own patients, the clinician may have difficulty in reversing the role of student-and-master when he consults a statistician. Aside from this difficulty, the clinician may be too frightened of mathematics to want to think about it or too embarrassed to admit how little he has understood of even an ap-parently good explanation.

For all these reasons, clinicians seldom demand that statistical consultants pro-vide an ample clarification and justifica-tion for their procedures. The consequence, for the statistician, is an underdeveloped skill in communication and the previously discussed hazard of intellectual arrogance. The consequence, for the clinician, is the condition described by Hogben[24] in his memorable indictment that "less than 1% of research workers clearly apprehend the rationale of the statistical techniques they commonly invoke." Hogben's remark can be further extended into the waggish defi-nition of a large-scale clinical trial as an elaborate exercise in which a clinician uses statistical procedures that he does not understand to draw conclusions from data that the statistician does not understand and has distorted to fit the statistical procedures.

6. Manners and morals

Clinicians have a long tradition of pro-viding service to the sick, regardless of the morality of the patient. The "good guy" and the "bad guy" are both regarded as entitled to the clinician's best efforts in medical care. The clinician does not re-ceive professional opprobrium when he treats a villain rather than a victim, nor is the clinician's scientific judgment ex-pected to be compromised by the act.

In the belief of many academic statistical consultants, however, any commercial or-ganization is obviously a "villain," and any consultant to such an organization is both perjured and prostituted by the work. An example of this attitude is the statisticians' rejection of Sir Ronald Fisher's doubts about the role of cigarette smoking in causing the many diseases of which it has been etiologically accused. Although unaware of specific evidence to disprove Fisher's contention that hereditary or constitutional factors might lead to both smoking and lung cancer, I can think of several rational counterarguments to Fisher's claim. Nevertheless, whenever I have heard Fisher's assertion raised in biostatistical enclaves, it is immediately dismissed not on a rational basis because of any logical or scientific demerits, but because Fisher had been employed as a consultant to the British tobacco industry.

In the current double standard of consultative "morals," a profit-making organization seems to be obviously evil, whereas a governmental or other nonprofit agency is obviously "on the side of the angels," no matter how committed the agency may be to supporting its bureaucracy, increasing its budget, and glorifying its policies. As a result of this double standard, statisticians who may not hesitate to impugn the motives and activities of governmental agencies concerned with military, socioeconomic, and political problems somehow manage to retain total faith in the selfless benignity of the academic-federal complex concerned with the biomedical and biostatistical activities of "health." Thus, when an academic statistical consultant defends the way his work has produced a possible mismanagement of millions of dollars in a huge medical project paid for by a governmental agency, he is obviously a dispassionate and unbiased critic. When another consultant is asked by an interested commercial agency to perform an objective review of the project, his conclusions (unless they agree with the original statistician) are obviously suspect because he was commissioned by a commercial agency.

This double standard of "morality" be-comes particularly important whenever a statistician's work must be subjected to critical review. Clinicians accused of malpractice could formerly often rely on being judged exclusively by the "standards of the community" and on being sheltered from adverse testimony by authoritative experts. In recent years, however, the standards of judgment have been expanded to a much larger scope than the practice in the "community" alone, and expert witnesses can readily be obtained from panels of various medical societies. Even if expert witnesses are unavailable, the doctrine of *res ipsa loquitur* may sometimes suffice to prove a plaintiff's point.

Although regularly applied to the suspected blunders of a clinician, the term "malpractice" is not used in the genteel vocabulary of statistical consultation. The harshest phrase that might be applied is "controversial." When a statistician's work in clinical research is regarded as controversial, however, the process of reappraisal contains some significant differences from the public litigation to which a clinical consultant may be exposed. A clinician's possible malpractice becomes judged by "laymen" rather than by a jury of his professional peers, whereas the main reviewers for a biostatistical controversy will usually be other statisticians, because authoritative clinical biologists may be considered too "lay" to participate. The criteria for judgment may include only the "standards of the community" because the reviewers may all share a common faith in the statistical ideologies of "experimental design."

In such circumstances, the objectivity of the statistical reviewers is of paramount importance for detection and removal of the intellectual errors that retard scientific progress. Nevertheless, if the integrity of R. A. Fisher was regarded as so easily purchased by an ancillary financial stipend from a commercial source, can any contemporary statistician be trusted to give crtical evaluation to activities sponsored by governmental or other nonprofit agencies that also give the statistician consultant-fees, grants to support his work, and even perhaps his basic salary?

Fortunately, clinical practice is relatively free of the type of professional paranoia that created the double standard of "morality" in statistical consultation. As statistical practitioners improve their methods, their stature, and their fears about how easily they can be bought," the attitude will probably vanish. Disagreements about statistical activities can then be argued on the basis of their rational quality, and not on whether the statistician's integrity is so fragile that it becomes compromised by the agency that pays him.

• • •

In all of these remarks, I have deliberately avoided the citation of specific research projects or of specific statistical consultants. To choose any individual investigations or people for particular comment would be unfair to the many available candidates, and besides, the general issues are difficult enough without the added problems of engaging in an *ad hominem* or *ad opus* argument.

Since attempts to create constructive criticism are necessarily aimed at what is defective, rather than what is laudable, my adverse remarks about certain statistical practices should not be regarded as derogatory to statisticians or to statistical principles. Just as the methodology of clinicians contains many deficiencies that have been described here and elsewhere,[10-12] the methodology of statisticians is also flawed, and the flaws should not be overlooked complacently during praise of the virtues. Statistical consultants have obviously made many positive contributions to clinical research. My admiration for some of the contributions and the people has been expressed elsewhere[13] or is sufficiently well known so that I believe I need not fear that the foregoing discussion has been offensive rather than merely provocative.

The picture of populational research also contains many bright components to contrast with some of the bleakness portrayed here. The existence of many highly successful large-scale clinical trials (particularly some of the older work in England and some of the recently published efforts by groups from the Veterans Administration in the United States) offers ample demonstration of the clinical and scientific illumination that is possible when knowledgeable clinical investigators collaborate with capable statistical advisors. These happy events, however, are not commonplace, and many of the unattractive situations described earlier have been the product of work by people who are regarded not merely as good statistical consultants, but sometimes as leaders in the field.

A thoughtful statistician could easily rebut this entire discussion by pointing out that most of the cited defects should really be blamed on the clinical investigators. The problems would not occur, the statistician might rightly say, if clinicians were better scientists. The clinician ought to be willing to think harder, to plan more effectively, and to avoid transferring his own intellectual obligations to a statistical consultant. The clinician, after all, is the principal investigator in the research. He is responsible for knowing what question to pursue in the project, for establishing a proper design for the pursuit, and for preserving the propriety of the design when it receives statistical implementation. The clinician must acquiesce in any of the statistician's recommendations for design and must acquire all of the data that the statistician analyzes. If the statistician creates a bad design, it has been approved by the clinician. And if the statistician's analysis of data resembles a futile attempt to process garbage, the clinician should have made greater efforts to refine the garbage and to isolate the fruit before the data were dumped on the statistician or entered into the computer.

This argument is quite correct, but the argument itself is an unacceptable excuse. If the clinician is allowed to escape from his responsibilities, they are inherited by the statistician who allows and abets the escape. By establishing himself as a connoisseur of the design of research, and by encouraging the clinician to believe that the scientific problems of design can be eliminated or solved by suitable attention to purely statistical principles, the statistician assumes the role of the authoritative consultant. Just as a good doctor does not blame his patients when things go wrong, a good consultant should either accept the responsibilities of being a consultant, or relinquish the authority. A statistician cannot offer himself as an expert on the design of research and then expect to place the onus on the clinical investigator when the research is badly planned.

A constructive approach to this problem would be for statistical consultants to stop acting as experts on the design of clinical research. The statistician is an authority on statistical analysis, not on the contents of clinical science. A statistician who is unfamiliar with the subtleties of clinical phenomena and who has had little direct exposure to the natural realities of science engages in self-delusion if he believes that his courses in "experimental design" have adequately prepared him for planning clinical research. As Zelen[41] has poined out, "The subject (of experimental design) as taught in most schools seems so far removed from reality that a heavy dose may be too toxic with regard to future applications." If the scholastic delusions about experimental design are also accepted by the clinician "patient," the statistician will act not as a wise consultant, but as an unwitting purveyor of statistical dogmas that may be clinically improper and scientifically destructive.

Rather than assume a consultative role for which he is unqualified, the statistician might contemplate a more productive way to use his talents. Instead of applying excellent but inappropriate statistical theories to poorly expressed clinical concepts, he can use his training in precision and quantification to improve the expression of the clinical concepts. Armed with the authority and prestige of a consultant, the statis-

tician can act as a stern protagonist in rehabilitating the clinician's intellect. By inquiring, goading, prodding, demanding, or using whatever tactics seem most effective, the statistician should insist that the clinician accept and confront all of his own scientific responsibilities. The clinician must delineate the objective of the research, specify the variables, harden soft data, establish appropriate criteria, and perform all the other scientific architectural necessities mentioned earlier and elsewhere[11-15] that he has thus far avoided. A thoughtful statistician can offer considerable aid to the clinician in these tasks, but neither biostatistics nor clinical science will make real progress if the focus of the "design" in research is diverted to the luxury of statistical strategies that neglect the scientific necessities.

For example, if a statistical consultant is asked to plan a therapeutic trial for a group of animals in which no one could tell the difference between a mouse and an elephant, the first act of science would be to establish suitable methods for identifying the different animals. If the investigators have not yet developed methods for making the distinctions, the consultant's first main job is to demand the attention, thought, and effort that will create such methods. If the consultant avoids this issue by designing a controlled, randomized, double-blind study of treatment—while still allowing the animals to be admixed and undifferentiated—he may create a satisfactory statistical plan but he produces poor science.

By making the clinician develop a clear account of his own knowledge about the ingredients of data and judgment that are needed for the proper study of sick people, the statistician will enlighten himself as well as the clinician. The enlightenment will be important in the current project and will be a valuable resource that the statistician can use in future projects. On the other hand, if the statistician rejects (or accepts) the mystical intuition of soft data and "clinical judgment," but fails to insist that the data be improved and that the judgment be dissected into logical constituents, neither the clinician nor the statistician will be intellectually advanced by their collaboration.

Regardless of whether the statistician decides to make more demands of the clinician, these problems can be helped if clinicians would make more demands of the statistician. Many defects of clinical practice have been improved because patients have decreased their former enchantment with the omniscience of medical doctors. Statisticians might also be more inclined to improve their own consultative attention to reality in clinical design, to suitability in statistical procedures, and to explanation in statistical analysis, if clinicians did not approach the consultation in so passive and servile a manner. In adopting a more "aggressive" pattern of behavior, the clinician should be impelled by a paramount respect for his own clinical wisdom, but must be ready to cooperate willingly when the statistician responds by "aggressively" demanding that the elements of the wisdom be appropriately stipulated.

Another positive step would be for statisticians to devote greater attention to the defects in their own education and conceptual ideology. There is no need for statistical practitioners to establish all of the licensure and other review procedures by which society guards itself against clinical malpractice, but a searching, and perhaps agonizing, reappraisal should certainly be given to the intellectual debility of the current curriculum for preparing a biostatistical consultant. The curriculum contains little or no exposure to biologic research or to the direct problems of clinical investigation, as witnessed at the sites where the work is performed. There is little or no opportunity for a "trainee" to observe a good consultant in action or to receive constructive criticism for an exercise in consultation. There is no encouragement to become familiar with the literature and other communicative media in the biomedi-

cal fields in which the future consultant will work. There is a plethora of courses in abstract theories that are not derived from, or cogent for, clinical realities, and there is a paucity of critical evaluation for the basic validity of many of the unproved ideologies that are promulgated as statistical methods.

As Ipsen[28] has pointed out:

> There are still too many medical questions that demand revision of statistical methodology for their solution. Statistics cannot be sold as a ready-made package to medicine. The optimal arrangement is to create an environment in which medical men and statisticians grow up together.

This environment cannot be found in the rarefied atmosphere of the statistician's office or in the clinically sterile publications of contemporary biometric literature. It can be found, however, in the clinical regions where the realities of research appear for creative, collaborative exploration by clinicians and statisticians. If, as Dyar and Gaffey[8] have said, "The major challenge to the statistician is to broaden himself," the broadening will require that he emerge from an isolated pursuit of statistical theories and that he stop regarding his consultative work mainly as an opportunity to disseminate statistical faith among the heathen.

To expand his own scientific horizon, the statistician will have to begin by acknowledging its limitations. For more than four decades, statisticians have believed that they became biostatisticians by inserting biologic data into standard statistical formulas. Since many of these formulas are based on assumptions incompatible with the phenomena of clinical biology, this belief is no more correct than the idea that a football player—wearing a helmet, shoulder pads, face mask, and cleats, and carrying a series of diagrams about use of the T-formation—becomes a tennis player by appearing on a tennis court. The strategy and tactics of a valid biostatistics must emerge from the scientific study of biology. The attempt merely to graft statistics onto clinical science, without appropriate attention to suitable integration with the realities of clinical science, should encounter the same rejection given to any other improperly planned transplantation.

Finally, instead of worrying so much about how to teach statistics to clinicians, statisticians might worry more about how to learn, understand, and incorporate the scientific clinical subtleties needed to make biostatistics meaningful and worthwhile. The biostatistician achieved his current medical status because clinical research is too important to be left to clinicians alone. To maintain and augment the vital clinical value of statistics, its practitioners should recall that biostatistics is also too important to be left to statisticians alone. An old maxim for clinical consultants has been, "physician, heal thyself." Biostatistical consultants might well heed the same advice.

References

1. Bernard, C.: An introduction to the study of experimental medicine, *translated by* Greene, H. C., published in paperback, New York, 1961, Collier Books. (The phrases cited here are on pp. 63, 165, and 222 of the paperback edition.) (Originally published in 1865.)
2. Bernard, C.: Ibid., p. 167.
3. Boardman, T. J.: Letter to the Editor, Biometrics 25:434, 1969.
4. Cameron, J. M.: The statistical consultant in a scientific laboratory, Biometrics 24:1027-1028, 1968. (Abst.) (Complete report, Technometrics 11:247-254, 1969.)
5. Cox, C. P.: Some observations on the teaching of statistical consulting, Biometrics 24:789-801, 1968.
6. Daniel, C.: Some general remarks on consulting in statistics, Biometrics 24:1029, 1968. (Abst.) (Complete report, Technometrics 11:241-245, 1969.)
7. Deming, W. E.: Some remarks on professional statistical practice, Biometrics 22:946-947, 1966. (Abst.)
8. Dyar, R., and Gaffey, W. R.: Current challenges to health statisticians, Amer. Statist. 23:(Dec.) 19-22, 1969.
9. Editorial: Significance of significant, New Eng. J. Med. 278:1232-1233, 1968.
10. Feinstein, A. R.: Scientific methodology in clinical medicine, Ann. Intern. Med. 61:564-579, 757-781, 944-965, 1162-1193, 1964.
11. Feinstein, A. R.: Clinical judgment, Baltimore, 1967, The Williams & Wilkins Company.
12. Feinstein, A. R.: Clinical epidemiology, Ann. Intern. Med. 69:807-820, 1037-1061, 1287-1312, 1968.
13. Feinstein, A. R.: Clinical biostatistics. I. A new name—and some other changes of the guard, CLIN. PHARMACOL. THER. 11:135-148, 1970.
14. Feinstein, A. R.: Clinical biostatistics. II. Statistics versus science in the design of experiments, CLIN. PHARMACOL. THER. 11:282-292, 1970.
15. Feinstein, A. R.: Clinical biostatistics. III, IV, and V. The architecture of clinical research, CLIN. PHARMACOL. THER. 11:432-441, 595-610, 755-771, 1970.
16. Feinstein, A. R.: Taxonorics. I. Formulation of criteria, Arch. Intern. Med., In press.
17. Feinstein, A. R.: What kind of basic science for clinical medicine? New Eng. J. Med., In press.
18. Fredrickson, D. S.: The field trial: Some thoughts on the indispensable ordeal, Bull. N. Y. Acad. Med. 44:985-993, 1968.
19. Gaines, W. J., and Langford, H. G.: Research on the effect of bloodletting in several inflammatory maladies, Arch. Intern. Med. 106:571-579, 1960. (Translation of a paper by P. Ch. A. Louis in Arch. Gen. Med. 321-336, 1835.)
20. Greenwood, M.: What is wrong with the medical curriculum? Lancet 1:1269-1270, 1932.
21. Greenwood, M.: Louis and the numerical method, *in* The medical dictator and other biographical studies, London, 1936, Williams and Norgate, Ltd., pp. 123-142.
22. Hardin, G.: The threat of clarity, Amer. J. Psychiat. 114:392-396, 1957.
23. Harshbarger, B.: Teaching of statistical consulting, Biometrics 24:455, 1968. (Abst.)
24. Hogben, L.: Chance and choice by cardpack and chessboard, An introduction to probability in practice by visual aids, New York, 1950, vol. I, Chanticleer Press, p. 5.
25. Hotelling, H.: The teaching of statistics, *in* Olkin I., editor: Contributions to probability and statistics (Essays in honor of Harold Hotelling), Stanford, Calif., 1960, Stanford University Press, chap. 3.
26. Huff, D.: How to lie with statistics, New York, 1954, W. W. Norton.
27. Hyams, L.: Letter to Editor, Biometrics 25:431-434, 1969.
28. Ipsen, J.: Statistical hurdles in the medical career, Amer. Statist. 19:(June) 22-24, 1965.
29. Kimball, A. W.: Errors of third kind in

statistical consulting, J. Amer. Statistic. Ass. **52**:133-142, 1957.

30. Melton, A. W.: Editorial, J. Exp. Psychol. **64**: 553-557, 1962.

31. Remington, R. D., and Schork, M. A.: Statistics with application to the biological and health sciences, Englewood Cliffs, N. J., 1970, Prentice-Hall, Inc.

32. Shimkin, M. B.: The numerical method in therapeutic medicine, Trans. Stud. Coll. Phys. Phila. **31**:204-215, 1964.

33. Skellam, J. G.: Models, inference, and strategy, Biometrics **25**:457-475, 1969.

33A. Sprent, P.: Some problems of statistical consultancy, J. Roy. Stat. Soc. (Series A) **133**: (Part 2) 139-164, 1970.

34. Trousseau, A.: Lectures on clinical medicine, *translated by* Cormack, J. R., London, 1869, The New Sydenham Society. (The phrases cited here are on pp. 34, 35, 37.)

35. Trousseau, A.: Ibid., pp. 34, 39, 40.

36. Tukey, J. W.: The technical tools of statistics, Amer. Statist. **19**:(Apr.)23-28, 1965.

37. Wallis, W. A., and Roberts, H. V.: The nature of statistics, New York, 1965, The Free Press. (Paperback edition.)

38. Walster, G. W., and Cleary, T. A.: A proposal for a new editorial policy in the social sciences, Amer. Statist. **24**:(Apr.) 16-19, 1970.

39. Yates, F.: Theory and practice in statistics, J. Roy. Stat. Soc. (Series A), **131**:(Part 4) 463-477, 1968.

40. Yerushalmy, J., and Palmer, C. E.: On the methodology of investigations of etiologic factors in chronic diseases, J. Chron. Dis. **10**: 27-40, 1959.

41. Zelen, M.: The education of biometricians, Amer. Statist. **23**:(Oct.) 14-15, 1969.

CHAPTER 11

Random sampling and medical reality

In modern clinical and epidemiological science, the ideas of *random* and *randomization* have begun to achieve a venerated status. They are regarded as fundamental essentials of the craft—a *sine qua non* somewhat like clean hands in the operating room or calibrated instruments in the laboratory.

The concept of a random sample is basic to almost all the tests of "statistical significance" that are constantly used for research data; and a randomized allocation of treatment is demanded as a scientific necessity of any properly designed therapeutic trial. Randomization, however, has also become a shield behind which any fallacies in the design of research can be sheltered or defended. For example, in responding to a citation of scientific defects in the methods used to identify the patients studied in a controversial clinical trial, a prominent statistician[1] recently wrote that "If one questions. . . . this matter of baseline differences, one must question the entire concept of the randomized therapeutic trial." Whenever any principle of research has become both sacrosanct and

tutelary, the time for reappraisal has surely arrived.

My purpose in this paper and in the next two installments of this series is to attempt such a reappraisal. I shall describe three distinctly different processes involving the ideas of *random* or *randomization*. Much of the current confusion about these ideas arises from a lack of attention to the three different processes, and from the subsequent failure to appreciate the problems created when the *random* concept that is suitable for one type of situation is inappropriately applied to another. The first of these processes deals with sampling to choose a small group from a large one. The second deals with testing the role of chance in certain numerical relationships. The third deals with allocating the maneuvers whose effects are studied in a research project. Although randomization can be applied in all three of these processes, the applications and the interpretation of results involve distinctly different types of reasoning. The rest of the discussion in this paper will be concerned with randomization in sampling. The problems of testing and allocating will be considered subsequently.

A. Basic principles in sampling

The purpose of random sampling is to choose a representative group of people

---

This chapter originally appeared as "Clinical biostatistics—XXII. The role of randomization in sampling, testing, allocation, and credulous idolatry (Part 1)." In *Clin. Pharmacol. Ther.* 14:601, 1973.

(or objects) from a delineated larger population. The preceding sentence contains three key ideas—*representative, delineated,* and *larger*—that need further discussion before we reach the idea of randomness itself.

The reason for observing a sample rather than the larger parent population is convenience. Although in many research projects we might like to observe the entire population, as is done during a national census, the act of getting the necessary observations for a large population may be so costly or so difficult that it would render the research impossible. Therefore, to allow research to take place, we regularly perform surveys to examine a smaller partial sample, rather than the entire population.

The reason for making the sample representative of the original population is extrapolation* (or generalization). In doing research we often want our conclusions to apply not to the sample alone, but to the original population from which the sample is drawn. The sampling process would usually be undesirable or futile if what we found pertained only to the particular group of people who constituted the sample. We must therefore find a way of getting a sample that truly represents the population from which it came.

In order to draw such a sample, the population itself must first be delineated. All members of the population must be listed in a way that allows each member to be eligible for selection in the sample. If any of the members have been omitted, we might later be able to "adjust" the results appropriately, but to make the adjustment we would have to know how many people were left out (and sometimes the reason why). If we could enumerate the omissions, however, we could add them to the included members and thus prepare a list of the entire population.

This full delineation of the population is the first requirement for sampling. Regardless of the particular method used for choosing the sample, we cannot be sure that the sample is representative unless the entire parent population has been listed or made available for selection. The delineation of the people to be sampled has a fundamental scientific purpose, however, beyond its statistical role as a list of subjects. In addition to their existence as potential "units" in the sample, the people have many individual personal characteristics. Some of these pre-sampling characteristics must be used to design the technique of sampling and to appraise the results.

1. The two types of observed variables. The ultimate purpose of sampling is to find out about certain target phenomena, such as blood pressure or political opinions, and to associate these phenomena with underlying characteristics of the observed people in such features as age, race, or place of residence. A diverse nomenclature has been created for these two different types of observed variables. In mathematical terms, the underlying variables are often called *independent,* and the target variables whose data are the main goals of the research are called *dependent.* The corresponding terms sometimes used in statistics are *sampling variable* and *criterion variable.*

These four terms are satisfactory for their corresponding roles in mathematical models, but not for their roles in describing the data of a sample. Variables cited mathematically as *dependent* may not depend biologically on those that are called *independent.* Furthermore, any variable observed in a sample can be regarded as a *sampling variable,* and the word *criterion,* amid its diverse meanings, does not connote the idea of a target or goal.

If the sampled population is followed forward in time as a cohort, we could talk about *initial-state* (or *baseline*) *variables*

---

*The word *extrapolation* has two meanings. In ordinary English, it means to "project by inference into an unexplored situation from observations in an explored field".[18] In the semantic jargon of Mathematics, it means "to calculate the value of a function lying beyond an interval from values within the interval".[18] I shall use *extrapolation* here in its first meaning, which is the one customarily employed in scientific literature. Mathematicians may prefer the alternative word, *generalization.*

and *subsequent-state* (or *response*) *variables,* but these terms cannot be used for the many samples that are obtained in cross-sectional surveys, where the two types of variables are noted concomitantly. Perhaps the best way of describing what is observed in a sample is provided by the words *underlying variable* and *target variable*—the two terms I shall use here. In the examples cited earlier, age, sex, or place of residence might be underlying variables, and blood pressure or political opinions would be target variables. If we wanted to know whether age and sex had any effects on place of residence, it would become a target rather than an underlying variable.

In sampling from human populations, the choice and distribution of underlying variables have paramount scientific importance because of a fundamental difference in the philosophic orientation of science and statistics. Scientific thinking is usually deterministic. The object is to be able to state that a certain effect always follows a certain cause. Statistical thinking is usually stochastic. The response is regarded as a "random variable" that occurs in some probabilistic relation to an associated independent variable. If a dropped apple strikes ground on 999 of 1000 falls, a statistician may be stochastically content to conclude that the event is not likely to arise by chance, but a scientist believes that all the apples should reach ground and will want to determine why that 1 apple in 1000 failed to do so.

Because of this difference in philosophic orientation, a statistician will accept the diverse numerical results found in a target variable, will call this diversity *variance,* and will deal with it stochastically. A scientific investigator, however, wants his results to be as deterministic as possible. He wants to reduce variance, not merely to measure it, and his method of reduction is by taxonomic classification.[6] He will use the underlying variables to classify the population into groups within which the variance is minimized.

For example, in a sample of 100 young adults, a history of menstrual periods might be found to occur in 40%, with a standard deviation of 49%.[*] A statistician might conclude that this sample is quite heterogeneous because of its high variance, but the populational rate would still be estimated as 40%. This estimation might be statistically correct, but it is scientifically unacceptable. After scanning the data for important underlying variables, the scientist might divide the sample into men and women. The high variance in the results would then disappear into none, if the sample were found to contain 40 women with a menstrual-history rate of 100%, and 60 men with a corresponding rate of 0%.

2. The two main applications of sampling. The data obtained in a sample are usually used for either *parametric estimation* or *analytic contrast.* In the estimation procedure, we simply want to know about the magnitude of the target variable. From what was found in the sample, we infer the true value or "parameter" in the parent population. If the target variable is an attribute—such as a history of menstrual periods, a political opinion, or death due to lung cancer—we want to learn its proportionate occurrence as a percentage in the sample. If the target variable is a dimension, such as height or serum cholesterol, we want to know its mean and standard deviation (although other expressions can be used). This type of estimation sampling is frequently used in social and political science. The product preferences of consumers are constantly estimated in marketing research, and voters' political preferences are regularly estimated for purposes of government or politics.

In most situations of clinical and epidemiologic research, the sample is used for analytic contrast, rather than for estimation. The goal is not to estimate the magnitude of the target variable in the parent population, but to contrast the results found in two different groups, which are defined according to some underlying characteristic. The implication of an analytic contrast is

---

[*]For a percentage, p, found in a random sample of size n, the standard deviation is $\sqrt{np\,(1\text{-}p)/(n\text{-}1)}$. Thus, $49 = \sqrt{100 \times 40 \times 60/99}$. We shall discuss shortly what is meant by a *random* sample.

that the difference in results is "caused" by the underlying characteristic. Thus, we might contrast the values for pulmonary function tests found in a group of smokers with the values found in a group of non-smokers. The collection of people investigated in this contrast might be obtained with a single sampling procedure, but once they are obtained, they are immediately divided into two groups according to the underlying variable, *smoking habit*. The pulmonary test results (as target variable) are then compared to see if a significant difference exists in those two groups.

Thus, in the samples obtained for estimation, the main questions to be answered about the target variable are *how many* or *how much*. In the samples obtained for contrast, the main questions to be answered are *how big is the difference* and *is the difference caused by the underlying variables*.

The mathematical interpretations used for estimating a parameter from a sample are seldom valid when the sample is used for analytic contrast, because the underlying variable is no longer a "passive" term of description. The particular characteristic noted in that variable has become an imposed maneuver in a type of cohort study. When we contrast the results of pulmonary function tests in smokers and non-smokers, we do not want to estimate a parameter. Our true scientific model is based on the idea that a population of healthy people, exposed and non-exposed to the maneuver of smoking, underwent certain responses in pulmonary function. We thus study the effects that follow the allocation of a principal maneuver (smoking) and its comparative maneuver (non-smoking) to two groups of people in a cohort. In this circumstance, we must consider not just whether the cohort was chosen in a representative manner, but also whether the compared maneuvers were representatively allocated to the two groups within the cohort.

Consequently, when a sample is considered for purposes of analytic contrast, rather than for parametric estimation alone,

there are two questions of representativeness, not one. The first question deals with choosing the people in the sample; the second deals with allocating the contrasted maneuvers to those people. The problems of allocating an investigated maneuver are substantially different from those of sampling a population, and will be reserved for subsequent discussion. The rest of this essay is concerned only with the type of sampling used for purposes of estimation.

B. Strategies in sampling

1. The method of selection. We now have a delineated population of N people, a selected list of underlying variables, and a target variable whose magnitude in that population is to be estimated from the results found in a sample. Let us assume for the moment that the sample is to contain n people. We now can talk about the sampling fraction, n/N. Thus, if we elect to sample 50 people from a parent population of 5000 people, we would choose a fraction of 1/100 or 1% of the population. In general, this fraction is expressed as a *1/k sample*, where k = N/n. We can now proceed to contemplate a method of choosing the sampled people in a manner that ensures their representativeness.

a. Systematic sampling. One simple and obvious method, so old that it was cited in the Bible,[2] is to engage in what is called *systematic* sampling. After each delineated person is assigned a consecutive serial number, we get our 1/k sample by starting with one of the numbers on the list and choosing every kth person thereafter. This systematic procedure—which is also called *fixed interval* sampling—would ordinarily work quite well, but it contains the hazard of distortion due to cyclic periodicity. This hazard would occur if the original list of the parent population were prepared in a ranking or some other arrangement that made every kth person different from the others. For example, in a list of military personnel arranged by platoons or companies, every 100th person on the list might be an officer. If we happened to start with an officer in a 1/100 sampling and if we collected every hundredth person on the list thereafter, the sample might exclude any enlisted men. Conversely, if we happened to start with an enlisted man, the sample might exclude officers.

b. 'Chunk' sampling. Probably the most common source of samples in clinical or epidemiologic research is a procedure in which the people are chosen as a "chunk" or "handy" group that is easily obtained or readily available.[3] Thus, instead of collecting 50 dispersed people as a 1/k sample from the delineated larger population, an investigator may pick a clump of 50 consecutive names somewhere on the list, or the first 50 people who are found in some particular geographic location, or 50 people whose last names begin with the letter M. Some investigators mistakenly use the term "at random" for these approaches, because the choice of the clump, the locale, or the alphabetical letter was done according to some "random" whim. Such a sampling, however, is at best haphazard (rather than truly random) and, at worst, the sample may be a severe distortion of the parent population it is supposed to represent. To continue our military illustration, the clump of 50 names may contain people who are all high-ranking officers; the geographic location of the sampling may be a sergeant's club; and the 50 people with surnames beginning with M may all belong to a single ethnic group.

c. The concept of randomness. We therefore want a method that can eliminate the hazards of fixed intervals, chunk selections, or any other form of choice that can be affected by human decisions. Such a method would depend on chance alone. When a selection is based only on chance, such as the fate of a ball spun in a perfect roulette wheel, the process is called *random.* The idea of using such a process to allocate treatment in experimental research was devised by R. A. Fisher,[11] but he was also (according to Kempthorne[12]) responsible for introducing randomization

as "the crucial element distinguishing modern sampling from that done early in this century."

In the term *random sample,* the word *random* really describes the process of selection rather than the sample. A random sample is chosen in a way that allows every member of the population to have an equal chance of being selected. Since chance alone is the only factor that affects a particular person's inclusion or exclusion, a random sample is also called a *probability sample,* and its properties can then be studied with statistical concepts derived from mathematical theories of probability.

There are several ways of achieving this type of randomness. One way is to write the serial number of each member of the delineated population on an otherwise identical card, to shuffle the cards well, and then to select the appropriate number of cards by dealing from the top of the "cut" deck or by blind entry into diverse portions of the deck. This has been the technique used for centuries in card games and in lotteries. The important constraint here is that the cards be well shuffled— a requirement that is not always fulfilled by human card shufflers or in lottery procedures.[*] Such alternative procedures as tossing a coin or dice can avoid the problems of shuffling and mixing, but the tosses can provide useful randomized choices only when 1/k is 1/2 or 1/6, respectively. Ordinary coins and dice would not be satisfactory if k is neither 2 nor 6 for our 1/k sample. A similar type of restriction would pertain if we used a roulette wheel.

A method that provides a probability sample while avoiding both of the difficulties just cited is the use of a table of random digits. The digits in such tables have been selected by techniques that seem consistent with chance alone, and the published tables have been checked

---

[*]A celebrated example of non-random sampling due to failure of suitable mixing for the "capsules" in a lottery occurred with the allocation of ranks to birth-dates in the U. S. "draft" procedures[10] of 1970. The error was not unique. It had also occurred in the U. S. draft lottery of 1940.

for their "random" reliability. An even more modern method of obtaining random digits is to have them generated by an appropriately tested computer program.[15]

The details of using random digits in sampling procedures are beyond the scope of this discussion, but one example can be cited for illustration. Suppose we wanted to achieve a 1/10 sampling. After entering a table of random numbers at some "randomly" selected page and location, we would assign each of the digits (0, 1, 2, . . . , 9), as they appear in successive order, to each member of our listed parent population. We would then, in some other "random" fashion, choose one of these digits, such as 4. The 1 in 10 sample would then consist of each populational member who received a 4 from the random number tables.

The main point to be noted is that a random selection must deprive the investigator of any element of choice, and must be achieved by a defined mechanical process: tossing coins or dice, shuffling cards, spinning wheels, or using random numbers obtained from an appropriate table or computer generator. For faithful reporting of research details, a scientific investigator who claims to be using a "random" technique in either sampling or allocating should always cite the particular mechanical process that was employed. Without such citations, a skeptical reader may wonder whether an allegedly "random" technique was truly random.

2. Tolerance, confidence, and sample size. If the sample has been drawn randomly, we can decide how large it should be by using a statistical application of probability theory. Although the principles of random sampling are usually cited in every textbook of statistics, the actual computation of sample size is seldom specified, and the subtle assumptions of the logic are seldom adequately emphasized.

In order to choose a sample size statistically, the investigator must make two judgmental specifications: a tolerance range and a confidence level. The tolerance range refers to the amount of error the investigator is willing to accept in the result. If the true populational parameter is 85 units, would the investigator be content with a value as low as 75 or as high as 95 in the sample, or does he want a much closer result, in the range of 84-86? This range of tolerance will depend on the purposes of the sampling. Thus, if we have no idea of whether the parameter is 8.5, 85, 850, or 8500 units, a sample value in the range of 75-95 might be a quite satisfactory approximation of where the true value lies. On the other hand, if the measurement deals with fine precision in machine tools, the range of 84-86 might be too wide, and the investigator might narrow the acceptable tolerance to a range of 84.8-85.2.

Having chosen the acceptable amount of error as a scientific judgment, the investigator now must make a different type of judgment based on statistical probability. What odds does he want as insurance against the chance that the acceptable tolerance will be violated by a misfortune in the luck of the draw, when random probability operates during the sampling? For most investigators, odds of 3 to 1 are much too risky and odds of 1,000,000 to 1 are much too cautious. The usual statistical decision is to take odds of either 19 to 1 or 99 to 1. These odds are called the *confidence level*.

At odds of 19 to 1, the chance we take is that the untoward event will occur once in twenty times, which can be expressed as a probability (or P value) of .05. Hence our "confidence" is that on 95% of occasions, the event will not occur. At odds of 99 to 1, P would be .01 and the confidence level would be 99%. The particular range of values about which we have this chosen level of confidence is called a *confidence interval,* and it is prefixed by the selected confidence level. Thus, for a statement that the "95% confidence interval" for the mean of a particular random sample is 84-86, the odds are 19 to 1 that the true mean lies in that interval.

(One of the major controversies that have still not been resolved in the basic foundations of statistics is the argument about the distinction between the *fiducial limits,* espoused by R. A. Fisher, and the *confidence interval,* espoused by J. Neyman. The point at contention in the dispute is esoteric, and for most practical purposes, the two procedures are similar.[13] In current fashions of statistical nomenclature, *confidence* has won the day, although the word *fiducial* would be scientifically preferable because its connotation of "faith" or "trust" is probably less misleading than the "assurance" implied by *confidence.*)

The range of values for a *confidence interval* is calculated from a sample as follows. If the sample contains n members, with a mean, $\bar{x}$, and a standard deviation, s, the confidence interval is the range spanned in the values from $\bar{x} - (ts/\sqrt{n})$ to $\bar{x} + (ts/\sqrt{n})$. The value for t is chosen from special tables based on the size of the sample and the magnitude of the confidence level. (It is the same t used in the well known t-test.) For the interpretation of a confidence interval, the word "confidence" is not used in its standard scientific sense. It does not refer to the accuracy of the result found in the individual sample or to the amount of confidence that can be given to the accuracy. It refers only to what would be expected to happen if the sampling were repeated over and over.

Thus, if we were to repeat the random sampling process an infinite number of times (placing the sampled people back into the parent population after each sample was drawn), *and* if we calculated a 95% confidence interval from each of those samples, *and* if we kept track of all of those intervals, *and* if we were somehow able to learn the true mean of the parent population, we would find that the true population mean was included in 95% of the intervals. This is the most rigorous mathematical explanation of a confidence interval. A somewhat simpler explanation is as follows: Suppose we calculated a 95% confidence interval from a single random sample, and then began drawing our infinite series of samples, calculating the mean for each of those samples. We would

find that 95% of those means fall within the boundaries of the original confidence interval. A third explanation, which is probably the simplest of all, is to say there is a 95% chance (odds of 19 to 1) that the true parametric mean will be found in the confidence interval calculated from the sample mean.

During these explanations, anyone who has done scientific research will have recognized that the concept of a confidence interval is based on an idea that is totally unrealistic. No investigator plans to repeat his sampling process an infinite number of times, and very few investigators plan to repeat it at all. The investigator is going to draw one sample. The results in that sample are what he will think about and use for drawing conclusions in his research. The "confidence" he wants to feel is in reference to the reliability of the sample whose data are before him. The "confidence interval," however, tells him nothing about the reliability of that particular sample; it tells him only what might happen if he drew many other samples. Its "confidence" is based on the results of indefinitely repeated sampling. It does not tell what happened in the single sample chosen for the survey. It does not indicate whether the sample mean is right or wrong; whether it is close to the true mean or far away.

At "95% confidence," the investigator knows that the chances are as high as 1 in 20 that the sample mean has exceeded the tolerable limit of error—but he does not know whether that calamity has occurred on this particular occasion. He knows that such calamities can occur on 4%, 1%, 0.5%, or 0.1% of the occasions on which samples are drawn, but he does not know whether it has happened now. He may be 95% confident that his sample results are "correct," but the confidence interval does not tell him whether, in this one instance, an unkind fate provided him with a sample drawn from the other 5% of instances in which the results are wrong.

This is the type of "sampling error" that we accept as a hazard of the random sampling process. With a 95% confidence interval, there is a 95% chance that fate will smile and give us acceptable results; there is also a 5% chance that fate will frown and ruin our work. Recognizing this hazard of the confidence limits for the tolerable error, we can now proceed to calculate a size for the sample.

One of the best simple discussions of the computation for sample size is provided by Snedecor and Cochran,[17] who offer the formula $n = t^2 s^2 / L^2$. In this formula, n is the sample size and s is the standard deviation found in the sample. L is the tolerance—the magnitude by which the sample mean is permitted to differ from the parametric mean in the parent population. The value of t^2 will vary according to the confidence level. Snedecor and Cochran[17] suggest that t^2 be simplified as 4 for a 95% confidence level and as 6.6 for a 99% level. If the data are expressed in proportions rather than means and standard deviations, the formula is $n = t^2 pq / L^2$, were p is the proportion of the target attribute, and $q = 1\text{-}p$.

Notice that these formulas for determining sample size require some strange activities. In order to use the formula, the investigator must have at least two pieces of information that cannot be known until the sample has been obtained and examined. One of these values is the sample size itself, which is needed for using the tables that provide the magnitude of 4, 6.6, or some other appropriate value for the t^2 associated with the chosen confidence level. The other required value is the standard deviation (s) or the proportion (p) that is to be found in the sample. Thus, in order to calculate the sample size, the formula requires us to know, in advance, the size and variance of the sample.

The way out of this dilemma is to guess. The guess for the value of t^2 is relatively easy. At a 95% confidence level, t^2 shows essentially little change as sample sizes increase upward from 20 (where $t^2 = 4.35$) to infinity (where $t^2 = 3.84$). The value of 4 is thus a good intermediate choice.

At a 99% confidence level, 6.6 is a conservative choice for sample sizes ranging from 20 (where $t^2 = 8.10$) to infinity (where $t^2 = 6.63$). As for guessing the variance that may be found in the sample, the investigator has no option but to rely on previous experience or lucky clairvoyance. After these two guesses have been made, the formula can be employed to yield a precise quantitative calculation for the size of the sample. (The amount of guesswork entailed in all this precise quantification may be one of the reasons that so few statistical textbooks demonstrate the actual calculation of sample size for estimating a parameter.)

A particularly important feature of the formula for sample size is that it makes no reference to N, the size of the parent population. This elimination of N is one of the most appealing and intriguing aspects of sampling theory. Regardless of whether the parent population is large or small, the sample size is determined by the guess about standard deviation in the sample, and by the choices of both a percentage for the confidence interval and an acceptable theoretical error for the result. Thus, if we wanted, with 95% confidence level, to come within 3 units of the true mean in a sample with standard deviation of 18, we could use the formula $n = 4s^2 / L^2$ to calculate the sample size as $4 \times 18^2 / 3^2 = 4 \times 324 / 9 = 144$.

C. The virtues and defects of random sampling

The random selection of a sample thus has two obvious virtues. Scientifically, it provides assurance that no subjective choices were used in the selection procedure. Statistically, it allows the results to be analyzed and the probability of "sampling error" to be quantified with principles based on mathematical theory. (The potential "sampling error" is the value of L calculated after the true values of s or p are found in the sample.)

The main defect of the random selection process is that it does not protect against inadvertent fortuitous distortion—or "the luck of the draw." As long as chance is permitted to operate, it will operate, and will occasionally produce samples that are greatly distorted. Thus, a hand containing 10, 12, or all 13 spades in a bridge game would obviously be a highly atypical sample, yet such hands regularly occur by chance alone. It is not very likely that someone using honest dice will toss eight consecutive 7's but the annals of gambling contain many such incidents. A truly random sample drawn from most military populations should contain many more enlisted men than officers—but the reverse can occur by chance alone. There is even a chance, allowing the random process to operate a large enough number of times, that a baby pecking at an electric typewriter may compose the 21st Psalm.

For a stochastically minded statistician, an event that can occur by chance for only 1 in 20 or 1 in 100 repetitions of the sampling process may be "infrequent" enough to allow formation of major inferential conclusions. For a deterministically minded investigator, however, these odds are unsatisfactory, particularly since they provide him with no safeguard against that one occasion in 20 (or even in 100) when chance has done him wrong, and has put major distortion into the single sample he drew for his research.

After discovering the distortion, the investigator might want to discard the sample, and repeat the project to draw another sample instead. In most forms of clinical and epidemiologic research, however, the project cannot be repeated. An enormous amount of time and effort was needed to assemble the people who constitute the sample. If it is badly distorted, the investigator is stuck with it. On this one time, which is 100% for the investigator's sample survey, he receives little solace from the statistician's assurance that chance would behave so unkindly only on 5% or 1% of other occasions.

The hazard of this type of misfortune can be regarded with equanimity in theoretical statistics, where a sampling procedure can readily be repeated an infinite number of times. The hazard is not acceptable, however, to an investigator who finds the reality of a sample survey much more difficult to consummate. For the one sample that the investigator is going to draw, he does not want to take the risk of 1 in 20, 1 in 100, 1 in 1000, or even 1 in 1,000,000 that the sample will be wrecked by fortuitous fate. He will want to take whatever precautions are needed to thwart the possible mischief of randomness. Furthermore, after the sample is drawn, he will want to have a method of checking what has happened, and, if substantial distortion occurred despite all the precautions, he will want to be able to eliminate or adjust for the effects of the distortion. We thus come to the most important *scientific* issue in sampling: the quantification of bias.

D. The quantification of bias

A non-representative sample distorts the characteristics of the parent population. Statisticians refer to such distortion as *bias*—a somewhat unfortunate term, because many scientists tend to think of bias* as an act of prejudice that is usually social and often deliberate, rather than a scientific distortion that is often subconscious or inadvertent.

These distortions of population characteristics can occur in two different ways: during the process of individual observation or during the process of assembling the group of objects that is observed. Observational bias occurs when inaccurate statements are made by the human or inanimate observers that produce the primary data. If these inaccuracies tend to go in the same direction, such as a consistently too high reading for blood pressure, the observations have received an error that is called *systematic bias.* (The

---

*Another problem of *bias* is that its verb creates, like *bus,* an orthographic debate about whether the past participle should be spelled with one or two s's. My own preference is *biased.*

Gaussian theory of randomly distributed errors in measurement depends on the assumption that the observational inaccuracies are equally distributed in both directions, and tend to cancel themselves out.)

The type of bias that mainly concerns us in sampling, however, is assembly bias rather than observational bias. We shall assume that our observational techniques are accurate. The problem is to assemble a group of people who will properly represent the parent population. For example, suppose we want to estimate the average blood pressure of a population containing white and black people. To avoid observational bias, we would want our blood pressure measurement to be accurate. To avoid assembly bias, we would want the sample to contain approximately the same proportion of white and black people as occurs in the parent population. This idea of proportionality is the key to the problem of measuring assembly bias.

If the parent population contains 70% whites and 30% blacks, we might be satisfied with a sample in which these percentages respectively are 68% and 32%, or 71% and 29%, but we would not be happy if the percentages were 85% and 15%, or 54% and 46%. In the last two situations, the sample would be substantially distorted in its constituent proportions.

The problem of disproportions that can create assembly bias is seldom discussed in most textbooks of statistics, although it is well known and thoroughly considered in the literature of sampling. A sequence of different scientific judgments is involved.

1. The formation of strata. The way that assembly bias is avoided or minimized in a sample survey is to demarcate a series of groups, or strata. The members of the sample are then chosen randomly from within each of the strata. The act of stratification in a cross-sectional survey has the same crucial scientific role that it plays in a longitudinal cohort study, as described earlier in this series.[7]

There are diverse ways of demarcating strata and choosing the number of people to be sampled in each stratum. The methods, which depend on the particular circumstances in which the survey is performed, are described in textbooks[14, 16, 19] devoted to sample surveys. The main point to be noted here is that stratification has been a fundamental ingredient of good sampling techniques because it helps eliminate assembly bias, increase specificity, and improve accuracy in the results.

2. The choice of important underlying variables. To demarcate strata, the investigator must choose certain characteristics as the elements that identify each stratum. For example, in the previously cited illustration of a survey of blood pressure, the strata were demarcated according to race, as white and black. Why not sex, age, height, familial patterns of disease, color of shoes, amount of education, place of residence, or income?

The answers to these questions were provided earlier in this series, during the discussion of the stratification process for cohorts.[7, 8] The selection of strata for a cross-sectional survey is quite similar, except that the underlying variables are regarded as *affector* rather than *predictor* variables. The object is to choose the underlying variables that can have major effects on the results in the target variable.

In the foregoing example, the target variable was blood pressure. In other instances, it could have been serum cholesterol, athletic ability, political opinions, or the occurrence of a myocardial infarction. In choosing the underlying variables that are potentially important for these targets we might decide that blood pressure can be affected by race; serum cholesterol by weight; athletic ability by height; political opinions by income; and myocardial infarction by familial patterns of disease. We might also believe that none of these target variables is particularly likely to be affected by color of shoes. After contemplating the underlying variables individually, we might decide that several of them may act concomitantly to affect the target variable. Thus, political opinions may depend on sex, age, and place of residence, as well as income.

In certain instances, the strata will be chosen not because they necessarily affect the target variable, but because the investigator wants to know the results in each stratum. Thus, with the current electoral college system for choosing a President of the United States, a political poll-taker trying to predict the outcome of the election would be sure to stratify the national results according to the data for each of the 50 states.

There are several ways to choose the individual underlying variables that can influence the target variable. If the population under scrutiny has been studied previously, quantitative evidence may exist to demonstrate which variables can have important effects. If such evidence does not exist, the important variables can be chosen by judgment or by ritual. In the judgment procedure, the investigator relies on previous experience and current wisdom. In the ritual procedure, the investigator chooses these variables according to certain traditional customs, regardless of whether or not the chosen variables have significant effects on the target.

Thus, the demographic variables of age, sex, and race are commonly chosen by ritual as the major underlying variables in epidemiologic and clinical surveys, regardless of the target variable, and regardless of whether the target variable is more importantly influenced by alternative variables. As discussed previously in this series,[4, 5] the important underlying variables that are often neglected are psychic distress and parental longevity in epidemiologic surveys of etiology; and co-morbidity and symptom severity in clinical surveys of therapy.

Finally, for some of the adjustments to be described later, the important underlying variables can be chosen after, rather than before, the sampling is performed. Just as the statistical values of the mean and standard deviation will be found after, rather than before, the sampled people are assembled, the scientific relationship of underlying and target variables will often be explored when the work of sampling is completed. For many sample surveys, in fact, the purpose of the research is to assemble suitable data with which the target effects of different underlying variables can be identified and quantified.

a. Suitable scope of variables. The investigator's scientific insight is challenged by the choice of underlying variables that will be checked for their potential importance. If the number of variables is too small, crucial variables may be omitted, and the investigator may fail to discern what was really vital. If the number of variables is too large, many of them will have trivial importance, and their inclusion in the data will serve only as a distraction of investigative energy. The investigator must therefore select a suitable scope for the variables by choosing enough different ones to cover the important topics and by avoiding the trivial ones that have relatively little value.

b. A quantitative mechanism for deciding importance. To decide whether one underlying variable is more important than another, the investigator will often use a simple quantitative mechanism: the difference noted in the target variable. For example, suppose the target variable in our survey is the political preference for Party A vs. Party B. In examining the relationship between this target variable and the underlying variable of sex, we find the following percentages of preference for Party A: among **men,** 51% and among **women,** 49%. In a similar examination for income, we find the following preference for Party A: among **high-income groups,** 70% and among **low-income groups,** 35%. In this situation, the 35% difference among income groups and the 2% difference among sex groups would suggest that *income* has a more important effect on political preference than *sex.* (In this example, the target variable was expressed in percentages and we compared the incremental percentages among groups. A similar tactic could have been used to compare means, rather than percentages, if the target variable had been expressed dimensionally.)

Although we might use certain statistical tests to confirm that the observed differences are probably not due to chance alone, it is the magnitude of the differences, rather than the size of the P value alone, that will determine the decision about the importance of variables. Here too, the investigator's judgment is based on scientific rather than statistical concepts of "significance."

3. *The formation of cogent strata.* After the potentially important variables have been chosen, they can be demarcated into groups or strata. These strata can be cited individually in an array of "substages," or certain substages can be combined to form composite strata. Thus, to create composite strata for the political poll noted earlier, we might find that *sex* and *income* can be combined to form groups with the following preferences for Party A: **high-income women,** 80%; **high-income men,** 60%; **low-income men,** 45%; and **low-income women,** 25%. The composite groups in this bivariate stratification are clearly more distinctive than what was noted earlier for the results with either variable alone.

In general, for a large survey sample, the investigator will use a substage technique, even though the process creates many different "cells" as the substages. For the relatively small samples studied in clinical cohort research, however, a large number of substages is unfeasible. Accordingly, various substages are combined to form a smaller number of composite strata for the cohort analyses.[7, 8]

Thus, based on the goal of the research and the available population, the investigator will choose the single strata, multiple substrata, or multivariate composite strata that produce the most effective demarcation of the data. These groupings form the *cogent* strata for the sampling. If formed in advance, they will be used for planning sample sizes within each stratum. If formed after the sampling has been completed, the cogent strata delineate the people who are counted in the proportions that can be used to demonstrate or reduce assembly bias.

4. *The measurement of bias.* The assembly bias in a sampling can be determined by comparing the proportions of its cogent strata with the proportions expected in the parent population. Thus, if the parent population contains 70% men and 30% women, a sample that has 40% men and 60% women is obviously biased with respect to sex. The amount of acceptable disproportion in strata will vary with the purpose of the survey and the magnitude of the target variable in the strata.

Suppose our target variable is survival rate, with values of 80% in men and 50% in women. The true survival rate in the above cited population would be 71% ($= [.70 \times .80] + [.30 \times .50]$). In the distorted sample, the rate would be 62% ($= [.40 \times .80] + [.60 \times .50]$). Thus, a distortion of 30% in the underlying variable lowered the rate of the target variable by 9%. As discussed earlier in this series,[4] the amount of bias in the target variable is equal to the product of two differences: Δ_r, the difference in target rates for the strata, and Δ_k, the difference in proportions of the strata. In the above example, $\Delta_r = .30$ ($= 80\% - 50\%$) and $\Delta_k = .30$ ($= 70\% - 40\% = 60\% - 30\%$). The product of $.30 \times .30$ is the difference noted in the target rate. The larger the disproportion in Δ_k, and the larger the difference for Δ_r, the larger will be the bias in the final results.

From the many variables that can be observed in a survey, myriads of different stratifications can be formed, and any or all of these stratifications can be used to demarcate the groups whose proportions will be checked for bias. The crucial feature of a test for bias, however, is that the stratification be demonstrated to be cogent. Otherwise, substantial bias can exist without detection.

For example, we may find that the preference for political Party A is 63% in a sample of people from population X, and 46% in a sample from population Y. We decide to check for bias by using sex as the stratification variable, and we find that the proportionate distribution of men and women was essentially similar in the two samples. If we then concluded that there was no bias in the samples, we would be wrong, because men and women alone did not produce cogent strata. If we had used a better stratification, based on income alone or on the combination of income and sex, we might have found a substantial bias in the sample. Thus, the sample from population X might have contained predominantly people of high-income levels, whereas low-income people predominated in the sample from population Y.

E. The prevention and removal of bias

Regardless of whether or not random selection was used, a sample that is found to contain substantial bias can be adjusted to remove or reduce the bias. A customary procedure for this adjustment is based on the same type of stratification that was used to identify the bias. Instead of expressing the results found in the entire sample, the investigator divides the sample into its cogent strata, and then expresses the results within each stratum. Suppose, for example, that the mean value of some estrogenic substance was found to be 75 units in a random sample of young adults. We later discover, however, that the sample of 100 people contained 30 men and 70 women instead of the 50:50 ratio that would have been correct for the parent population. We therefore list the data within strata, and find that the mean value in the 30 men was 40 units, whereas the mean value in the 70 women was 90 units.

This expression of results for the individual strata will often suffice to tell us what we wanted to know, but we may still want to cite the data as a single value for the sample. We therefore multiply the strata-specific results by certain factors that provide "standardization." If our sample had represented the parent population, it would have contained 50 men and 50 women. Assuming that these people had the same strata-specific values found in our actual sample, the mean result would have been $[(50 \times 40) + (50 \times 90)] \div 100 = 65$ units. This 65 units would be the standardized sex-specific value for our sample.

This type of adjustment, based on a *post-stratification* performed after the sample is obtained, is a conventional part of the methods used in epidemiologic research. It regularly is expressed in such phrases as *age-standardized* or *age-and-*

sex standardized death rates. The population used as reference for the standardization can be obtained from the data of a national census, or by other methods that are beyond the scope of this discussion.

A better way of dealing with this problem in sampling bias, of course, is to keep it from happening. A cautious investigator, who respects both science and chance, will not take the risk, however small, that his careful planning and hard work will be vitiated by sheer bad luck. He will rely neither on randomization alone to prevent bias nor on subsequent statistical adjustments to remove it. To protect against outrageous fortune, he will draw his sample by *pre-stratification*.

In this technique, the population is not lumped together for randomized choices; instead, it is divided into cogent strata. A separate random sample, having appropriate size, is then drawn from each of the strata. For example, suppose we want to draw a 1/100 sample for a population consisting of 20% young adults, 60% middle-aged adults, and 20% old adults. If age is a cogent feature of this population (and if the standard deviations in each age group are similar despite the differences in means), we would like the sample itself to have the same proportionate age distribution as the population. A shift of 5% in two of the groups by chance could badly distort the results. Thus if fate gave us 15% young adults, 55% middle-aged adults, and 30% old adults in the sample, the old group would be twice as large as the young one, instead of being equal-sized. To avoid this hazard, we can sample separately within each stratum, taking a 2/1000 sample in the older and younger groups and a 6/1000 sample for middle age. We emerge with a sample of the desired size of 1/100 [= (2/1000) + (6/1000) + (2/1000)], but the sample is now both randomly chosen and properly distributed.

The technique of *stratified random sampling* is one of the basic methods used in modern survey research, particularly for social and political science. The stratification technique can be applied with diverse modifications that are described in textbooks devoted to sampling,[14, 16, 19] but the basic principle remains the same. Before the sampling begins, we divide the population into suitably delineated groups, and we sample within those groups.

These problems in bias are well known in the domain of political and social science, particularly for investigators who perform the types of sample surveys used for political poll taking. In these domains, the investigator usually wants to estimate the magnitude of a selected target variable, such as certain political or social opinions, in a large population. In epidemiologic and clinical medicine, however, the investigator often wants to contrast the difference in results found in two groups: an exposed and non-exposed; a diseased and non-diseased; or a treated and a non-treated.

When epidemiologists and clinicians study the effect of a principal maneuver vs. a comparative maneuver, the main emphasis is on the difference in the effects of the two maneuvers rather than on the individual results for each maneuver. In social or political surveys, however, an imposed maneuver is often not a part of the research plan, and instead the investigator merely wants to find out what is happening. For this purpose, the validity of representation in the sample is crucial. If the clinician or epidemiologist is wrong, it may take years for the error to be detected and corrected. If the political poll taker is wrong, however, the error is discerned soon thereafter, on Election Day. Consequently, the methods of accurate sampling receive particularly careful attention among political and social scientists.

The methods seldom receive adequate attention, however, in textbooks of medicine, epidemiology, or biostatistics. Perhaps the main reason for this inattention to sampling is that the basic methods for preventing or removing potential sources of bias must be chosen with scientific rather than statistical judgment. No statistical theories can be used to recognize the important variables that must be examined in a research project.

Nevertheless, an investigator who neglects making suitable provision for assembling the necessary data to explore important bias is doubly delinquent. He entrusts his research and his readers to the faithful but sometimes mistaken hope that bias will be removed by the statistical act of random sampling; and he fails to perform the necessary scientific observations for which no amount of statistical theory can be substituted. Just as enlightened scientists today find wry amusement in condemning the many mistaken concepts and procedures that have existed throughout the centuries of medical history, future historians will surely encounter a plethora of analogous transgressions when reviewing the sampling procedures used in present-day epidemiology and clinical medicine.

All of the many epidemiologic investigations devoted to causal factors in disease have depended on chunk samples, regardless of whether the samples were followed forward as cohorts, backward as trohocs,[9] or in a cross-sectional "prevalence" approach. *All* of the many investigations devoted to therapeutic surveys and trials of diverse diseases have also depended on chunk samples taken from the groups of patients conveniently available in the medical centers where the investigators worked.

For these research activities, the investigators have not fulfilled the basic requirement of a fully delineated population from which to sample; and the "samples" have been obtained by a convenient intake procedure, not by random selection from the population that they allegedly represent. Since all of these intake groups can be substantially distorted by bias in the diverse transitional and chronologic transfers that made the people available to the investigator, the results cannot be extrapolated unless the bias was suitably identified and the results appropriately adjusted. As noted earlier[4, 5, 7] in this series, this challenge has seldom received adequate attention. Instead of searching diligently for better scientific methods to identify and remove sources of major bias, the investigators have often become diverted by the allure of two types of mathematical manipulations: calculating standardized adjustments and performing tests of "statistical significance."

In hoping that the standardized adjustments will take care of the bias, the investigator may concentrate on the mathematical processes of stratification, regression, or discriminant analysis while neglecting the scientific process of searching for the cogent variables associated with major bias. Because the mathematical adjustments cannot identify important variables that have been omitted, the adjustment process may yield calculations that embellish the fundamental bias without affecting it.

The second type of mathematical allure consists of testing for "statistical significance." When a contrast is found to be "statistically significant," the investigator may be deluded into believing that the content of his explanation rather than the magnitude of his numbers has been rendered acceptable. Regardless of how the "significance" tests are used, however, they depend on mathematical ideas about randomization. Some of those ideas are similar to what has just been discussed, but others are quite different. The randomization principles used in statistical tests will be the topic of the next paper in this series.

References

1. Cornfield, J.: The University Group Diabetes Program. A further statistical analysis of the mortality findings, J. A. M. A. **217**:1676-1687, 1971.
2. David, F. N.: Games, gods, and gambling. A history of probability and statistical ideas, London, 1962, Griffin & Co., Ltd.
3. Feinstein, A. R.: Clinical biostatistics. VII. The rancid sample, the tilted target, and the medical poll-bearer, CLIN. PHARMACOL. THER. **12**:134-150, 1971.
4. Feinstein, A. R.: Clinical biostatistics. X. Sources of 'transition bias' in cohort statistics, CLIN. PHARMACOL. THER. **12**:704-721, 1971.
5. Feinstein, A. R.: Clinical biostatistics. XI. Sources of 'chronology bias' in cohort statistics, CLIN. PHARMACOL. THER. **12**:864-879, 1971.
6. Feinstein, A. R.: Clinical biostatistics. XIII. On homogeneity, taxonomy, and nosography, CLIN. PHARMACOL. THER. **13**:114-129, 1972.
7. Feinstein, A. R.: Clinical biostatistics. XIV. The purpose of prognostic stratification, CLIN. PHARMACOL. THER. **13**:285-297, 1972.
8. Feinstein, A. R.: Clinical biostatistics. XV and XVI. The process of prognostic stratification, CLIN. PHARMACOL. THER. **13**:442-457; 609-624, 1972.
9. Feinstein, A. R.: Clinical biostatistics. XX. The epidemiologic trohoc, the ablative risk ratio, and 'retrospective' research, CLIN. PHARMACOL. THER. **14**:291-307, 1973.
10. Fienberg, S. E.: Randomization and social affairs: The 1970 draft lottery, Science **171**:255-261, 1971.
11. Fisher, R. A.: The arrangement of field experiments, J. Ministry Agriculture **33**:503-513, 1926.
12. Kempthorne, O.: The randomization theory of experimental inference, J. Am. Stat. Ass. **50**:946-967, 1955.
13. Kendall, M. G., and Stuart, A.: The advanced theory of statistics. Vol. 2. Inference and Relationship, ed. 2, London, 1967, Charles Griffin & Co., Ltd.
14. Kish, L.: Survey sampling, New York, 1965, John Wiley & Sons, Inc.
15. Landis, J. R., and Feinstein, A. R.: An empirical comparison of random numbers acquired by computer-generation and from the Rand tables. In press, Comp. Biomed. Res., vol. 6, August, 1973.
16. Slonim, M. J.: Sampling, New York, 1966, Simon & Schuster, Inc. (Paperback.)
17. Snedecor, G. W., and Cochran, W. G.: Statistical methods, ed. 6, Ames, Iowa, 1967, Iowa State University Press.
18. Webster's New Collegiate Dictionary, Springfield, Mass., 1951, G. & C. Merriam Company, Publishers.
19. Yates, F.: Sampling methods for censuses and surveys, ed. 3, London, 1960, Charles Griffin & Co., Ltd.

CHAPTER 12

The rancid sample, the tilted target, and the medical poll-bearer

Scientists are often quite skeptical about the polls taken to sample public opinion in politics. The data are highly subjective; the results are sold commercially; the percentages are usually cited without indication of the sample sizes that went into the denominators; the qualifications of the investigators are usually unstated; and the forecasts have been shockingly wrong in at least three well-remembered national elections—in the United States in 1936 and 1948, and in England in 1970.

In contrast to this skepticism about political polls, scientists often give limitless credence to another type of poll: the epidemiologic survey. Such surveys are seldom regarded as *polls,* although every study of incidence and prevalence of disease, every calculation of mortality rates for different diseases, and every statistical assessment of "causal association" in human malady is exactly analogous to a political poll. From the general total population (or "universe"), a smaller population (or "sample") is selected; the people in that sample are interrogated or examined to obtain data; and the conclusions drawn from the ana-

lyzed data are then applied (or "extrapolated") to the larger universe.

The results of these epidemiologic medical polls are usually received with considerable confidence. The data are often based on objective laboratory tests; the results are presented in the scientific literature; the sample sizes are generally stated and are sometimes immense; and the investigators usually hold advanced academic degrees. Besides, having forgotten some of the old classic epidemiologic blunders in investigations that discovered low-altitude atmospheric conditions to be the "cause" of cholera,[8] and that found pellagra to be an infectious and possibly hereditary disease,[2, 32] modern scientists do not vividly recall any recent examples of egregious epidemiologic error.

As the medical pollster of our era, the statistical epidemiologist leads a charmed scientific life. People can respect him for the erudition of his training and the majesty of his numbers—and he need seldom worry about being proved wrong. Unlike a laboratory experiment or a clinical treatment, which can usually be repeated and tested elsewhere, the epidemiologist's work can almost never be duplicated. Other investigators can rarely take the time and effort to find a similarly large population of people and to examine those people in the same way. Moreover, unlike the "universe"

Under the same name, this chapter originally appeared as "Clinical biostatistics—VII." In Clin. Pharmacol. Ther. 12:134, 1971.

of the political pollster, which demonstrates its true condition by notations made in ballot boxes on Election Day, the condition of the epidemiologist's "universe" is never revealed. No one except census takers ever gets data for the entire general population, and census takers do not study disease.

A statistical epidemiologist thus works in extraordinary scientific isolation. Unlike the political pollster, the epidemiologist has no "election day" to tell him immediately whether his poll was correct, or whether he has produced gross errors that need reappraisal and rectification. Since his work is seldom repeated, and since his actual "universe" can seldom be observed, he can commit the most flagrant violations of scientific methodology without having either to fear that his results will be directly refuted, or to hope that his mistakes will be openly detected. Sheltered from the harsh realities of scientific verification, an epidemiologist must exercise constant vigilance to avoid the many pitfalls into which other polltakers have traditionally stumbled.

The purpose of this discussion is to note three of those pitfalls, and to compare the way they are managed today by our contemporary political and medical pollsters. One of the pitfalls deals with the validity of the sampling procedure, and the other two, with bias and error in the collected data.

1. Validity of the sampling procedure

People were using sampling techniques to make decisions long before medicine, epidemiology, or statistics became formal intellectual disciplines. When an orchard is judged from a few of its apples, a barrel of wine from a glass, or a loaf of bread from a slice, the judge performs a sampling exercise in which the character of a whole is decided from examination of a representative part. Although sampling of a "part" is often done to save the time and effort that would be needed to examine the entire "whole," the sampling procedure in the instances just cited was also necessary to

conserve material. The value of the testing would be negated if the judge had to bite all the apples, drink all the wine, or eat all the bread in order to reach a conclusion.

In epidemiologic studies, however, the observed population is not consumed or destroyed by the examining procedure, and if necessary, every member of the entire population could be examined. Such a "total sampling" is attempted, for example, during our decennial national census. For many other types of epidemiologic investigation, however, a total sampling is not feasible because the investigator has neither the massive facilities of a national census nor the many trained personnel needed to get medical data. Thus, although an epidemiologist might prefer to examine the entire population to which his work refers, he cannot do so because of practical realities that would keep him from ever completing his research if he tried to reach everyone. He therefore turns to sampling as a methodologic compromise: a necessary evil that he accepts because it is expedient and because, without it, he could not work.

The investigator buys the compromise at a price that is usually called *sampling error*. This error represents the difference between the result obtained from the sampled population and the true result that would have come from examination of the entire population. Since the entire population cannot be examined in most epidemiologic surveys, the true result cannot be known, so we can never really determine the actual value of the sampling error. Instead, the epidemiologist obtains only one real value: the results noted in the selected sample. Everything else thereafter is "estimated." From the observed results in the sample, we estimate a sampling error, and from that estimation, we estimate the condition of the "universe" population from which we have sampled. The fundamental link in this chain of estimations is our guess about the sampling error. How good is the method of estimating that error? How do we decide whether an estimate is right or wrong?

For many years, statisticians have convinced themselves and their clients that the theories of probability provide an excellent method of estimating the sampling error. According to these theories, which are discussed in most statistical textbooks and which can be expressed in a neat mathematical formula,* the larger the size of the sample, the smaller will be the sampling error. Thus, a sampling of 2,000 people should yield a "standard error" about 1/10 the size of that found with a sampling of 20 people. With a sampling of 2,000,000 people, the "standard error" should be negligible.

The quantitative comfort of these statistics is generally achieved, however, by overlooking a distressing qualitative fact: the calculated estimates are valid only if based on a "probability sample." Such a sample, which is also called a *random sample,* is one in which every member of the sampled population has the same chance of being included as any other member. W. E. Deming[6] has given the following description of some of the rules of getting a random sample:

> A probability survey is carried out according to a statistical plan embodying automatic selection of the elements (for) which information is to be obtained. In a probability sample, neither the interviewer nor the elements of the sample have any choice about who is the sample. . . . A probability sample will send the interviewer through mud and cold, over long distances, up decrepit stairs, to people who do not welcome an interviewer; but such cases occur only in their correct proportions. Substitutions are not permitted: the rules are ruthless.

A sample is nonrandom if selected by any methods other than those just cited. Whenever a nonrandom technique has been used, the investigator (and reader) must beware that a bias has been exerted against choosing certain members, or groups of members, of the original population. For example, we could immediately determine that a sampling of the general American population is nonrandom and biased if it contains only white people, or significantly more men than women, or disproportionately large numbers of people with a college education.

The unpleasant necessity for a random sample precludes the direct calculation of a simple "sampling error" in the ethereal manner provided by statistical theories. If the sample has been demonstrated to be truly random, its *stochastic error** can be calculated according to probabilistic concepts. If the sample is nonrandom, however, the calculation of a stochastic error is inappropriate because the rules of probability do not apply. Although such probabilistic calculations are often performed and presented as the "sampling error," the main problem to be considered is the *selectional error* imposed by the nonrandom sampling.

Most of the major errors in contemporary sampling are due to problems in selection. For example, in an excellent discussion of "misuses of statistics," Wallis and Roberts[30] present 67 brief "case reports" of various types of statistical blunders, most of which were due to defects not in quantification but in the manner of choosing the sample. Unlike a stochastic error, a selectional error may be magnified rather than minimized by a large sample. Furthermore, a selectional error can thwart any attempt to draw conclusions from a survey, because we may have no idea of how the true state of the base population was distorted by the nonrepresentative sampling procedure. Unless we can demonstrate that such

---

*If N people have been sampled, with p found to be the proportion of people who plan to vote for a candidate, and with q the proportion who plan to vote the opposite way, the "standard error" is $\sqrt{\dfrac{pq}{N}}$. If p and q remain the same as the size of the sample is increased, the amount of error decreases in inverse proportion to the square root of N.

*According to Kendall and Buckland,[18] "the adjective 'stochastic' implies the presence of a random variable." Because of the implication of randomness, the term *stochastic* seems more appropriate to describe the ideas used for calculating this type of error, than such alternate terms as *arithmetical, mathematical, numerical, probabilistic, quantitative,* or *statistical.*

distortions were avoided, an entire investigation may be vitiated by the hazards of selectional error in sampling.

Nevertheless, these hazards are seldom thoroughly discussed in most epidemiologic and statistical publications. After a brief mention of the need for random sampling, the text is quickly turned to an intense exposition of the principles of probability used in calculating stochastic error. There is little or no discussion of how to determine whether a sample is random, what happens if it is not, and what methods can be used to assess the magnitude or consequences of the selectional error in nonrandom samples.

There are many reasons why the problems of "rancid" samples are so disregarded by both statisticians and epidemiologists. In learning about sampling, a statistician can either concentrate on an imaginary universe, where all samples are made random by proclamation, or else he can work with a simple biologic domain—such as agricultural plots, brewery vats, and fruit flies—where the "population" is nonhuman, reasonably homogeneous, and subservient to whatever sampling choices the investigator wants to make. In these idyllic circumstances, the statistician need not worry about the diversity and freedom of human populations.

An epidemiologist's research environment is less idyllic, since the "material" of his investigations consists of people, who are both heterogeneous and nonsubservient. In fact, because people can usually choose to accept or reject the offer to be "sampled," the subjects of most epidemiologic surveys must be acquired by *intake* rather than by sampling.[12] An epidemiologist who allowed himself to become too concerned about the possible defects of nonrandom sampling, however, might have to stop all research activity. He might be overwhelmed by the difficulties of obtaining truly random samples of people, while simultaneously obtaining data of high scientific quality. Thus, in order to do research and to apply statistical tactics for numerical estimations, an epidemiologist often condones the disconcerting fact that his samples are not random.

These methodologic flaws are seldom recognized by the person who reads the results of an epidemiologic survey. Impressed by the magnitude of the numbers and confused by the mathematics of the estimations, the reader may omit any critical attention to the sampling procedures. Besides, a clinical reader's natural skepticism may be sated by the care and apparent humility with which epidemiologists report their calculations of a "sampling error." The reader may assume that any investigator who is so aware of his errors and who can quantify them so precisely must surely have exercised suitable precautions in selecting his sample. Unlike a statistical epidemiologist, however, a political pollster cannot rely on having credulous readers and an unexamined universe. Election Day reveals reality, and when reality contradicts the pollster's prediction, a defective sampling procedure becomes identified, and its causes must be sought.

Among the many ways in which a "rancid" sample can be chosen, two have become particularly famous as sources of horrendous error in political poll taking.

A. The "chunk" sample. A *chunk* sample* is chosen not for its representation of the general population, but for the investigator's convenience. Instead of trying to get a random selection of the population into the sampling, the investigator deals with a group of people who happen to be readily available.

The classic example of chunk sampling occurred in the famous United States presidential poll of 1936, conducted by the *Literary Digest* magazine. The poll was regarded as surely accurate because, according to statistical theory, it had essentially no stochastic error in sampling: the poll contained the awesome number of 2,000,000

---

*According to W. E. Deming,[6] this term was first used by the demographer, Philip M. Hauser, to distinguish "a convenient slice of a population."

people. Unfortunately, those 2,000,000 people constituted a group obtained by chunk sampling. Questionnaires were sent to all subscribers of the magazine and also to a collection of people randomly chosen from the names listed in telephone directories throughout the nation.[20] The result of the poll was a prediction of a "landslide" victory for the Republican candidate, Alfred M. Landon. What happened on Election Day was just the reverse: the Democrat, Franklin D. Roosevelt, carried all but two states.

As statisticians analyzed this polling catastrophe, which led to the demise of the magazine soon thereafter, they quickly discovered how chunk sampling had produced the error. In 1936, a depression year, people who could afford to maintain telephones or subscriptions to literary magazines were much more likely to be in a higher income group, and thus Republican, than the rest of the voting population. Hence, despite the "random sampling" from the telephone books, the pollsters arrived at the fallacious prediction of a Republican "landslide."

B. The "volunteer" sample. A *volunteer* sample, like a chunk sample, is also chosen for the convenience of the investigator; it consists of a self-selected group of people who have responded to a questionnaire or to a call for volunteers.

The *Literary Digest* presidential poll just cited was flawed not only by chunk sampling, but also by volunteer sampling. The magazine's subscribers and the people chosen from the telephone book were sent questionnaires, and the results of the poll were calculated from the returned questionnaires.[20] Since the Democrat, Roosevelt, was already in office, unhappy Republicans were more likely than contented Democrats to express their displeasure by completing and returning the questionnaire. In this way, the volunteer aspect of the sampling was another reason for its erroneous results.

From the blatant error of this disastrous poll, the political polltakers learned two important lessons: a chunk sample is un-

satisfactory because it does not represent the general population, and a volunteer sample is unsatisfactory, even if solicited randomly, because the investigator is uncertain about the way that the nonresponding group may affect the results by failure to appear in the sample. Both types of "rancid" sampling may produce distortions by introducing bias that cannot be quantified because the investigator does not know the condition of the universe beyond the sample. Sensitized by these errors, political polltakers now go to great lengths to avoid chunk sampling and to seek appropriate representatives of the general population of voters. The pollsters also avoid mailed questionnaires, and get their data instead by direct personal interviews.

These lessons do not yet seem to have permeated the ranks of medical pollsters. Until the United States National Health Survey[23] was established a few years ago, the political pollsters were the only investigators who had developed a mechanism for getting an approximately random sample of our national population. Epidemiologic and other surveys of medical topics have almost all come from samplings that were either chunk, or volunteer, or both. Consequently, amid the hundreds of published medical surveys that depend on sampling techniques, it is difficult to find even one that has the elementary scientific virtue of a random sampling. Illustrations of "rancid" samples abound in both the clinical and the epidemiologic literature, and the ones I shall cite here are themselves a chunk sample of what is available, i.e., I am already familiar with them and shall not take the trouble to find a more representative collection.

A chunk sample is the source of the "range of normal" calculated for most of the new chemical, chromosomal, and other tests developed in hospital laboratories during the past 15 years. The sampled "normal" population in these studies usually consisted of hospital personnel: technicians, medical students, house officers, and a few cooperative secretaries. Such a group obviously does not represent the world outside the hospital because the sampled people are younger and different in many other features than the rest of the "normal" population.

People who have life insurance policies are both a chunk and a volunteer sample of the general population. They were given a medical screening before the policy was issued, and consequently can be expected to be a somewhat healthier group than the noninsured. Moreover, members of the insured population had to decide to apply for a policy and had to be able to afford it; thus, they may represent a somewhat higher income level than the rest of the population and, if diseased at the time they applied for insurance, they may have sought the policy because of unstated features of illness known to the applicant but not detected during the screening examinations. For these and other reasons, data taken from life insurance rosters will tend to exclude people with severe, overt disease and those who are healthy but poor. The rosters may also have disproportionately large numbers of subtly diseased people who have masqueraded as "normal." The analysis of data from such rosters can be used with commercial success by the life insurance companies in calculating actuarial rates, but because of the defects in sampling, the data are not suitable for scientific descriptions of the general population.

A population of people in the armed forces is also epidemiologically biased by both chunk and volunteer sampling. The population contains a predominance of men, many of whom were volunteers, and they had to pass specific physical and mental examinations before being admitted to the armed forces. Nevertheless, military groups have often been used in epidemiologic surveys of the health hazards of various demographic features, and in recent studies of the range of normal in electrocardiograms and other tests. A population of veterans of the armed forces is also epidemiologically biased by the same features that governed their entrance into military service and by other features that determined their survival while in the service.

A surprisingly fertile source of examples of defective epidemiologic sampling techniques is the Surgeon General's report on "Smoking and Health."[27] Each of the "prospective" epidemiologic surveys cited in that report depended on a group of people collected by chunk sampling, by volunteer sampling, or by both. In one of the best known of these surveys, the sampled population consisted exclusively of British medical doctors who had answered questionnaires. In another celebrated survey—with a "sample" of more than 2,000,000 people—the basic data came from questionnaires answered by friends of volunteer workers in various branches of the American Cancer Society. Such surveys are already flawed because their selected population was chunk sampled, but the use of questionnaires adds even more uncertain bias to the results. Since non-smokers could fill out the questionnaires more easily than the smokers, who were asked many details of their smoking habits, a disproportionate number of smokers failed to return the questionnaires.

Sampling bias is rampant throughout clinical medicine in clinicians' characterizations of disease. The investigated group of patients may not truly represent the "disease" because of features that led the patients to be referred to a particular doctor or to assemble at the hospital where the survey is conducted. For example, at a large private referral institution, such as the Mayo Clinic, the patients must be able to afford the costs of individual attention and must be well enough to travel there; at a municipal "charity" hospital, such as Bellevue in New York City, the patients will generally come from the lowest socioeconomic strata of society and will often be brought moribund by public ambulance; at a public clinic that does not hold evening sessions, the patients will differ from those who consult a private physician at night. Although all of the patients seen in these diverse circumstances may have the "same" disease, they may have different forms of the disease and may differ in many other characteristics that make the sampling of disease seen at one locale inapplicable to what is seen elsewhere.

An awareness of epidemiologic aspects of sampling is also strikingly absent in the work of psychiatrists, who regularly characterize certain diseases according to the personality and family structure of diseased patients referred because of profound psychiatric problems; such characterizations often do not apply to patients with the same disease who were not referred for psychiatric help. Clinical psychologists and other investigators have often studied the symptomatic reactions of paid "normal" volunteers to various types of stressful circumstance, but the investigators have not established whether the people who volunteer for such experiments are really representative of the general population. In one recent investigation,[19] many such volunteers were shown to have major psychic disturbances.

Certain hazards of nonrandom sampling may be avoided if the investigator can assign the "maneuver" whose effects are being observed. Thus, in a therapeutic trial, the different modes of treatment can be allocated randomly to the patients. In such circumstances, the investigator can generally conclude that the compared treatments were given in an unbiased manner. Nevertheless, he is still unable to extrapolate the therapeutic results to other people with the same "disease" unless the observed patients were demonstrated to be a random sample of people with that disease. For conventional epidemiologic surveys, however, the investigator cannot assign the "maneuver" randomly.[11] Instead, he seeks to characterize the effects of ontogenetic, pathogenetic, or other maneuvers that were imposed by nature or self-selected by the members of the observed population. In collecting various types of intake from this population, the epidemiologist then hopes that the "sample" will somehow represent a random assignment of the maneuver.

The results of a "rancid" epidemiologic sample are not vitiated merely because the sample was easy and convenient for the investigator to obtain. The vitiation, if any, will depend upon the particular entity that is being tested, and the particular factors of preselection that helped create bias in the sample. For example, if an investigator wants to measure the change of blood pressure that occurs in healthy middle-aged men responding to a cold pressor test, the results may be the same in a sampling of men taken from a laborer's clubhouse as in a group from a country club. The results in these two groups might be quite different, however, if the entity under examination is the type of automobile or house owned by the individual samplees.

This relationship between the type of people in the sample and what is assessed in those people determines the scientific propriety of the results. The investigator must constantly beware that some inapparent features of preselection in the sample have created a bias in the relationship between what is assessed and the people in whom it is assessed. In the foregoing example, the economic difference between laborers and country club members would be immediately apparent as a bias affecting their ownership of automobiles and homes. Although this economic difference seemingly should not influence the responses of the two groups to a cold pressor test, we cannot be certain *a priori* that this physiologic reaction is not altered by other subtle differences in the two groups. Thus, the selected laboring men might have come predominantly from one ethnic group, and the country club members might have come mainly from another, and these two different ethnic groups might have fundamental genetic or constitutional differences that alter their cold pressor responses.

The subtle bias exerted by preselection in a nonrandom sample is not always grossly evident in the sample or in the data, and the bias is seldom detectable by any simple statistical techniques. Occasionally, the defect in sampling is made apparent by comparing certain characteristics of the sampled population with those of the general population. For example, in one of the surveys of smoking cited earlier, the friends of the American Cancer Society workers had a much higher educational level, and those who smoked had a much *lower* death rate than the general American population. For the most part, however, if a truly random sampling cannot be obtained, the investigator (or reader) has no choice but to use logic and medical judgment for evaluating the validity or "rancidity" of the selected population, and for estimating the way that the existing bias may distort the results of the investigation.

In certain types of clinical surveys, the results can be subsequently confirmed or refuted with direct clinical observations. Such future assessments are possible when the survey deals with the "range of normal" for a paraclinical test, or with the characteristics of patients with a particular disease. For example, if the "range of normal" for a chemical test was initially determined in an age-restricted sample of hospital personnel, and if the test ordinarily shows increasingly higher values as people grow older, many healthy elderly people will at first be regarded as abnormal when the test comes into general use. After an "epidemic" of these inexplicable abnormalities, however, clinicians may either recognize the fallacy of the initial sampling, or may pragmatically extend the boundaries of the initial "range of normal." Similarly, when Buerger, reporting on his sample of patients observed at New York's Mount Sinai hospital, stated that thromboangiitis obliterans (Buerger's disease) occurred almost exclusively in Jews, his erroneous epidemiologic conclusion could be detected and corrected when clinicians elsewhere found the disease in members of other ethnic groups.

The most difficult type of survey to verify is an epidemiologic assessment of cause for a noninfectious disease. What we would want to check is the attack rates of the disease for people exposed and not exposed to the alleged causal agent. Unfortunately, the routine activities of medical practice bring clinicians into contact mainly with the people who become diseased. Clinicians seldom get adequate or complete samplings of the people who are exposed or not exposed to the alleged cause. There is, in fact, no one who routinely inspects the exposure of the populations with the kind of care that clinicians (and pathologists) can routinely give to the groups who emerge diseased. For a particular survey, an epidemiologist assembles the "exposed" and "nonexposed" people as part of his sampling procedure, but his work is seldom checked thereafter. Thus, the validity of the sampling becomes a critical feature of the subsequent causal reasoning applied to the data. If the sample does not accurately represent the general population, the results may lead to plausible but erroneous conclusions about the cause of the disease.

2. Bias in detection of target

In a poll of political opinion, the investigators usually seek only one main type of data: the subject's political beliefs. In epidemiologic surveys, however, at least two main types of data are needed for the comparisons. To provide the numerators and denominators of the compared ratios (or rates), the epidemiologist must have data for the "initial state," which indicates the characteristics of the populations who enter the denominators, and data for the "subsequent state" that is counted in the numerators.

For example, when we say that the mortality rate for coronary artery disease has gone up between 1920 and 1960, our denominators for the two compared rates consist of census data about the number of people alive in 1920 and in 1960. Our two numerators contain the number of people

during each of those years who died with "coronary artery disease" listed as the cause of death. In epidemiologic surveys of etiology for lung cancer, the compared rates depend on denominator populations consisting of smokers and nonsmokers; the numerators contain the people from each population who were reported to have died with lung cancer.

In all of these ratios, the numerator population is determined from detection of a particular target in the subsequent state. In the two examples just cited, the respective targets were coronary artery disease and lung cancer. Since epidemiologic comparisons depend on the values for ratios, rather than for denominators alone, an elemental requirement of science would be that the numerators as well as the denominators be determined without bias. Unless the compared populations have had the same likelihood of detection of target in the numerators, the comparisons may have no more scientific validity than results that contain bias in the denominators.

Suppose we wanted to determine the occurrence of disease X in two groups of people, Group A and Group B, and suppose that disease X requires special examination procedures to be identified. If Group A receives more of these examinations than Group B, the rate of disease X may be higher in A than in B not because of any inherent differences in Group A, but because the detection of the target was "tilted" in the two groups. The hazard of this type of "tilted target" must be considered whenever the numerator of a ratio depends on a disease that is frequently undetected during life. For example, according to necropsy studies, about 50 per cent of people with coronary artery disease,[3] and about 20 per cent of people with lung cancer,[15] do not receive these diagnoses while alive. Since thrombophlebitis is seldom a fatal disease, it can often occur mildly and transiently in episodes that escape diagnostic detection because the victim does not seek medical attention. Consequently, if we were planning to use any one of these three diseases as the numerators in a scientific survey, we should ascertain that the compared denominator populations were exposed to the same frequency and intensity of such procedures as electrocardiograms, chest x-rays, routine physical examinations, and other appropriate diagnostic tests.

Within the past 25 years, political poll-takers have twice been badly stung by neglect of the bias caused by "tilted targets." Although reasonably random samples were used for the denominator populations in polls taken before the United States national election of 1948 and the British national election of 1970, the careful sampling procedures were sabotaged with errors caused by two different types of tilting in the target data.

In the recent British election, the polled voters seemed more inclined to vote Labor than Conservative, but the pollsters did not ascertain whether the two groups of potential voters had the same intention of carrying their beliefs to the target of expression at the voting booths. When Election Day came, the Conservatives won because their supporters were more diligent than those of Labor in reaching the target ballot box. As a result of the spectacular error in the predictions for this election, we can expect future political pollsters to inquire not merely about the opinions of the electorate, but also about the likelihood that the potential voters will actually vote. In the American election of 1948, the target was tilted in a different manner. Because one of the candidates (Thomas E. Dewey) seemed to hold a commanding lead over his rival, the pollsters did not continue testing beyond late September and early October. By the time Election Day arrived in early November, however, many voters apparently changed their minds, and cast ballots contrary to opinions previously expressed in the polls.[26] In a stunning "upset," Harry S Truman won the election. Consequently, political pollsters (at least in the United States) now continue their activities as close to Election Day as possible.

Perhaps the single greatest flaw in contemporary epidemiologic concepts and methods is the neglect of possible problems caused by a tilted target. Although the idea of random sampling has been developed and promulgated as a method for removing bias from the denominators, no substantial methodologic attention or investigation has been given to the possible distortions caused by bias in the numerators. Both of the cited problems in the tilted targets of political polls—the unequal registration of target and the temporal change of opinion —have many counterparts in epidemiologic surveys. These two scientific hazards have been discussed in greater detail elsewhere[12] and will be only outlined here.

The problems of unequal registration occur in groups of people followed concurrently whenever an initial feature of one of the groups or of the "causal agent" produces a disparate intensity of medical examination in the two groups. For example, an unequal frequency and scope of the examinations used to detect disease in compared groups may be responsible for some of the differences in the rates of coronary artery disease found in executives versus laborers, in the rates of lung cancer in smokers versus nonsmokers, and in the rates of thrombophlebitis for women who use "the pill" versus other forms of contraception. Executives are generally more likely than laborers to receive routine electrocardiograms and other periodic "checkups." Because of the development of chronic cough, smokers may be more likely to receive chest x-rays than noncoughing nonsmokers. The increased medical attention needed for renewing prescriptions or checking other hormonal problems may create more routine examinations for women taking the "pill" than for women using other forms of contraception. Although all of the targets in disease detection may be tilted in these groups for the reasons cited, the existence of the tilts has never been investigated, and the possible magnitude of the bias in these and other epidemiologic surveys is currently unknown.

The effects of temporal changes in opinion create a different problem in tilted targets. The problem occurs whenever mortality rates for a particular disease are compared in nonconcurrent populations, observed in different years or eras. The mortality rates for different diseases are based on the data reported in death certificates, but a death certificate does not list diseases; it lists the diagnoses made by clinicians. The "vital statistics" derived each year from death certificates do not indicate annual changes in rates of disease; they indicate a changing rate of diagnosis.[10]

Since a clinician examines not a "disease" but the clinical condition of a patient, most contemporary names of "disease" depend not on observed evidence, but on inferences, interpretations, or technologic expansions of the actual bedside evidence. Consequently, the "diseases" reported on death certificates will vary both with the diagnostic fashions popular among clinicians during any particular era in medicine, and with the diagnostic tools and tactics available for assigning names of "disease" to the observed clinical conditions. If the criteria and techniques of diagnosis can be shown to remain the same as time progresses, then the annual statistical tabulations may actually reflect an altered natural occurrence of the disease. But if the concepts and technology of diagnosis should change with time, the changing rates of many "diseases" noted on death certificates may be an artifact of target tilting, due to temporal changes of diagnostic opinion, rather than to new conditions of nature.

A simple example of this distinction is the disappearance of the disease *dropsy*, which was held responsible for so many deaths a century ago, but which seldom seems to kill anyone today, according to modern mortality data. The clinical condition of dropsy is still present in abundance, of course, but it is now called by other names, and its fatalities are usually attributed to some form of cardiac, renal, or hepatic disease. The modern changes from *dropsy* to *congestive heart failure* or other

names illustrate an alteration solely in the fashion of diagnostic nomenclature, but many other diagnostic changes are due to the new technologic agents that have been developed, with increasing frequency during the past half century, for identifying "disease." Such procedures as roentgenography, biopsy, endoscopy, exploratory surgery, electrocardiography, electroencephalography, chemical measurements, immunologic reactions, the various assessments of microbial agents, and the entire phantasmagoria of contemporary laboratory tests are almost all a product of the past 50 years, increasingly available and increasingly used during the past few decades.

These new diagnostic adjuncts can be expected to have both an immediate and a delayed effect on the occurrence rates of the "diseases" that they identify. The immediate effect is on the "diseases" diagnosed at the medical centers where these tests are usually first developed and adopted; the delayed effect takes place over many years as the new adjuncts are slowly disseminated into use by practicing physicians in the communities beyond the medical centers. The availability and dissemination of these new diagnostic procedures will often differ from one year to the next, and certainly from one decade to the next, creating major changes in the clinical opinions that are offered as names of "diseases."

The temporal changes in diagnostic tactics are particularly important in death certificate data, since the clinician's final statement on the certificate is seldom subjected to revision or confirmation by necropsy. Necropsy is performed for only about 20 per cent of deaths in the United States today[22]; it does not always yield a clear diagnostic answer when performed; and its results do not always appear on the death certificate, which is usually filled out before the necropsy is done. Consequently, the "vital statistics" used in so much of epidemiologic reasoning depend mainly on the diagnoses made by practicing clinicians.

Although temporal alterations in standards can greatly affect the way that clinicians "vote" when identifying "disease," no major surveys have been done to study the changing incidence and prevalence of the intellectual fashions, paraclinical tests, and diagnostic criteria that so greatly influence which "diseases" will be designated, when, and where. Even when epidemiologists acknowledge that the availability of new diagnostic tests may change the occurrence of certain "diseases," the temporal *dissemination* of the tests from academia to community is not considered.

The Surgeon General's report[27] provides another useful example of the limited awareness of some of these hazards. According to that report, the rising incidence of lung cancer between 1947 and 1960 could not be due to any new identification tests because "there were no significant advances in diagnostic methods" during that period.[28] The presumptive reason for this statement is that exfoliative cytology techniques were first described in 1945. What is ignored in the statement, however, is not the mere existence of a test, but its dissemination. Exfoliative cytologic studies of sputum were not in use at many hospitals until at least a decade after Papanicolaou introduced the test. As the sputum "pap" smear became disseminated to practicing doctors, it would help identify many cases of lung cancer that had previously escaped detection. The dissemination of a new test, rather than its mere existence, could thus lead to a rising annual incidence of a disease. This possibility, and many other aspects of changing diagnostic rates for disease, are regularly overlooked in the type of reasoning used in the Surgeon General's report.

The hazards of tilted targets are not unknown to people who work with clinical rather than general populations. In a celebrated account of the error that is now known as "Berkson's fallacy", Berkson[4] showed that differential bias in the rates of hospital admission could cause spurious associations in the concurrence of diseases. Thus, if gallstones are found more often in hospitalized diabetic patients than in a "control" hospital population, we can not conclude that gallstones and diabetes are associated. We would first have to demonstrate equality of target detection: did members of the general (or the "control") population have the same prevalence of opportunities and tests for detecting gall-

stones as members of the hospitalized diabetic population?

Another classic error, based on neglect of Berkson's fallacy and on failure to check for a tilted target, occurred during a major statistical study of a necropsy population.[24] Patients who died with and without cancer at necropsy were carefully matched for sex, race, and date of death. Because active tuberculosis was recorded in 6.6 per cent of the cancer patients but in 16.3 per cent of the noncancer group, the investigators concluded that tuberculosis was antagonistic to cancer. Extensive efforts were then instituted to use tuberculin in treating neoplastic disease. This old "blooper" seems to have been forgotten by the many epidemiologic investigators today who engage in similar acts of retrospective "matching." As Mainland[21] describes the denouement[25] of the situation,

Then a serious flaw was thought of—the possibility that cancer killed its victims quicker than did many of the other diseases, and therefore gave a person less time to develop florid tuberculosis such as was found in members of the noncancerous group. The concept of a cancer-tuberculosis antagonism was quickly dropped; but we ought not to forget the story, because the biostatistician responsible for the research method and the conclusions was one of the most penetrating thinkers in his field.

The fallacies created by tilted targets have thus become painfully evident to political pollsters, to pathologists, and to clinicians. Although epidemiologists may privately acknowledge the hazard, it is not given major attention in epidemiologic textbooks, in the literature of epidemiologic research, and in such analytic reviews as those contained in the Surgeon General's report. A century ago, convinced of the therapeutic value of blood-letting, many clinicians argued that therapeutic trials or other proofs of the procedure were not necessary. Epidemiologists today seem equally convinced that no tests or precautions need be taken to ensure against the distortions introduced by a tilted target. In clinical medicine, the value (or lack of value) of the old therapeutic doctrines was demonstrated as soon as satisfactory scientific studies were done. In epidemiology, some of the current doctrines may also become altered when chronic diseases are investigated with satisfactory scientific methods that arrange for the effects of bias to be assessed in the numerators as well as in the denominators of the compared statistical ratios.

3. Reliability of data

An additional defect of the polling techniques used in the Dewey-Truman presidential election of 1948 was the pollsters' assumption that the "undecided" vote would be split for each candidate in the same proportion as the "undecided" ballots.[26] Since Dewey held the lead among "decided" voters in the poll, his share of the "undecided" group would presumably maintain a margin of victory. On Election Day, however, Truman was the choice of most of the "undecided" voters, who had apparently been reluctant earlier to express what seemed to be an unpopular belief. As a result of this problem, the interviewers in political polls now use many additional questions to assess the reliability of the replies they receive.

The issue of reliability in data is the last of the major scientific defects that beset contemporary epidemiologic statistics. Although most scientific investigators will ordinarily go to great lengths to check the reliability of the data with which they work, a corresponding concern has not been evident in epidemiologic surveys. When the data are obtained from mailed questionnaires, the investigators seldom determine whether the questions were understood or correctly answered by the recipients. A second set of identical questionnaires is rarely mailed to determine whether the repeat responses are consistent with those received in the first set. When the data are obtained from death certificates, such target variables as the diagnoses of disease are not thoroughly checked for accuracy. From time to time, an effort is made to verify certain diagnoses re-corded on death certificates, but the efforts have always been biased toward the detection of false positive diagnoses only.[10] Thus, when lung cancer appears on a death certificate, investigators may seek substantiating evidence to ensure against a false positive diagnosis, but the investigators do not explore the problem of *false negative* diagnoses. As noted earlier, about 20% of lung cancers found at necropsy have not been diagnosed during life. Nevertheless, epidemiologists have not performed careful tests to note the way that their data may be distorted by the occurrence of lung cancer in people for whom the diagnosis was *not* recorded on the death certificate.

These problems in reliability of data are major scientific hazards for the many epidemiologists and statisticians whose analytic work depends on the mortality data assembled by the Bureau of Vital Statistics. An epidemiologist who performs direct populational surveys may not always be as scientifically careful as Deming[6] recommends, but at least he does active research. He must design a questionnaire, find a population, get the questions to the people, receive their responses, and evaluate the responses. By contrast, an analyst of mortality data need not make any plans for collecting information and need not even leave his desk. All he has to do is wait for the Bureau of Vital Statistics to receive and tabulate death certificates, whose design is standardized and whose preparation is a traditional obligation of clinicians. Passively receiving the Bureau's tabulations about rates of death, the epidemiologist becomes a poll-bearer, rather than a poll-taker.

One obvious source of unreliable data in these poll-bearing activities is the unequal skills of the diverse clinicians who fill out the certificates. Instead of carefully checking this source of unreliability, epidemiologic statisticians often regard it as being unimportant. The belief is based on the assumption that the vicissitudes of the clinical data-recorders will create random errors, with cancelling effects in all directions. This assumption might be acceptable if the data were free from any systematic sources of general bias. At least three main sources of systematic bias, however, destroy the blithe assumption that the only problem to be considered (or ignored) is the diverse diagnostic skills of clinicians.

One such source has been discussed earlier in this essay and elsewhere[10]: the changing standards of criteria, technology, and concepts of disease from one era to the next. Another source of bias is the bizarre oscillations in disease categories imposed by changes in the hierarchial ratings and coding rubrics assigned to the diagnosed diseases each decade by statisticians.[7, 10, 16, 29] The third major source of systematic bias is the excessive rigidity and general inadequacy of the death certificate as a "questionnaire." William Farr, who is generally regarded as having founded modern "vital statistics" a century ago, was vigorously opposed to inflexible classification procedures that did not allow for adequate description of doubt. Said Farr,[9] "The refusal to recognize terms that express imperfect knowledge has an obvious tendency to encourage reckless conjecture." Farr's advice seems to have been unheeded by his successors.

In its current format, the death certificate appears to have been deliberately designed to produce a specious specificity. It makes no request for evidence or criteria for the cited diagnoses; it allows no room for honest doubt; and it demands a statement not only of the disease regarded as *the* cause of death, but also a list of the contributing diseases, arranged in their sequential order of lethality. Every clinician who has ever filled out a death certificate is thus familiar with the problems of the "undecided voter."

In many instances, a definite disease has not been identified, and, in many other instances, a single cause of death cannot be selected from the array of diagnoses. Even when necropsy is performed, the issue of "cause of death" is seldom easily resolved. Although newspapers and magazines often describe isolated cases that were brilliantly "solved" in the morgue, no exciting articles are published about the much more frequent situations in which a specific single cause of death cannot be identified. Sometimes no cause is evident; sometimes there are too many candidates; sometimes death was due to a conditon—such as cardiac arrhythmia or diabetic acidosis—requiring detection with special functional or chemical tests that cannot be applied in the routine morphologic examinations at necropsy; sometimes a leading suspect is present, but the actual mechanism of death is uncertain. The selection of *the* cause of death is an extraordinary difficult task, particularly for patients with chronic diseases. A good clinician or pathologist can often identify most of the diseases that were present, but he can seldom say exactly what was *the* precise cause of death. He often does not know; nor does anyone else.

A clinician (or a pathologist) may thus be unable to decide which disease caused death in a patient who had widespread cancer of the colon, advanced cerebral arteriosclerosis, multiple myocardial infarctions, and diffuse bronchopneumonia. Reluctant to make a choice, the clinician is not permitted by the death certificate to be an undecided voter. He is obligated to choose *a* cause of death, so he picks one, and, depending on his arbitrary choice, the patient enters the statistical lists as a case of either heart disease, stroke, cancer, or something else.

Difficult as the problem may be for a pathologist who has the open body before him, the situation is much worse when the death certificate must be filled out, as most of them are, in circumstances distant from the diagnostic paraphernalia of a major medical center. The clinician is often not exactly *certain* of any diagnosis, let alone an exact cause of death. Yet he is not permitted to state, when necessary, that the patient died of uncertain but apparently natural causes, nor can the clinician make any other allowances for doubt in listing the sequence of lethal diseases. The rigid form of the death certificate is there, with all its structured spaces, and each space must be filled in as demanded, with a particular disease cited as *the* cause of death, and with an order of succession for the "contributory" diseases. If the clinician fails to fill in all the exact demands of the form and does not precisely state the cause of death, the surviving family may think him stupid, the insurance company may delay payment, and the funeral director may even refuse to accept the body.

So the clinician often make a guess. Generally an intelligent, educated, thoughtful guess; a guess that seems as reasonable and as consistent as possible with the diagnostic concepts of the era; a guess that may often be right or often wrong—but a guess. Anyone who has ever experienced the realities of clinical medicine knows about these guesses, and about the way they may be biased by the fashions of the doctor's training and his environment.[1, 10] The results of this guesswork continue, however, to be assiduously collected, industriously tabulated, and avidly analyzed, and the product is called "vital statistics."

A death certificate today is a documentation of the name, age, and sex of a person, and the time and place of an event; the certificate provides a civilized passport to the disposal of a dead body, but not a scientific identification of disease. Until major improvements are made in the collection, organization, and standardization of the data, the information about individual diseases cannot be used in serious scientific activities. Nevertheless, without careful assessment of the multiple human and technologic fashions that can distort the cited diagnoses and "causes" of death, the certificates have been confidently used as the basis for gauging the changing frequency of diseases, for major statistical studies of various "causal associations," and for new epidemiologic surveys seeking etiologic explanations for different geographic rates of chronic disease. As the mortality rates for various diseases rise and fall in different countries at different years,

it is impossible to decide how much of the change is due to nature, to technologic changes, to preventive measures, to therapeutic advances, to fashions of opinion, or to inconsistent guesses and conclusions by that undecided voter: the clinician.

• • •

Not all modern epidemiologists perform "research" in the manner described here, and many new surveys have been carried out with methods that improve or remove the cited defects. Some of the new "active" investigators have even openly acknowledged the scientific disparity between preaching and practice in the older, "passive" epidemiologic research. According to Wright and Acheson,[31]

> If the field epidemiologist is to maintain his integrity, he must be prepared to admit that, as often as not, the circumstances underlying the judgments made by him and his colleagues do not quite come up to the standards which he himself may indicate to be desirable in his teaching.

Regardless of the efforts being made in new investigations, the vast bulk of existing epidemiologic statistics about incidence, prevalence and causes of chronic disease has been assembled with the apparent philosophy of "better bad data than none." For many major activities in medical science, epidemiologic statisticians have preferred to work with quantitative data rather than with unquantified recollections alone, and have hoped that "good judgment" would be used in recognizing and evaluating the defects of the data.

The hope that good judgment will remedy poor science has been a wishful dream throughout all of medical history, and the annals of medical history are filled with the ruins of the dream. In the evaluation of clinical therapy, clinicians for centuries used a fallacious philosophy of *post hoc ergo propter hoc* to justify all the blood-letting, blistering, purging, and puking that were once regarded as the basic staples of treatment. In concepts of the etiology of disease, clinicians used the same *post hoc* or other defective philosophies to create beliefs in the angry gods, unfriendly demons, deranged humors, contagious miasmas, visceral inflammations, dystonic blood vessels, defective teeth, and toxic organs that have incorrectly— from ancient to modern times—been held responsible for causing disease.

During the past few decades, the fallacies of *post hoc* reasoning in therapy have come under scientific reappraisal. Clinicians have recognized the need for appropriate comparison and quantification, and have begun to apply scientific methods in both surveys and trials of therapy. The methods still require many clinical and statistical improvements, but the defects of the old approaches have been amply recognized, and the need for better scientific methods is well accepted.

The fallacies of *post hoc* etiologic reasoning have received neither the same recognition nor commensurate efforts at improvement. Although Koch's postulates could be used several generations ago to provide experimental evidence for causes of infectious disease, a different methodology has been needed for the chronic diseases that are prime targets of contemporary research. This methodologic vacuum has been filled by statistical procedures.

What is at stake here is not such specific issues as whether coronary disease is caused by physical inactivity, lung cancer by cigarette smoking, or thrombophlebitis by the "pill." The main issue is whether clinicians, mindful of their long history of erroneous therapeutic and etiologic reasoning, are to be led uncritically into a new philosophy in which diverse characterizations of disease and causal "proofs" are based on elaborate numerical analyses of bad scientific data.

In diagnostic activities, clinicians have now begun to use extraordinary precision for identifying diseases. In therapeutic activities, clinicians have begun to use scientific procedures for assembling suitable evidence, and have begun to recognize that in treatment, as in guerrilla warfare, success cannot be gauged from body counts alone. But in epidemologic activities, clinicians have accepted the results of body counts assembled without scientific verification of either the procedures or the data.

To obtain satisfactory medical data from a valid random sampling of a human population is an extraordinarily difficult and almost heroic epidemiologic task. Because the task is so formidable, it has been approached with convenient but defective techniques of sampling and data collecting. Although the results have been widely accepted, thoughtful medical scientists will be uneasy about the wisdom of allowing the heroic diagnostic and therapeutic advances of the past few decades to be accompanied by less than heroic epidemiologic research.

The acquisition of a truly random sample is almost impossible for a large general population. With appropriate ingenuity and effort, however, satisfactory samples can be attained from random choices within suitably selected strata and clusters of the population.[6] The problems of death certificates cannot be solved merely by statistical manipulations of the data and by decennial shufflings of the terms used in coding. The certificate itself must be changed to correspond to clinical realities, and connoisseurs of modern clinical and pathologic diagnosis should be enlisted to help explain those realities to the coders and other statistical personnel.[10, 17] Perhaps the most easily removed of the existing difficulties are the defects due to target tilting and unverified data. These problems can be solved as soon as epidemiologic investigators recall that valid evidence—rather than statistical theory, magisterial computation, or imaginative conjecture—is the primary principle of scientific research.

The obliteration of science during the collection of numbers was deplored a half century ago by Major Greenwood,[14] one of the founders of modern epidemiology:

Because the results of their labour are useful, the compilers and analysers of these statistics are no more entitled to rank as scientific investigators than are the equally useful artisans who manufacture our laboratory apparatus.

Modern investigators who regard scientific method as a fundamental necessity in epidemiology will also note the recommendation of Bradford Hill[5]:

One need not accept as final what some third party can give or chooses to give. . . . One must go seek more facts, paying less attention to technique of handling the data and far more to the development and perfection of methods of obtaining them.

For such investigators, the main challenges of scientific epidemiology will be found not in the speculator's arm chair, the questionnaire-collector's mail room, the tabulator's annual volumes, the statistician's desk calculator, or the computer aficionado's terminal. The challenges will be to develop suitable strategies for choosing a proper sampling of population, persuading and examining the selected people, validating the tests and other procedures for gathering data, maintaining liaison with the population during the follow-up period, and performing satisfactory examinations of the subsequent state.

Additional incentive can come from the classical exhortation of Francis Galton[13]:

It is the triumph of scientific men to rise superior to . . . superstitions, to desire tests by which the value of beliefs may be ascertained, and to feel sufficiently masters of themselves to discard . . . whatever may be found untrue.

When Galton made that remark many years ago, he was urging the use of statistical methods in epidemiologic science. His remark still pertains today; but the need is for scientific methods in epidemiologic statistics.

References

1. Anderson, D. O.: Geographic variations in deaths due to emphysema and bronchitis in Canada, Canad. Med. Ass. J. **98**:231-241, 1968.
2. Barrett-Connor, E.: The etiology of pellagra and its significance for modern medicine, Amer. J. Med. **42**:859-867, 1967. (Edit.)
3. Beadenkopf, W. G., Abrams, M., Daoud, A., and Marks, R. V.: An assessment of certain medical aspects of death certificate data for epidemiologic study of arteriosclerotic heart disease, J. Chron. Dis. **16**:249, 1963.
4. Berkson, J.: Limitations of the application of fourfold table analysis to hospital data, Biometrics Bull. **2**:47-53, 1946.
5. Bradford Hill, A.: Observation and experiment, New Eng. J. Med. **248**:995, 1953.
6. Deming, W. E.: Some theory of sampling, New York, 1966, Dover Publications. (Paperback.)
7. Dorn, H. F.: Mortality, *in* Lilienfeld, A. M., and Gifford, A. J., editors: Chronic diseases and public health, Baltimore, 1966, Johns Hopkins Press, pp. 23-54.
8. Farr, W.: Influence of elevation on the fatality of cholera, J. Stat. Soc. **15**:155-183, 1852.
9. Farr, W.: *Quoted in* Greenwood, M.: The medical dictator, and other biographical studies, London, 1936, Williams and Norgate, Ltd.
10. Feinstein, A. R.: Clinical epidemiology. II. The identification rates of disease, Ann. Intern. Med. **69**:1037-1061, 1968.
11. Feinstein, A. R.: Clinical biostatistics. II. Statistics versus science in the design of experiments, CLIN. PHARMACOL. THER. **11**:282-292, 1970.
12. Feinstein, A. R.: Clinical biostatistics. IV. The architecture of clinical research (continued), CLIN. PHARMACOL. THER. **11**:595-610, 1970.
13. Galton, F.: Quoted *in* Inside cover of each issue of Ann. Hum. Genet.
14. Greenwood, M.: Is statistical method of any value in medical research? Lancet **2**:153-158, 1924.
15. Heasman, M. A.: Accuracy of death certification, Proc. Roy. Soc. Med. **55**:733, 1962.
16. Israel, R. A., and Klebba, A. J.: A preliminary report on the effect of eighth revision ICDA on cause of death statistics, Amer. J. Public Health **59**:1651-1660, 1969.
17. James, G., Patton, R. E., and Heslin, A. S.: Accuracy of cause-of-death statements on death certificates, Public Health Rep. **70**:39, 1955.
18. Kendall, M. G., and Buckland, W. R.: A dictionary of statistical terms, ed. 2, New York, 1960, Hafner Publishing Co.
19. Lasagna, L., and von Felsinger, J. M.: The volunteer subject in research, Science **120**:359-361, 1954.
20. Likert, R.: Public opinion polls, Scientific American **179**:7-11, 1948.
21. Mainland, D.: Elementary medical statistics, ed. 2, Philadelphia, 1963, W. B. Saunders Company.
22. National Center for Health Statistics, Division of Vital Statistics, United States Department of Health, Education, and Welfare: Vital Statistics of the United States, vol. I: Mortality, Washington, D. C., 1963, United States Government Printing Office.

23. National Center For Health Statistics: Cycle I of the Health Examination Survey; sample and response. Vital and Health Statistics. PHS Pub. No. 1000—Series 11. No. 1. Public Health Service Washington, April, 1964, United States Government Printing Office.

24. Pearl, R.: Cancer and tuberculosis, Amer. J. Hyg. **9:**97-159, 1929.

25. Pearl, R.: A note on the association of diseases, Science **70:**191-192 (August 23), 1929.

26. Rogers, L.: The pollsters, New York, 1949, Alfred A. Knopf.

27. Surgeon General's Advisory Committee On Smoking and Health. Smoking and Health 1964. United States Department of Health, Education and Welfare, Public Health Service Publication No. 1103.

28. Surgeon General's Advisory Committee On Smoking and Health. Smoking and Health 1964. United States Department of Health, Education and Welfare, Public Health Service Publication No. 1103. p. 140.

29. Van Buren, G. H.: Some things you can't prove by mortality statistics, *in* Vital Statistics—Special Reports, Department of Commerce, Bureau of the Census, **12:**191, 1940.

30. Wallis, W. A., and Roberts, H. V.: The nature of statistics, New York, 1965, The Free Press. (Paperback edition.)

31. Wright, E. C., and Acheson, R. M.: New Haven survey of joint diseases. XI. Observer variability in the assessment of x-rays for osteoarthrosis of the hands, Amer. J. Epidem. **91:** 378-392, 1970.

32. Yerushalmy, J.: On inferring causality from observed associations, *in* Ingelfinger, F. J., Relman, A. S., and Finland, M., editors: Controversy in Internal Medicine, Philadelphia, 1966, W. B. Saunders Company, pp. 659-668.

CHAPTER 13

Ambiguity and abuse in the twelve different concepts of 'control'

Sir Ronald Fisher began his classic book,[8] *The Design of Experiments*, by pointing out that a critic who refuses to accept the conclusions of an experiment can take "two lines of attack." In one approach, the critic believes that the results have received a faulty interpretation. In the second approach, the experiment itself is regarded as "ill designed."

After deciding that the first approach—criticism of interpretation—belonged to "the domain of statistics," Fisher seemed to regret that the second approach—criticism of design—was often employed by people who were not "professed statisticians" and whose main qualification was only "prolonged experience or at least the long possession of a scientific reputation." Fisher complained that "technical details are seldom in evidence" when a "heavyweight authority" attempts to discredit the design of a research project by making assertions such as "his *controls* are totally *inadequate*."

Fisher may have been quite justified in disparaging an expert who makes disparaging remarks without citing the justification of "technical details," but where can either an expert or a novice find an account of the details that define an adequate *control*? Such details are obviously crucial for scientific plans and interpreta-tions, but the details are not presented in the writings of "professed statisticians." The concept and choice of a control receive almost no discussion in Fisher's work, and the word *control* does not appear in either the index or the table of contents for any of his three epochal books[7-9] on statistics and research.

The challenge has also not been accepted by Fisher's successors. Despite his warning that "the statistician cannot excuse himself from the duty of getting his head clear on the principles of scientific inference," and despite the many subsequent statistical publications devoted to the "design of experiments," a clearheaded account of the principles of *control* has not yet appeared in the statistical literature. The word *control* constantly occurs in diverse statistical discussions, but the concept of control is still defined ambiguously, and the concept is often applied imprecisely or erroneously.

According to Kendall and Buckland's dictionary,[10] which usually serves as an arbiter of statistical terms, *control* can be employed in at least two different statistical senses. One of these ideas is stated as follows: "If a process produces a set of data under what are essentially the same conditions and the internal variations are found to be random, then the process is said to be statistically under control. The separate observations are, in fact, equivalent to random drawings from a

Under the same name, this chapter originally appeared as "Clinical biostatistics—XIX." In Clin. Pharmacol. Ther. 14:112, 1973.

population distributed according to some fixed probability law." This statistical idea refers to the regulation of a process, and is applied most often as part of the reasoning (to be discussed later) that laboratory workers use for an entity usually called *Quality Control*.

The second definition of *control* ". . . concerns experimentation for the testing of a new method, process, or factor against an accepted standard. That part of the test which involves the standard of comparison is known as the control." This statistical idea refers to comparison, and is the concept that most research workers would use in describing the role of a control when different investigative maneuvers are contrasted.

In addition to these two definitions, Kendall and Buckland describe three other usages of *control*. Two of these occur in the terms *control chart* and *control limits*, both of which are applied during procedures used for testing quality control. The third additional idea, called *control of substrata*, is ". . . a term used in sampling inquiries to denote the employment of . . . factors which are being used in a scheme of multiple stratification." According to this idea, when we divide survey data that have been cited for two baseline (or "initial state") variables, we would control the substrata if we express the results according to groups demarcated with both variables. For example, if the baseline variables were *age* and *sex*, our controlled substrata might be expressed as **young men, young women, old men,** and **old women.**

The statistical dictionary thus provides at least three distinctly different ideas for *control*: the quality with which a process is performed; the maneuver that is compared in an experiment; and the characteristics of the objects compared in a survey. With these three different ideas to create ambiguity in the use of *control*, it is not surprising that the term is applied with so much confusion. Unfortunately, however, Kendall and Buckland have

omitted many other ways in which the word *control* is used in clinical science and biostatistical analysis. The idea of *control* is actually applied in at least twelve different ways rather than three. In the rest of this discussion, I shall describe the diverse uses of the term *control*, and I shall cite some of the points that weighty authorities might make about its abuse. A few of the points are statistical, but most of them rest on straightforward concepts in biology and clinical science.

Perhaps the most direct way to demonstrate these ideas is in reference to the "architectural" model that was proposed earlier in this series[3, 4] to describe a research project, and to develop certain scientific principles in the choice of "controls." In that model, the *initial state* of an entity is exposed to a *maneuver* and undergoes a response observed in the *subsequent state*. With this model in mind, we can proceed to the different ways in which the idea of *control* appears in the architecture of clinical research.

A. The idea of regulation

Four of the twelve different uses of *control* occur in reference to the idea of regulating, governing, or choosing a particular entity. The concept of comparison is not included in these applications of the term.

1. Control of the maneuver. This type of control is what distinguishes an experiment from a survey. In an experiment, the investigator "controls"—i.e., governs, decides, assigns, or chooses—the maneuver to which each investigated entity is exposed. In a survey, the maneuver is chosen by nature or by man, but not by the investigator. Thus, a therapeutic trial is an experiment, because the clinical investigator assigns the treatment to each patient. A survey of therapy is not an experiment, because the treatments were chosen *ad hoc* by other doctors or by patients, or by both. Almost all of the contemporary epidemiologic investigations of alleged causes of disease—such as diet, urban living, smoking, and oral contraceptive pills—have been performed not as experiments, but as surveys in which the investigated maneuver was usually self-selected.

If the investigator controls the assignment of the maneuver, he can make the assignment by randomization, thereby allowing subsequent application of statistical inference based on random allocation. If the investigator does not control the maneuver, its allocation occurs with all of the possible bias that can enter human decisions. The differences found thereafter may be caused by the initial bias, rather than by the effects of the compared maneuvers. The differences found in these circumstances cannot be properly assessed with tests based on probabilistic statistical inference, and one of the scientist's main jobs in analyzing survey data is to seek out the bias and make suitable adjustments for it. This potential bias in allocation of the maneuver is not removed by selecting a "random sample" of population, since this aspect of randomness refers to choice of the population, rather than assignment of the maneuvers. Thus, if tense people are likely to die young and also selectively move to urban regions, we shall find a higher death rate in urban rather than rural locations, regardless of whether or not the urban-rural sample of population was chosen randomly.

Many of the fallacious statistics contained in so many epidemiologic and clinical surveys today are due to confusion about this type of control. The statistician who learned about research from courses in *experimental design* may not be familiar with the many potential sources of major bias that can occur in a non-experimental *survey*, in which the investigator did not control the assignment of the maneuvers. Instead of urging the investigator to search for bias and to correct the data accordingly, the statistician may accept the distorted results as if they were experimental data. He may then massage the data with tests of significance, relative risk rates, logistic function analyses, and other tactics that are statistically inappropriate and

scientifically misleading if the basic information has been distorted by unrecognized bias.

2. Quality control. The regulation of a process evokes three different uses of the word *control*. In the procedures of "quality control"—which refers to the first of the definitions cited by Kendall and Buckland—the process is used to produce a particular entity, such as a barrel of beer or a measurement of serum cholesterol. To determine how well the process is being performed, the investigator uses certain well-defined statistical tactics.

For a tangible product, such as beer, the assessment depends on measuring the size, shape, or some other dimensional property of the finished product. If the individual products have similar values for this measurement, the results are regarded as consistent, and the process is regarded as having high quality. An analogous procedure is used if the "product" is a measurement itself. Such measurements are the principal event that occurs in modern laboratory medicine, where quality control of the numerous chemical, microbiologic, and other technologic tests has become a paramount scientific challenge.

The approaches used in meeting this challenge are heavily dependent on statistical principles, and a thoughtful account of the procedures has recently been published by Roy Barnett.[2] From a repeated measurement of the same specimen of material, the laboratory personnel can determine the mean and standard deviation, and can prepare *control charts* that show the upper and lower *control limits* for the measurement. The personnel can also develop procedures for determining "external quality control" when the same specimen is measured at different laboratories.

This is the type of activity for which statistical principles are applied magnificently, since the process of measurement was the stimulus for the original ideas that led to development of theories about the disperson of "errors" in measurement, and that produced the shape of the frequency distribution now known as a "normal" or Gaussian curve. Although developed for the variations found in the process of measuring objects, these statistical principles were later applied to describe the variability of the objects themselves. The new application of the principles has now become traditional, but has also become a source of major problems[5] in clinical epidemiologic research. We can safely assume that multiple measurements of a single specimen of serum glucose will have a "normal distribution" and we can safely accept the mean of those values as the "correct" measurement. We cannot safely assume, however, that single measurements of multiple specimens of serum glucose from a group of people will be "normally distributed," nor can we safely assume that a "normal range" for the people who provided those specimens will be determined by Gaussian statistics.

These problems, which are beyond the scope of this discussion, create major difficulties in clinical activities. In trying to interpret a single measurement for a patient, the clinician must contemplate the variability of the laboratory's quality control, as well as the variability encountered in human populations. To cope with the latter forms of variability, the clinician must consider some of the many other types of control that are not expressible in statistical formulations.

3. Control of the disease process. This type of *control* refers to the adequacy with which a program of therapy produces certain desired effects in the "activity" of a patient's disease. In hypoglycemic treatment of diabetes mellitus, for example, the purpose is to keep the blood sugar or urine sugar regulated within certain boundaries. When such regulation occurs, the sugar (or the patient) is said to be in "good control." A similar phrase is used in referring to maintenance of a "remission" in a patient with acute leukemia, or to the lowering of serum cholesterol in a patient with hyperlipidemia.

The description of this type of control often occupies an unusual position in the architecture of a research project. The control is expressed as a variable having such categories as **good** or **bad, rise** or **fall,** and **in remission** or **active,** but the variable is not a baseline characteristic noted in the initial state, and it is often not the principal target event noted in the subsequent state. Thus, in a study of hypoglycemic agents for patients with diabetes mellitus, the main target events might be vascular complications, and the concomitant regulation of blood sugar would be an ancillary variable in the subsequent state. In a previous discussion,[6] I suggested the term *synchronous variable* for the citation of this type of regulation. It refers to an entity that is noted after onset of the main maneuver (such as therapy), and before or during the occurrence (or nonoccurrence) of the events that are the main target variables.

In other situations, the regulation of the disease process may be the principal target of the maneuver. Thus, the production (rather than maintenance) of a remission is often the main goal of treatment for acute leukemia, and the reduction of "disease activity" may be the prime target in patients with rheumatic fever or rheumatoid arthritis.

4. Control of the environment. This topic refers to the investigator's ability to govern the environment in which the research maneuvers are administered. The experimenter in the laboratory can "control" the cages in which the animals live, can ascertain that they are given and ingest the assigned medication, and can make them appear for all of the planned examinations and procedures. The investigator who deals with human populations has no such options, and must contend with the possible bias caused by migration or loss of patients, and by noncompliance with either the prescribed maneuver or with the schedule of follow-up examinations.

The difficulties that can occur between the inception of the maneuver and the observation of the subsequent state have been discussed elsewhere[6] as problems in "intrusion." Among the most striking of these problems are those that arise when an effective oral medication is spuriously deemed ineffective because patients failed to take it; when compliance requires an unusual psychic resolution that may distort the characteristics and outcome of the self-selected group of people who are able to comply; and when the detection of the target event in compared groups of people is distorted by inequalities in the frequency and intensity of the diagnostic procedures used to detect the target.

The performance of compliance and of target detectability can also often be expressed as synchronous variables. Although the control of these environmental features of research is another aspect of "regulation," any of the synchronous variables cited here or in the previous section can become a member of the "control strata," described later, that are used for comparing results. Many crucial analyses in clinical or epidemiologic research may depend on appropriate division of the population according to compliance with the maneuver; changes in sugar, cholesterol, or white blood count; or the frequency and intensity of diagnostic tests. Nevertheless, as discussed previously,[6] these synchronous variables are generally ignored in most statistical "models" of experimental design for clinical research. The stratified gradations in this type of "control" may be completely neglected in many statistical reports, or the synchronous results may be analyzed in an unsatisfactory retrograde manner.[6]

B. The idea of comparison

The next five types of *control* all depend on the concept of comparison. The confusions in usage arise because the comparisons are based on different elements in the research architecture. Some of the comparisons refer to the maneuver; others, to the initial state of the objects under investigation; others, to the subsequent state; and yet others to the transitions between initial and subsequent state.

1. The control maneuver. This is the sense in which most scientific investigators think about *control*. It refers to the maneuver that is compared with the principal maneuver—the saline injection vs. the ACTH; the placebo vs. the active drug; the high dose vs. the low; non-smoking vs. smoking; urban vs. rural life.

The choice of appropriate control maneuvers is a sophisticated, subtle act of scientific reasoning. As described previously,[4] a proper choice requires suitable attention to a complex array of "technical details." These details include: the *potency* of dosage or other procedures with which the maneuvers are administered; the *relativity* with which comparative maneuvers are chosen to demonstrate efficacy or efficiency; the *internal accompaniment* provided by the ancillary ingredients or excipients of a pharmaceutical agent, or the anesthesia and other concomitants of surgery; the *external accompaniment* provided by postoperative recovery rooms and solicitous medical personnel; and the *concurrency* with which comparative maneuvers precede, parallel, or follow the principal maneuver. In view of the scientific complexity, it is not surprising that investigators sometimes choose control maneuvers that are "totally inadequate" and that statisticians may not recognize the defects.

A classic example of an unsatisfactory control maneuver occurred in a highly publicized recent experiment[1] designed by a pathologist collaborating with a statistician. Warm air containing cigarette smoke was pumped into the tracheostomy of beagle dogs, who were then examined for pulmonary lesions. Every intelligent layman to whom I have described this experiment has promptly selected the appropriate control maneuver. Warm air (devoid of cigarette smoke) should have been pumped into the tracheostomy of the control dogs. Nevertheless, in the actual experiment, the comparative maneuver consisted of insertion of a tracheostomy tube alone, without anything else.

The decision that a particular comparative maneuver is inadequate cannot be made with any statistical reasoning and is apparently sometimes not evident to experienced investigators. By considering the stated principles[4] of potency, relativity, accompaniment, and concurrency, a reviewer can often quickly discern what may be wrong, but the application and interpretation of those principles will usually rest on a mixture of judgment, wisdom, and common sense.

2. *Size of the control group.* The "control group" consists of the entities who receive the comparative (or control) maneuver. These entities might be the rats who get the saline injection, the patients who receive placebo, or the dogs who get (or failed to get) warm air blown into a tracheostomy.

An important scientific principle of research is that the groups receiving the control maneuvers and the investigative maneuvers be qualitatively similar before the maneuvers are instigated. This qualitative aspect of similarity depends on the control of strata, as described in the next section. The quantitative similarity of groups is a different issue, however. Ordinarily, we would like the compared groups to have the same number of members. This equal-size principle is intuitively appealing and also has the numerical virtue of being most likely, *ceteris paribus*, to produce "statistical significance" in the results.

On certain occasions, however, particularly when multiple maneuvers are being compared in the same experiment, some of the groups may be made proportionately larger or smaller than others. For example, if a single placebo group acts as the "control" for four treatment groups, we might make the placebo group substantially larger than any of the others. If a single medication is being given at two dosage levels, we might make each dosage group half the size of the other groups so that the results for the two dosages can be combined into a single full-size group for that medication.

The planning of deliberate inequalities in the size of compared groups is one of the statistical subtleties of experimental design. Regardless of why the inequalities are chosen, the investigators who make

such plans are scientifically obligated to describe their reasons and justifications. Without such descriptions, the readers of a published report cannot discern whether a gross imbalance in the size of compared groups is due to perceptive planning, capricious plodding, or an unforeseen disaster that the investigators hope will pass unnoticed.

An interesting example of an unexplained gross imbalance in sample sizes occurred in the aforementioned investigation[10] of smoking dogs. The group that "smoked" through a tracheostomy contained 86 dogs. The "control" group that had a tracheostomy alone contained 8 dogs. The investigators provided no statement of how and why this bizarre disparity occurred.

3. *Control of the strata.* This type of control refers to the last meaning cited by Kendall and Buckland.[10] If we were comparing treatment X vs. treatment Y in patients with diabetes mellitus, we would "control" for sex if we divided the patients into men and women, and analyzed the results of the two treatments separately in each sex group.

Readers of previous papers in this series should immediately recognize that this type of "control" is achieved by stratifying the patients according to characteristics that are present in the baseline initial state, before the maneuver is imposed. The purpose of prognostically predictive or other forms of stratification is to achieve qualitative similarity in the compared groups. This type of stratification is used to avoid or reduce the bias that may occur when maneuvers are not assigned randomly or when the randomization does not produce equal proportions of important strata in the people assigned to the compared maneuvers.

Attention to this type of "control" has been strikingly absent from most general statistical textbooks and works devoted to "experimental design." One reason is that a statistician who thinks only about experiments, but not surveys, will obviously have no incentive to contemplate the sources of bias that enter a survey. A second reason is the basic fallacy of the currently accepted statistical "model" of experiments.

This model, which depends on the effects of only a single maneuver, is inadequate for the common clinical and epidemiologic situations in which a maneuver of human intervention or pathogenesis is imposed on an underlying maneuver of nature (or of man).

The purpose of the stratification is to identify what was done by the underlying maneuver—to separate the people according to their different degrees of baseline susceptibility for the target event that may later follow the imposed maneuver. If the stress, parental longevity, severity of clinical condition, or other features that create this susceptibility are not appropriately identified and separated, the investigator courts an intellectual disaster. He may attribute, to the imposed maneuver, results that are really due to the unrecognized underlying maneuver. This error is the data analyst's equivalent of the *post hoc ergo propter hoc* folly into which clinical reasoning has so often been seduced throughout the centuries.

Because the current statistical "model" of "experimental design" is concerned with one maneuver, rather than a dual maneuver, statisticians have had no major intellectual incentive to consider the need for two types of "control": a control that compares the overt imposed maneuvers, and a control that creates strata to "equalize" the previous effects produced by the antecedent underlying maneuvers. The literature of modern "science" thus becomes filled with large amounts of clinical and epidemiologic data that are misleading or worthless, because no attempt was made to perform the control stratifications that could help remove the diverse forms of selection bias, susceptibility bias, detection bias, compliance bias, chronology bias, and other forms of bias that permeate contemporary statistics.

An excellent example of this problem appeared in a recent survey[11] published in the *British Medical Journal*. A stellar array of investigators reported that "the children known to have been treated by physicians specializing in the treatment of leukaemia in childhood have survived

considerably longer than the others" who were treated "in the country as a whole." For this type of conclusion, a reader would surely want to know about the bias introduced by interiatric referral patterns. Were the compared patients equal in their clinical severity of illness? Were the children who were "healthier" and more likely to tolerate both the travel and the chemotherapy generally referred to the specialist physicians, whereas the sicker or moribund children were kept at home to be treated "in the country as a whole"?

A stratification according to clinical severity of illness would therefore be expected in this type of survey. In other forms of cancer, such stratifications are regularly attempted with the "staging systems" that are used in an effort to distinguish severity of illness or other major prognostic differences among patients with the same age and the same neoplastic cell type. The leukemia "working party" stated that they "had taken care to eliminate bias so far as possible from the . . . comparisons." This "care" consisted of stratifying the children with acute leukemia according to age and cell type. The patients were not staged according to the clinical severity of illness or according to any of the prognostic features that might militate for or against referral to a specialist.

Unfettered by the absence of randomization and by neglect of a major source of selection bias, the investigators nevertheless concluded that "there is good reason to believe that the improvements in survival" were due to "the availability of special facilities and expertize." The investigators also recommended that "it would seem desirable . . . that children with acute leukaemia should be referred, where this is feasible, to a centre specializing in the treatment of the disease." The chairman of the "working party," in a previous publication,[12] made the remark that "practising clinicians have not always taken kindly to the statistical approach to medical problems in which patients are considered as units in a more or less homogeneous whole." The absence of suitable stratifications is one of the main reasons for the scientifically unacceptable clinical conclusions that emerge when the prognostic heterogeneity of patients is ignored and left uncontrolled.

4. The epidemiologic "case-control." In all of the comparisons discussed so far, the scientific reasoning proceeded in a forward direction, from cause toward effect. The comparisons dealt with the initial condition, the maneuvers, and synchronous changes that accompanied the maneuvers —but the populations were all being followed from their initial state toward their subsequent state.

A quaint tradition among chonic disease epidemiologists calls for a total reversal of the direction of scientific logic. Instead of pursuing a cohort group in the customary sequence of cause → effect, the epidemiologic investigator may begin with a population in whom the effect has already occurred. By historical or other methods of inquiry, the epidemiologist then follows the "cases" backward toward the putative cause. Thus, to determine whether contraceptive pills lead to thrombophlebitis, most scientists would assemble a population of pill-takers and non-pill-takers, follow them forward, and determine the rate with which the people in each group develop thrombophlebitis. Many epidemiologists, however, would start with people who already have thrombophlebitis, and would then determine the proportion who had taken the pill.

In this situation, the epidemiologist is confronted with the problem of getting a group of people for comparison. The people cannot be chosen in the customary scientific manner, on the basis of receiving or not receiving the investigated maneuver, because the investigation is being conducted in a backward direction. The patients are chosen according to the "effect," not the "cause," but the control groups used in scientific research are selected from the "initial state," not from the "subsequent state." Nevertheless, with a majestic display of antipodal scientific logic, epidemiologists will choose a *contrast* group from "subsequent-state" people in whom the effect has not occurred. For example, in a study of the allegedly evil effects of oral contraceptive pills, the eligible contenders for this contrast group would be people who do not have thrombophlebitis.

To add a semblance of scientific veneer to this retroverted scientific procedure, epidemiologists usually engage in various forms of "matching." Members of the contrast group are usually matched to the case group according to features of age, sex, and other data that were conveniently available to the investigator. The result is then called a "case-control" group. The tortuous reasoning used for this unique form of "control," and the many biases it ignores or creates, will be discussed in greater detail in a later installment of this series.

5. *The control value.* We now turn to a different type of "comparison": the *before* value of a *before-and-after* pair of values that form a transition variable. For example, we can measure the baseline level of serum cholesterol and call it the "control value." We then treat the patient with a lipid-lowering agent, and, after a period of time, we measure cholesterol again. The change between the two values of cholesterol then becomes the transition that is analyzed. The change is expressed as an increment (or decrement) if we subtract the control value from the new value; or as a proportion or percentage if we divide the new value by the control value. In this situation, the control value is not used for comparison in a scientific sense. It serves merely as a numerical ingredient in the subtraction or division by which we calculated the change that is the value of the transition variable.

Many investigators seem to believe, however, that this type of control value has a stronger role in comparison, and can substitute for the "control" provided by a comparative maneuver. I remember one instance several years ago when an august professor wanted to test the effect of a certain surgical procedure on a particular chemical in blood. He planned to measure the level of the chemical before surgery and after surgery, and he intended to hold the surgery responsible for any changes. When members of the institution's research committee insisted that he examine a "control group," he claimed he did not need one because the pre-surgical values were alone satisfactory. The patients would act as their "own controls."

The failure of prominent clinical academicians to understand what is meant by a controlled comparison might be excused by the fact that many clinicians have had so little training in research methods. It is more difficult to find a suitable excuse, however, when exactly the same confusion appears among statisticians, and when this confusion becomes the instructions offered in statistical textbooks devoted to the design and analysis of research data.

The quotation below is taken directly from a prominent, internationally known textbook of statistics. I have found an analogous example in another textbook of biostatistics. I shall not cite either textbook by name here because my investigation of the literature is incomplete. Had I done the research more thoroughly, I might have found similar examples in many other leading statistical books. The exact text of the "example" in that book is as follows:

> A certain stimulus is to be tested for its effect on blood pressure. Twelve men have their blood pressure measured before and after the stimulus. The results are shown in Table 8-3. Is there reason to believe that the stimulus would, on the average, raise the mean systolic blood pressure?

From the data contained in the cited table, the authors calculate the difference in the before-and-after values for each patient, perform a paired t-test, and find that t is only 1.09. Because this value is below the level of "statistical significance," the authors state that "we do not have sufficient evidence to conclude that the stimulus increases blood pressure." The implication is that if t were only high enough to be "significant," we would have satisfactory evidence for that conclusion.

This is precisely the type of defective scientific reasoning that clinicians are urged to avoid by getting consultative help from statisticians. The paired t-test might allow the investigator to conclude that a "significant" change had or had not occurred in the two pairs of readings, but no scientist would conclude that the imposed stimulus was responsible for the change. To reach the latter conclusion, we would require a

"control" maneuver, not merely a "control" value. The change observed by the statisticians may have been due to anxiety, the experimental setting, a flaw in the equipment, or many other causes other than the observed "stimulus." Nevertheless, in a renowned textbook of statistics, this blatant error in research design has been supplied to students as a fundamental example of how to perform a paired t-test.

C. The control period

The last three types of *control* refer to neither regulation nor comparison, and are produced by exactly the same phrase: *control period.*

1. Stabilization. In many experimental situations, a time interval of observation is used before the research maneuver is imposed. The main purpose of this interval is to allow the observed values of data to "stabilize" into the result that will be called the baseline or "control" value. For example, in the blood pressure experiment just cited, the baseline value may have been a single reading taken just before the stimulus was imposed. Alternatively, the patient may have been observed during a control period of several days or weeks. From the many blood pressure values obtained during that interval, the investigators then chose (or calculated) what was used as the baseline value. The calculation may have produced a mean, median, mode, or some other derivative of the data observed during the entire control period, during a period of apparent equilibrium, or during the few readings that preceded the imposition of the stimulus.

This sound scientific procedure is marred only by the frequent failure of investigators to report the details of how the "baseline" value was chosen from the values observed during the control period.

2. Qualification. A second usage of *control period* is in reference to a time interval during which the investigator tests a person's eligibility or qualification for admission to a research study. During this period the patient may be called upon to demonstrate such features as compliance with the proposed protocol, ability to remain free of diabetic ketosis on diet alone, etc. This type of "qualification trial" is a reasonable procedure in many research projects. Its main hazard is that it can create substantial bias in the ultimate results. The people who fit the qualifications for compliance or other standards may not be a representative sample of the general population of people who have the condition that is under investigation.

3. Washout. The last usage of *control period* is in reference to the "washout" interval that is often necessary between the successive therapeutic agents administered in a cross-over trial. The patient may receive placebo or no treatment during this interval. This type of control period is somewhat analogous to the first type in that its purpose is to restore stabilization. The main hazard of the washout period is that it is sometimes too short, or omitted when necessary. A frequent problem—particularly when subjective symptoms are an important variable—is the decision about whether the patient should receive placebo or no treatment during the washout.

• • •

The main purpose of this essay has been to point out the confusion that exists about the term *control,* and to specify some of the "technical details" whose absence was so distressing to R. A. Fisher. The lack of specific information about what constitutes an "adequate control," however, does not seem to have inhibited statistical dissertations devoted to the "design of experiments." Nor has the absence restrained "heavyweight authorities" in the domain of statistics from delivering oracular conclusions about the interpretation of epidemiologic surveys, clinical trials, or laboratory experiments in which the crucial controls were either omitted, malconceived, or otherwise scientifically unsatisfactory.

Of the twelve different types of control cited here, eleven are best discerned, noted, chosen, and evaluated with principles that are inherently scientific and that require no

knowledge of statistical theory. Even in the twelfth type, the statistical principles used in *quality control* require no mathematical sagacity more profound than familiarity with a mean, a standard deviation, and a Gaussian distribution. Because statisticians are obviously confused about the topic of control, clinical and epidemiologic investigators are obligated to clarify the issues and to educate our colleagues about these arcane aspects of scientific research.

The statistician who was "raised" to think only about experiments will not appreciate the bias that can occur in surveys where the populations were self-referred and the maneuvers were self-selected. The statistician who regards experimental design as an exercise in analysis of variance and Latin squares cannot appreciate the issues of potency, relativity, accompaniment, and concurrency that are needed to choose a control maneuver. The statistician whose research model makes provision only for a single maneuver cannot appreciate the need for controlling strata in the common research situations that involve a double maneuver. The statistician who mistakes a control value for a control group may have difficulty supplying helpful advice to the people who consult him for guidance in designing research.

Sir Ronald Fisher[8] said that "the statistician cannot evade the responsibility for understanding the processes he applies or recommends." In exchange for the many useful tactics that statisticians have brought to science, the least that scientific investigators can do is to help statisticians understand the processes and meet the responsibility.

References

1. Auerbach, O., Hammond, E. C., Kirman, D., and Garfinkel, L.: Effects of cigarette smoking on dogs. I. Design of experiment, mortality, and findings in lung parenchyma, Arch. Environ. Health **21:**740-753, 1970.
2. Barnett, R. N.: Clinical laboratory statistics, Boston, 1971, Little, Brown & Co.
3. Feinstein, A. R.: Clinical biostatistics. II. Statistics vs. science in the design of experiments, CLIN. PHARMACOL. THER. **11:**282-292, 1970.

4. Feinstein, A. R.: Clinical biostatistics. III-V. The architecture of clinical research, CLIN. PHARMACOL. THER. 11:432-441, 595-610, and 755-771, 1970.

5. Feinstein, A. R.: Clinical biostatistics. XII. On exorcising the ghost of Gauss and the curse of Kelvin, CLIN. PHARMACOL. THER. 12:1003-1016, 1971.

6. Feinstein, A. R.: Clinical biostatistics. XVII. Synchronous partition and bivariate evaluation in predictive stratification, CLIN. PHARMACOL. THER. 13(Part 1): 755-768, 1972.

7. Fisher, R. A.: Statistical methods and scientific inference, ed. 2, Edinburgh, 1959, Oliver & Boyd, Ltd.

8. Fisher, R. A.: The design of experiments, ed. 8, New York, 1966, Hafner Publishing Co.

9. Fisher, R. A.: Statistical methods for research workers, ed. 14, Edinburgh, 1970, Oliver & Boyd, Ltd.

10. Kendall, M. G., and Buckland, W. R.: A dictionary of statistical terms, ed. 3, Edinburgh, 1971, Oliver & Boyd, Ltd.

11. Report to the Medical Research Council from the Committee on Leukaemia and the Working Party on Leukaemia in Childhood. Duration of survival of children with acute leukaemia, Br. Med. J. 4:7-9, 1971.

12. Witts, L. J., editor: Medical surveys and clinical trials, ed. 2, London, 1964, Oxford University Press, p. 5.

CHAPTER 14

The epidemiologic trohoc, the ablative risk ratio, and 'retrospective' research

About two years ago, in a journal that may seldom be seen by the readers of this series, there appeared[13] a remarkable public rebuke to the epidemiologic fraternity. Dr. John P. Fox, who is co-author of a new textbook of epidemiology,[14] wrote a note "to call attention to and correct a surprising error in a report . . . (that) presumably was produced by . . . several persons highly distinguished as epidemiologists." Dr. Fox pointed out that the authors of the cited report had made incorrect use of the terms *prospective* and *retrospective.*

Like every domain of science, Epidemiology contains certain basic conceptual ideas, and the terms that express these ideas become the fundamental vocabulary of the domain. Investigators trained in other forms of research may not fully understand those ideas when applying them in another domain, and may misuse either the corresponding words or the associated concepts. For example, in reporting the results of therapy, clinicians regularly confuse the epidemiologic nuances that distinguish *incidence* from *prevalence,* and *mortality rates* from *fatality rates.* Converse-

ly, epidemiologists analyzing general mortality rates for different causes of "disease" regularly confuse the clinical nuances that distinguish a *diagnosis* listed on a death certificate from the true occurrence of a *disease.*[8]

The misuse of *prospective* and *retrospective* by epidemiologists themselves is unexpected, however, because these terms are fundamental to any scientific reasoning about populations—a subject on which epidemiologists are regarded as experts. Furthermore, the ideas of "looking forward" and "looking backward" are expressed directly in those words, in contrast to the arbitrary meanings that have been created to distinguish *incidence* from *prevalence,* and *mortality* from *fatality.* The confusion about *prospective* and *retrospective* seems to arise not from any arbitrarily created distinctions, but from the unfortunate custom of using the terms to describe two different and sometimes conflicting concepts of research. One concept refers to the directional pursuit of a population; the other refers to the method used for collecting research data.

The basic unit of epidemiologic research is a person who has a particular condition. When groups of persons are under investigation, the *prospective-retrospective*

Under the same name, this chapter originally appeared as "Clinical biostatistics—XX." In Clin. Pharmacol. Ther. 14:291, 1973.

terminology has been applied for two different research activities: (1) the chronologic direction in which each person is followed in relation to that condition, and (2) the way the investigator gets the data that describe each person's observed and other conditions. In an earlier paper[10] in this series, I discussed the conflicting ambiguity and scientific confusion caused by the two sets of concepts, and I suggested that the best way to remove the difficulties was to discard the words *prospective* and *retrospective*. We could then use two new sets of terms to describe the two different concepts.

A. The two sets of terms

1. The collection of data. An investigator can assemble research data in two basic ways. In the first way, the person under study was originally observed by people who were not performing a specific investigation, and who reported the observations in routine records. Afterward, to get the research data, the investigator extracts the information available in those records. In the second way, the investigator makes special plans beforehand for the techniques with which each person is to be examined and the data recorded. The first way of collecting research data can be called *retrolective*, and the second way, *prolective*.

The ability to use special procedures for acquiring the primary data will depend on whether the research was planned before or after the persons under surveillance reached the locale at which their condition was to be observed. For example, suppose we want to study the growth achieved in the first year of life for premature babies born in our hospital during 1965. If we decide in 1964 to begin this research the following year, we can make advance plans for performing suitable examinations to collect the data from birth onward for all appropriate children. If, however, we decide in 1973 to do this same research project, we cannot make any advance plans, because the conditions we want to study were noted at our hospital eight years

earlier in 1965. Therefore, to do the research, we would have to rely on the information entered in the hospital's medical records. From the hospital's diagnostic registry, we would find the names of all premature babies born in 1965. From each baby's medical record and from supplemental *ad hoc* communications, we would collect the necessary data about birth weight and subsequent growth.

Regardless of whether the research was done prolectively or retrolectively, we would attempt to assemble the same group of patients and to follow that group in the same chronologic direction from birth onward. The main tactical difference would be in the methods used for collecting the research data.

2. The direction of populational pursuit. The other set of terms would refer to the temporal direction in which a group of people is followed. The direction can be either forward or backward. For example, suppose we want to know whether oral contraceptive pills predispose to thromboembolism. In forward research, we would assemble a group of women who use the pill and another group who use other forms of contraception. We would then follow the two groups forward and note the rate at which they develop thrombophlebitis. In backward research, we would assemble a group of women who have developed thrombophlebitis and another group who do not have thrombophlebitis. We would then note the proportionate frequency with which the two groups had previously used oral contraceptives.

Both types of research could be done prolectively or retrolectively, according to the methods used for assembling data. The distinguishing feature of the two cited projects would be the direction of populational pursuit, rather than the way in which the research data were collected. In the first project, the population is followed forward, from "cause" toward "effect." In the second project, the population is followed backward, from "effect" toward "cause."

The word *cohort* has been established to describe a group of people who are pursued in the forward (or "prospective") direction that characterizes scientific research. Thus, to assess the growth rate of premature babies in the projects described earlier, our first project would have involved a *prolective cohort,* and the second, a *retrolective cohort.* In studying the development of thrombophlebitis in pill-takers or non–pill-takers, we would perform cohort research, regardless of whether the data are obtained prolectively or retrolectively. In studying the antecedent use of contraceptive pills in people with or without thrombophlebitis, however, we would *not* be examining a cohort.

Regardless of how the data are collected, a cohort population is usually divided into two or more groups. The main division is done to compare the principal maneuvers under investigation. If the principal maneuver is an alleged cause of disease, the cohort may be divided into an "exposed" and "non-exposed" group, and the exposed group may be further divided into degrees of exposure. Thus, if cigarette smoking is the putative pathogen under study, the cohort may be divided into non-smokers, light smokers, moderate smokers, and heavy smokers. If the investigated maneuver is a therapeutic intervention in the course of a disease, the cohort is divided into a treated and a "control" group, or into groups who have received different forms of treatment. We might then refer to an exposed cohort and a non-exposed cohort, or to a treated cohort and a control cohort. A second form of division for a cohort is the separation into strata that may be different in prognosis, compliance, ancillary response, or detectability of target event. Regardless of how the first or subsequent divisions are created, the key feature of cohort research is that the groups are followed forward, in a scientific direction, from "cause" toward "effect."

There is currently no word to describe the population that is followed backward in the opposite of cohort research. The term "retrospective" may describe the direction of the research, but it does not provide a name for the different groups under study. The term *cases* or *case-group* is sometimes used for the people in whom the "effect" has already occurred, and the term *case-control* is applied for the people who are in the "non-effect" group. These terms are not particularly specific, since the word *case* can imply almost anything, rather than the occurrence of an "effect." A good substitute for the *cases* or "effect" group is *probands,* a term that has been employed by Taube in several excellent analyses.[24-26] The only difficulty with *probands* (or its alternative, *propositi*) is that the word has been almost wholly preempted by geneticists. Almost 40 years ago, Sir Ronald Fisher[11] was using *proband* during statistical analyses of genetic phenomena, and the word has often been applied in a genetic sense since that time. Despite the genetic connotation, however, *probands* refers to a group of people with an identified disease, and the term could be quite satisfactory for our purposes here. It might still be chosen by epidemiologists who prefer it to the alternatives that follow.

A new word that might be created to describe a group of diseased people is *morbery,* formed from the Latin *morb-* (disease) and *-ery* (collection). This word has no genetic associations, but it has the disadvantage of implying the existence of a disease—and this type of research may not always begin with an "effect" that is a distinctive disease. (We might be studying the "causes" of unemployment by backward pursuit of antecedent characteristics in a group of unemployed people.)

Regardless of how we label the people who do or do not have the "effect," none of the terms just cited conveys the idea of a backward direction, analogous to the forward direction connoted by *cohort.* In quest of a word for a group of people followed in a chronologically backward direction, I have searched unsuccessfully through several dictionaries, a few variants of Roget's *Thesaurus,* and some Greek and

Latin lexicons. The best I can do at the moment, until some philologic connoisseur comes up with a better idea, is to reverse the word *cohort*, and to propose *trohoc* as the name for a group of people who are followed backward from "effect" (or "non-effect") toward "cause." The "effect" group would form a *case, proband,* or *morbery* trohoc, and the "non-effect" group would be the *control* or *contrast* trohoc.

Thus, in the timing of data collection for a research project, the words "prospective" and "retrospective" would be replaced by *prolective* and *retrolective*. In the directional pursuit of a population, the words "prospective" and "retrospective" would be replaced by *cohort* and *trohoc*.

B. The problems of trohoc research

Clinicians often have difficulty in understanding what may be wrong with the scientific direction of trohoc research. From the many conceptual errors that have prevailed at different times in medical history, we know of the problems doctors have had merely in distinguishing a cause from an effect, without the added burden of distinguishing the direction of reasoning. A more substantive source of difficulty, however, is that clinicians are unfamiliar with trohoc research because it seldom occurs as part of clinical investigation. A clinical investigator will usually either do experiments confined to the laboratory or will perform surveys and trials of clinical therapy. With either of these two forms of research, the clinical investigator follows a cohort forward from an imposed "cause" to an observed "effect." Accustomed to this standard direction of scientific thinking, the clinician may become uncomfortable, uncertain, or logically confused when he encounters a complete reversal of that direction. If the retroversion is accompanied by a barrage of mathematical formulas and statistical tabulations, the clinician may promptly withdraw from the epidemiologic melee, returning to the security of more familiar forms of science while hoping that the epidemiologic experts will know what they are doing and will do it right.

And yet, as Fox pointed out,[13] the experts can be wrong. In the instance about which Fox complained, the term *retrospective* was erroneously applied by epidemiologists to a "prospective" study of a cohort of people whose data were obtained retrolectively from medical records. This type of error in scientific thinking can be eliminated as a younger generation begins to outgrow or avoid the confusion transmitted by its elders. A much greater source of real or potential error in scientific research, however, is the trohoc investigations to which the term *retrospective* might be correctly applied.

These potential errors seldom receive sufficient emphasis when students are taught about the trohocs investigated in "analytic epidemiologic" studies. The difficulties of a backward direction may be mentioned in passing, but the instructor or the textbook usually dwells mainly on such things as relative risk ratios and other statistical manipulations of the data. The possibility that the data might be immensely distorted or wholly erroneous does not receive intensive discussion, perhaps because retroverted trohoc research has been the standard practice of leaders in the field.

At a time when all other basic aspects of medical education have come into question, however, a reconsideration of scientific validity in epidemiologic trohocs would not be out of place. A prime challenge is to arrive at a way of illustrating what might be wrong with the way that the backward procedure works, and with the data it provides. For this purpose, I shall draw an analogy from the game of baseball, with apologies to readers in countries where the game is unfamiliar.

Suppose we suspected that right-handed batters among professional baseball players were worse hitters than left-handed batters, and we wanted to get data to test this suspicion. In the prospective cohort approach that has been used for more than a century in the science of baseball statistics, we would determine the number of times that each type of batter came to bat, and the number of times that were followed by a hit or an out.° We would then calculate each batter's "batting average" as a rate of hits per times at bat. To make our decision about left-handed versus right-handed batters, we would compare the overall batting averages in the two groups.

To construct a table showing the results, we would put the batters in the rows, as the independent variable used for the "sampling," and the hits and outs in the columns, as the subsequently observed phenomena. The table would contain the following numbers:

	Number of hits	Number of outs
R.-handed batters	a	b
L.-handed batters	c	d

The "batting average" percentages to be compared would then be a/(a+b) vs. c/(c+d).

In the trohoc approach, we would not consider the times at bat or even what occurred during the game. Instead, we might consider a particular location in the ball park, such as center field. Whenever a batted ball came into center field, we would determine whether it was a hit or an out. We would then ask the center fielder to inquire and let us know whether the batter had been right- or left-handed. We would then construct the following table:

	R.-handed batters	*L.-handed batters*
Number of center field hits	a'	c'
Number of center field outs	b'	d'

The rows of this table contain the center field hits and outs that were the basis for our "sampling"; the columns contain the subsequently observed "handedness" of the batters; and the interior letters are chosen to correspond with their presumptive counterparts in the preceding table.

Because we derived our data from cen-

°In accordance with statistical custom in these matters, a walk or a sacrifice hit would not count as a time at bat.

terfield hits and outs, rather than from all the batting events, we cannot use a'+b' and c'+d' to represent times at bat. We can contemplate only the proportions of hits and outs that were associated with the two types of batters. Thus, we could calculate the proportion of R.-handed hits as a'/(a'+c') and compare the result with b'/(b'+d'), which is the proportion of R.-handed outs. If the first proportion was substantially lower than the second, we would conclude that R.-handed batters are worse than L.-handed batters.

Anyone who understands the game of baseball should immediately recognize what is wrong with these trohoc statistics. We have not compared true batting averages (or rates); we have looked only at the proportion of hits and outs in balls batted to the center field region. More importantly, our station in center field gave us a highly restricted view of what was going on; we have no idea about the number of times at bat that culminated as strikeouts, walks, bunts, infield singles, line-drive infield outs, pop-ups, foul-outs, or batted balls that become either hits or outs in left field or right field. Our view was entirely limited to events in center field. If we are sure that the events occurring in R.-handed and L.-handed batters are equally represented by what takes place in center field, our restricted observational focus may be valid, but the only way we can decide about such equal representation and validity would be to get results with a cohort approach, which we have not used.

To translate this baseball analogy into trohoc tactics for studying cause of disease, we need merely substitute a medical center for center field; a person with disease *D* as a "hit" and a person without disease *D* as an "out"; exposure to the putative cause of disease as a R.-handed batter and non-exposure as a L.-handed batter. With these translations, an epidemiologist using medical-center data, assembling a diseased trohoc and a "case-control" group, and noting exposure or non-exposure to the alleged "cause" in both groups, performs the same type of analysis just cited for baseball.

If a statistician ever tried to analyze baseball batting in this manner, the sports pages of the nation's newspapers would be filled with howls of derision. Suppose the statistician, stung by public laughter, decides to improve the analysis, but he remains unwilling or unable to leave his observation post in center field. His "improvement" consists of keeping center field as the source of data, but he will try to eliminate some of the problems by "matching."

Whenever a hit or out appears in center field, he gets the center fielder to indicate not merely the batter's handedness, but also the batter's age and height. With these additional data, the statistician divides age into groups of **old, middle,** and **young** and height into **short, medium,** and **tall**—so that each batter can fall into one of nine categories for "matching." Each ball batted to center field by a R.-handed batter from one of these nine categories is then matched with a ball batted by a L.-handed batter from a similar category. The proportions of "hits" versus "outs" are then compared statistically within each of the nine categories, and a series of mathematical "adjustments" are later employed to combine the nine groups into a single final comparison.

This type of matching would probably revive and expand whatever derision had subsided after the initial statistics were presented. The original error would not have been properly corrected. Instead, it would have been elaborated with a series of cumbersome scientific and mathematical trappings. Having chosen to do nothing about the inappropriateness of an exclusively center-field site for examining what takes place in a baseball game, the statistician could at least have based the "matching" on the cogent features that can affect a batter's likelihood of "success." Among such features are the batter's general prowess as a **hitter** (e.g., pitchers are known to be poor hitters and should be

separated from non-pitchers); and also the corresponding left- or right-handedness of the pitcher who threw to each batter. Since age and height are not known to have particularly strong effects on the batting ability of an active professional baseball player, the choice of age and height as matching variables, rather than the more important features just cited, served to betray the statistician's unfamiliarity with subtle but important nuances in the game of baseball.

Consequently, the statistician's proposed matching would be regarded as a futile mathematical exercise that would manipulate the numbers without providing clarity or understanding. Nevertheless, when an analogous type of matching is performed in epidemiologic trohoc research, a reader is likely to approach the results with admiration for the statistical "refinements," and a student is likely to be taught the procedure as a basic method to be used for investigating causes of disease.

C. Sources of bias in trohoc research

In the statistics of epidemiology, as in baseball, a procedure that merely creates matches, without identifying, adjusting, or reducing bias, can be a counter-productive activity. During the past few decades, the annals of epidemiologic investigations into causes of disease have contained many instances of such "matchless" matchings. The persons under study may be subdivided according to age, race, sex, occupation, income level, and numerous other demographic variables—but not according to major factors responsible for hidden bias that can substantially distort the results. As noted earlier[9] in this series of papers, three major sources of "transition bias" can profoundly alter the composition and outcome of the populations exposed or non-exposed to alleged causes of disease. In susceptibility bias, an underlying factor (such as psychic stress or parental longevity) can influence an outcome event (such as coronary disease or early death), but can also affect a person's decision to self-select the alleged causal agent (such as a particular pattern of dietary intake or smoking). In compliance bias, the long-term outcome of a maneuver is affected by the person's adherence, or ability to adhere, to the chosen maneuver. In detection bias, the identification of a target event (such as coronary disease, lung cancer, or thrombophlebitis) can be distorted by inequalities in the frequency and intensity of examination procedures needed to diagnose the event.

All three of these major sources of transition bias have been almost totally neglected in the data assembled in contemporary epidemiologic research. Having verbally acknowledged the possible presence of such bias, the investigator often makes no effort to assemble the data that might help confirm or refute the effects of the bias.

A simple example of this problem occurred with the recent flurry of publicity about the rising rate of death due to cancer in American blacks. The epidemiologic speculations about causes for this rising rate have been concerned with the possible roles of diet, occupation, or even racism. Before embarking on all these speculations, no one seems to have given any attention to the possibility that the compared rates are erroneous, and that the recent rise is due mainly to better methods of disease detection. As blacks have increasingly received better medical care, and also as they have increasingly moved from rural to urban settings, they have increasingly been better exposed to the diagnostic procedures that would lead to detection of many cancers that formerly would have escaped identification. The rates of death due to those cancers would rise accordingly. This obvious possibility seems to be constantly overlooked as epidemiologists analyze the causes of a 'change' in mortality rates, without analyzing the bias due to changes in the detection procedures associated with possibly 'better' rather than 'worse' medical care.

In cohort research, an alert investigator could easily inquire about factors that can create bias in susceptibility, compliance, or detection, but these sources of "transition bias" have not been considered and tested in most cohort studies devoted to causes of disease. When the research is performed with a trohoc, however, the investigation of such bias is much more difficult. The prime problem is a lack of knowledge about the population from which the trohoc arose. Without such information, the rates of transition bias cannot be correctly discerned, even if the investigator makes efforts to assemble the data that would describe differences in susceptibilty, compliance, or target detection of the compared groups. In making such efforts, however, the trohoc investigator would try to use the information for "matching" or stratified adjustments that may reduce the bias. The investigator has no assurance that the adjustments will be effective, but the efforts are necessary to provide as much vigorous science as can be applied to the fundamentally unscientific direction of trohoc research.

Another major form of bias, however, is impossible to test in trohoc research. Within a trohoc population, there is no way in which an investigator can assemble suitable data or perform suitable adjustments to deal with the existence, magnitude, or effects of *chronology bias*.[10] Despite the illusion that the trohoc investigator has observed the "effects" of exposure or non-exposure to a "cause," what has actually been observed are the conveniently available survivors of the antecedent cohort population. The investigator has no idea, and has no way of getting any idea from the trohoc itself, of the way in which the original cohorts were chronologically distorted by death, by referral, or by migration before the members of the cohorts emerged as members of the available trohoc groups. As Mantel and Haenszel[19] have noted, "The retrospective study picks up factors associated with becoming a diseased or a disease-free *subject,* rather than simply factors associated with presence or absence of the disease."

D. Criteria for validity in trohoc research

Since trohocs are so relatively easy to find and examine, this form of research will doubtlessly continue to appeal to investigators and to appear before readers. Besides, the trohoc approach will sometimes be the best or the only way to check certain hunches about etiology, or to determine whether a cohort project is worth doing. For these reasons, a statement of the scientific standards needed for trohoc research would be useful to the investigators who design such studies and to the readers who judge the results.

The effects of transition bias and chronology bias can destroy the validity of the research by altering the observed groups so that they do not represent the correct populations or events. Unless suitable data have been obtained, examined, and analyzed to rule out such bias, or to make suitable adjustments for it, an investigator has no scientific assurance that the research is valid. The need for representative groups has been acknowledged by almost all the epidemiologists and statisticians who have discussed the analysis of trohoc data. The discussions have contained no direct instructions about how to check for "representativeness" by examining specific data related to susceptibility bias, compliance bias, detection bias, or chronology bias, but nevertheless, the general problems of bias have received abundant public warning.

As Harold Dorn[5] pointed out,

> The most serious defect of the case-history method is that it provides no basis for judging the validity of the observations obtained by its use. . . . If valid inferences are to be drawn from a sample, two requirements must be fulfilled: the sample must be representative of the population to which inferences are to be drawn; and the data collected must be of sufficient reliability and validity to answer the hypotheses to be tested. It is essential to fulfill both requirements. . . . Too frequently there is a temptation to relax both requirements because it is cheaper, more convenient or quicker to use readily available data even though these may be of doubtful validity and cannot be referred to any known population.

To improve validity in trohoc studies, Dorn suggested that the examined group be obtained as new cases occurring in a defined population, and that more than one type of "control group" be tested. Mantel and Haenszel[19] made the following comments, which include the concept of detection bias:

> The fundamental assumption underlying the analysis of retrospective data is that the assembled cases and controls are representative of the universe defined for investigation. This obligates the investigator not only to examine the data which are the end product but also to go behind the scenes and evaluate the forces which have channeled the material to his attention, including such items as local practices of referral to specialists and hospitals and the patient's condition and the effect of these items on the probability of diagnosis or hospital admission. . . . Any factor which increases the probability that a diseased individual will be hospitalized may mistakenly be found to be associated with the disease.

As precautions against bias, Mantel and Haenszel[19] suggested the use of dual control groups—chosen from both hospital and general populations. Also, when hospital controls are chosen, they should be ". . . drawn from a wide variety of diseases or admission diagnoses." Furthermore, "interviews should be conducted without knowledge of the identity of cases and controls to guard against interviewer bias." Finally, the investigators should establish, "precisely and in advance, the method by which controls are selected for study. . . . The rule should be rigid and unambiguous to avoid creating effects by subconscious selection and manipulation of controls."

These requirements were accepted and augmented in a later paper by Cornfield and Haenzel.[3] In describing several "potential sources of error in retrospective studies," these workers stated,

> A basic assumption . . . is that it is possible to enumerate all new cases of a disease, or a representative sample of them, without having to observe all the individuals in the population from which they arise and watching for cases to develop. This assumption might be correct if (1) all new patients with the disease sought medical attention, (2) all medical sources to which such patients might go were completely canvassed, and (3) an effective system for reporting such cases was in operation. In practice these conditions may be far from satisfied. . . .

> A second and closely related assumption which also requires careful examination is that the sample of individuals not developing the disease sup-

plies an unbiased estimate of the prevalence of the characteristic under study among the entire nondiseased population of interest. Most retrospective studies are content to select a "control" group . . . and to assume that the prevalence of the characteristic in that control group is an unbiased estimate of the required proportion.

Cornfield and Haenszel also proposed "several ways of guarding against the possibility of error":

First of all, controls may be drawn from a wide variety of disease or admission diagnoses. If the prevalence of the characteristic under study varies widely among the groups, the possibly unrepresentative nature of at least some of them is strongly indicated. . . .

A second possible way . . . is to draw the control sample from the general population and not from other disease groups available in the hospital. This introduces (however) a possible source of incomparability in the responses of the patients with disease and the controls, since the same question may elicit different responses when asked in radically different situations. . . . The use of both general population and a variety of hospital controls provides a quite general (but not foolproof) safeguard against error from this source.

. . . Another potential source of error . . . may arise (from) . . . conscious or unconscious bias in response. . . . The interviewer who believes, for example, that lung cancer is caused by excessive smoking might be more zealous in questioning a lung cancer patient who gave a nonsmoking history than he would be in questioning a control. A patient's own preconceptions may also influence the answers.

From the Dorn-Mantel-Cornfield-Haenszel statements, we can derive at least five requirements for scientific credence to be given to the results of a retrospective trohoc investigation. These requirements constitute some of the fundamental criteria for validity in trohoc research:

1. An unbiased method for getting information about the presence or absence of the alleged "cause."

2. A group of "cases" who are representative of people who have the disease under investigation.

3. A "control" group chosen from a wide variety of diseases or admission diagnoses at the hospital.

4. An additional "control" group chosen from the general population.

5. A rigorously specified method, established before the work begins, for selecting the members of the "control" group(s).

Fulfillment of these five principles cannot guarantee the removal or reduction of transition bias and chronology bias, but the principles can be accepted as part of the minimal standards for scientific performance in trohoc research. We shall later note the attention (or inattention) given to these principles when statistical procedures are applied to trohoc data.

E. The concept of 'relative risk'

The calculation of a "relative risk" is frequently performed in modern epidemiology. To illustrate the circumstances, suppose that F people have been exposed to a particular "risk factor" and that E of those people later develop a particular target event (or disease). The incidence rate, or "risk," of the event in the exposed people is $p_1 = E/F$. Note that the people "at risk" are placed in the denominator of this fraction, and that the occurrence of the event is placed in the numerator. If F' people have *not* been exposed to the risk factor, and if E' of those people develop the target event, their incidence rate or "risk" of getting the event is $p_2 = E'/F'$. Thus, we might find (if suitable data were available) that cancer of the lung is noted to develop in 205 of 1,000,000 smokers per year and in 86 of 1,000,000 non-smokers per year.[*]

We now have the individual risk rates for the exposed and non-exposed groups. These two rates could be compared in two different ways. The first way is to inspect both of them directly, as we have just done. The second way is to convert them into a single value by performing a calculation that eliminates their individual values. This calculation can also be done in two ways. The first is a subtraction. Thus, we might say that the incremental risk of lung cancer in smokers is 119 (= 205-86) per million per year. The second method of calculation

---

[*]These numerical rates are based on the estimates provided on page 1271 of Reference 2.

is to form a ratio by dividing the two rates. This ratio is called the *relative risk*. Thus, we might say that the relative risk of lung cancer in a smoker is 2.38 (= 205/ 1,000,000 ÷ 86/1,000,000).

Although the concept of a relative risk has achieved considerable popularity among modern epidemiologists, the conversion of two different statistical rates into a single ratio is an old strategy, having been used by Quetelet[21] more than a century ago. The strategy has also been employed throughout the years for various other clinical purposes, most commonly in laboratory tests.

Because of some obvious disadvantages, the strategy has been increasingly abandoned by many clinical investigators. For example, the ratio of concentrations of serum albumin and serum globulin (expressed as an A/G ratio) was a favorite laboratory calculation for many years, but is seldom employed today. The reason is that the values of the two individual components are obscured when converted into the single value of the ratio. Thus, the A/G ratio may be abnormally low because of a marked decrease in A or a marked increase in G. Although these two causes of a low A/G ratio are distinctively different, the distinctions are obliterated when the result is expressed merely as a single A/G ratio. Consequently, most thoughtful clinicians today prefer to examine the albumin and globulin values separately, rather than an ambiguous single ratio.

When the ratio-of-rates strategy is applied to a laboratory test, there are no major problems of bias in the numbers that form the numerators and denominators of each of the two rates. The main hazard is that the contributions of the different components will be lost or confused. When a ratio of rates is used for the data of different groups of people, however, the result is fraught with all of the types of transition bias and chronology bias that can affect each of the two denominators and two numerators that become reduced

to a single number during the calculations.

The problems created by such distortions were, paradoxically, not particularly important when Quetelet was calculating relative risks from the data available a century ago. The denominators in such data consisted of an entire population enumerated by census; whereas the usual groups studied in modern epidemiologic cohorts consist of a conveniently available "chunk sample," such as physicians, military veterans, or employees of a particular industry. The "factors" that delineated Quetelet's "risks" were either geographic regions or age—neither of which caused difficulty in identification and both of which could be adjusted for their contributions to transition bias. For the risk factors studied in modern epidemiology, however, major types of susceptibility bias, compliance bias, and detection bias will be associated with such self-selected maneuvers as dietary intake, smoking, and use of oral contraceptive pills.

The numerators in Quetelet's data consisted of deaths, rather than deaths attributed to a particular disease, so there was no problem in detecting the target, or in adjusting for secular changes in diagnostic techniques. Furthermore, because Quetelet's death data were cited annually for the population alive at the beginning of each year, there were no major problems in chronology bias. In modern epidemiologic research, however, the deaths are related to the beginning of exposure to a causal agent, but the research is seldom, if ever, based on the type of *inception cohort* required to avoid chronology bias in such research.[10] For example, of the seven "prospective" groups cited in the U. S. Surgeon General's report[27] on Smoking and Health, *none* was investigated as an inception cohort. All seven groups contained a cross-sectional assembly of available survivors who were still alive many years after inception of the smoking (or non-smoking). In commenting on the problems of chronology bias in such research, Mac-Mahon[18] emphasized that "at least half of the relevant association (the cause) had operated prior to the time of the study, and . . . the follow-up period has been so short . . . that one may wonder how many of the subsequently identified cases were not in fact already affected at the time of the first questionnaire."

Even if all these sources of bias could be suitably identified, however, and even if the bias could be suitably eliminated or "adjusted," the relative risk ratio would still contain a fundamental flaw that is irredeemable. To form the ratio, the magnitude of the individual risks is ablated, i.e., removed, destroyed, extirpated. If actual rates for the compared risks are 1 in 5 versus 1 in 10, we would get exactly the same relative risk ratio as if the compared risks were 1 in 5,000,000 versus 1 in 10,000,000. Thus, for the lung cancer data cited earlier, the relative risk ratio was 2.38, based on rates of 205/1,000,000 and 86/1,000,000. This ratio would still be 2.38 if the corresponding rates were individually a thousand times higher, i.e., 205/1,000 and 86/1,000, or a thousand times lower, i.e., 205×10^{-9} and 86×10^{-9}.

Deprived of the values of the individual risk rates, a reader who relies on the relative risk ratio has no idea of just how great the actual risk may be. Thus, although smoking may seem almost 2.5 times more "risky" than non-smoking for the development of lung cancer, an objective observer examining the data may appraise the result somewhat differently when he compares the individual rates of 205 per million versus 86 per million. Since the difference in these two rates is 119 per million, a smoker's chance of getting lung cancer is incrementally higher by about 1 in 10,000 than the chance of a non-smoker. From the standpoint of public health authorities, this increment may warrant major preventive action for a general population involving millions of people. From the standpoint of an individual smoker, however, the increment of individual risk may not be great enough to counterbalance the pleasures the smoking provides.

Regardless of whatever be the merits of the data used to indict the neoplastic potential of cigarette smoking, the main point to be noted here is that scientific decisions must rest on factual data, not on statistical calculations that ablate or obscure the basic facts. For this reason, when an investigator reports a ratio of relative risk, without providing a statement of the individual rates that comprise the ratio, the result can be called an *ablative risk ratio*.

F. The ablative risk ratio in trohoc research

The ablative risk ratio has achieved its greatest current popularity in trohoc re-search dealing with causes of disease. The classical fourfold table in trohoc research would be constructed as follows:

	Exposed	Non-exposed
Diseased	a	c
Non-diseased	b	d

If these data were based on cohorts taken from a general population, we could readily calculate the rates of disease in the exposed and non-exposed groups. Such rates cannot be calculated in a trohoc population, however, because the sums a + b and c + d, which are needed for the denominators, have no real meaning in trohoc groups. These sums are wholly contrived values formed by the cases included in the arbitrary selection of diseased and non-diseased people that form the trohoc. The only possibly meaningful sums in the trohoc table are a + c, the sum of members in the chosen diseased group, and the counterpart "control" sum, b + d. Hence, from what is available in the trohoc table, we cannot calculate the correct risk ratio, which would be $a/(a + b) \div c/(c + d)$.

By an intriguing maneuver in statistical reasoning, however, a different type of ablation was brought to the apparent rescue of what would otherwise be an obvious scientific fallacy. Cornfield[2] pointed out that if b (the size of the non-diseased group in a general population) was much larger than a (the size of the corresponding diseased group), the ratio $a/(a + b)$ was essentially equal to a/b. Similarly, if d was substantially larger than c in the general population, then $c/(c + d)$ was essentially equal to c/d. This reasoning cannot be faulted for the data of a general population. For most major diseases (including lung cancer and thrombophlebitis), the number of non-diseased people in a general population will be substantially greater than the number of those who are diseased. With this reasoning, the risk ratio for a general population could be expressed as $a/b \div c/d$ or ad/bc. Because of the way the terms are taken from the fourfold table, this ratio is also sometimes known as the *odds ratio, relative odds ratio, cross ratio,* or *cross product ratio.*

When this reasoning, which applies to a cohort of the general population, is transferred to an epidemiologic trohoc, the statistical effect is splendid. We need no longer pay any attention to the (a + b) and (c + d) terms that were meaningless in the trohoc. These terms do not appear in the odds ratio, which depends only on the individual values noted for a, b, c, and d in the trohoc population. The odds ratio used for "relative risk" in a trohoc thus becomes a doubly ablative procedure. The ephemeral denominators, which were not determined, are ablated together with the individual risk rates, which were also not determined.

The result is quite pleasing statistically, since it provides a single number that can be subjected to diverse manipulations with mathematical theories about estimation, variance, and "significance." The result is less pleasing medically because it fails to show the individual risk rates. The result is quite unpleasing scientifically, however, because its validity is so open to suspicion. To transfer our reasoning from the cohort of general population to the trohoc group, we had to make the assumption that the composition of the trohoc was adequately representative of the general population. For this assumption to be tenable, we would need evidence to establish that the five criteria of validity have been fulfilled and also to rule out the possibility of distortion by sources of transition bias and chronologic bias that are not considered in the five points of those criteria. An investigator who wants to apply the odds ratio to a trohoc is therefore scientifically obligated to demonstrate the validity of this assumption—but as we shall see later, this obligation is seldom heeded.

G. Calculations of bias in a trohoc

A simple mathematical illustration can demonstrate the distortions produced by a single form of bias: detection bias. Let us assume that a general population can be divided into a proportion, e, of people who are exposed to an alleged cause of disease. The proportion of non-exposed people will be 1-e. Let us further assume that the rate of disease in the exposed people is p_1, and the rate in non-exposed people is p_2. We will then have the following numbers of people in the population: exposed and diseased = p_1e; exposed and non-diseased = $(1-p_1)e$; non-exposed and diseased = $p_2(1-e)$; and non-exposed and non-diseased = $(1-p_2)(1-e)$. Suppose now, however, that a differential bias exists in the rate of detection of the disease. In people who are both exposed and diseased, the rate of detection, d_1, is substantially higher than the rate, d_2, with which the disease is detected in people who are non-exposed. The numbers of people with detected disease in the cited population will therefore be as follows: exposed and diseased = p_1d_1e; and non-exposed and diseased = $p_2d_2(1-e)$. For non-diseased people, the numbers will remain: exposed and non-diseased = $(1-p_1)e$; and non-exposed and non-diseased = $(1-p_2)(1-e)$.

If a trohoc population is assembled, the relative risk (or odds) ratio will be calculated as:

$$R = \frac{p_1d_1e}{p_2d_2(1-e)} \times \frac{(1-p_2)(1-e)}{(1-p_1)e}$$

$$= \frac{p_1}{p_2} \times \frac{d_1}{d_2} \times \frac{1-p_2}{1-p_1}$$

If p_2 and p_1 are relatively small in relation to the general population, $1-p_2$ and $1-p_1$ are both essentially equal to 1. We can then approximate the value of R as

$$\frac{p_1}{p_2} \times \frac{d_1}{d_2}$$

Thus, although true relative risk is p_1/p_2, the relative risk found in the trohoc will be inflated by a factor of d_1/d_2.

In an excellent recent paper in *Biometrics*, Peacock[20] has described a general formulation for calculating the effects of major bias that have been neglected in both cohort and trohoc research. With simple, readily understood examples, Peacock shows how a relative risk can be shifted from 4.07 to 3.35, and (in the same data) how an

Table I. *Fulfillment of criteria for validity in two trohoc investigations*

Requirement for validity	Methods used in the cited investigations	
	First reference[23]	Second reference[17]
1. Unbiased interviewing	Yes	Yes
2. Representative group of diseased patients	Patients consisted of male veterans from region of Chicago, and veterans from other regions, referred to a special 'cancer center'	Men referred to special institute for treatment of cancer
3. 'Control' group chosen from wide variety of diseases	'Controls' consisted of patients with 'other tumors' outside the respiratory and digestive tract	'Controls' consisted of 'noncancer' patients with symptoms originally suggestive of cancer
4. Additional control group from general population	None obtained	None obtained
5. Predetermined method of selecting 'controls'	'Controls' chosen *after* inspection of results for patients with diverse diseases	Method and timing of selection not described

odds ratio can be shifted from 6.45 to 5.31, merely by changes in the way the investigated population is assembled. According to Peacock, "the size of a relative risk depends on the prevalence of other risk factors in the population and the magnitude of the risks associated with these other risk factors. Where suitable corrections are not made for this, relative risks from different studies cannot be compared." Peacock's comments about other risk factors apply equally well to the bias factors that have been cited here. Peacock concludes that "No amount of mathematical manipulation can compensate in this context for inadequate epidemiologic information."

H. The adequacy of epidemiologic information

If the risk ratios calculated in trohoc research can be so easily distorted by diverse sources of bias, an investigator's first scientific responsibility is to demonstrate that such bias is absent. This responsibility has seldom received adequate attention during statistical or other analyses of the numbers assembled in trohoc data. The absence of such attention can be noted by inspecting the way in which the five criteria of validity were checked or fulfilled in several prominent reports published by some of the foremost exponents of trohoc research.

The first report to be inspected is the one[2] in which the "relative risk ratio" was adapted for trohoc research. In that report,

two previous trohoc studies[17, 23] of patients with lung cancer were used to supply illustrative data for the calculations. The author of the statistical analysis, after warning about the dire scientific consequences of failure to satisfy the criteria, made no comment about whether or not those two studies had complied with the criteria. By reviewing the original references, however, we can note in Table I how well the five principles were fulfilled.

As shown in Table I, each of the two investigations chosen to illustrate the introduction of the relative risk ratio fulfilled only one of the five criteria for validity. A population that contains men only, veterans only, or people referred to cancer centers can not be regarded as representative of people with cancer. Control groups chosen from people with "other cancers" or from people suspected of cancer cannot be regarded as representative of a wide variety of diseases, and the hospital groups certainly do not represent a general population outside the hospital. The method of selecting control patients was not described in one report and was obviously biased in the other.

Another popular application of trohoc research has been in the alleged causal relationship between oral contraceptive pills and thrombophlebitis. The five points of the criteria for validity will be inspected here for three of the most prominent trohoc studies, two of which were done in the United Kingdom[16, 28] and one in the United States.[22]

1. In none of these three studies was there a distinct statement to confirm that the interviewing was done without bias. The diagnoses of disease were obviously known to the practitioners interviewed in one project[16] and were probably also known to the medical students used as interviewers in another.[22]

2. In none of the three studies could the diseased population be regarded as representative of the diverse clinical spectrum of ambulatory and hospitalized women with thromboembolic phenomena: In one study,[16] the "cases" were obtained exclusively from death certificate diagnoses of thromboembolism, and in the other two studies,[22, 28] the diseased population was drawn only from hospitals. The hospital groups were further constricted by the exclusion of patients with "superficial thrombophlebitis" or with predisposing or precipitating conditions. The only women accepted in all three studies were married, although some unmarried women were later accepted at an unstated time "in the course of the (U.S.) study." The clearly unrepresentative nature of the U.S. cases of "idiopathic thromboembolism" is demonstrated by the fact that student nurses constituted 26 of the 175 patients under investigation.

3 and 4. In one of the U.K. investigations,[16] 'controls' were drawn from the 'general population' but not from people with other diseases. In the other U.K. investigation and in the U.S. study, controls were drawn from people hospitalized with other diseases but not from the general population. The other diseases consisted of acute medical or surgical conditions (such as trauma), and entities for which elective surgery was planned.

5. In all three investigations, a specified method was described for choosing "controls," but no statement was made about whether the specifications were formulated before the work began and whether they remained unaltered as the work progressed.

Thus, in all three of the most prominent trohoc studies of thromboembolism and the 'pill,' at least two of the five criteria for scientific validity were grossly violated.

In pointing out the massive scientific defects of trohoc research, the late Harold Dorn referred to it as ". . . the most unproductive method yet devised for studying the natural history of disease."[4] He later noted that the major defense of trohoc research seemed to rest on the somewhat similar results found in ". . . a comparison of retrospective and prospective studies of the relation of smoking to cancer of the lung."[5] The scientific validity of the data regarding smoking and lung cancer has long been regarded with suspicion because the investigators have failed to check two underlying sources of major bias that could have created the same distortions in both the trohoc and cohort studies. One such bias is in target detection. Because of cough, the smokers might be much more likely than non-coughing non-smokers to receive the X-ray, cytology, and other examination procedures needed to diagnose lung cancer. The other source of bias is in susceptibility. Although R. A. Fisher[12] proposed that a constitutional (and possibly genetic) factor might lead to both smoking and lung cancer, a simpler common factor that can predispose to both smoking and reduced longevity is psychic stress, which has never received satisfactory investigation in the epidemiologic appraisals of smoking and its consequences. The proper assessment of both these currently uninvestigated sources of bias is of crucial scientific importance for the indictment against cigarettes because the etiologic capacity of cigarettes has never been checked (nor can it be checked) with a controlled trial in which smoking or non-smoking is randomly assigned to a general population.

If the validity of existing trohoc research

is to be defended, therefore, the defense would require data more scientifically impeccable than the existing studies of smoking. No such additional defense has been offered, and, furthermore, in at least two other topics of epidemiologic research, careful studies of cohorts (or subsequent trohocs) have shown the fallacy of the initial conclusions derived from trohoc data.

One such refutation was provided in studies of the "validity of the reported association between various factors and cancer of the cervix," where Dorn[5] demonstrated "the lack of agreement between the relative risk of cervical cancer obtained from the retrospective interviews and incidence rates, as well as the variation in the estimates of relative risk among the retrospective studies."

A more recent refutation has occurred for the topic of thrombophlebitis and oral contraceptive pills. Formerly, the only existing argument against the conclusions of the trohoc studies was contained in arrays of "prospective" cohort data[6, 7] that had been collected without the use of "control" groups, and that had been combined without intensive regard for the comparability of the populations whose results were pooled. Because the cohort data were also open to suspicion, the trohoc investigators had been able to offer vigorous rebuttals against the refutation of their claim for the high risk ratio of thrombophlebitis in pill-takers.

At long last, however, there has now been conducted a controlled, randomized, cohort study[15] of oral and non-oral contraception in a group of almost 10,000 women in the reproductive age group. The results showed almost identical rates of incidence of thrombophlebitis: 1.81 per 1,000 women in the oral group and 1.62 in the non-oral control group. The relative risk ratio of 1.12 found in the scientifically designed cohort trial can be contrasted with the misleadingly higher analogous ratios found in the previous trohoc investigations. These ratios

were 4.4 in the U.S. study, 2.9 in one of the U.K. studies,[*] and 8.6 in the other.[*]

•   •   •

In presenting a thoughtful description of concepts, methods, and pitfalls in trohoc research, Cornfield and Haenszel[3] offered the following plea:

Sweeping condemnation of the retrospective method or uncritical acceptance of the results . . . are equally to be avoided. The frame of mind which condemns any method that could lead to error under some conceivable set of circumstances, without also considering whether those circumstances have in fact arisen, is unlikely to be satisfied with any result outside the field of pure mathematics. The contrary frame of mind, which accepts a method simply because it will yield an answer without consideration of how much in error the answer could be, is scarcely likely to be any more productive.

The plea seems entirely proper. There are clearly certain forms of research questions for which trohoc approaches will be necessary because cohort studies either cannot be done or are too expensive and time-consuming. The trohoc approach to research should not receive a "sweeping condemnation" merely because it has so enormous a potential for error due to hidden bias, and merely because it has been demonstrably erroneous in two major epidemiologic issues. There is no reason, however, for a careful scientist to give "uncritical acceptance" to the results of research that contains gross violations of the principles of scientific investigation. What is obviously needed is for the scientific quality of methods in trohoc research to receive the attention that has so long been diverted mainly into mathematical theories.

It is the obligation of a scientific investigator—not of his audience—to consider sources of bias and to assemble suitable data that can help demonstrate whether bias is present or absent. A reader can not

---

[*]The U.K. investigators did not actually express the relative risk values, but the results can be calculated as odds ratios from Inman and Vessey's[16] Table II ($2.9 = 25 \times 64 \div 50 \times 11$) and from Vessey and Doll's[28] Table IV ($8.6 = 26 \times 106 \div 32 \times 10$).

consider "whether those circumstances (of bias) have in fact arisen" if the investigators have made no effort to assemble, analyze, and report the necessary information. An elemental requirement of any statistical appraisals of trohoc research would be the demonstration of fulfillment (or lack of fulfillment) for the basic criteria of validity stated by the statistical proponents of such studies. The five criteria should also be expanded to include a sixth, concerned with appropriate investigation of bias due to differences in susceptibility, compliance, and target detection. Harold Dorn has contended that "if this assumption (about validity) cannot be made, the data should be discarded."[4] Even an apparent confirmation of one set of trohoc results by another trohoc study does not make the conclusions acceptable. As Dorn pointed out, "Reproducibility does not necessarily establish validity, since the same mistake can be made repeatedly."[4]

A useful summary of the problem was provided in remarks written by Jerome Cornfield[1] more than 30 years ago.

. . . The data yielded by mere collections of cases are not without value; they may give the investigator greater insight into his subject; they may strengthen his intuitive grasp; they may possess a high order of intrinsic interest. The one characteristic they lack, however, is the ability to provide statements of a known order of accuracy about a parent population.

. . . The possibilities of bias are always present in even the most well-conducted of surveys and are frequently beyond control. Consequently they must always be explored and the possible necessity of weighting to reduce the resulting bias constantly kept in mind.

The statistics for trohoc research have now been well developed, and trohoc investigators appear to be aware of the need to seek and correct for sources of bias. This backwardly directed form of research cannot become scientifically acceptable, however, until the investigators actually look for major sources of bias, rather than the minor ones that can be conveniently examined in demographic data.

Harold Dorn demanded[5] that adequate epidemiologic investigation must be

. . . obtained by a persistent search rather than by a quick walk through a hospital ward as if one were picking up flotsam by casually strolling along the beach. Nature guards her secrets well and throws up deceptive camouflages. . . .

To unravel the tangled skein of causation of disease . . . requires the utmost persistence, a profound skepticism of the obvious, an alertness for the selective factors that have produced the most readily available subjects for study, the ability to penetrate beneath the surface of the observations, a strong distrust of what is said or seen . . . and a willingness to spend long hours upon the development and perfection of methods of making observations. . . .

Modern scientists can accept the investigative ease of looking backward and the lure of simplistic statistical analysis—but the intellectual cost is high. The work itself must be done with the hard-headed thinking, properly chosen variables, and rigorously collected data that confer scientific credibility.

References

1. Cornfield, J.: On certain biases in samples of human populations, J. Am. Stat. Assoc. **37**:63-68, 1942.
2. Cornfield, J.: A method of estimating comparative rates from clinical data. Applications to cancers of the lung, breast, and cervix, J. Nat. Cancer Inst. **11**:1269-1275, 1950-1951.
3. Cornfield, J., and Haenszel, W.: Some aspects of retrospective studies, J. Chron. Dis. **11**:523-534, 1960.
4. Dorn, H.: Some applications of biometry in the collection and evaluation of medical data, J. Chron. Dis. **1**:638-664, 1955.
5. Dorn, H.: Some problems arising in prospective and retrospective studies of the etiology of disease, N. Engl. J. Med. **261**:571-579, 1959.
6. Drill, V. A., and Calhoun, D. W.: Oral contraceptives and thromboembolic disease, J. A. M. A. **206**:77-84, 1968.
7. Drill, V. A.: Oral contraceptives and thromboembolic disease. I. Prospective and retrospective studies, J. A. M. A. **219**:583-592, 1972.
8. Feinstein, A. R.: Clinical epidemiology: II. The identification rates of disease, Ann. Intern. Med. **69**:1037-1061, 1968.
9. Feinstein, A. R.: Clinical biostatistics: X.

Sources of 'transition bias' in cohort statistics, CLIN. PHARMACOL. THER. **12**:704-721, 1971.

10. Feinstein, A. R.: Clinical biostatistics: XI. Sources of 'chronology bias' in cohort statistics, CLIN. PHARMACOL. THER. **12**:864-879, 1971.

11. Fisher, R. A.: The effect of methods of ascertainment upon the estimation of frequencies, Ann. Eugen. **6**:13-25, 1934.

12. Fisher, R. A.: Smoking. The cancer controversy, London, 1959, Oliver & Boyd, Ltd.

13. Fox, J. P.: Prospective studies defined: A comment on a report on the use of hospital data in epidemiologic research, Am. J. Epidemiol. **91**:231-232, 1970.

14. Fox, J. P., Hall, C. E., and Elveback, L. R.: Epidemiology. Man and disease, Toronto, 1970, The Macmillan Company.

15. Fuertes-de la Haba, A., Curet, J. O., Pelegrina, I., and Bangdiwala, I.: Thrombophlebitis among oral and nonoral contraceptive users, Obstet. Gynecol. **38**:259-263, 1971.

16. Inman, W. H. W., and Vessey, M. P.: Investigation of deaths from pulmonary, coronary, and cerebral thrombosis and embolism in women of child-bearing age, Br. Med. J. **2**:193-199, 1968.

17. Levin, M. L., Goldstein, H., and Gerhardt, P. R.: Cancer and tobacco smoking, J. A. M. A. **143**:336-338, 1950.

18. MacMahon, B.: Epidemiologic methods in cancer research, Yale J. Biol. Med. **37**:508-522, 1965.

19. Mantel, N., and Haenszel, W.: Statistical aspects of the analysis of data from retrospective studies of disease, J. Nat. Cancer Inst. **22**:719-748, 1959.

20. Peacock, P. B.: The non-comparability of relative risks from different studies, Biometrics **27**:903-907, 1971.

21. Quetelet, M. A. (1849). Quoted in Reference 20.

22. Sartwell, P. E., Masi, A. T., Arthes, F. G., Greene, G. R., and Smith, H. E.: Thromboembolism and oral contraceptives: An epidemiologic case-control study, Am. J. Epidemiol. **90**:365-380, 1969.

23. Schrek, R., Baker, L. A., Ballard, G. P., and Dolgoff, S.: Tobacco smoking as an etiologic factor in disease. I. Cancer, Cancer Res. **10**:49-58, 1950.

24. Taube, A.: On statistical practice in retrospective studies, Acta Soc. Med. Ups. **72**:237-245, 1967.

25. Taube, A.: Matching in retrospective studies; sampling via the dependent variable, Acta Soc. Med. Ups. **73**:187-196, 1968.

26. Taube, A., and Hedman, B.: On the consequences of matching in retrospective studies with special regard to the calculation of relative risks, Acta Soc. Med. Ups. **74**:1-16, 1969.

27. U. S. Surgeon General's Advisory Committee on Smoking and Health. Smoking and Health, 1964, U. S. Department of Health, Education and Welfare, Public Health Service Publication No. 1103.

28. Vessey, M. P., and Doll, R.: Investigation of relation between use of oral contraceptives and thromboembolic disease, Br. Med. J. **2**:199-205, 1968.

CHAPTER 15

On the sensitivity, specificity, and discrimination of diagnostic tests

In 1947, Yerushalmy[18] introduced the terms *sensitivity* and *specificity* as statistical indexes of the efficiency of a diagnostic test. The sensitivity of the test would indicate its capacity for making a correct diagnosis in confirmed positive cases of the disease. The specificity would indicate the capacity for correct diagnosis in confirmed negative cases.

These concepts need not be restricted to diagnostic tests alone and can be applied to a variety of tests used for identifying clinical conditions. The relationship between clinical conditions and the results of tests is commonly shown in the following "fourfold" table:

	CONFIRMED CONDITION	
RESULT OF TEST	*Positive*	*Negative*
Positive	True positive	False positive
Negative	False negative	True negative

In this table, the column headings denote the patient's confirmed condition; the row headings denote the result of the test; and the four interior "cells" denote whether the patient has been correctly or falsely diagnosed as either positive or negative. According to Yerushalmy's delineation, *sensitivity* would be the number of true positive cases divided by the total number of confirmed positive cases, which is the sum of true positive plus false negative cases. *Specificity* would be the number of true negative

cases divided by the total number of confirmed negative cases, which is the sum of true negative plus false positive cases.

Yerushalmy introduced these terms while performing studies of observer variability among radiologists; and his work was an important contribution to the scientific growth of epidemiology. He helped shatter some of the complacency with which unverified diagnostic statements have been accepted and tabulated in epidemiologic statistics, and his indexes of sensitivity and specificity provided a quantitative method for expressing the problems. The indexes have now become widely applied as statistical tools in the analysis of clinical epidemiologic data. The phrase *sensitivity and specificity*, like the phrase *range of normal*, is now an established part of the mathematical concepts that constantly appear in medical statistics.

Like the statistical concepts associated with *range of normal*[8], however, the conventional mathematical ideas associated with *sensitivity* and *specificity* are inadequate for the real world activities of clinical medicine. One of the main problems is in temporal direction. A clinician wants to use the test predictively; the epidemiologic indexes are often constructed in the wrong chronologic direction, emanating from a "backward" rather than "forward" viewpoint. A second problem arises from oversimplification. Not all diagnoses can be dichotomously cited as either *yes* or *no*; among the other categories to be considered are *probably yes, prob-*

Under the same name, this chapter originally appeared as "Clinical biostatistics—XXXI." In Clin. Pharmacol. Ther. 17:104, 1975.

ably no, and *uncertain.* A third problem is caused by clinical imprecision in the idea of a "diagnostic test". Some diagnostic tests are used to detect the existence of a particular disease, whereas others are used to confirm it. The statistical expression of the test's "ability" will be inadequate unless the purpose of the test is suitably considered. The greatest problem of all, however, arises from neither the unsatisfactory direction of the arithmetic nor the clinical naiveté of the mathematics. The problem is caused by inadequate choices of "control" groups. The patients whose conditions are tested during the evaluation procedures are seldom selected in a way that will determine the true discrimination of the test.

A. Temporal direction

1. Choice of symbols. To discuss chronologic and certain other issues in the mathematics, we need to have some symbols for the four groups of people who appeared in the "cells" of the foregoing table. The choice of these symbols creates a problem of its own. There may be a great deal of observer variability among physicians practicing medicine, but there is even more "symbol variability" among the investigators who discuss sensitivity and specificity.

In Yerushalmy's original paper, he used no symbols. Subsequent authors[1, 3, 11, 13−17] have chosen diverse arrangements of two-letter or one-letter expressions to provide a magnificently creative array of such symbols as α, β, a, b, R, K, ρ, $f_1(\rho)$, $f_2(\rho)$, p, $1 - p$, $1 - b$, ϵ, η, ρ^+, ρ^-, p_{ij}, cf, Se, In, and $P[R|Y]$. In the absence of any national or international efforts at standardization of this statistical babel, an author newly entering the field is free to choose whatever symbols he wishes. I shall use the a, b, c, d symbols that are reasonably familiar to most clinicians looking at the contents of a fourfold table.

The numbers of people present in the four cells of the table cited earlier will thus be listed as:

RESULT OF TEST	CONFIRMED CONDITION	
	Positive	*Negative*
Positive	a	b
Negative	c	d

I shall also use *s* to represent the sensitivity of the test and *f* to represent the specificity. With this convention, the sensitivity of the test is

$$s = \frac{a}{a + c},$$

and the specificity of the test is

$$f = \frac{d}{b + d}.$$

2. Predictive use of a test. At the time a test is first evaluated, its proponents usually assemble a population of people whose condition was known to be positive or negative. When the test was performed in these people and when the numerical frequencies of the data were arranged in the fourfold pattern of the table, the investigators calculated the indexes of sensitivity and specificity. If the results seemed sufficiently encouraging, the test might be accepted into general clinical usage. The troubles would then begin.

The original investigators started with a population whose condition had already been confirmed, but the clinician who later uses the test starts with patients whose condition is unknown. The purpose of the test is to predict (or identify) what the patient's condition really is. In receiving the result of the test, an investigator therefore wants to know its predictive accuracy, not its sensitivity or specificity. He wants to know how well the test would perform for an unknown patient, not its capacity in people who really did not need the test because their correct diagnosis had already been established. If the test result is positive, is the patient's actual condition likely to be positive? If the result is negative, is the actual condition likely to be negative?

To answer these two questions, we need a different set of indexes. In the sensitivity-specificity calculations, the denominators were chosen on the basis of what was found after the diagnoses had already been confirmed. For clinically useful indexes, we would want the denominators to depend on the predictions made by the test. We would therefore want to have an index of positive accuracy—denoting how often the test was correct when its result was positive. We would also want an index of negative accuracy for the correctness of negative results.

If we denote positive accuracy by v, and negative accuracy by g, these indexes would be expressed respectively as

$$v = \frac{a}{a + b} \text{ and } g = \frac{d}{c + d}.$$

An alternative complementary approach is to consider the "false positive rate", $1 - v$, which is the number of false positives divided by the total number of positive results in the test; and the "false negative rate", $1 - g$, which is the number of false negatives divided by the total number of negative results.

With either set of approaches, the denominators now contain the sums of either the positive results or the negative results of the test. We have avoided the denominator "criss-cross" that occurs when negative and positive results are combined for calculating sensitivity and specificity. The positive accuracy and the false positive rates of the test are based on the total of true positive and false positive results; the negative accuracy and the false negative rates are based on the total of true and false negatives.

To illustrate the predictions with some numbers, let us assume that the original investigator assembled 50 patients known to be positive and 100 patients who were confirmed as negative. After the test was performed, the results were as follows:

RESULT OF TEST	CONFIRMED CONDITION	
	Positive	*Negative*
Positive	45	10
Negative	5	90

For these data, the sensitivity of the test is $45/(45 + 5) = 90\%$; and the specificity of the test is $90/(90 + 10) = 90/100 = 90\%$. In its predictive value, however, the test has a positive accuracy of $45/(45 + 10) = 45/55 = 82\%$; and a negative accuracy of $90/(90 + 5) = 90/95 = 95\%$.

The false positive and false negative rates would give these data an even more meaningful clinical expression. In the cited example, the false positive rate is 18% ($= 100\% - 82\%$); and the false negative rate is 5% ($= 100\% - 95\%$). These distinctions demonstrate that a test with equally high rates of sensitivity and specificity can give substantially different rates of false positive and false negative results when it is applied in clinical practice.

3. *Effect of population ratios.* We can now get ready for another dismaying discovery. Suppose the original investigator had gotten different numbers of patients in the two groups he assembled for the evaluation. Suppose he had applied the test to 20 patients who were known to be positive and to 200 patients who were the known negative "controls". Since the sensitivity and specificity of the test are presumably its inherent properties, they would have remained intact at 90% each. After the test was performed, the fourfold table of results would show the following:

RESULT OF TEST	CONFIRMED CONDITION	
	Positive	*Negative*
Positive	18	20
Negative	2	180

In these data, the sensitivity of the test ($= 18/20$) and the specificity ($= 180/200$) are each 90%. A dramatic change has occurred, however, in the test's predictive value. The positive accuracy rate is only 47% ($= 18/38$), so that a false positive result occurred in more than half the people who were diagnosed by the test. On the other hand, the negative accuracy has improved to 99% ($= 180/182$) so that only 1% of the patients were false negatives.

We now recognize not only that the sensitivity and specificity of a diagnostic test will fail to indicate its predictive value, but also that the predictive value will depend entirely on the ratio of confirmed positive and confirmed negative people to whom the test was applied. This ratio is best noted by contemplating the prevalence rate of the confirmed positive condition. This prevalence rate equals the number of confirmed positive cases divided by the total number of cases under study.

For readers who are willing to endure some algebra, the relationships can be symbolically shown as follows. Let N be the total number of people for whom the test is evaluated. Let P be the prevalence rate (or proportion) of people whose confirmed condition is positive. [$P = (a + c)/N$]. The ingredients and totals of our fourfold table would then be numerically expressed as follows:

People with confirmed condition positive	$= PN$
People with true positive results	$= sPN$
People with false negative results	$= (1 - s)PN$
People with confirmed condition negative	$= (1 - P)N$
People with true negative results	$= f(1 - P)N$
People with false positive results	$= (1 - f)(1 - P)N$

The rate of positive accuracy of the test would be

$$\frac{sPN}{sPN + (1 - f)(1 - P)N} = \frac{sP}{sP + (1 - f)(1 - P)}$$

The rate of negative accuracy of the test would be

$$\frac{f(1 - P)N}{f(1 - P)N + (1 - s)PN} = \frac{f(1 - P)}{f(1 - P) + (1 - s)P}$$

In the first numerical example, we had 50 confirmed positive cases and 100 negative controls, so that $P = 50/(100 + 50) = 1/3$. With $s = f = 0.9$, we then have a positive accuracy of $(0.9)(.33)/[(0.9)(.33) + (0.1)(.67)] = .30/[.30 + .07] = .30/.37 = 82\%$. The negative accuracy would be $(.9)(.67)/[(.9)(.67) + (.1)(.33)] = .60/[.60 + .03] = .60/.63 = 95\%$.

In the second numerical example, we had 20 confirmed positive cases and 100 negative controls, so that $P = 20/[20 + 200] = .90$. With $s = f = 0.9$, the positive accuracy is $(.9)(.09)/[(.9)(.09) + (.1)(.91)] = .081/[.081 + .091] = .081/.172 = 47\%$. The negative accuracy is $(.9)(.91)/[(.9)(.91) + (.1)(0.9)] = .819/[.819 + .009] = .819/.828 = 99\%$.

By looking at the algebraic symbols for these expressions, we can note that P appears in the numerator of the expression for positive accuracy. If P is large (i.e., a value close to 1), the tested population will contain a preponderance of confirmed positive patients and very few negative "controls". With this large value of P, the value of $1 - P$ will be small (i.e., a value close to 0), and so the positive accuracy of the test will approach a value of 1 (i.e., 100%). Conversely, since $1 - P$ appears in the numerator of the expression for negative accuracy, this expression will take on its highest value when P is very small (approaching 0), so that $1 - P$ is essentially equal to 1.

By altering the prevalence rate of confirmed positive cases in the tested population, an investigator can thus make the results show almost any values that he wishes to achieve for positive or negative accuracy, regardless of whatever be the sensitivity and specificity of the test. For example, suppose the test is not much better than tossing a coin, having a sensitivity and specificity each equal to 50%. Let us choose 100 positive people and 10 negative "controls" for evaluation. The results will show 50 true positives, 50 false negatives, 5 false positives and 5 true negatives. The test will therefore have a good "batting average" for positive accuracy [$= 50/(50 + 5) = 50/55 = 91\%$] but a bad one for negative accuracy [$= 5/(50 + 5) = 9\%$]. On the other hand, if we chose our evaluation group to contain 10 confirmed positive people and 100 negative "controls", these batting averages would be exactly reversed, with a 9% positive accuracy and a 91% negative accuracy.

If the test is being used to diagnose a disease, the value of P will indicate the prevalence of the disease in the tested population. With a very high prevalence of the disease, a test with a sensitivity and specificity that are no better than tossing a coin might thus have excellent predictive accuracy. If the disease has a very low prevalence in the tested population, the same test will have high accuracy for the negative prediction of "excluding" the disease.

A different type of distress will occur when a test of apparently high sensitivity and specificity is removed from its evaluation in a hospital population and is applied for diagnostic screening in a general population. Suppose an investigator reports a sensitivity of 0.95 and a specificity of 0.85 in a new diagnostic test for cancer. When we apply this test in screening, we can expect the prevalence of cancer to be about 150 per 100,000 patients, so that $P = .0015$. By substituting in the previous formula, we can promptly determine the rate of positive accuracy of the test. Since $s = 0.95$, $f = 0.85$, and $P = .0015$, the rate of positive accuracy will be $(.95)(.0015)/[(.95)(.0015) + (.15)(.9985)] = (.00143)/[.00143 + .14978] = .00143/.15120 = .00942 = 0.9\%$. Thus when the test gives a positive result, the likelihood will be less than 1% that the patient actually has cancer!

The problems caused by these differences in the prevalence of a tested condition have been thoroughly discussed by Vecchio[17] and by Sunderman and Van Soestbergen.[16] Both of these authors' presentations contain tables showing the extraordinarily wide range of values that can occur for "false positive" and "false negative" results of a diagnostic test whose sensitivity and specificity are evaluated in populations with different prevalence rates of the disease.

4. Alternative pattern of "sampling". In the foregoing procedures, the investigator who evaluated the test did his "sampling" from the confirmed cases. He began by choosing one group of people who were known to be positive for the disease (or target condition) and a "control" group of people who were known to be negative. Since these groups were selected by the investigator, he could determine their size and would thereby set the prevalence rate of the disease.

An alternative method of getting the tested population is for the investigator to choose the groups according to the results of the test. He would select one group of people with positive results in the test and another group with negative results. He would then determine the actual conditions in the two groups, and calculate the rate of false positives and false negatives. In this circumstance, the size of the two groups chosen by the investigator would determine the rate of a positive result in the tested population, and we would encounter a different arrangement of the algebraic phenomena.

Let R = the proportion of people with a positive test result, so that $R = (a + b)/N$. Assuming that the test has a fixed sensitivity and specificity, and letting $J = s + f - 1$, we can go through an array of mathematical manipulations (which I shall spare the reader here) to show the following result:

$$\text{Rate of positive accuracy of test} = \frac{s}{J}\left[1 + \frac{f - 1}{R}\right]$$

$$\text{Rate of negative accuracy of test} = \frac{f}{J}\left[1 - \frac{1 - s}{1 - R}\right]$$

To check this calculation, consider the second numerical example cited earlier, where $s = f = 0.9$ and where we had 38 positive test results and 182 negative test results, so that $R = 38/(38 + 182) = 38/220 = 0.173$. Substituting into the formula just cited, we find that the positive accuracy of the test is $[.9/.8][1 - (.1/.173)] = [1.125][.422]$

$= .474 = 47\%$. The negative accuracy of the test is $[.9/.8][1 - (.1/.827)] = [1.125][.8791] = .989 = 99\%$. These results are the same as what we obtained before with the formulas based on values of P, rather than R.

The two formulas just listed will indicate how the rates of positive and negative accuracy can be affected by the choice of R. The algebra is more complex than the arrangements noted earlier for P, but a scan of the associated values of s, f, and J will usually suggest an appropriate choice of R to create suitable effects on the rates of positive or negative accuracy.

Thus, regardless of whether the investigator gets his evaluation groups by choosing cases from the confirmed condition of the patients or from the results of the test, he can arbitrarily alter the calculated rates for false positive and false negative values. Sensitivity and specificity therefore indicate properties that are unaffected by numerical caprice in the respective sizes of the groups used to evaluate a test. This statistical constancy is the desirable feature that has made these two indexes achieve such widespread acceptance. As we shall see later, however, sensitivity and specificity depend on much more than numerical ratios alone. The basic issue is the clinical composition of the tested groups, not just their sizes.

B. Summary indexes

The next major problem occurs as a result of the statistical penchant for "data reduction". Rather than having two different expressions, such as *sensitivity* and *specificity* or *false positive rate* and *false negative rate*, we might prefer to combine the two expressions into a single index. Several statistical indexes of association can be used to create a single value that "summarizes" the results found in a fourfold table. The available indexes include[10] such splendid algebraic eponyms as Guttman's λ, Yule's Q, Yule's Y, Pearson's C, and Tschuprow's T, as well as the $\emptyset$ coefficient and the coefficient of tetrachoric correlation.

Two other indexes, however, have become particularly popular for summarizing the results of a fourfold table dealing with the sensitivity and specificity of a diagnostic test. One of these is called an index of "validity". It is determined as $(a + d)/N$, and it represents the total

Table I. *Palpation vs. thermometry for measuring temperature* *

Temperature estimated by palpation	Actual temperature			Total
	≥ 39° C (major fever)	38-38.9° C (minor fever)	No fever	
≥ 39° C (major fever)	15	3	3	21
38-38.9° C (minor fever)	19	43	15	77
No fever	3	55	993	1051
Total	37	101	1011	1149

*Table rearranged from data presented by Bergeson and Steinfeld.[2]

number of correct predictions divided by the total number of predictions. From our previous symbols, we can recall that a = sPN and d = f(1 − P)N. The index of validity will therefore be the sum of sP and f(1 − P). The constituents of this sum clearly indicate how the "validity" of the test can be altered by the way that the investigator chooses P, the prevalence of the positive condition. To get a high validity score, the investigator need merely choose a high or low value of P according to the relative magnitudes of s and f.

Another summary index, introduced by W. J. Youden[19] (and sometimes called "Youden's J"), has an algebraic structure that ultimately becomes equal to the sum of sensitivity plus specificity minus 1. Since this index has the advantage of being unaffected by the choice of P, Youden's J is a preferred way of combining sensitivity and specificity into a single value.

No matter how a summary index is contrived, however, it will suffer from two major disadvantages:

1. By combining everything into a single value, we lose track of whether the diagnostic test is better in sensitivity or specificity. For example, if Youden's J has a value of 0.55, we would have no idea of whether the sensitivity is 0.95 and specificity is 0.60; or vice versa.

2. More importantly, in using any of the fourfold summary indexes, we accept the idea that the results of the evaluation procedure can readily be listed in a fourfold table. According to this idea, the presence of the disease can be expressed as a simple *yes* or *no*, and the results of the diagnostic test can also be expressed in the same dichotomy. This double-dichotomy arrangement creates a gross and often erroneous oversimplification of the reali-

ties of clinical diagnosis. In many circumstances, the disease cannot be cited as definitely present or definitely absent, and the diagnostic test may yield the result of *maybe* (or *uncertain*) rather than *yes* or *no*. If both the presence of the disease and the results of the test are cited in a 3-category rating scale, however, the calculations of sensitivity and specificity become much more complicated; and the summary index must deal with a ninefold rather than fourfold table.

To avoid these complexities, the data analyst may try to compress a table with nine or more cells into one that contains only four cells. For this compression, the data analyst gets to draw two arbitrary lines that determine the dichotomous "break points" for the consolidations that form the rows and columns of the new table. The arbitrary choice of these lines can strikingly alter what happens to the sensitivity and specificity of the test.

To illustrate the problem, let us consider Table I, which contains data taken from a recent report in which Bergeson and Steinfeld[2], working in a Child Care Clinic at the Johns Hopkins Hospital, tried to determine whether the fever discerned with a thermometer could be detected equally well by a nurse's palpation of the child's forehead or chest. The ninefold arrangement in Table I shows the bivariate frequencies of the data obtained with each method of examination, using a 3-category scale for reporting the result as **no fever, minor fever** (38-38.9° C) and **major fever** (≥ 39° C). The investigators decided to categorize the results of palpation according to three designations: *correct, too high,* and *too low.* Correct results, shown in the three downward diagonal cells of the table, occurred in 15 + 43 + 993

= 1051 cases. In 21 cases (= 15 + 3 + 3), the palpation method gave a falsely high result; and in 77 cases (= 55 + 3 + 19), palpation yielded a falsely low result.

The investigators laudably made no effort to calculate a dichotomous sensitivity and specificity for the "palpation test". In many other similar circumstances, however, such calculations would have been performed with one of at least three different ways of compressing the Bergeson-Steinfeld data. One approach would be to draw perpendicular dichotomous lines at fever vs. no fever. With this approach the numbers in Table I would become:

RESULT OF PALPATION	ACTUAL CONDITION	
	Fever	*No fever*
Fever	80	18
No fever	58	993

The second arrangement would be to draw the dichotomous lines at major fever vs. non-major fever. With this arrangement, Table I would become:

RESULT OF PALPATION	ACTUAL CONDITION	
	Major fever	*Not major fever*
Major fever	15	6
Not major fever	22	1106

A third arrangement depends on a previous decision about clinical tactics. Let us decide that we will always use a thermometer to take the patient's temperature if palpation indicates the intermediate condition of **minor fever**. Furthermore, for purposes of using palpation as a "screening test", let us assume that we are not really interested in circumstances where the thermometer shows only **minor fever**. What we really want to know is the reliability of palpation in "screening" for major fever. With these assumptions, five cells are removed from the original nine-fold table, and it reduces to the following four-fold table:

RESULT OF PALPATION	ACTUAL CONDITION	
	Major fever	*No fever*
Major fever	15	3
No fever	3	993

We can now calculate the sensitivity and specificity of palpation, as shown in three different arrangements of the same basic set of data.

In the first arrangement, s = 58% (= 80/138) and f = 98% (= 993/1011). The false positive and false negative rates are 18% and 6%, respectively. In the second arrangement, s = 41% (= 15/37) and f = 99% (= 1106/1112). The respective false positive and false negative rates are 29% and 2%. In the third arrangement, s = 83% (= 15/18) and f = 99.7% (= 993/996). The false positive rate is 17%; and the false negative, 0.3%. We can thus get three different sets of values for sensitivity and specificity, or for false positive and negative rates, according to the way we decide to dichotomize the data. If the original table had contained more categories in both directions—so that the results were arranged in a 4 × 4 or even larger pattern of cells—the opportunities for disagreement would be even greater when the data were doubly dichotomized.

In addition to this difficulty, a separate problem that arises in the construction of any "two-way" contingency table—no matter how many cells it contains—is the assumption that the entity being evaluated is the univariate result of a single test. Many medical diagnoses depend on an aggregate of the results found in several different variables, not just in one. For example, in acute myocardial infarction, the clinical diagnosis would depend on certain combinations of symptoms, electrocardiographic data, and laboratory tests. In acute rheumatic fever, the Jones diagnostic criteria call for an enumerated collection of entries from certain "major" and "minor" manifestations. A test procedure based on input from just one variable is obviously inadequate for determining the sensitivity and specificity of these complex diagnoses. We would need to use an expression that contains multivariate constituents. An example of such a variable would be *fulfillment of composite criteria for diagnosis of acute myocardial infarction*. The categories of this variable could be expressed in terms such as **yes** or **no** (or **uncertain**).

This method of citing the result of a multivariate diagnostic procedure would allow us to use a 2-way table for comparing the enumerated data of whatever method was employed to confirm the patients' correct diagnoses. On the other hand, because the constituent multivariate elements are lost in a single expression such as **yes** or **no**, we would have no direct way of determining the causes of erroneous results when they occur. To track down the sources of false positive and false negative diagnostic errors, we would have to go back and start with each of the multivariate constituents.

C. Relationship of index and purpose

Both of the statistical difficulties that have just been mentioned could be overcome (or at least reduced) with a more sophisticated set of mathematical indexes for expressing the relationships. Instead of using Youden's J, or the "index of validity", or any other indexes that depend on doubly dichotomous data in a four-fold table, we could use indexes of association that allow the variables to have polytomous (more than two) categories. Such indexes would include Kendall's tau, Goodman and Krushkal's G, Cicchetti's statistic[4], and some of the various "kappa" statistics described by Fleiss[9] or the "lambda" statistics described by Hartwig[12]. (If worst came to worst, or perhaps to best, we could simply enumerate the results according to the proportions that were too high, correct, and too low). To consider the correlation between multivariate constituents of data and the patient's confirmed condition, we could use some of the diverse correlation coefficients that can be derived from multiple linear regression or discriminant function analysis.

These statistical improvements in managing multicategory or multivariate data, however, will not solve a more fundamental problem in describing the effectiveness of a test. What seems to be almost wholly overlooked in clinicostatistical strategies for calculating a test's effectiveness is the purpose for which the test is used.

1. The three types of diagnostic test. Diagnostic tests are employed for at least three different purposes: discovery, confirmation, and exclusion. During various types of "screening" procedures, we use a *discovery test*. Examining people who seem healthy, with no clinical complaints to suggest the presence of a particular disease, we often search for that disease in a clinically "silent" form. Examples of such discovery tests in lanthanic patients are the uses of a serum calcium measurement for hyperparathyroidism, a fasting blood sugar for diabetes mellitus, or a rectal examination for rectal cancer.

A *confirmation test* is employed in situations where we have strong suspicions that the disease is present. The purpose of the test is to verify this suspicion. The performance of bronchoscopy with microscopic examination of biopsy tissue is a confirmation test for lung cancer; and a glucose tolerance test provides confirmation for diabetes mellitus.

An *exclusion test* is usually employed to "rule out" the presence of a disease when it is suspected. Such a test is usually too expensive or inconvenient to be employed merely for discovery purposes during routine "screening". For example, a stool guaiac examination might be used for the screening discovery of colonic cancer, but a more elaborate roentgenographic or colonoscopic examination would be needed to "rule out" the disease if its presence is suspected. Certain exclusion tests are cheap enough and convenient enough to be used for screening purposes. Thus, when an appropriate skin test for tuberculosis is negative, the presence of active disease can usually be excluded, although a positive test will neither discover nor confirm active tuberculosis.

Some tests are good for only one of these three purposes. Some are good for two. Some can be used for all three. For example, the performance of sigmoidoscopy, together with biopsy and histologic examination when appropriate, can generally be used to discover, confirm, and exclude cancer of the rectum. A glucose tolerance test can be used to confirm and to exclude the presence of diabetes mellitus, but is generally too inconvenient for purposes of screening discovery. The histologic examination of tissue from a bronchoscopic biopsy is an excellent way to confirm lung cancer, but cannot be used to exclude the disease or to discover it during routine screening.

Since diagnostic tests are employed for these different purposes, the statistical indexes of efficiency should be arranged accordingly.

2. Requirements of detection and confirmation. In a discovery test, we want reasonably high sensitivity. If the disease is present, it should be found, even at the risk of getting a high rate of false positive results. [We are willing to take this risk because a discovery test, when positive, is usually followed by a confirmation test]. In an exclusion test, we want the sensitivity to be even higher than in a discovery test. Unless the sensitivity is 1 or close to 1, the risk of a false negative result would keep us from being confident that a negative test has excluded the disease.

The discovery and exclusion tests are thus both intended to have a high sensitivity for detecting the disease when it is present. To get the particularly high sensitivity that is sought in an exclusion test, we must be willing to pay the appropriate clinical price. Thus, to test urine for sugar is a good, cheap, convenient way of "screening" for the discovery of diabetes mellitus, but the urine test will regularly give some false negative results. To measure fasting blood sugar is a more expensive and less convenient discovery procedure, but it is more diagnostically effective because it has a lower false-negative rate than the urine test. If we want to rule out diabetes mellitus with certainty, however, we cannot rely on either of these procedures. We would have to use the much more expensive and cumbersome mechanism of the glucose tolerance test, which, in this instance, would be both an exclusion and a confirmation test.

By contrast, in a confirmation test, we want extremely high specificity, with few or no false positive results. If the test shows that the disease is present, we want to be sure that it is present. We would have no real objection to occasional false negative results, since the confirmation test will probably be ordered after an exclusion test was used to find any cases that might otherwise be missed as false negatives.

3. Combinations of tests. A single test can seldom be excellent for the goals of both detection and confirmation. With rare exception, the same procedure cannot be sensitive enough to find all cases of the disease while simultaneously being specific enough to avoid false positive identifications. For example, the chest X-ray is a quite sensitive but non-specific way of finding lung cancer. Almost all patients with lung cancer have abnormal roentgenograms, but not all people with positive roentgenograms

turn out to have lung cancer. Conversely, a positive bronchoscopic biopsy is a quite specific but non-sensitive way of identifying lung cancer. The bronchoscopic biopsy almost never gives false positive results, but it regularly will miss lung cancers that are located at inaccessible sites.

For these reasons, many diagnostic tests are regularly used in tandem. A high sensitivity test is used to find the disease; and a positive result is followed by a high specificity test that will confirm the diagnosis by "excluding" its possible falsehood. Because of these tandem arrangements, the best statistical appraisal of the results will depend on a suitable arrangement of the paired tests. In such an arrangement, the result of the pair might be called *negative* if the detection test is negative; and the paired result would be called *positive* only if both the detection test and the confirmation test are positive. The positive and negative results of this kind of paired arrangement would have both high specificity and high sensitivity.

D. Choice of the tested populations

There are important clinical reasons for trying to solve some of the problems that have just been discussed. Perhaps the most important reason is that this form of correlation between the result of a test and the patient's actual condition is the best way of making clinical sense out of the statistical chaos that now exists in demarcating the "range of normal"[8]. If "normality" is determined purely on a univariate basis, according to arbitrary statistical boundaries for a distribution of data, the demarcation will indicate the zone of customary values for the test, but not their clinical connotations in health or disease. If the demarcated zone is to have these clinical connotations, the demarcations must be established in direct correlation with an actual condition of health or disease. This type of correlation can be achieved and evaluated only through the type of bivariate arrangements we have been discussing.

The discussion so far has been concerned, however, only with the defects of existing clinico-statistical strategies and with ways of improving the defects. Unfortunately, these mathematical improvements will not solve the really fundamental biostatistical problems of diagnostic tests. Like so many other sophisticated statistical procedures, the complex indexes of association produce elegant but superficial algebra. The indexes can provide useful methods of quantitative expression for what has been observed—but the calculations are totally dependent on what is submitted as the observed data. And the fundamental biostatistical problem lies in the choice of the populations that are the sources of the data.

1. The role of clinical suspicion. If we are going to use a test for different diagnostic purposes, it must be evaluated in groups of people who suitably represent the different diagnostic challenges. These people cannot be chosen merely according to whether or not they were demonstrated to have the disease in question. Since the preceding clinical suspicions will affect the choice of a test and the evaluation of the test's performance, the tested population must at least be divided according to the existence of clinical suspicions. We would thus choose one group of people who constitute the ordinarily healthy population for whom the test would be used, during "screening", as a detection test. The second group of people would have medical conditions that aroused our suspicion of the disease and that made us want to confirm it or exclude it.

The customary fourfold diagnostic table would thus be converted into the following "eightfold" table:

RESULTS OF TEST	ACTUAL CONDITION	
	Positive	*Negative*
Screened population:		
Positive	a′	b′
Negative	c′	d′
Suspected population:		
Positive	a″	b″
Negative	c″	d″

If these populations are going to approximate reality, we would want P, the prevalence of the actual disease, to be low in the screened population and high in the suspected population.

When the test results are correlated with the patients' actual condition, we would calculate at least two sets of values for sensitivity and specificity—one set for the screened population and another set for the suspected population. Thus, instead of a single value for sensitivity [which would be $(a' + a'')/(a' + c' + a'' + c'')$], we would determine two separate values: $a'/(a' + c')$ for the screened population and $a''/(a'' + c'')$ in the suspected population. Two analogous calculations would be done for specificity, using the respective b and d values in the screened and suspected populations.

2. The role of pathologic derangement. By inspecting this eightfold arrangement of data, we can begin to see why a particular test might have not one set of values for sensitivity and specificity, but several different sets. Suppose a positive result in the test depends on the disease having produced a certain level of pathologic derangement. When this level of derangement occurs, the diseased persons almost always develop symptoms that arouse suspicions of the disease. In such suspected patients, the test will therefore have high sensitivity. On the other hand, if the disease is present without having reached the prerequisite level of pathologic derangement, the patient may be asymptomatic and part of a screened population. In such a population, the diagnostic test may have low sensitivity.

Once we begin to contemplate a pathologic derangement[7], rather than the particular entity that is called a "disease", we can also recognize the causes of many false positive or disproportionately positive results that can destroy the value of a diagnostic test. For example, suppose the positive result of a particular diagnostic test really depends on a derangement in the patient's nutritional status, but suppose we want to employ this test for the diagnosis of cancer. For the evaluated population, we choose the diseased group from hospitalized patients with cancer, and the non-diseased group from healthy technicians, secretaries, and other staff personnel. Since patients whose cancer is severe enough to require hospitalization are often malnourished, the results of their test are usually positive. Since the staff personnel are well nourished, their test results are negative. We emerge from the evaluation process with the belief that we have found an excellent new diagnostic test for cancer: the sensitivity and specificity values are quite high.

After the test begins to be applied, we may be chagrined to discover that it really has low sensitivity and low specificity. The test fails to detect the neoplasms of asymptomatic well-nourished patients with cancer; and it gives false positive diagnoses of cancer for malnourished patients with stroke, chronic cardiopulmonary disease, or certain enteropathies. Because we failed to include such patients in the original test population, we did not discover the inefficiency of the test until after it became clinically popular.

3. Surrogate vs. pathognomonic tests. The term *pathognomonic* is usually applied to a clinical manifestation that uniquely indicates a particular condition. For example, the palpation of spontaneous movement within a suitable sized suprapubic mass in a woman would be pathognomonic of pregnancy. This term can also be used for paraclinical procedures that either delineate, demonstrate, or otherwise identify a particular disease. For example, the histologic findings in an appropriate tissue specimen will be pathognomonic of cancer or hepatitis; a specified set of values in a glucose tolerance test will be pathognomonic of diabetes mellitus.

In a *surrogate* test, we examine an entity that will be used to represent or approximate the disease we want to identify. Examples of surrogate tests are pap smears for cancer, serum glutamic oxalic transaminase (SGOT) for hepatitis, chest X-ray for tuberculosis, electrocardiogram for myocardial infarction, or urine sugar for diabetes mellitus.

A pathognomonic test is seldom evaluated for sensitivity and specificity. We may worry about observer variability when a pathologist interprets a tissue specimen; or about the standards of glucose ingestion, specimen timing, and chemical measurement when a laboratory performs a glucose tolerance test; but we are not concerned that the test itself may be misleading.

It is the surrogate tests that create the main problems of sensitivity and specificity. A surrogate test does not identify the disease; it identifies something else that we hope will denote the disease. We often use surrogate tests because they are simpler, cheaper, and more convenient than the corresponding pathognomonic test. The surrogate test may also be more sensitive. For example, a measurement of serum alkaline phosphatase may detect metastatic

cancer that has been missed by a liver biopsy; and a positive chest X-ray can detect tuberculosis that has not shown tubercle bacilli in the microscopic examination of sputum. To compensate for these advantages, surrogate tests often produce false results and the problem of evaluating sensitivity and specificity.

Because the procedure is a surrogate test, it depends on a pathologic entity that is different from the one we are trying to diagnose. To contemplate sources of false positive and false negative results, we must therefore contemplate the mechanisms that might "trigger" a test into errors of omission or commission. These mechanisms will consist of alternative pathologic derangements or clinical conditions. Thus, inflammation may create a false positive pap smear for cancer; and inaccessibility of the desquamated cells may make the pap smear falsely negative. The electrocardiogram may fail to show a myocardial infarction if taken too early after the acute attack and may give false positive results because of some other myocardopathy. Many chemical tests give falsely high results in response to alternative diseases and drugs; and the results can be falsely lowered under other appropriate clinical conditions.

4. The process of discrimination. For all these reasons, a proper evaluation of the surrogate procedures that are called *diagnostic tests* would require them to receive several different challenges in discrimination. The test must be able to discriminate among a variety of pathologic derangements that might simulate either the target disease or an entity in the clinical and paraclinical spectrum of that disease. The various groups of patients who enter the evaluated population must be selected according to their suitability for providing these challenges. If patients are chosen merely because they do or do not have the target disease, the discrimination of the test will not be adequately evaluated.

The choice of patients to provide appropriate challenges will depend on both the medical spectrum of the disease and its diagnostic comorbidity. The medical spectrum[5] of the disease refers to the array of clinical and paraclinical laboratory abnormalities that it can produce. The diagnostic co-morbidity of the disease consists of other diseases that might be mistaken for it. Diagnostically co-morbid diseases are usually entities occurring in the same topographic location of the body or producing somewhat similar morphologic or other paraclinical abnormalities.

For example, the medical spectrum of primary lung cancer would indicate patients with hemoptysis, with major weight loss, and with abnormal chest roentgenograms. The spectrum of diagnostic co-morbidity for lung cancer would include patients with non-neoplastic pulmonary diseases (such as tuberculosis and chronic bronchitis) and with metastatically neoplastic pulmonary lesions. To evaluate the discrimination of a proposed new test for lung cancer, we would therefore want to challenge the test with patients who represent different parts of the medical and co-morbid spectrum.

Our investigated population might thus include the following groups of people: asymptomatic patients with lung cancer; patients with lung cancer and only primary symptoms, such as hemoptysis; patients whose lung cancer symptoms include such systemic effects as major weight loss; patients whose lung cancer manifestations include such metastatic effects as hepatomegaly or bone pain; asymptomatic patients with other causes of pulmonary disease; hemoptytic patients with other pulmonary disease; patients with major weight loss due to other diseases; and patients with hepatomegaly or bone pain due to other diseases.

In a more general statement of principles, the populations used to evaluate the discrimination of a diagnostic test for Disease X should consist of representatives from the following groups of people:

1. Patients with Disease X who are asymptomatic.

2. Patients with Disease X who are symptomatic with a diverse collection of manifestations that cover the medical spectrum of the disease.

3. Patients without Disease X who have other diseases that have produced overt manifestations similar to those in the medical spectrum noted in Group 2.

4. Patients without Disease X who have other diseases that can mimic Disease X's pathologic derangement by occurring in a similar location

or by having similar paraclinical dysfunctions.

The sensitivity of a test used for discovery purposes in "screening" will depend on its capacity to identify patients in Group 1. The test's sensitivity for exclusion purposes will depend on its performance in identifying members of groups 1 and 2. The specificity of the test will depend on its avoidance of false positive results in groups 3 and 4. These four groups would seem to be a minimum demarcation of the necessary comparisons, but additional subgroupings would be needed in appropriate circumstances.

The complexity of these arrangements may seem distressing, but they are ultimately less distressing than the continued proliferation of diagnostic tests whose inadequacies escape initial evaluations because the initial evaluations did not contain suitable challenges. The oversimplification of the existing tactics for getting "control" groups and calculating statistical indexes has led to the spawning of many tests that are grossly unsatisfactory for clinical purposes.

To deal with clinical reality requires a confrontation with clinical complexity. The new arrangements proposed here are both feasible and analyzable after the appropriate data have been assembled. The performance of such complex analyses is not at all a novel idea. It has been, in fact, performed for many years during a generally unquantified procedure called *clinical judgment*[5]. With increasing advances in technology, clinicians will increasingly have to evaluate the costs, risks, and diagnostic discrimination of new diagnostic tests. If these evaluations are to provide sensible clinical science, the subtleties and complexities of clinical judgment must be acknowledged, adapted, and incorporated into the plans for choosing the patients who are tested and for quantitatively expressing the results.

References

1. Bennett, B. M.: On comparisons of sensitivity, specificity and predictive value of a number of diagnostic procedures, Biometrics **28**:793-800, 1972.
2. Bergeson, P. S., and Steinfeld, H. J.: How dependable is palpation as a screening method

for fever? Clinical Pediatr. (Phila.) **13:**350-351, 1974.

3. Berkson, J.: "Cost-utility" as a measure of the efficiency of a test, J. Amer. Stat. Assn. **47:**246-255, 1947.

4. Cicchetti, D. V.: A new measure of agreement between rank ordered variables, Proc. Am. Psychol. Assoc. **7:**17-18, 1972.

5. Feinstein, A. R.: Clinical judgment (reprinted edition), Huntington, N. Y., 1974, Robert E. Krieger Publishing Co.

6. Feinstein, A. R.: The pre-therapeutic classification of co-morbidity in chronic disease, J. Chronic Dis. **23:**455-469, 1970.

7. Feinstein, A. R.: An analysis of diagnostic reasoning. I. The domains and disorders of clinical macrobiology, Yale J. Biol. Med. **46:**212-232, 1973.

8. Feinstein, A. R.: Clinical biostatistics. XXVII. The derangements of the range of normal, CLIN. PHARMACOL. THER. **15:**528-540, 1974.

9. Fleiss, J. L.: Statistical methods for rates and proportions, New York, 1973, John Wiley & Sons, Inc.

10. Freeman, L. C.: Elementary applied statistics: For students in behavioral science, New York, 1965, John Wiley & Sons, Inc.

11. Greenhouse, S. W., and Mantel, N.: The evaluation of diagnostic tests, Biometrics **6:**399-412, 1950.

12. Hartwig, F.: Statistical significance of the Lambda coefficients, Behav. Sci. **18:**307-310, 1973.

13. Mantel, N.: Evaluation of a class of diagnostic tests, Biometrics **7:**240-246, 1951.

14. Muic, V., Petres, J. J., and Telisman, Z.: Validity of a diagnostic test designated by a single function, Methods Inf. Med. **12:**244-248, 1973.

15. Nissen-Meyer, S.: Evaluation of screening tests in medical diagnosis, Biometrics **20:**730-755, 1964.

16. Sunderman, F. W., and Van Soestbergen, A. A.: Laboratory suggestions: Probability computations for clinical interpretations of screening tests, Am. J. Clin. Pathol. **55:**105-111, 1971.

17. Vecchio, T. J.: Predictive value of a single diagnostic test in unselected populations, N. Engl. J. Med. **274:**1171-1173, 1966.

18. Yerushalmy, J.: Statistical problems in assessing methods of medical diagnosis, with special reference to X-ray techniques, Pub. Health Rep. **62:**1432-1449, 1947.

19. Youden, W. J.: Index for rating diagnostic tests, Cancer **3:**32-35, 1950.

SECTION THREE
PROBLEMS IN MEASUREMENT

In discussing the methods used for assembling and analyzing data, we begin with the assumption that the basic information is (or will be) there, awaiting the statistical manipulation. For many activities in medical research, however, the main challenges are in the data, not in the analysis. This aspect of research architecture requires decisions about what data to get and what methods to use for the process of measurement that converts an observed entity into an item of data. Statistical strategies are seldom pertinent for these challenges, because the mathematical models are concerned with numerical methods of analysis, not with scientific methods of mensuration.

The four papers in this section deal with a few of the many important problems in clinical measurement that require clinical rather than statistical solutions. For one set of solutions, clinical investigators need an intellectual liberation from the entrenched but erroneous doctrine that data can be "hard" only if expressed in dimensional numbers. The persistence of this fallacious doctrine has been abetted by an unbalanced emphasis on parametric forms of statistical analysis and by the scientific aberration that occurred many years ago when Gaussian ideas about the variance of different measurements for a single entity became applied to the distribution of single measurements for different entities. A separate set of solutions will involve remedial action for the inappropriate use of the word "normal" to describe the shape of a statistical curve, and for misguided attempts to establish medical normality solely according to statistical locations.

Statistical proposals for the assessment of safety and efficacy have been scientifically unsatisfactory because of the failure to delineate what is meant by "safety" or by "efficacy." The many published reports of adverse drug reactions have not been accompanied by a reproducible operational identification of adverse drug reactions; and efficacy is constantly appraised with techniques that do not encompass the wide spectrum of phenomena requiring consideration. To accomplish a large-scale surveillance of the effects of therapeutic agents, careful attention will be needed for many complex issues in clinical specifications and clinical analyses for the populations to be observed, the methods of observation, and the differentiation of effects. These issues are usually disregarded or oversimplified when the investigators hope that the problems will be solved mainly with mathematical inspirations or computerized extravaganzas.

CHAPTER 16

On exorcizing the ghost of Gauss and the curse of Kelvin

At any era in the history of science, the further advance of science has been retarded by certain fundamental concepts that were enlightening when introduced, but that later, after persisting too long, became barriers to future progress.

In his perceptive book, *The Structure of Scientific Revolutions,* Thomas S. Kuhn[27] has used the term *paradigms* for these fundamental concepts, which he defines as "universally recognized scientific achievements that for a time provide model problems and solutions to a community of practitioners (of science)." As examples of change in such paradigms, Kuhn cites the transitions from Ptolemaic to Copernican to Keplerian theories of astronomy; and from Aristotelian to Newtonian to Einsteinian concepts of dynamics. An example in the history of biomedical science would be the successive basic alterations in ideas of cardiac physiology from pre-Galenic times to Galen to Harvey to modern beliefs.

Kuhn notes that contemporary paradigms have important roles as stimuli to the growth and development of the "normal science" of an era, but he also points out

Under the same name, this chapter originally appeared as "Clinical biostatistics—XII." In Clin. Pharmacol. Ther. 12:1003, 1971.

the way that creative research becomes stultified when adherence to an outdated paradigm produces "a strenuous and devoted attempt to force nature into the conceptual boxes supplied by professional education."[29] When nature refuses to remain in those boxes, "anomalies, or violations of expectations, attract the increasing attention of (the) scientific community . . . (to) . . . the emergence of crises that may be induced by repeated failure to make an anomaly conform."[28]

The initial response to a crisis is resistance, as the defenders of the old paradigm devise "numerous articulations and *ad hoc* modifications of their theory in order to eliminate any apparent conflict."[32] Eventually, however, after "normal science repeatedly goes astray . . . the profession can no longer evade anomalies that subvert the existing tradition of scientific practice."[32] The crisis becomes intolerable and a "scientific revolution" occurs, producing a new paradigm, "a new set of commitments, a new basis for the practice of science."[30]

My object in this essay is to call attention to two outdated paradigmatic concepts that have been stifling the intellectual growth of clinical biostatistics. One of these concepts—an extension of ideas often attributed to Carl Gauss—is the belief that the observed data of clinical medicine can usually be expressed with "normal" distributions for "continuous variables" having a "variance" that can be calculated from the observations. The second concept —an extension of beliefs stated by Lord Kelvin—is the idea that scientific data must be expressed objectively in the form of dimensional measurements. Both of these concepts provided major enlightenment when they first became accepted as paradigms; both have now led to major intellectual crises that remain unsolved by various *ad hoc* modifications of the basic paradigms; and both are now being used to substitute for enlightened thought or to thwart it.

1. The ghost of Gauss

As technologic devices of measurement began to proliferate during the 19th century, scientists became confronted by a phenomenon that we now call "observer variability." Repeated measurements of the same object did not yield identical results. The disagreements immediately provoked the question of how to choose a *correct* value from among the diverse measurements. The obvious answer to this question was to designate the mean of the measurements as *correct*. With this assumption, the amounts by which values differed from the mean would be regarded as *errors*. The magnitude of individual deviation from the mean could be calculated for each of the n measurements; the individual deviations could be squared (to remove negative signs); the squared deviations could be added together; and the sum could be divided by n to provide a "mean" of the squared deviations that was called the *error variance*. The square root of this error variance was designated as the *standard deviation*.

One of the great statistical contributions of Carl Friedrich Gauss was to notice that these errors in measurement were usually distributed in a specific pattern of symmetry. The most commonly repeated single value was usually the mean itself; small errors on either side of the mean were next most frequent; large errors were uncommon, although present in about equal frequency on both sides of the mean; and extremely large errors were rare. When the frequency of the individual measurements was graphically plotted against their values, the result was a symmetrical "bell-shaped" or "cocked-hat" curve, with its apex at the value for the mean.

The name "normal" was given to the pattern of frequencies shown in this curve, and it has become the familiar "normal distribution" on which so much statistical reasoning has depended during the past century. The important intellectual advances that have come from this reasoning are too well known to need recapitulation here. What is less apparent, however, is the enormous obstacle that this reasoning now imposes to progress in clinical biostatistical research.

A. The ambiguity of 'normal.' The decision to call this type of curvilinear symmetry a "normal distribution" was a reasonable act of mathematical nomenclature. The word "normal" has often been applied in various aspects of mathematics and the natural sciences. In clinical medicine, however, the word *normal* had already been established, long before its statistical usage, in reference to a quite different connotation: the distinction between health and disease. The definition of this distinction is an issue too fundamental and complex for further discussion here. Suffice it to say that the word *normal* has two entirely different meanings in its two types of usage. Statisticians refer to the shape of a curve; clinicians refer to a state of well-being.

The extensive medical problems created by the confusion between these two ideas about *normal* will be reserved for a later paper in this series. For the moment, however, we can note that clarity of thought in clinical biostatistics would best be served if the bell-shaped curve had another name. The adjective *campaniform*, which has been proposed[46] for the curve's configuration, might be a satisfactory "generic" designation, but a commemorative eponym seems more appealing. The phrase *Gaussian curve* is readily understood and has already been used by many writers, although it perpetuates the same type of historical "injustice" created by the many medical eponyms in which the commemorated person is the man who first popularized a phenomenon, rather than the man who first described it. The earliest account of the bell-shaped curve was by Abraham De-Moivre, not by Gauss.[45]

B. The choice of a 'normal range.' Another major problem in *normality* is the choice of a "normal range." The problem has at least three components: (1) should the idea of normality depend on the characteristics of a state of health or on the value of a numerical measurement; (2) what is the appropriate population whose individual medical characteristics or numerical measurements (or both) will be used to determine normality; and (3) by what method should boundaries be demarcated to create a *range?*

These questions have been increasingly debated in recent years, particularly as a "range of normal" has been sought for the abundance of new paraclinical data produced by the increasing medical use of chemical technology. My own contributions to this debate will be deferred for a later paper, but I have borrowed part of my title here from the title of an excellent recent discussion ("Health, Normality, and the Ghost of Gauss") by Elveback, Guillier, and Keating.[10]

C. The logical alteration of 'variance.' In the original development of Gaussian statistics, the term *variance* referred to inconsistencies in observation. When the same object had received a series of non-identical measurements, the deviations from the "correct" mean would be the source of *error variance*. The term *error* was thus attached to *variance* in the 19th century in order to connote disparities in the act of mensuration, and the term *error variance* referred to the size of the discrepancies. Thus, in the sequence of OB-

JECT → ACT OF MEASUREMENT → VALUE, the mean and the variance referred to the values per act of measurement. Since only a single object had been measured, the variance clearly did not refer to the object itself.

During the 20th century, however, the original logic of variance has been altered, so that variance may now refer to the objects themselves, as well as to the measured values. We can therefore talk about the variance of the data regardless of whether we get 30 repeated measurements of the same object, or a single measurement for 30 different objects. In the first kind of variance, however, we refer to the process of measurement, whereas in the second, we usually ignore the mensurational activity and refer to a characteristic of the measured object. From variance per measured value, the term has been altered into variance per measured object. For example, when we repeatedly measure the value of sodium in a single specimen of serum, we get the variance of the laboratory procedure; but when we look at the single values of serum sodium for a group (or "sample") of people, we get the variance of the people.

One obvious problem of ambiguity in this double usage of the same term is caused by the persistence of the phrase *error variance* in some statistical textbooks. The phrase may be appropriate in reference to a process of measurement, but the term *error* is improper and confusing when it prefixes a *variance* that refers to a group of people. The reader may be misled into believing either that the measured values are themselves incorrect (a point that is seldom at issue), or that something was wrong about the people who deviated from the mean. Aside from this semantic difficulty, however, the logical alteration of variance has had profound effects on the use and abuse of modern statistics.

(1) The distinctions of quality control and populational variance. When the many chemical tests performed in modern clinical laboratories are checked for "quality control," a traditional Gaussian calculation is

applied to values obtained in repeated measurements of the same specimen. The variance of these multiple values helps indicate the reproducibility and precision of the test.

When an array of results is assembled for specimens from a group of patients or for successive specimens from the same patient, however, the calculated variance contains an admixture of variances arising not only from the differences in the specimens but also from the vicissitudes of the test. Nevertheless, when the data for two such specimens are compared, most clinicians usually decide that one value is higher or lower than the other without considering the amount of variation attributable to the test. The necessary adaptations, which are beyond the scope of this essay, are particularly well discussed in an intriguing new book by Roy Barnett.[2] The main point to be noted here is that the variations in people, as discerned from a test, cannot be properly interpreted without considering the variations in the test itself.

(2) Homogeneity of sample. In the days when variance always depended on the measurements of a single object, statisticians did not have to worry about the homogeneity of the objects being measured. The sampled object was "homogeneous" unto itself. When measurements are performed for a group of objects, however, the issue of homogeneity becomes fundamental to the scientific validity of the group.

In order to apply any statistical calculations that depend on a group of objects, we must first decide that the objects can be considered collectively as a *group*. If the objects are sufficiently homogeneous, they can readily be combined for the calculation of a collective mean and variance. If the objects are too heterogeneous, however, the collective values of mean and variance may produce statistical gibberish. For example, we might have no objection to calculating the mean and variance for the height of a group of people, but we might greatly demur from such calculations if the group contained people, mice, elephants, and gerbils, or if the group was confined to people but comprised a mixture of newborn infants, adult pygmies, and professional basketball players.

The complex problems of defining and determining homogeneity will be reserved for a later paper in this series. The only point to be noted now is that a "chicken-and-egg" type of problem has been created by the frequent use of *variance*—in its newer, logically altered meaning—as a measure of homogeneity. Do we first decide that a group is homogeneous and do we then determine the variance, or do we first measure the variance and then decide that the group is homogeneous?

The classical statistical approach to this question is to determine homogeneity from the calculated variance. If the *co-efficient of variation*, which is the ratio of the standard deviation divided by the mean, is below 10%, the group is often regarded as reasonably homogeneous. Statistical strategies and tactics are permeated with the idea that homogeneity is determined from *post hoc* calculation rather than from *a priori* classification. In most textbooks and other statistical literature, the term "homogeneity" rarely appears alone, and is generally used in the context of *homogeneity of variance.* Diverse "corrections" and other adaptations have been developed for statistical inferences and tests in circumstances where the variance is not "homogeneous."

The classical scientific approach to this question, however, is to regard homogeneity as an issue in taxonomy, not in statistics. Scientists usually make an *a priori* judgment about homogeneity before we measure, not afterward. We decide, as an act of taxonomic classification and diagnostic identification, whether our observed objects are mice or elephants, newborn babies or professional basketball players. We do not rely on measurements and calculations for these issues in identification. For example, if a group of objects had a mean weight of 15.1 pounds with a standard deviation of 0.2 pounds, a classical statistician might conclude that the objects were quite homogeneous because their co-efficient of variation is only 1.3%.* This conclusion might be entirely justified with respect to the weight of the objects, but a classical scientist would demand more description of the objects before drawing any conclusions about their homogeneity. He might then discover that the group consisted of littermates chosen from kennels of large cats, small dogs, and huge birds.

In certain forms of scientific classification, the available categories of taxonomy may not be satisfactory for decisions about homogeneity. Thus, the classical taxonomy of biology is adequate for distinguishing different four-legged animals as mice, dogs, cats, cows, horses, or elephants, and for distinguishing different species among these animals. The available taxonomy of human chronology and occupations is adequate for distinguishing newborn babies from professional basketball players. But classical taxonomy has not been equally satisfactory for distinguishing different species of such entities as bacteria or worms. A form of *numerical taxonomy*[6, 38] has now been developed to make such distinctions by calculations based on the measured values of different physical and chemical properties of these entities.

In the classification of clinical phenomena, many important problems of heterogeneity have been overlooked during the statistical attention to variance as an exclusive index of homogeneity. Among such problems are the inadequacies of the current taxonomy of disease, which cannot be remedied merely by calculations or by reshufflings of categories of coding for the diseases.[11] The prognostic inadequacy of diagnostic nomenclature also cannot be improved by statistical tactics alone, and the improvements will require careful consideration of important variables that have been omitted from current classifications.[11] These improvements will not occur, however, if the intellectual problems of medical

taxonomy remain neglected, and if Gaussian variance continues to be regarded not only as a description of a group, but also as a primary index of homogeneity.

D. The idea of continuous variables. Perhaps the most intellectually pernicious current residue of Gaussian statistics is the abstract mathematical concept of continuous variables. One of the basic tenets of the mathematical expression for the Gaussian curve and of the statistical reasoning based on this expression is that the variables are continuous. A variable is regarded as *continuous* if it can take on additional values that lie within any defined interval of values, no matter how small the interval becomes. For example, serum sodium can be regarded as a continuous variable. If we could measure it as finely as 136.75 or 136.76 meq./L., it can still assume the values of 136.752 or 136.753 within that interval. If our measuring device were precise enough to identify the latter two values, serum sodium could still be 136.7528 or 136.7529, and so on.

All the mathematical concepts of analytic geometry and the calculus depend on continuous variables, as do most of the concepts of mathematical statistics. As soon as statistics leaves its theoretical origins and enters the world of reality, however, a new symbol is necessary to indicate that the real world does not permit such niceties in measurement. This symbol is the Σ sign that is the traditional emblem of statistical activities. If the measurements used in statistics were minute enough to be truly continuous, we would not need the Σ sign. To calculate the sum of values for a continuous variable, x, that had different frequencies at each value, we would say that x had a "density function," $f(x)$, which represented the frequency of x at each point as it "moves" continuously along its curve. The sum of the values of x would then be expressed as $\int x f(x) dx$, using the integral sign ($\int$) for sums of continuous variables.

In both biologic and statistical reality, however, we cannot determine $f(x)$ and

---

*$1.3\% = \dfrac{0.2}{15.1} \times 100.$

the idealized continuous values of x. Instead we note the actual metric values of x at a series of i points, and we count the corresponding frequencies. We express those metric values as x_i, the frequencies as f_i, and the sum of the values for x as $\Sigma f_i x_i$. Furthermore, when we draw a graph to show the pattern of these frequencies, we do not draw a continuous curve. Instead, we draw a "frequency polygon" that connects the observed points with straight lines. Alternatively, we do not draw a line at all, and we construct a bar-graph called a "histogram."

This distinction between the ideal and real metric values of a continuous variable would be merely pedantic were it not for another crucial feature that differentiates clinical biology from the statistical models that have been proposed for it. Many important clinical variables are discrete rather than continuous. They are expressed in specific categorical terms that may be numerical or verbal. Some of these discrete variables are also metric, in that they can be expressed on a ranked scale with equal intervals between adjacent ranks. Illustrations of discrete metric variables are number of children or number of previous myocardial infarctions.

Many other important clinical variables, however, are not even metric. They are expressed as discrete categories in "scales" of values that are either ordinal, nominal, or existential. An ordinal scale contains such values as *none, mild, moderate,* and *extreme* for the variable, severity of chest pain, or such values as *0, 1+, 2+, 3+,* and *4+* for the variable, briskness of patellar reflex. Although an ordinal scale is demarcated into ranked values, the interval between any two adjacent ranks is not measurably equal. A nominal scale contains unranked values such as *male* and *female* for the variable, sex; or *doctor, lawyer, merchant,* and *other* for the variable, occupation. An existential scale contains such unranked values as *yes* and *no,* or *present* and *absent,* for the variable, presence of chest pain, or for the variable, presence of

rheumatic fever. An existential scale can be converted to ordinal rankings with such gradations as *definitely present, probably present, uncertain, probably absent,* and *definitely absent.*

A statistical paradigm that depends on continuous metric variables will frequently produce biologically peculiar results when the paradigm is applied to variables that are either metrically discrete or non-metric. Some of the peculiarities have occurred so often that the classical mode of calculation may be abandoned in favor of an alternative expression. Thus, rather than saying that the average American family has 2.3 children, we would avoid calculating a mean that creates the strange 0.3 child, and we would state, instead, that American families have a median of 2 children. When a variable is expressed nominally, neither a mean nor a median can be used for calculating a summary of the values, and the result would be stated as a mode or proportion. Thus, we might note that chest pain is the most common (i.e., the mode) presenting complaint among patients in a coronary care unit, or that chest pain appeared in 76% of such patients.

In many other instances, however, a suitable alternative expression has not yet been developed, and *ad hoc* modifications are still being proposed for the anomalies produced by an unsatisfactory statistical paradigm. For example, to predict survival from the many variables that describe a patient's initial state, the main paradigm offered by modern statistics is a technique called multiple linear regression. For clinical reasoning, this technique has many defects that have been described elsewhere.[25] I shall here cite only two of the statistical difficulties. Since the regression technique depends on numerical data, it cannot accommodate existential or nominal variables, which are not expressed in numerical values. Accordingly, the *ad hoc* modification is to assign arbitrary numbers as "values" for these variables, so that *absent* may become *0* and *present, 1;* or *male* may become *2* and *female, 3.* An additional problem of the multiple regression procedure is that its array of numerical co-efficients, when applied to the data for a particular patient, may sometimes yield a *negative* value for the predicted survival. The *ad hoc* modification for this anomaly is to apply a "logistic" correction that makes the regression procedure always yield a positive value.

As long as the tactics are otherwise successful, a gerrymandered statistical procedure need not create any major biologic difficulties. The main scientific hazard of the continuous-variable paradigm occurs when a devotion to such variables becomes the basis for rejecting or disdaining data that are discrete, rather than continuous. Such attitudes can arise from either intellectual inertia, intellectual prejudice, or both. In the customary educational background of a statistician, the contemplated variables are usually continuous, so that he becomes most comfortable intellectually when dealing with continuous data. To avoid the "discomfort" of discrete data, the statistician may then advise his clinical consultees to eliminate discrete variables in favor of continuous metric data. With these substitutions of variables, the research may become altered from its true objectives. The easily measured continuous variables may yield statistically comfortable and numerically precise results that answer the wrong questions.

The intellectual inertia that leads to these inappropriate substitutions could not have been sustained for so long a time, however, without an additional source of support. No scientist would persistently discard or fail to analyze important data merely for the convenience of statistical calculations. The attitude that encourages a displacement of discrete data by continuous variables has required intellectual reinforcement not just from statistical ideology, but from the paradigms of science itself. The prejudice against discrete data has been incorporated into scientific thinking for almost a century, and is epitomized in the doctrine of William Thompson, later knighted as Baron Kelvin.

2. The curse of Kelvin

About 90 years ago, a time when the work of Charles Darwin was drastically altering some fundamental paradigms of human biology, when the concepts of Rudolf Virchow had led to the new paradigms of medical histopathology, and when Francis Galton was performing the magnificent analyses that would culminate in the development of biometry as a distinctive new intellectual discipline, a recurrent exhortation was being offered to physicists. The exact words of Lord Kelvin's theme, as Kuhn[26] has noted, appear in diverse forms, but the basic sentiment is: "When you cannot express it in numbers, your knowledge is meagre and unsatisfactory." This theme, which was later repeated by many other eminent researchers, including Galton, has become one of the paradigms of modern science.

For physicists, chemists, astronomers, and other workers in the contemporary "natural science," Kelvin's exhortation seemed entirely appropriate. During that era, a burgeoning technology had begun to produce many new instruments with which to measure physical and chemical phenomena. Scientists were avidly working to create those instruments and to apply them in measurements. Kelvin's exhortation was also promptly accepted and implemented by biologists who could apply the new instruments to study similar phenomena in the fluids, excreta, tissues, and cells of biologic organisms. The exhortation was also happily received by biometricians who were seeking numerical measurements with which to develop the principles and data of their infant discipline.

An important feature of Kelvin's doctrine was that it demanded numbers, but did not discriminate among three different ways in which numbers could be obtained. The two principal sources of numbers are mensuration and enumeration. In mensuration, the number is observed as a dimension on an established continuous scale of values. In enumeration, the number is obtained by counting a group of identified entities. In mensuration, the number is "continuous," and in enumeration "discrete." A third way of getting numbers is to divide one of the principal types of numbers by another. Thus, a *mean* is usually created by dividing a mensuration by an enumeration; and a *proportion,* by dividing one enumeration by another enumeration.

For example, we can use numbers to say that a particular man weights 70.21 kg., has 4 children, and belongs to a club of which 20% of the members are board-eligible doctors. Each of these citations contains a numerical statement, but the first number is a dimensional mensuration, the second is a counted enumeration, and the third is a proportionate ratio or percentage. All three of these numbers provide quantification in whatever setting they are used, but the numbers arise from distinctively different basic forms of description. In one form of citation, the basic observation is itself a number on a dimensional scale. In the other form of citation, the basic observation is a verbal description whose "units" are nouns, adjectives, verbs, or adverbs. We use such words to stipulate that an entity is a *child* or a *board-eligible doctor,* and we then quantify that stipulation by counting a group of verbally described entities, or by expressing the counted group in proportionate percentages of some other counted group.

An individual object can therefore be described in dimensions or in words. A group of objects can be quantified by calculating a mean for the dimensions, or by determining a count or ratio for what is represented by the descriptive words. Statistical data could thus be achieved from either a route of dimensional mensurations and calculated means, or a route of verbal descriptions, counted enumerations, and fractional proportions.

In the general interpretation given to the Kelvin doctrine, however, the latter route was rejected. A populational quantification by counts and ratios of verbal data would have provided numbers that were just as "numerical" as dimensional means

and standard deviations, but the desideratum chosen for "science" was to achieve a dimension at the basic level of observation. The concept of quantification was limited to the concept of metrification.

With this constricted interpretation of Kelvin's "numbers," the rush toward dimensional measurement began and has continued. During the stampede, many clinical biologists and biometricians apparently forgot that Darwin's and Virchow's major scientific advances had not required the use of numbers, and that Galton's biometry was based mainly on describing phenomena and counting them, not on dimensional mensuration. Furthermore, during Kelvin's lifetime, bacteriology and radiography* were introduced as new disciplines of observation, producing data that were scientifically fundamental, precise—and verbal.

Although these triumphs of verbal description might have been expected to reduce the alacrity with which mensurational pursuits became a prime goal of biomedical research, the allure of measured dimensions was too great. Technology was available to provide the measurements, and Gaussian-type "continuous" statistics were available to manipulate the numbers. The current interpretation of Kelvin's doctrine has now become so well established as a scientific paradigm that its fundamental basis is almost never questioned, despite the major problems and anomalies it has caused.

For clinicians and for social scientists, the consequences of Kelvin's exhortation have been more of a curse than a comfort. The variables that are most important to practicing clinicians and sociologists are usually expressed in nominal, existential, or (at best) ordinal form and can not readily be converted to dimensional metric measurements. There is no technologic device or natural scale of dimensions[22, 40] with which a physician can metrically measure such entities as chest pain, back pain, dyspepsia, abdominal cramps, dyspnea, dysuria, or

---

*The arrival of x-rays was greeted with surprise and shock by many members of the scientific community. Lord Kelvin at first regarded them as an elaborate hoax.[31, 42]

other discomforts encountered in the daily work of clinical medicine. There is no technologic device or natural scale of dimensions that can be used by a psychiatrist to metrically measure love, fear, anxiety, hostility, or depression, or by a sociologist to metrically measure the diverse attitudes and exchanges that occur in social interactions. To achieve mensurational numbers for approval by scientific colleagues, a clinical or sociologic investigator would have to abandon his precision in the use of words, and would have to replace the discrete data of verbal description with variables that could be cited in metric units. The effect of these replacements has been wryly summarized by Frank Knight in the remark, "If you cannot measure, measure anyhow."[24]

The new metric variables could be obtained in two different ways. The first was to use laboratory technology, when possible, for dimensional appraisal of entities that might correspond to those previously cited in verbal descriptions. Thus, a measurement of vital capacity or some other test of pulmonary function might replace a verbal account of the severity of dyspnea. The second method was to contrive a "scale" of numerical values that would provide a seemingly metric expression for a non-physical quality, such as intelligence, that had no counterpart in technologic tests.

A. The 'metrics' of psychology and sociology. Since laboratory technology offered almost no dimensional variables that corresponded to the non-physical phenomena of behavioral or sociologic research, psychologists and sociologists began to create new numerical "scales" for "measuring" such entities as intelligence, anxiety, and family inter-relations. By assigning arbitrary grades to the answers received in questionnaires or interviews, and by combining these grades in diverse manners, the investigators could express the results in ranked numbers.[3, 5, 33, 41, 43]

The main difficulty with these scales has been their validation. How could the investigator determine that a scale actually measured what it purported to measure? If the previous verbal descriptions were inadequate so that intelligence and anxiety were themselves ambiguously specified, with what could the investigator correlate his scale to validate it? For example, do current tests of "intelligence" place too high a premium on vocabulary and arithmetic, at the expense of imagination and creativity? When intelligence is assessed exclusively in the analytic framework of multiple-choice answers to a question, do we neglect the importance of an ability in logical synthesis that might be demonstrated only with an "essay" type of response? How do we decide that one particular scale for "anxiety" or for "personality inventory" is better or more accurate than another scale?

The difficulty of validating scales for non-physical phenomena has been a major scientific handicap for workers in psychology and sociology. Some of the contrived scales have been highly effective (or at least widely accepted), but most of them have never received a primary validation, many new scales are "validated" only in correlation with an accepted (but unvalidated) old scale, and many others have been non-productive exercises of the "quantophrenia" described by Sorokin.[39] (The passion for contrived but unvalidated measurements was tellingly satirized by R. E. Dickinson,[9] who suggested a scale for assessing feminine beauty: "The unit proposed is the milli-helen, the quantity of beauty required to launch exactly one ship.")

Even if all the problems of contrived metrification had been solved, however, scientific progress in the quantification of sociology and clinical psychology would still be handicapped by almost insurmountable difficulties in selection of the population to be measured. As indicated in preceding papers[15, 17, 18] of this series, the validity of an investigated population may be destroyed if it consists of a non-random or chronologically diffuse cross-section, or if it is examined in a backward etiologic direction instead of being pursued forward as a cohort. Although clinicians can constantly observe cohorts of patients who are offered therapy and followed thereafter, sociologists do not ordinarily "treat" their subjects, and psychologists (or psychiatrists) have not studied therapy with the same fervor that has been devoted to the etiology of psychic ailments. Consequently, many sociologic populations have consisted of "cross-sections" that could not be chosen randomly, and psychologic populations have often consisted of psychically ill people who were followed in a backward direction toward etiology and "psychodynamics." When psychologists have attempted to perform forward studies of pathogenesis, the members of the cohort have usually consisted of "healthy" volunteers, "chunk groups," or other "rancid" samples.[15] These epidemiologic difficulties have outweighed any major advances obtained from the creation of metric scales by psychologists and sociologists. The full scientific potential of the scales cannot be exploited until satisfactory methods have been developed for getting suitable cohorts and other appropriate populations for investigation.

B. The 'metrics' of clinical medicine. In ordinary medical activities, a clinical investigator is spared many of the problems that his psycho-social colleagues encounter in non-physical phenomena and in cohort availability. The symptoms and signs observed as clinical data can generally be related to "physical" entities, and clinicians constantly treat patients who become cohorts for studies of the course and therapy of disease. With satisfactory techniques of classification and investigation, the treated cohorts could be analyzed in a manner that would remove or adjust the bias accrued during their non-random collection.[17, 18]

Given the opportunity to study the clinical data and therapeutic cohorts of "organic" disease, physicians could have been expected to make major intellectual improvements in the scientific assessment of therapy. The major therapeutic advances of the past few decades, however, have been technologic, not intellectual. The advances have occurred in the surgical tactics and pharmaceutical agents of treatment, not in the scientific design and analysis of therapy. Clinicians have finally learned that therapy must be "controlled" and quantified, but have not yet developed satisfactory methods for choosing suitable "controls" and for quantifying the appropriate variables. Clinicians have begun to accept and utilize the statistical concept that planned therapeutic experiments require a randomized allocation of treatment, but equal attention has not been given to the scientific concept that the treated patients and their clinical responses must be adequately identified. The consequences of the unsatisfactory methods of investigation are evident in the therapeutic controversies that exist today at every level of treatment from such minor ailments as the sprained back and common cold to major ailments such as diabetes mellitus, myocardial infarction, fracture of the hip, and peptic ulcer, to catastrophic ailments such as cancer. The abundance of statistical data and even randomized trials has produced many numerical "confidence intervals," but few therapeutic numbers about which thoughtful physicians could feel clinically confident.

Many of the problems have been due to the clinician's abdication of his own responsibilities by delegating the design of research to statisticians whose abstract "models" have been inadequate for the realities of clinical biology.[14] But an equally important source of problems has been the clinician's failure to emulate the metric creativity of his psycho-social colleagues. A discipline of *clinimetrics* has not been established to correspond to *psychometrics* and *sociometry*. Clinicians have become metrically oriented, but not while observing patients. The metric data have come from paraclinical tests of patients' blood, urine, and other substances observed in the laboratory.

If clinicians had respected their clinical

observations, a collection of suitable "scales" would have been created, tested, and validated for identifying the existence or assessing the severity of such phenomena as pain, digestive distress, dyspnea, and all the other "physical" symptoms encountered in medical practice. The scales, by now, could have been standardized in direct clinical activities, and would be available today for therapeutic surveys and trials. Instead, however, clinicians have evaded the scientific challenges of their own observational data. Rather than confronting and solving the problems of clinical data, clinicians have substituted the plethora of metric data available from paraclinical technology. An array of dimensional numbers far beyond the fondest expectations of any Kelvinistic dream has been provided by the technologic ability to measure the constituents of diverse fluids; to assess the physiologic magnitudes of structural volume, mechanical pressure, electrical conduction, and muscular contraction; and to count the uptake of radioactive substances. All of these phenomena are generally observed, however, not in the patient, but in substances derived from the patient and examined by methods other than clinical skills. To achieve the phantasmagoria of metric data in modern medicine, clinicians have shifted their medium of observation from the patient in the bed to the substance in the lab.

This deliberate dehumanization of the observed variables was inspired by the quest for "better science" and it has produced results that are often scientifically excellent. Nevertheless, the absence of suitable attention to patients has produced major defects in both therapeutic science and therapeutic care. Some of the most crucial aspects of clinical therapy can be discerned only in the patient and cannot be appropriately measured with paraclinical data. Neither the initial state nor the subsequent state of a treated patient are properly identified if the analyzed variables do not include such clinical features as iatrotropy, co-morbidity, and the cluster, sequence, and chronometry of symptoms.[11]

A patient's performance in an isolated laboratory test of exercise does not indicate his dyspnea or angina pectoris in the circumstances of daily life. The assessment of roentgenographic tumor size, white blood count, and survival time does not indicate whether a patient with cancer is alive and vibrant, or miserable and vegetating. The assessment of electrocardiographic changes, angiographic anatomy, or digitalis intake does not indicate a patient's cardiac function.

In these examples and in numerous other instances of the data needed for evaluating modern therapy, the necessary verbal variables of clinical observation have been replaced by numerical data from paraclinical variables that provide the right measurement for the wrong entity. The consequences of this "substitution game" have been inadequate clinical science, because neither the pre-therapeutic nor post-therapeutic state of the patient is sufficiently specified; and dehumanized clinical care, because the patient himself is deliberately ignored as an important source of information for analysis.

The basic reason for avoiding the verbal descriptions of clinical data has been that they are subjective, "soft," and non-reproducible. Much of this difficulty could be promptly removed, however, if clinicians gave serious attention to improving the methods of observation and classification for the data. By shunning the intellectual seduction of inadequate metric substitution, by establishing suitable taxonoric criteria[12] for interpretation of the "soft" data, by identifying the observational details necessary for the interpretations, and by analyzing and reducing the inconsistencies with which these details are observed, clinicians could preserve the important "soft" data while "hardening" their scientific quality. The various nominal, existential, or ordinal categories of classification for these data would then produce the necessary scales of clinical medicine.

Many such scales have been created in recent years. Some of them are used for diagnostic (or "screening") identification; and others deal with grading the severity of an entity either for prognostic or therapeutic purposes. Among such scales are: the various ratings of mental and physical impairment issued by committees of the American Medical Association[7]; the "Apgar score" of the condition of newborn babies[1]; and the "Katz index" of independence in activities of daily living.[23] Other recent scales have dealt with the severity of such entities as tetanus,[34] asthma,[4] the neonatal respiratory distress syndrome,[20] osteoarthritis of the knee,[21] and alcoholism.[37] After many previous "statistical" investigations of clinical course and treatment, scales (or "criteria") have finally been proposed for such scientific fundamentals as the diagnosis of lupus erythematosus,[8] the severity of renal disease,[35] and the quality of survival in patients with breast cancer.[36]

These and other new scales are all based on categorical arrangements of information that is primarily verbal. Although the proposed scales represent important scientific progress, the progress is scant and overdue. Almost none of the scales has been directly validated, either in construction or in application, because no satisfactory scientific and statistical strategies have been developed for the validations. For example, no penetrating analyses have been given to the issue of whether a composite scale is best created by "additive weights" or by "Boolean clusters." In addition, almost all the scales refer to the patient's condition at a single point in time. Satisfactory scales have not been established for grading *transitions* in severity from one state to another. The scope of the scales is still greatly restricted. Many important clinical phenomena, including the assessment of what is really accomplished in the care of patients,[19] have not yet received appropriate investigation and scales for evaluation. A further significant problem is that many major therapeutic trials have been (or are now being) performed with the necessary scales either omitted or abjured. For example, in the celebrated UGDP

study,[44] the conventional clinical scale for diabetic neuropathy was replaced by a metric measurement performed with a biothesiometer. In exchange for the statistical satisfaction of these measured dimensions, however, the investigators had to accept the scientific chagrin that later came when the biothesiometric baseline data could not be obtained for more than half the cohort, and when the measured results in the toes were found to be non-reproducible.[16]

All of the necessary work in "clinimetrics" will require intensive attention and thought from clinicians who respect the basic scientific importance of the subject and who have the trained observational skills to study it. The work cannot be done by statisticians or other personnel who lack familiarity with the clinical nuances of both the observational procedures and the data. The process of analyzing and validating the results can be greatly aided, however, by statisticians who are enlightened enough to welcome the intellectual challenges of categorical data, perceptive enough to encourage the clinical investigators to grapple with the problems, and wise enough to avoid misleading the investigators into the specious allure of metric substitutions.

In using verbal data to yield discrete categories that can be enumerated and quantified with proportionate ratios, clinicians can fulfill the larger meaning of Kelvin's doctrine about the need for numerical expressions. But a sublime paradox of modern technology can enable the demand for numbers to be satisfied even at the fundamental level of description. At about the same time that Kelvin's exhortation was achieving wide popularity, Herman Hollerith introduced a punch card system with which data could be coded for mechanical processing. First used for the United States census of 1890, the coding system has now evolved into the familiar Hollerith (IBM) cards that are used today for managing data with a digital computer. The tactics of expressing discrete data with numerical "co-ordinates" and coding digits have been described elsewhere,[13] and will not be further discussed here. The main point to be noted now is that such verbal data as "substernal chest pain, provoked by exertion, relieved by rest" can be faithfully and precisely represented when a coding number like *137406* is entered appropriately into the columns of a Hollerith card.

The sublime paradox of computer automation, therefore, is that its system for coding data offers clinicians the opportunity to re-humanize clinical science instead of using the inanimate technology to potentiate further dehumanization. By restoring attention and standardization to crucial clinical data that have hitherto been neglected because they could not be expressed numerically, the Hollerith coding system can permit the patient rather than the laboratory to gain supremacy as the center of attention in clinical science. As a group of coding digits, the number *137406* has no more dimensional connotation than a telephone number or a zip code, but it provides a numerical expression for a precise verbal description, it has six meaningful digits (in contrast to the three "significant figures" that usually suffice for metric measurements), and it can serve as a prophylactic agent for avoiding the transmogrified data of "metric madness." Since the remedy for this chronic biostatistical malady is now available, the only real problems that remain are the entrenched intellectual inertia and constricted paradigmatic allegiance that prevent clinical investigators from recognizing the opportunity, grasping its challenge, and creating the necessary changes.

• • •

The curse of Kelvin can be exorcised, therefore, by recognizing the paramount importance of clinical observations, by augmenting the precision with which the observations are made and verbally described, by developing operational criteria to convert the descriptions into precise categories, and by using computer coding techniques to express those categories in numerical digits. The ghost of Gauss can be eliminated by transfer to a new spiritual home

in the *Gaussian curve,* and the term *normal* can then be liberated and returned to its primordial medical meaning. This transfer, however, will not remove the poltergeist of neo-Gaussian *variance,* an ambiguity that has confounded the fundamental differences between an intellectual process of classification and an observational process of measurement. The scientific distinctions that separate *homogeneity* and *homogeneity of variance* will be discussed later in this series.

The computer's capacity for calculation also offers the opportunity to remove another neo-Gaussian eidolon: the appraisal of "significance" according to abstract inferences based on observed variance. An entirely new approach to statistical decisions has been made possible by the computer's ability to perform randomizations of data in a *Monte Carlo* procedure. The new statistical paradigms provided by Monte Carlo concepts will also be reserved for discussion at a later date.

References

1. Apgar, V.: Proposal for new method of evaluation of newborn infant. Anesthes. Analg. **32:** 260-267, 1953. (Further details reported in J. A. M. A. **168:**1985, 1958.)
2. Barnett, R. N.: Clinical laboratory statistics, Boston, 1971, Little, Brown & Company.
3. Buros, O. K., editor: Personality tests and reviews, Highland Park, N. J., 1970, The Gryphon Press.
4. Chai, H., Purcell, K., Brady, K., and Falliers, C. J.: Therapeutic and investigational evaluation of asthmatic children, J. Allergy **41:**23-36, 1968.
5. Church, C. N., and Ratoosh, P., editors: Measurement: Definitions and theories, New York, 1959, John Wiley & Sons, Inc.
6. Cole, A. J., editor: Numerical taxonomy. Proceedings of a colloquium held in the University of St. Andrew's, September, 1968, London, 1969, Academic Press, Inc.
7. Committee on Rating of Mental and Physical Impairment (American Medical Association). The committee has issued 13 publications dealing with different body systems. A list appears in the most recent publication in: J. A. M. A. **213:**1314-1324, 1970.
8. Diagnostic and Therapeutic Criteria Committee of the American Rheumatism Association

Section of the Arthritis Foundation. Preliminary criteria for the classification of systemic lupus erythematosus, Bull. Rheum. Dis. **21**:643-648, 1971.

9. Dickinson, R. E.: A letter in *The Observer*, Feb. 23, 1958. Quoted in: Atkins, H. J. B.: The three pillars of clinical research, Br. Med. J. **2**:1547-1553, 1958.

10. Elveback, L. R., Guillier, C. L., and Keating, F. R.: Health, normality, and the ghost of Gauss, J. A. M. A. **211**:69-75, 1970.

11. Feinstein, A. R.: Clinical judgment, Baltimore, 1967, The Williams & Wilkins Company.

12. Feinstein, A. R.: Taxonorics. I. Formulation of criteria, Arch. Intern. Med. **126**:679-693, 1970.

13. Feinstein, A. R.: Taxonorics. II. Formats and coding systems for data processing, Arch. Intern. Med. **126**:1053-1067, 1970.

14. Feinstein, A. R.: Clinical biostatistics. VI. Statistical "malpractice"—and the responsibility of a consultant, CLIN. PHARMACOL. THER. **11**:898-914, 1970.

15. Feinstein, A. R.: Clinical biostatistics. VII. The rancid sample, the tilted target, and the medical poll-bearer, CLIN. PHARMACOL. THER. **12**:134-150, 1971.

16. Feinstein, A. R.: Clinical biostatistics. VIII. An analytic appraisal of the University Group Diabetes Program (UGDP) study, CLIN. PHARMACOL. THER. **12**:167-191, 1971.

17. Feinstein, A. R.: Clinical biostatistics. X. Sources of 'transition bias' in cohort statistics, CLIN. PHARMACOL. THER. **12**:704-721, 1971.

18. Feinstein, A. R.: Clinical biostatistics. XI. Sources of 'chronology bias' in cohort statistics, CLIN. PHARMACOL. THER. **12**:864-879, 1971.

19. Gilson, J. S.: Urgently needed: A way to measure how much we really help patients, Resident Staff Physician **17**:139-145, 1971.

20. Gomez, P. C. W., Noakes, M., and Barrie, H.: A prognostic score for use in the respiratory-distress syndrome, Lancet **1**:808-810, 1969.

21. Gresham, G. E.: A method for the evaluation and classification of symptomatic and functional status in osteoarthritis of the knees, Arthritis Rheum. **13**:320, 1970.

22. Hamilton, M.: Measurement for what? Proc. Roy. Soc. Med. **63**:1315-1319, 1970.

23. Katz, S., Ford, A. B., Moskowitz, R. W., Jackson, B. A., and Jaffe, M. W.: Studies of illness in the aged. The index of ADL: A standardized measure of biological and psychosocial function, J. A. M. A. **185**:914-919, 1963.

24. Knight, F.: Quoted in footnote, p. 34, ref. 26.

25. Koss, N., and Feinstein, A. R.: Computer-aided prognosis: II. Development of a prognostic algorithm, Arch. Intern. Med. **127**:448-459, 1971.

26. Kuhn, T. S.: The function of measurement in modern physical science, *in* Woolf, H., editor: Quantification, Indianapolis, 1961, Bobbs-Merrill Co., pp. 31-63.

27. Kuhn, T. S.: The structure of scientific revolutions, ed. 2, Chicago, 1970, University of Chicago Press, p. viii.

28. Ibid. p. ix.

29. Ibid. p. 5.

30. Ibid. p. 6.

31. Ibid. p. 59.

32. Ibid. p. 78.

33. Nunnally, J.: Tests and measurements: Assessment and prediction, New York, 1959, McGraw-Hill Book Co., Inc.

34. Phillips, L. A.: A classification of tetanus, Lancet **1**:1216-1217, 1967.

35. Report of the Council on the Kidney in Cardiovascular Disease (American Heart Association). Criteria for the evaluation of the severity of established renal disease, Circulation **44**:306-307, 1971.

36. Schottenfeld, D., and Robbins, G. F.: Quality of survival among patients who have had radical mastectomy, Cancer **26**:650-655, 1970.

37. Shelton, J., and Hollister, L. E.: Quantifying aleoholic impairment, Mod. Med. **37**:188-189, 1969.

38. Sokal, R. R., and Sneath, P. H. A.: Principles of numerical taxonomy, San Francisco, 1963, W. H. Freeman & Co.

39. Sorokin, P.: Fads and foibles in modern sociology, Chicago, 1956, Henry Regnery.

40. Stevens, S. S.: Mathematics, measurement, and psychophysics. *in* Stevens, S. S., editor: Handbook of experimental psychology. New York, 1951, John Wiley & Sons, Inc., pp. 1-49.

41. Stouffer, S. A., Guttman, L., Suchman, E. A., Lazarsfeld, P. F., Star, S. A., and Clausen, J. A.: Measurement and prediction, Princeton, N. J., 1950, Princeton University Press.

42. Thompson, S. P.: The Life of Sir William Thomson Baron Kelvin of Largs, London, 1910, The Macmillan Company. (Cited on p. 59 of ref. 27.)

43. Torgerson, W. S.: Theory and methods of scaling, New York, 1958, John Wiley & Sons, Inc.

44. University Group Diabetes Program. A study of the effects of hypoglycemic agents on vascular complications in patients with adult-onset diabetes. Part I: Design, methods, and baseline characteristics. Part II: Mortality results, Diabetes **19**:(Suppl. 2) 747-830, 1970.

45. Walker, H.: Studies in the history of the statistical method, Baltimore, 1929, The Williams & Wilkins Company.

46. Zilversmit, D. B.: The impact of rigid definitions on scientific thinking, Perspect. Biol. Med. **7**:227-247, 1964.

CHAPTER 17

The derangements of the 'range of normal'

According to certain contemporary standards, the basketball player Wilt Chamberlain is grossly abnormal. At more than seven feet, his height is at least five standard deviations away from the mean. Yet no one, except possibly a basketball opponent, has proposed that Chamberlain's normality be restored by amputating his legs.

This outrageous vignette helps illustrate the confusion that can arise from the current chaos of medical publications dealing with the "range of normal". Despite all the proposed new units of measurement and all the calculations spawned by computers, the concept of a "range" has not been suitably defined in either data or population, and the medical meaning of "normal" has been lost in the shuffle of statistics.

A. The meaning of 'normal'

In a series of masterly papers, E. A. Murphy[35-38] has demonstrated the ambiguity and inconsistency with which the concept of "normal" is applied in modern medicine. Murphy has noted at least seven different meanings[37] for the word *normal*. For most practical purposes, these meanings can be divided into two groups: the isolated and the correlated. In the isolated meanings, the idea of normal is univariate, emerging from the direct partition of an array of numbers that are the values of a single variable, such as height, age, or serum cholesterol. In the correlated meanings, the idea of normal is bivariate. The values for the single variable (height, age, or serum cholesterol) are regarded as normal or abnormal according to the way they relate to some other variable, such as state of health, genetic fitness, or prognostic expectations.

In the isolated approach, the zone of normality is delineated according to what is found to be conventional, customary, average, or habitual in the array of numerical values. With this approach, we might use such expressions as "he normally begins work at 9 AM" or "families these days normally have two children". When the isolated approach receives rigorous quantification, the demarcation of *normal* becomes an act of pure statistics. After the array of numbers is assembled, a statistical principle is used to choose the boundaries of the groups that will be included or excluded as *normal*.

In the correlated approach, the idea of normal is medically referred to some innocuous, harmless, or ideal situation of health. If the particular number implies a current state of ill health, it is usually called *abnormal*; if it implies the hazard

Under the same name, this chapter originally appeared as "Clinical biostatistics—XXVII." In Clin. Pharmacol. Ther. 15:528, 1974.

of some future ailment, the number may be called a *risk factor*. For example, the current standards of normality in blood pressure were established in a correlated rather than univariate manner. The decision that a diastolic blood pressure of more than 90 or 95 mm/Hg. is abnormal was based on the relationship between these values and the occurrence of future vascular complications. The decision did not depend on a purely statistical partition of an array of blood pressure values for a large population. Similarly, a temperature of 101° F. is regarded as abnormal, not because of its position in a univariate frequency distribution, but because of the clinical "abnormalities" that are directly associated. A person in otherwise excellent health, with a barrage of unremarkable laboratory tests, might be deemed to have an "abnormal" level of serum cholesterol if it is high enough to be regarded as a "risk factor" for future coronary artery disease. A person with sickle cell trait could go through a medically uneventful lifetime, but might be regarded as "abnormal" because of the potential genetic hazard to subsequent offspring.

These correlated approaches are the traditional way in which physicians have used the words *normal* and *abnormal*. The words imply a direct medical relationship to a past, present, or future state of health. This semantic strategy seems eminently sensible to any thoughtful practicing physician, but it has some major drawbacks in an era of quantitative technology.

One of the main problems arises from the non-dimensional characteristics of most medical diagnoses. Many (perhaps most) of the major diseases in modern medicine are diagnosed by observation and verbal description, not by mensuration. All of the disease entities that are expressed in morphologic terms (*coronary occlusion, carcinoma, pulmonary emphysema, hepatic cirrhosis, cerebral arteriosclerosis, cholelithiasis, prostatic hypertrophy, femoral fracture*, etc.) are ultimately diagnosed by gross or microscopic examination of anatomic structures, not by dimensional measurements of chemical substances. The clinician gets prime help in these diagnoses from the verbal descriptions of the roentgenologist, histopathologist, or cytologist—not from the dimensional numbers of the clinical chemist. The disease entities of psychiatry also depend for diagnosis either on clinical observations or on special psychometric tests that are unrelated to clinical chemistry. Certain organic diseases often contain a dimensional measurement among the diagnostic constituents. Thus, a change in the level of streptococcal antibodies or serum transaminases may be part of the elements used, respectively, for diagnosis of rheumatic fever or myocardial infarction. But the diagnostic criteria also include many other morphologic and clinical observations that are not expressed dimensionally. In all of these diagnostic circumstances, a single dimensional value is alone insufficient to decide that the candidate disease is absent and that the patient is therefore "normal".

A second problem has been the frequent lack of quantification in prognosis. Only in recent years have clinical epidemiologists begun to perform the long-term follow-up studies that would allow an outcome to be quantitatively correlated with an antecedent state. The current research that has delineated "risk factors" for diverse diseases is still primitive in scientific quality of data, in epidemiologic scope of data, and in scientific procedures for analysis.

Perhaps the greatest problem, however, is the many types of relations that can go into the correlations. The data employed for medical decisions about normality are often multivariate, rather than merely bivariate. Before deciding that a particular measured value is abnormal, a clinician may want to consider its reproducibility (if the test is repeated), its duration, its previous levels, its association with other abnormalities, and its therapeutic or other consequences for the patient. A diastolic blood pressure of 96 mm/Hg. might be ignored if it appears only sporadically in a middle-aged adult and might be regarded as desirable if found in a healthy septuagenarian. A temperature of 101° F could be greeted happily if the patient's previous temperature was 105° F. The occurrence of asymptomatic sickle cell trait might be a welcome genetic event in a family where most members have suffered from sickle cell disease. In at least two proposed definitions of normality, the determinant factor is a clinical action, rather than a diagnostic label. Elkins, Pagnotto, and Brugsch,[9] in considering guidelines for inorganic lead and mercury in urine, divided the range of values into three zones where the action indicated was none, a periodic check, or medical surveillance. Cochrane and Elwood[7] have suggested that the upper limit of normal would be the point "below which treatment does more harm than good".

In these and many other examples of the medical approach to normality, the doctor incorporated elements from diverse types of data into the final judgment. Because these judgments are often not clearly specified (or are too complex to be readily stated in simple statistical terms or in an algorithmic flow chart), contemporary medical seekers of scientific precision and quantification have been frustrated. If the concept of meaningful medical correlation was to be preserved, modern strategies of quantitative analysis could not be readily employed for studying or expressing normality.

The most straightforward scientific reaction to this difficulty would be to confront it directly. Investigators would have to develop better strategies for dealing with non-dimensional data, better research for determining "risk factors", and better specifications for the constituents of clinical judgment. There was an easier way out, however. The problems could be avoided rather than confronted. If the idea of medical correlation were abandoned, there would be no need for improving the medi-

cal information to which the numerical values were related. The dimensional data obtained in laboratories could be analyzed in a univariate manner, eliminating any direct association with medical phenomena. The data were there; the statistical techniques were available; and the digital computers were willing and hungry. To insist on meaningful medical correlation would preserve the difficulties and would create an intolerable barrier to quantitative "scientific" progress. And so the correlation was abandoned. The concept of normality was transferred from multivariate clinical decision to univariate statistical partition.

B. The meaning of a 'range'

In the univariate approach to normality, the main challenge is to choose a statistical mechanism for demarcating two boundaries: an upper and lower limit. The zone spanned between these limits is called the *range of normal.* For example, the range of normal for a fasting blood sugar value might be listed as 70-110 mg/100 ml. This particular citation of a range is usually chosen by a purely statistical method that contains no provision for at least three other ranges whose variations must also be considered: the type of population included in the data; the intra-personal fluctuations of the individual people; and the analytic variability (or quality control) of the test that provided the data.

Even when normality is converted to a univariate statistical strategy, therefore, the problem remains multivariate. There are four different ranges to be contemplated: statistical, epidemiologic, intra-personal, and mensurational. Of these four ranges, however, only the statistical range receives major attention in most current strategies of normality.

1. Statistical Principles.

a. Demarcation of a zone. The usual statistical partition of the zone called the "range of normal" depends on three arbitrary judgments about proportions, location, and symmetry. With the first judgment, we decide that 1 in every 20 values (95% of the total array) are sufficiently uncommon to be regarded as "abnormal", i.e., beyond the "normal" zone. In the second judgment, we decide that this 95% zone of normality will be located in the central portion of the ranked array of numbers, rather than at one of the extremes. In the third judgment, we decide to place the 95% in the exact center of the distribution, so that the remaining 5% of the values are divided symmetrically, with 2.5% at one end and 2.5% at the other.

These judgments are completely arbitrary. As Murphy[37] points out, the strategy "contrary to popular opinion . . . is *not* a recommendation of statisticians, and . . . has no support from statistical theory". Nevertheless, the strategy is entirely consistent with statistical theory and is readily derived from it. The choice of proportions comes from "tests of statistical significance", which are based on the idea that 5% of events are sufficiently infrequent to be called "significantly" uncommon. The idea is expressed with the use of "P $\leqslant$ .05" as the boundary of "statistical significance." At this level of probability, the uncommon event is regarded as sufficiently unlikely to warrant major inferential decisions.

The choices of location and symmetry come from the Gaussian (or "normal") curve[14] that is constantly employed to illustrate statistical reasoning. This bell-shaped curve is regularly marked with a vertical line near each end. The central 95% of the values of the population are contained between the two lines, so that 2.5% of the population is symmetrically distributed beyond each line. The sum of these two outlying groups is the "highly unusual" or "extraordinary" portion of the total distribution.

Regardless of the intrinsic merits of this statistical reasoning, it has been taught to anyone who has ever learned about "significance tests", and it was easily transferred to the demarcation of normality. The proportions would be 95% "normal"

and 5% "abnormal". The "common" 95% group would be placed in the center of the distribution and called the *range of normal*. The "uncommon" 2.5% zones, symmetrically placed on either side, would be the *abnormal*. This operational strategy seems quite direct, but it requires a peculiar assumption about people, an uncertain assumption about data, and another decision about a demarcational mechanism.

The peculiar assumption about people was to regard the outer 5% of the population as *abnormal*. Many of the arrays of data assembled for these analyses are obtained from people who were deliberately chosen as medically healthy or "normal". Having been selected for their normality, the people might be expected to remain "normal" after the numerical analyses, but the statistical procedure is remorseless. No matter how medically "normal" the people may have been, 5% of them must emerge as "abnormal" after the statistical partitions.

(The consequences of this peculiar assumption become particularly bizarre if the population has received a series of "screening" tests, and if a range of normal is determined independently for each test.[5, 46, 47] Of the 95% of people who were "normal" on the first test, 95% will be "normal" on the second, so that only 90% [$=95\% \times 95\%$] of the original population will be "normal" on both tests. If 10 tests are done and if the abnormalities do not overlap, only 60% of the population [$=(95\%)^{10}$] will emerge as "normal". Sackett[45] has pointed out that a patient who receives an average of 20 different laboratory tests has only "about one chance in three of being classified as normal for all his results even if he is perfectly healthy". Alternative tactics of adjusting for "multivariate normality"[20] have now been proposed as a way of dealing with this issue. Since the adjustment is still based on the idea that 5% of medically normal people will arbitrarily be called abnormal, the consequence of the adjustment is to restore simple peculiarity to what would otherwise be egregiously bizarre.)

The uncertain assumption in the statistical strategy was to divide the abnormal 5% symmetrically on either side of the centrally normal 95%. Why an equal break of 2.5% and 2.5%? Why not 1% and 4%, or 3% and 2%? How do we know that abnormality and its implications are equally distributed among the low and high values? The answer to this question is that on a purely statistical basis we do not know—and so an even split seems the best thing to do.

After these two assumptions were made, the next step was to find a mechanism for demarcating the central 95%. Since the idea of the central 95% had come from concepts of Gaussian statistical distributions, the Gaussian curve seemed the appropriate strategy to use. Furthermore, a great convenience of the Gaussian curve was that the central 95% could easily be calculated from the two main statistics* of this curve: the mean and the standard deviation. These two statistics might have been calculated for other purposes, but once the calculations were completed, the central 95% "range of normal" could be obtained as a simple arithmetical bonus. For Gaussian curves, a zone that spans two standard deviations on either side of the mean will encompass 94.63% of the observed values.

This zone is sometimes erroneously designated[46] as "95% Confidence Limits." The concept of a *confidence limit* refers not to the actual distribution of data, but to the location of the *mean* of the population whose data were analyzed. As the size

of the analyzed group increases, so that larger amounts of data are included, the standard deviation and the 95% "range of normal" for the population may increase or remain the same, but the 95% confidence limit for the mean will become substantially smaller.

The Gaussian strategy for marking the central 95% zone seems intuitively acceptable and would produce no major problem if medical data were regularly distributed in a Gaussian manner. In clinical reality, however, most data are not Gaussian. Many examples of non-Gaussian medical distributions had been noted long before the technologic explosion of the past few decades, but the examples have proliferated enormously in recent years as modern new tests have been developed for chemical and physical measurements, and as the new tests have been applied to general populations. Instead of showing a Gaussian symmetry, the curves of frequency distribution for medical data are often substantially skewed, and the shape of the peaks may make the curve leptokurtic (too tall), platykurtic (too short), bi-modal (two humps), or otherwise deformed from the classical "bell shape".

When the distribution contains such aberrations, a central 95% "range of normal" cannot be calculated with the usual statistical (or *parametric*) techniques used for a Gaussian curve. Aside from the basic mathematical theory that would be violated by such calculations, the results are often biologically bizarre. For example, in 265 children and adolescents, the duration of "activity" in an episode of acute rheumatic fever[13] was found, by standard parametric calculations, to have a mean of 109 days, with a standard deviation of 57 days. The "normal range" for a rheumatic episode would therefore be 223 days at the upper end and –5 days at the lower end. An imaginative data analyst might claim some profound undiscovered meaning for those negative five days, but a biologic scientist would recognize the result as silly. Similarly, the range of normal values for fasting blood sugar would

*The word *statistics* serves as the name of an entire intellectual discipline, but the same word is also used for certain numerical entities that are regularly calculated from the raw data subjected to statistical procedures. Thus, the mean is a *statistic*, the standard deviation is a *statistic*, the variance is a *statistic*, etc. If the data have been obtained from an entire population, rather than from the "sample" usually observed by investigators, and if the populational data have a Gaussian distribution, the mean, standard deviation, and variance of the population are its *parameters*. The term *parametric* is often used for statistical procedures in which the distribution of populational data is assumed to be Gaussian.

take on a negative lower boundary if the range were based on parametric calculations from the widely skewed curve usually found in a hospital population.

This apparent conflict between a statistical paradigm and biologic reality has generally been managed by an *ad hoc* modification of the usual procedures.[14] With careful choice of a method of mathematical transformation, we can often convert the original data into a new set of values that have a Gaussian distribution. Thus, instead of working with the original measurements, we may work with their logarithms, square roots, arc sines, or some other derived value that provides a Gaussian curve for the transformed data.

The justification for such arbitrary transformation is that the original data were themselves measured with an arbitrarily chosen scale. For example, it is a purely arbitrary act to measure height on a scale that is linear, with intervals of equal length between any two points on the scale. We could just as arbitrarily have decided to express height in logarithmic rather than linear units. An instance of a common biologic measurement that is actually logarithmic, but that is expressed as though it were linear, is the value for pH. Another widely employed transformation is our method of expressing biologic antibody titers as the reciprocal of their true values: we often talk about an Antistreptolysin 0 titer of 250, but the actual value is 1/250.

Since there is nothing mathematically sacred about the arbitrary units of biologic measurement, there should presumably be no reluctance to transform the units into a new scale that will provide a Gaussian pattern for the data. The difficulty with many of the transformations, however, is that they are alien to the basic units with which a biologist has learned to think. In dealing with logarithms, cube roots, or other conversions that make the data attain a Gaussian distribution, the investigator may lose track of whatever biologic meaning is under scrutiny. After using the arc sine of his data to find a Gaussian

mean and standard deviation, and after re-converting the appropriate arc sine values back to the original data, the investigator may get a statistically acceptable "normal range" for his results, but he may then be somewhat bewildered when he tries to explain them.

A series of tactics have been proposed to avoid transforming the data while still adjusting for non-Gaussian distribution.[1, 26] These "indirect methods" for estimating a range of normal include such procedures as truncated normal distributions; replacing the mean by the mode; taking averages of normals; and preparing composite distributions. After performing a pragmatic evaluation of the indirect methods, Amador and Hsi[1] concluded that they were "quite inaccurate, because the estimated means were shifted significantly toward pathologic values and the estimated standard deviations were unacceptably wide".

At this point in the discussion, someone who has not yet been "educated" into idolatrous acceptance of traditional statistical paradigms might pose a simple common sense question: "If you want to know the central 95% zone of the data, why not find it directly?" In the direct approach, there would be no calculations of means and standard deviations. The observed values of the data would be ranked in ascending order from lowest to highest. We would then note the particular values that demarcate the first 2.5% and the last 2.5% of the ranked group. For example, if 999 values are ranked from lowest to highest, the 95% central zone will fall between the values of the 25th-ranked and the 975th-ranked observation. If the array of ranks does not allow a boundary value to be demarcated exactly, a suitable choice can be made between two adjacently ranked values that span the boundary.

Suppose we want to find the 2.5% percentile point for a distribution that contains 50 ranked values. None of the 50 ranks occurs exactly at the 2.5% demarcation. To resolve this problem we use the following procedure. We know that the median (i.e., fiftieth percentile point) of a distribution containing N ranked values is defined to be the value whose rank is 50% of N+1. Similarly, the 2.5 percentile point of a distribution containing 50 values is defined to be the rank that is 2.5% of 51. This would be the rank that is 1.28 in the sequence. There is no such rank, but we can assume that if it existed, its value would lie 0.28 of the actual distance between the first and second ranked values. Thus, if the first ranked value were actually 27 units and the second were 33 units, the 2.5% percentile point would be at 27+(.28)(6) = 27+1.68 = 28.68 units. An analogous process could be used to find the 97.5% boundary point.

This ranking procedure for determining the central 95% range of a distribution has existed for many years and has impeccable credentials in both statistics and biology. The procedure is called the "percentile technique". It was statistically proposed by Thompson[49] and developed by Wilks.[50] It was biologically explored further by Herrera[24] and has been particularly well described by Mainland.[30, 31] The procedure is simple, realistic, and direct, requiring no transformations of data and no assumptions about the distribution of frequencies or Gaussian parameters. For Gaussian data, the percentile technique produces the same 95% range that would emerge from the parametric calculations; and for non-Gaussian data, the technique produces a result that is biologically sensible and easily comprehended.

Nevertheless, the percentile technique is not mentioned in several standard textbooks used for teaching statistics to medical people, and when mentioned in the books, the technique is usually quickly crossed over en route to a more extensive discussion of the Gaussian paradigms. Since clinicians do not receive adequate instruction in using the percentile procedure, it seldom appears in general medical literature[15] and it has not been used for calculating the "range of normal" in most of the tests reported in the past few decades. Consequently, prominent general medical journals have begun to publish papers calling the profession's attention

to the defects of Gaussian standards, and urging adoption of a better "modern" method that has existed for more than 35 years. One of the best recent papers on this topic was by Elveback, Guillier, and Keating.[12]

Since the percentile technique is so obviously superior to its Gaussian predecessor, a common sense question would be to ask why the inferior Gaussian procedure has endured so long and remained so popular. Although a simple explanation is that the scientific community has always resisted a change in paradigms,[14] the reasons for such behavior are usually much more complex. I shall try here to identify two of those reasons.

By describing a distribution according to the number of observations, the mean, and the standard deviation, a statistician immediately gets an idea about variance. Since the concept of variance is the basis for so many other contemporary statistical paradigms, and particularly for parametric "tests of significance", the abandonment of the Gaussian procedure would strike at many more fundamental ideas than the mere calculation of a "range of normal". The percentile technique provides nothing more than this range, and therefore does not have the statistical versatility that is offered by the calculated Gaussian values. A physician, who wants only a range and who has no interest in "parametric estimation", is served perfectly well by the percentile technique. A statistician, who may want to be able to estimate parameters even when they are biologically unnecessary or absurd, prefers a technique that provides "variance".

Probably the main reason for current resistance to the percentile technique, however, is the act of calculation itself. A mean and standard deviation could readily be determined for many years if the appropriate keys were pushed on a conventional desk-calculator, but the percentile procedure does not involve classical acts of statistical calculation. Since the observed values must be ranked in ascending order of magnitude, and since an ordinary desk calculator cannot perform rankings, a statistician who wanted to use the percentile technique had to do the rankings himself. For large amounts of data, the manual ranking procedure was too oppressive to be appealing, no matter how receptive a statistician might be to new and improved paradigms.

With the modern availability of computers, however, this calculational oppression has vanished. Using a suitably programmed desk calculator or an office "terminal" connected to a large computer, a statistician can now obtain the percentile values just as easily as he formerly calculated the mean and standard deviation. In fact, if he makes the right plans, he can get both the parametric and the nonparametric results simultaneously during a single "run" of the data.

As these new computational devices become increasingly available and increasingly used by a new generation of data analysts, the old excuse about difficulty in calculation will no longer be tenable. The failure to use percentile techniques will then be attributable only to professional recalcitrance and intellectual inertia.

b. The unit of expression. As the variety of different laboratory tests has soared, clinicians have had difficulty trying to remember the different numerical boundaries that delineate the range of normal for each test. The usual pragmatic approach to this problem is for the clinician to carry a card that lists all the boundaries or for the laboratory to cite the appropriate range of normal adjacent to the result for each test. In recent years, however, proposals have been made to achieve a common unit of expression for all results. The diverse dimensional scales would be abandoned, and all results would be expressed in terms of standardized units of normality or aberration from normal.

The systems proposed to free the physician's mind from what has been called "conversion drudgery" have received such titles as probits,[18] normal quotient units,[25] standard deviation units,[21] statens and stanines,[6] clinical units,[28] physician liberation units system,[27] and system of organizing relevant tests.[42] In all these systems the value of any test is referred to its deviation from a central reference point. The differences in the systems arise mainly from the choice of the reference point (mean or median) and the tactic used for expressing the deviation.

These systems have at least two fundamental flaws. Because they are inapplicable whenever a laboratory test is expressed in non-dimensional scales, they offer no way of citing morphologic data or quantitative data (such as antibody titers) that are listed in arbitrary ordinal categories. More importantly, for those clinicians who prefer to exercise judgment in correlative interpretation of the results, the systems create unfamiliar new units that impair usage of the background of experience on which the judgments depend.

The main apparent advantage of the systems is that they would free the clinician from the burden of remembering the ranges for diverse forms of data. This is a spurious burden, however. Any clinician who orders the tests can readily keep a list of their customary ranges available to him, and any laboratory that issues results can print the ranges adjacent to each result. The new standard-unit systems may actually add to the clinician's mnemonic problem by forcing him to remember how the standard units were calculated so that he can re-convert them for purposes of clinical correlation. Furthermore, if the standard units are determined without regard to any of the epidemiologic, intra-personal, or mensurational variations to be discussed later, the clinician may have no direct way of contemplating the effect of these variations as he assesses the result of the test.

2. Epidemiologic scope. Perhaps the greatest defect in all current expressions of the range of normal—regardless of whatever units are employed—is the absence of information about the reference population.[29] The recipient of data about this range has no idea of the people on whom it was determined. Were they all medically "normal", and how was their normality established? Were they a group of hospital in-patients or out-patients? If so, how might their clinical abnormalities affect the results? Were their age, sex, and other biologic features similar to those of the person for whom the range of normal will pertain? Is the range of normal for certain tests in young women different from that of elderly men? If so, were the data listed separately for each biologic category? Were there enough people in each biologic category for the results to be numerically cogent?

Almost none of these questions receives a satisfactory answer in most current approaches to the range of normal. The zone is calculated or published as an accomplished fact, and the reader is left to divine the constituents with which the fact was accomplished. As Files, van Peenen, and Lindberg[17] have noted, "different subpopulations vary enough in mean values and breadth of frequency distribution so that age and sex differences are sometimes reversed". In addition to age and sex, the properties that delineate important subpopulations may include living habits and the presence of certain clinical conditions. For example, Hamburger[22] has pointed out that the customary ranges noted for tests of thyroid function have "no meaning without defining the patient population in terms of thyroid abnormality, medications, and quantitative data on iodine ingestion". Oppenheimer[40] has commented on the unexpectedly low values of serum protein-bound iodine that can occur in euthyroid patients with chronic disease. Such patients would obviously need separate calculations when a range of normal is determined for the serum PBI. In assessing laboratory values for a pregnant patient, obstetricians might want to use a range based on healthy women who have not merely the same age and race, but also the same trimester of pregnancy.

An important but generally ignored epidemiologic issue is the propriety of determining a "range of normal" from the data assembled in a hospital laboratory. Since the population who provided the data will include many diseased people, the "unedited" results clearly cannot represent a range of medical normality. On the other hand, if the results are "edited" so that only healthy people are included in determinations of the "range", the data analyst will have to confront the challenge of choosing and applying diagnostic criteria for "healthy". In certain statistical theories[25] that have been elegantly demolished by Elveback,[10, 11] the problem of clinically identifying healthy people is replaced by the faith that mathematical analysis alone will serve to make the distinction between good and ill health. An alternative argument, offered with reasonable justification, is that the laboratory's results should not be edited, because they represent the hospital population and will be applied to other hospital patients. If this approach is used, however, the demarcated zone surely does not delineate a range of health, and should not receive the medically misleading designation of *normal*.

The one epidemiologic strategy that has no mitigating justification is a procedure that has been used for years by many clinical investigators. An investigator develops a new diagnostic test, measuring substance X in the serum. To determine the normal range for X, the investigator assembles blood from some apparently healthy people. They usually consist of himself and his laboratory technicians, some itinerant house officers, several cooperative secretaries, a few indentured medical students, and an orderly who happened to pass the lab that morning. From the mean and standard deviation of the values found in this highly restricted group of people, the investigator calculates, publishes, and disseminates the "range of normal" for X. As this range becomes applied in general usage, many people are unexpectedly found to be "suffering" from a deficit or surplus of X. They then receive elaborate, expensive "workups" that produce no useful explanation for the "abnormality". Eventually someone looks up the original paper and discovers the grossly unsatisfactory epidemiologic scope of the group used for establishing the "normal range". A new group—including people much older and younger than the investigator's convenience sample—is assembled and tested. Suddenly the "normal range" becomes considerably expanded and the previous "abnormalities" vanish.

Most good medical editors today would not tolerate this pernicious scientific practice in the original proclamation of the range of normal for a new test, but the tactic still gets used and published. A striking recent variation on this theme has occurred during the contemporary development of chromosome studies. For several years, genetic investigators performed such analyses only on people with obvious clinical abnormalities. The correlations between the chromosomal and clinical abnormalities were excellent until someone had the idea of doing the tests on some healthy people and determining a range of normal. To the shock and chagrin of the genetic fraternity, a relatively high incidence of chromosomal "abnormalities" was found[41] in babies with no congenital malformations or other clinical defects.

3. Intrapersonal range. Another range that must be considered in establishing a range of normal is the scope of physiologic variation within a particular person. This intrapersonal variability can occur at a relatively fixed level that changes with recurrent cyclic periodicity; or the level itself may be distinctly altered as the person grows older. The fluctuations may be due to circadian rhythms,[48] seasonal patterns, aging, or such features[2] as eating, exercise, emotion, pain, and posture.

Although mathematical procedures[23] can be employed in an attempt to separate this type of physiologic variation from the mensurational (or "analytic") variation discussed in the next section, the main point to be noted here is that intrapersonal variation cannot be used in any calculations unless its existence is recognized. If clinicians and investigators do not think about the intrapersonal "range of normal", no data will be assembled to demonstrate its effects and to allow the effects to be suitably adjusted during the arithmetic of normality. For example, within the same person, the electrocardiogram[51] may show substantial daily variation; major diurnal fluctuations[2] can occur in serum albumin and in volume of urinary excretion; serum iron[2] can vary both diurnally and menstrually; uric acid may show both diurnal and hebdomadal patterns[44]; the neutrophil count may have long-term cyclical oscillation[34]; and serum cholesterol levels may be affected by exercise[33] and by posture.[43]

Fortunately, Cotlove, Harris, and Williams[8] have found that healthy people are generally more chemically stable than the mensurational variability of the chemical tests themselves. Nevertheless, certain individual people might have wide intrapersonal fluctuations that must be contemplated when decisions are made about whether or not a single value lies in the normal range. These fluctuations become particularly important when the decision deals not with the normality of a single value, but with the magnitude and possible causes of a change observed in serial values. Without such awareness, a therapeutic agent may be credited or blamed for having produced a change that was entirely within the customary range of variation for that patient.

4. Mensurational variability. The last range of variation to be cited here arises from the test itself. Although often called *analytic variability*, this type of fluctuation is better named as *mensurational variability*, since the word "analytic" has so many other meanings in biostatistics. The stability of mensuration has been particularly well studied by clinical chemists,[3, 4, 32] possibly because the research is done, within the confines of the laboratory, on specimens whose epidemiologic and clinical sources need not be considered during the analysis of data. The mathematical strategy depends on finding the variations that occur when the same test is applied repeatedly to the same specimen in the same or in different laboratories.

An abundant literature exists on the subject of quality control, and I shall not attempt to summarize it here. The statistical problems have been well discussed by Barnett[3] and by Grams, Johnson, and Benson.[19] The mensurational issues have been well covered in a stellar symposium whose proceedings were edited by Benson and Strandjord.[4] (This book is one of the best, most readable "transcribed conferences" that I have ever encountered. Each paper is excellent, and the associated discussion is clear and pungent. Among the plethora of good things in the book, some irreverences that may appeal to readers of this biostatistics series are David Seligson's indictment of the accuracy of multi-channel automated techniques, and Murray Young's application of the word *eolithism*—"a piece of junk like a spear, accidentally adapted to a use which is suggested by its form"—in reference to some of the machinery and practices employed in medical laboratories.)

The main point to be noted here is that every test has its own range of variability. Consequently, the data of a particular patient cannot be catalogued as "normal" or "abnormal" unless provision is made for the additional variability of mensuration.

C. Conclusions

In the absence of accepted agreement about solutions for these problems, any author can offer suggestions on what might be done. My own proposals would be as follows:

1. The phrase *range of normal* should be abandoned. It no longer has any real meaning and it produces nothing but confusion. The phrase is semantically misleading if the calculated *range* includes values obtained from diseased people, and is medically improper if the boundaries of *normal* are truncated to exclude parts of the entire scope found in healthy people.

2. The best medical way of establishing these ranges is to correlate them directly for their separate roles in diagnosis, prognosis, and therapy. Different boundaries may be needed for each of these three different kinds of clinical decision. The correlations will be best achieved not with Bayes theorem or with other abstract statistical theories, but with data directly assembled at the appropriate portions of "flow chart" algorithms that are suitably constructed for the clinical decisions.[16]

3. The ideal situation described in the preceding paragraph will not become reality for many years. Until that time, some other mechanism will be needed to demarcate the ranges used in contemporary medical reasoning. A univariate statistical approach, if employed appropriately, can provide satisfactory boundaries.

4. The percentile technique is the best univariate statistical strategy available for this purpose and should replace Gaussian calculations, which are both archaic and erroneous for medical data. The percentile technique is already widely used in pediatrics for describing growth patterns of children, and can be readily adapted to other aspects of medicine. The adaptation is facilitated by the increased availability of digital computers for ranking data and performing ancillary calculations.

5. The percentile technique can be used without establishing a specific "range". A patient's individual result can simply be reported for its absolute value and its percentile ranking. Such reporting would eliminate the need for arbitrary demarcation of a "range" and for artificially constructed scales containing standardized units of deviation.

6. If clinicians insist on maintaining an analog of a "range of normal", it can be called the *customary range* or *customary zone*. This zone need not occupy 95% of the distribution. It can cover 90%, 97%, or 99% of the distribution, although many clinicians may want to preserve the 95% tradition. Since the zone

has no direct clinical correlation, it can be demarcated symmetrically. Thus, a *95% customary range* would span the interval between the 2.5% and 97.5% percentile values.

7. The data used for determining this customary zone should preferably be derived from healthy people, but could be taken from a hospitalized population as long as the source is clear. The reporting laboratory should always indicate the particular population from which the customary values were calculated. Whenever possible, these values should be at least sex-specific and age-specific for the particular patient; and when necessary, the values should also be adjusted for their specificity in pertinent clinical conditions. Programs for a computer to prepare such reports can readily be created. An excellent illustration of the appearance of the reports has been presented by Elveback.[10, 11]

8. The laboratory reports should also indicate the range of mensurational variability for each test and should mention any tests for which major intrapersonal variations can frequently occur. If these descriptions would occupy too much space on individual reports, they can be assembled into a single document that is made available to clients of the laboratory. This document would replace current cards or charts of the "range of normal" for diverse tests.

The availability of digital computers offers clinicians and clinical chemists a magnificent opportunity that is currently being neglected. Most clinical laboratories using computers for data processing have merely automated a defective status quo by calculating "ranges of normal" with Gaussian statistics. A more important role for computers, however, is to improve rather than simply automate the status quo. To achieve this improvement, the computer should do new things. It can expedite the long overdue conversion from Gaussian to percentile methods of reporting. It can create ranges that have epidemiologic specificity. And it can easily

produce constant reminders of intrapersonal and mensurational variability.

The great statistician Jerzy Neyman[39] once referred to statistics as a "servant of all sciences". Nowhere is the opportunity for this service greater than in efforts to correct the current derangements of the *range of normal*.

References

1. Amador, E., and Hsi, B. P.: Indirect methods for estimating the normal range, Amer. J. Clin. Pathol. **52**:538-546, 1969.
2. Annotation. Interpretation of laboratory tests, Lancet, pp. 1091-1092, May 20, 1967.
3. Barnett, R. N.: Clinical laboratory statistics, Boston, 1971, Little, Brown & Company.
4. Benson, E. S., and Strandjord, P. E., editors: Multiple laboratory screening, New York, 1969, Academic Press, Inc.
5. Best, W. R., Mason, C. C., Barron, S. S., and Shepheard, H. G.: Automated twelve-channel serum screening, Med. Clin. North Amer. **53**:175-188, 1969.
6. Casey, A. E., and Downey, E.: Further use of statens in the recording, reporting, analysis, and retrieval of automated computerized laboratory and clinical data, Amer. J. Clin. Pathol. **53**:748-754, 1970.
7. Cochrane, A. L., and Elwood, P. C.: Laboratory data and diagnosis, Lancet, p. 420, February 22, 1969.
8. Cotlove, E., Harris, E. K., and Williams, G. Z.: Biological and analytic components of variation in long term studies of serum constituents in normal subjects, Clin. Chem. **16**:1028-1032, 1970.
9. Elkins, H. B., Pagnotto, L. D., and Brugsch, H. G.: Confusion concerning "normal" values in biologic analysis, N. Engl. J. Med. **286**:1268-1269, 1972.
10. Elveback, L. R.: How high is high? A proposed alternative to the normal range, Mayo Clin. Proc. **47**:93-97, 1972.
11. Elveback, L. R.: The population of healthy persons as a source of reference information, Hum. Pathol. **4**:9-16, 1973.
12. Elveback, L. R., Guillier, C. L., and Keating, F. R.: Health, normality, and the ghost of Gauss, J. Amer. Med. Assn. **211**:69-75, 1970.
13. Feinstein, A. R., and Spagnuolo, M.: The duration of activity in acute rheumatic fever, J. Amer. Med. Assn. **175**:1117-1119, 1961.
14. Feinstein, A. R.: Clinical biostatistics. XII. On exorcising the ghost of Gauss and the curse of Kelvin, Clin. Pharmacol. Ther. **12**:1003-1016, 1971.
15. Feinstein, A. R.: Clinical biostatistics. XXV. A survey of the statistical procedures in gen-

eral medical journals, CLIN. PHARMACOL. THER. **15**:97-107, 1974.

16. Feinstein, A. R.: An analysis of diagnostic reasoning, Yale J. Biol. Med. **46**:212-232 and 264-283, 1973; and **47**: In press, March, 1974.

17. Files, J. B., van Peenen, H. J., and Lindberg, D. A. B.: Use of "normal range" in multiphasic testing, J. Amer. Med Assn. **205**:94-98, 1968.

18. Finney, D. J.: Probit analysis—a statistical treatment of the sigmoid response curve, Cambridge, England, 1952, Cambridge University Press.

19. Grams, R. R., Johnson, E. A., and Benson, E. S.: Laboratory data analysis system: Section II. Analytic error limits, Amer. J. Clin. Pathol. **58**:182-187, 1972.

20. Grams, R. R., Johnson, E. A., and Benson, E. S.: Laboratory data analysis system: Section III. Multivariate normality, Amer. J. Clin. Pathol. **58**:188-200, 1972.

21. Gullick, H. D., and Schauble, M. K.: SD unit system for standardized reporting and interpretation of laboratory data, Amer. J. Clin. Pathol. **57**:517-525, 1972.

22. Hamburger, J. I.: Normal ranges de-emphasized, N. Engl. J. Med. **281**:331, 1969.

23. Harris, E. K.: Distinguishing physiologic variation from analytic variation, J. Chronic Dis. **23**:469-480, 1970.

24. Herrera, L.: The precision of percentiles in establishing normal limits in medicine, J. Lab. Clin. Med. **52**:34, 1958.

25. Hoffman, R. G.: Statistics in the practice of medicine, J. Amer. Med. Assn. **185**:864, 1963.

26. Keyser, J. W.: The concept of the normal range in clinical chemistry, Postgrad. Med. J. **41**:443-447, 1965.

27. Langdon, D. E., and Leeper, C. K.: Physician liberation units system, N. Engl. J. Med. **283**:1413, 1970.

28. Lo, J. S., and Kellen, J. A.: A proposal for a more uniform output in laboratory data, Clin. Chim. Acta **41**:239-245, 1972.

29. McCall, M. G.: Normality, J. Chronic Dis. **19**:1127-1132, 1966.

30. Mainland, D.: Elementary medical statistics, ed. 2, Philadelphia, 1963, W. B. Saunders Company.

31. Mainland, D.: Remarks on clinical "norms", Clin. Chem. **17**:267-274, 1971.

32. Mefferd, R. B., and Pokorny, A. D.: Individual variability reexamined with standard clinical measures, Amer. J. Clin. Pathol. **48**:325-331, 1967.

33. Mirkin, G.: Labile serum cholesterol values, N. Engl. J. Med. **279**:1001, 1968.

34. Morley, A. A.: A neutrophil cycle in healthy individuals, Lancet, pp. 1220-1222, December 3, 1966.

35. Murphy, E. A.: A scientific viewpoint on normalcy, Perspect. Biol. Med. **9**:333-348, 1966.

36. Murphy, E. A., and Abbey, H.: The normal range—a common misuse, J. Chronic Dis. **20**:79-88, 1967.

37. Murphy, E. A.: The normal, and the perils of the sylleptic argument, Perspect. Biol. Med. **15**:566-582, 1972.

38. Murphy, E. A.: The normal, Amer. J. Epidemiol. **98**:403-411, 1973.

39. Neyman, J.: Statistics—servant of all sciences, Science **122**:401-406, 1955.

40. Oppenheimer, J. H.: An unsolved problem: Low serum PBI values in patients with chronic disease, J. Chronic Dis. **22**:129-131, 1969.

41. Ratcliffe, S. G., Stewart, A. L., Melville, M. M., and Jacobs, P. A.: Chromosome studies on 3500 newborn male infants, Lancet, pp. 121-122, January 17, 1970.

42. Reece, R. L., and Hobbie, R.: Diagnosis in *PLUS* and *SORT*, N. Engl. J. Med. **284**:1387-1388, 1971.

43. Reece, R. L.: Effect of posture on laboratory values, N. Engl. J. Med. **289**:1374, 1973.

44. Rubin, R. T., Plag, J. A., Arthur, R. J., Clark, B. R., and Rahe, R. H.: Serum uric acid levels: Diurnal and hebdomadal variability in normoactive subjects, J. Amer. Med. Assn. **208**:1184-1186, 1969.

45. Sackett, D. L.: The usefulness of laboratory tests in health-screening programs, Clin. Chem. **19**:366-372, 1973.

46. Schoen, I., and Brooks, S. H.: Judgment based on 95% confidence limits: A statistical dilemma involving multitest screening and proficiency testing of multiple specimens, J. Clin. Pathol. **53**:190-193, 1970.

47. Sunderman, F. W., Jr.: Expected distributions of normal and abnormal results in multitest surveys of healthy subjects, Amer. J. Clin. Pathol. **53**:288-291, 1970.

48. Tedeschi, C. G.: Circadian challenges in "quality control". Biochemical rhythms and spacial phenomena, Hum. Pathol. **4**:281-287, 1973.

49. Thompson, W. R.: Biological applications of normal range and associated significance tests in ignorance of original distribution forms, Ann. Math. Stat. **9**:281, 1938.

50. Wilks, S. S.: Statistical prediction with special reference to the problem of tolerance limits, Ann. Math. Stat. **13**:400, 1942.

51. Willems, J. L., Poblete, P. F., and Pipberger, H. V.: Day-to-day variation of the normal orthogonal electrocardiogram and vectorcardiogram, Circulation **45**:1057-1064, 1972.

CHAPTER 18

How do we measure 'safety' and 'efficacy'?

The phrase *safety and efficacy* has become an accepted pharmacologic slogan. Whenever journal editors, sanctioning committees, advertising managers, legislative inquirers, or practicing physicians engage in the evaluation of drugs, this slogan usually serves as a label for the evidence to be presented and for the goal to be attained.

The confirmation of this slogan has become an increasingly important scientific challenge in the pharmacologic activities of clinical research and practice. For new drugs to be made available to the public, their safety and efficacy must be demonstrated, according to law, in "adequate and well-controlled clinical investigations." New "guidelines" for these investigations are now being constructed by members of the FDA and pharmaceutical industry. For drugs that have long been on the market, continued tenure has been reviewed and sometimes revoked after recent reappraisals by committees of the National Academy of Sciences and National Research Council.

During these activities, the procedures of evaluation are based on an act of faith. We believe that satisfactory methods exist for determining safety and efficacy. Ac-

cordingly, if the desired attributes have not been demonstrated for a particular drug, we conclude either that the drug is "bad" or that the methods were not properly applied.

My purpose in this essay is to show that our act of faith is a delusion. The methods do not exist. There are no satisfactory standard procedures for assessing the safety and efficacy of drugs. Despite general acceptance, the existing techniques are oversimplified, naive, and grossly inadequate for the needs of clinical medicine.

The main difficulty is due to a classic type of scientific error: the development of precise techniques for attaining a goal that is itself unspecified. A series of statistical procedures and designs have been established for demonstrating safety and efficacy, but no satisfactory operational definitions have been created for either *safety* or *efficacy*. Both these words represent abstract concepts that can readily be defined during informal conversation or with formal recourse to a dictionary. But when either (or both) of these concepts is to be used as the specific target of a scientific investigation, a citation from conversation or a dictionary is unacceptable. The concepts must be expressed in operational terms.

As S. S. Wilks[35] has pointed out, "The

Under the same name, this chapter originally appeared as "Clinical biostatistics—IX." In Clin. Pharmacol. Ther. 12:544, 1971.

first requirement (of quantification in science) . . . is that making a measurement must be an *operationally definable process* . . . (achieved) by specifying a set of realizable experimental conditions and a sequence of operations to be made under those conditions." For an abstract concept, the operational process described by Wilks would today be called an *algorithm*—a demarcated succession of intellectual strategies and decisions that are performed under certain stipulated conditions.

There is a major logical disparity between an ordinary definition and an algorithmic identification. An ordinary definition often follows a logical direction from cause toward effect. An algorithmic identification often goes in the opposite sequence, from effect toward cause. For example, we can define thrombophlebitis of the calf by describing the anatomy of the muscles and veins, the thrombus, the associated inflammatory reaction, and the clinical symptoms and signs. But a quite different order and succession of reasoning would be necessary to describe the operational identification (or clinical algorithm) that could be used to conclude that a patient with pain in the calf had thrombophlebitis. In the first instance, the reasoning was pathogenetic; in the second, diagnostic. Similarly, we could state pathogenetically that nausea can be produced during digitalis toxicity; but we would need a much more complex array of statements to decide that a patient's nausea was caused by digitalis toxicity.

The algorithms of an operationally definable process are a scientific necessity for converting substantive, abstract, or judgmental concepts into precisely delineated entities that can be identified reproducibly. Without operational definitions, such tangible substances as *glucose* and *carcinoma*, such measurable dimensions as *1 cm.*, such concepts as *anxious*, and such judgments as *improving* or *moribund* would remain vague, uncertain, and nonreproducible. For *glucose, carcinoma,* and *1 cm.*, the operational definitions are uni-

versally standardized, having been established, respectively, by chemists, by pathologists, and by the National Bureau of Standards. For *anxious, improving*, and *moribund*, universal standards of identification do not exist, and the operational definitions called "criteria"[12] must be established whenever these terms are used in scientific investigation. Similarly, for *safety* and *efficacy* to be used as the scientific or legal desiderata of therapeutic trials, the terms must be operationally defined. The algorithmic stipulations for *safety* and *efficacy* need not always contain numerical dimensions, but the specifications must be sufficiently clear and direct to operate as a scientific "instrument" for separating what is safe or efficacious from what is not.

But no such operational definitions have been established. In many textbooks of pharmacology,[2, 6, 7, 14, 16, 17, 19, 21, 26, 27] the terms *safety* and *efficacy* do not even appear amid the many discussions of mode of action of drugs. When a definition is offered, the contents are often vague or imprecise, culminating in phrases—such as *better, adverse reaction,* or *side effect*—that are themselves left operationally undefined. Even in books that contain sections on therapeutic trials[3, 5, 15, 32, 34, 38] or in symposia devoted to pharmacologic quantification,[23, 29, 37] no algorithmic specifications are presented for identifying safety or efficacy.

In the absence of suitable scientific specifications, clinicians performing "statistically designed" therapeutic trials have hoped that safety and efficacy could somehow be demonstrated with careful methodologic attention to such statistical tactics as randomization, double-blind procedures, hard data, and numerical analyses. These methods offer a precise intellectual weapon for aiming at a target, but they do not indicate the target. None of the statistical tactics provides *operational* identifications for either "safety" or "efficacy."

Because the basic elements have been scientifically and statistically neglected, the evaluation of safety and efficacy in the treatment of patients today is in a state of intellectual chaos. In most current statistical approaches to therapeutic trials, the many different ideas and goals of *efficacy* are neither identified properly nor assessed adequately. The concept of *safety* is generally expressed so nebulously that "effects" often cannot be distinguished from "side effects," or desirable habituation from unwarranted abuse. The idea of *treatment* is often reduced to a superficial pharmacologic exercise that excludes the role of the most consistently powerful therapeutic agent in medicine: the clinician. And the *patient* who is presumably the beneficiary of all these activities may be deliberately ignored as a source of information, or may be deliberately described with a collection of data so dehumanized that a reader unaware of the "material" under investigation might be unable to discern whether the results came from people, dogs, or rats.

A. Problems in efficacy

According to the doctrines of current statistical faith, efficacy of a drug should be easy to appraise. With tables of random numbers, we allocate therapy to a "treated" group and a "control"; with double-blind techniques, we ensure "objective" observations; with a dimensionally measured endpoint, we obtain "hard" data; and with an array of mathematical tests, we demonstrate "statistical significance." We might have some difficulty in finding and managing a suitable group of patients for the trial, but the basic methods are there. All we have to do is apply them.

This simplistic belief, which has been used as the premise for many statistical evaluations of clinical therapy, unfortunately does not indicate how much of an effect is to be regarded as "effective," does not provide for disparities or contradictions among multiple effects, does not distinguish a pharmacologic from a therapeutic effect, does not differentiate among a diversity of therapeutic actions and environments, and does not allow decisions about

the kinds of patients to whom the results will apply.

1. The distinction of a difference. Perhaps the most deleterious consequence of using conventional statistical theory in modern clinical science has been the widespread fantasy that a *statistically significant* difference is a *significant* difference.

A statistical "test of significance" indicates only whether an observed numerical difference can readily be attributed to chance alone. The test does not indicate whether the difference itself is significant, and does not authenticate, validate, or annotate the meaning of the difference. "Statistical significance" can be achieved by a trivial difference if it occurs consistently, or by a meaningless difference if the sample size is large enough. Conversely, if the sample size is too small, a difference of major importance will not be "statistically significant."

The intellectual pollution produced by these tests and by the abuse of the word *significance* is too enormous and deeply entrenched for thorough discussion here. The issue will be contemplated in greater detail in a future paper in this series. The main point to be noted now is that despite extensive dissertations about the α and β levels used for determining "statistical significance," statistical textbooks give little or no attention to Δ, the amount of difference that makes a distinction.

Suppose we performed a trial of anti-inflammatory agents, using an end-point based on the length of time required for cessation of redness in an induced skin lesion. In 18 patients receiving Drug X, the mean duration of redness is 10.4 days, with a standard deviation of 0.2 days. In 19 patients receiving Drug C (the "control"), the mean duration is 10.7 days, with a standard deviation of 0.5 days. For these data, the value of "Student's" t is 2.31, and P is statistically significant at <0.05. Is this "statistical significance" meaningful? The answer to this question depends on what we wanted to know clinically. If we were searching for an agent that promptly suppressed the inflammation, anything that took longer than 2 or 3 days might be worthless. If we wanted to find an agent that was substantially faster than the control, a difference of one-third of a day in the two agents might also be unimportant. The difference that was "statistically significant" might thus be clinically trivial.

As another example, consider a trial of drugs for weight reduction. With Drug Y, 23 patients lose a mean of 2.1 pounds with a standard deviation of 4.7 pounds, whereas 21 patients who receive Drug Z lose a mean of 8.4 pounds with a standard deviation of 10.2 pounds. For these data, t is 2.61, and P is "statistically significant" at <0.02. Inspecting this result for "significance," and noting that the mean value for Drug Z is four times as much as the mean for Y, we might conclude that this difference is meaningful as well as "significant." Nevertheless, the issue of clinical importance depends on information that has not yet been stated: the initial weight of the patients. As soon as we learn that the average baseline weight of both of the tested groups was 300 pounds, we might conclude that both drugs were ineffectual. In such patients, a mean loss of either 2.1 pounds or 8.4 pounds is an insignificant amount of weight reduction, regardless of the "statistical significance" of the difference.

To illustrate a different aspect of these principles, consider a therapeutic trial of 200 patients, with improvement occurring in 49 of 100 patients treated with Drug W, and in 50 of 100 patients treated with Drug V. Noting the small increment of 1 per cent between 49 per cent and 50 per cent, we would conclude that the difference was clinically unimportant. Suppose we now conducted the same therapeutic trial with a sample size of 50,000 rather than 200 patients. If we encountered the same difference of 49 per cent improvement for Drug W and 50 per cent for Drug V, we might still be unimpressed by the difference of 1 per cent. Never-

theless, in the second trial, with 50,000 patients, the 1 per cent difference is "statistically significant" ($\chi^2=5.0$; $P<0.05$), whereas in the first trial of 200 patients the identical increment of 1 per cent is not "significant" ($\chi^2=0.02$; $P>0.75$).

A converse example of this same issue occurs if we consider a therapeutic trial in which the improvement rate is 30 per cent for 30 patients receiving Drug W and 60 per cent for 30 patients receiving Drug Z. The difference of 30 per cent in the two rates for these 60 patients seems important clinically. Furthermore, if the trial had been conducted on only 40 patients, and if we had observed the same percentages of improvement—30 per cent for 20 patients with Drug W and 60 per cent for 20 patients with Drug Z— we would still be clinically impressed with the difference of 30 per cent. Nevertheless, in the first trial this difference was "statistically significant" ($\chi^2=5.4$; $P<0.05$), whereas in the second trial, the identical difference was not "significant" ($\chi^2=3.3$; $P>0.05$).

Why has the concept of Δ—the amount of difference that makes a difference— been so neglected in statistical discussions of "significance"? Probably the main reason is that Δ cannot be selected with an act of statistical reasoning. The selection requires scientific judgment about the clinical or biologic meaning of the difference. Since this judgment is not a statistical inference, it is ignored in discussions of "statistical inference." Because the term *significance* has been usurped for these statistical concepts, however, the more basic, fundamental meaning of "significance" has been lost in a maze of α, β, χ^2, t, and P values.

How large a value for Δ is significant? If we were unimpressed by a difference of 0.3 days, 8.4 pounds, or 1 per cent in the foregoing examples, what values or percentage would we have accepted? Although we regarded a 30 per cent difference as clinically important, would we still have thought so if the difference was

20 per cent or 10 per cent? There are no fixed answers to these questions. They require arbitrary judgments that must be adapted appropriately to each situation.

If standard answers are to be created for these questions, a consensus must be established for each of the arbitrary judgments. But no efforts have been made to establish, or even to consider, such a consensus. In most other branches of scientific activity, authoritative committees have met to debate and decide issues that require arbitrary judgments. Meetings of this type have been the basis for the medical terms used internationally for anatomic and biochemical nomenclature, for the standardization of diverse laboratory tests, and for establishment of the diagnostic criteria used in such diseases as rheumatic fever[1] and rheumatoid arthritis.[31] In therapeutic science, however, no such committees or workshops have been assembled. Despite diverse symposia devoted to the "design" of clinical trials, various meetings to create "guidelines" for testing drugs, and many other statistical conclaves devoted to "therapy," the fundamental issue of Δ has been persistently ignored. Panels of knowledgeable, authoritative clinicians have not met to discuss and create the appropriate principles.

One of the basic scientific barriers to evaluations of therapeutic efficacy, therefore, is the absence of any standardized method or concepts for deciding what is *good,* and what or how much is *better.* An elaborate series of mathematical principles has been developed to demarcate what is "significant" statistically, but no comparable clinical principles have been established to indicate what is significant therapeutically.

2. The evaluation of multiple effects. Another fundamental problem ignored in current statistical doctrines is the assessment of multiple responses to therapy. Since a patient can have many different responses to treatment, a thorough appraisal of the therapeutic effects requires a careful evaluation of the multiple separate responses. Suppose the patient's peripheral edema disappears while his dyspnea grows worse? Or his sedimentation rate falls dramatically while his arthritic fingers remain useless? Or he loses weight successfully while becoming habituated to amphetamines? Or the size of his cancer shrinks while he becomes constantly nauseated and miserable? Or the treatment provides a slight degree of relief but is extremely inconvenient and expensive? How do we assess these conflicting, contradictory effects?

Statistical theory provides no useful help in answering these questions, and actually creates some major impediments, because the theory is deliberately geared for single rather than multiple responses. The existing statistical tactics of "multiple regression" are devoted almost exclusively to associations between the multiple variables of the patient's *initial* state and the response in a single target variable, but the tactics are not applicable to multiple *targets.* The tests of "statistical significance" thus depend mainly on the response observed only in a *single* variable.

To make use of the tests, a clinical investigator must accept their severe intellectual restrictions, which force him into a choice of two unhappy alternatives. The first, which is regularly used in most trials of therapy, is to ignore all the multiple variables of response, and to concentrate on only a single variable as the basis for determining "statistical significance." The second alternative is to create a single "index" of response by combining diverse components of the multiple variables. The statistical tests are then applied to the single "variable" created in this composite index.

The construction of composite indexes involves judgments[9, 10] even more subtle and difficult than the choice of Δ for a single variable, and the problems are not susceptible to easy solution by any of the decision-making tactics of statistical theory. The problems of these judgments can be avoided by avoiding a careful clinical analysis of all the pertinent phenomena, and by basing the statistical tests on isolated single variables—such as the mortality rates or survival times used in recent large-scale trials of treatment for diabetes mellitus, coronary artery disease, or cancer. But if the totality of posttherapeutic phenomena are to be assessed, as exemplified in recent trials of treatment for rheumatoid arthritis,[24] enormous attention and thought must be given to the creation of a satisfactory composite index.

Here, too, authoritative connoisseurs must be assembled to discuss the issues, and to make suitable decisions about how the multiple constituent variables can be combined and "weighted" in a sensible manner. But here, too, the issues of composite indexes for multiple variables have been generally neglected. Amid all of the recent meetings, "guidelines," and other public pronouncements about the efficacy of drugs, no intellectual procedures have been developed to create specific composite indexes or specific principles for scientific evaluation of the many different concomitant effects that occur when patients are treated.

3. *Pharmacologic versus therapeutic efficacy.* The two problems just cited refer to the evaluation of a single response and to the assessment of multiple responses. All the remaining problems to be discussed here deal with the types of responses that are chosen for appraisal. Among these distinctions, another important principle omitted from many considerations of *efficacy* is the difference between the pharmacologic and the therapeutic action of a drug.

The pharmacologic action of a drug is demonstrated by its particular pattern of uptake, distribution, metabolism, and excretion in the human body. In the course of that pharmacodynamic pathway, the drug may affect the function of certain chemical or physiologic systems in the body. Thus, pharmacologically, an anorexigenic agent may reduce appetite, an antilipemic agent may lower serum lipids,

a parasympatholytic agent may reduce intestinal contractility, and an antihypertensive agent may lower blood pressure. One of the roles of pharmacologic research is to demonstrate that these effects occur, and to explore the mechanisms by which they are produced.

Therapeutically, however, a drug is often used for clinical purposes quite different from those noted as pharmacologic effects. These clinical goals may require that the drug be pharmacologically effective, but the goals are not expressed or assessed in the same terms used for indicating pharmacologic efficacy. Thus, an anorexigenic agent is used therapeutically for weight reduction; an antilipemic agent is used therapeutically to prevent or reduce atherosclerosis; a parasympatholytic agent, to relieve intestinal pain; and an antihypertensive agent, to prevent diverse vascular complications and to prolong life. The methods and indexes employed to assess anorexia, serum lipids, intestinal contractility, and blood pressure are quite different, however, from the procedures used to assess weight reduction, atherosclerosis, abdominal pain, and vascular complications.

Furthermore, although the main pharmacologic action of a drug can usually be observed promptly, the clinical goals of therapy may be immediate, short-term, or long-term. Thus, in the treatment of an obese patient, an anorexigenic agent may be used pharmacologically to suppress appetite and in short-term therapy to produce weight reduction, but the long-range goal of treatment is maintenance of the reduced weight. Similarly, although the pharmacologic and short-term therapeutic aims of antihypertensive treatment are to lower blood pressure, the long-range goal is to reduce or prevent strokes, myocardial infarction, renal failure, or other vascular complications.

Since these different goals require different acts of observation and decision, the methodologic procedures used for determining pharmacologic efficacy can seldom be used to demonstrate therapeutic efficacy. Three entirely different sets of investigative designs, indexes, and populations might be needed to show whether a drug is effective pharmacologically, in short-term therapy, or in long-term therapy. Although the terms *Phase 1, Phase 2,* and *Phase 3* are regularly used to denote the investigations in which a new drug is first tested for safety and pharmacologic efficacy, the ideas of a *Phase 4, Phase 5,* or more advanced therapeutic goals are generally omitted from pharmacologic discussions, and the term *efficacy* is regularly used without specification of which type of efficacy is under consideration.

4. The peritherapeutic responses of the patient. The targets of therapy are usually a patient's direct medical responses—manifested in the "soft data" of such symptoms[25] as pain, dyspnea, or other types of discomfort, or in the "hard data" obtained from objective tests of the patient's blood, urine, feces, tissue specimens, roentgenograms, or electrophysiologic tracings. Because adequate attempts are seldom made to improve the "hardness" of "soft" data, the uniquely human responses of pain, discomfort, or incapacitation are often deliberately omitted from assessment because the data are regarded as too "soft" for scientific attention. Consequently, many investigations of therapy depend on objective, precise, "hard" data that may be irrelevant or inadequate for the clinical goals. The report of changes in tissue, blood, urine, or feces provides "hard data" and a methodologic unity for evaluating pharmacologic effects in both animals and man, but clinical attention to the treatment of a patient requires an appraisal of such distinctively human data as angina pectoris, headache, digestive distress, abdominal cramps, and insomnia. These issues, which have been discussed in greater detail elsewhere[9, 25] can be exemplified by the many trials of chemotherapy in which the "hard" data of survival time are used as the only index of "palliation" for patients who have ad-

vanced cancer, with no assessment of the effects on the patient's symptoms or general functional state.

Even when "soft" clinical phenomena are evaluated in addition to the "hard" data, however, the appraisals are still confined to direct medical responses. The many personal or peritherapeutic responses of patients are almost wholly ignored in current concepts of *efficacy*. These peritherapeutic responses are manifested by the patient's relative ease or difficulty in attempting to maintain a prescribed regimen. For example, most patients would prefer to receive an oral preparation than an injection; if an injection must be repeated daily, most patients would rather take a self-administered hypodermic regimen than an intravenous preparation given by a physician. A diet or medication that tastes good is more appealing than one prepared without gustatory concern. A long-acting drug that can be taken once daily is usually easier to remember than a regimen requiring multiple daily doses. An inexpensive drug is obviously more desirable than a costly one. Other peritherapeutic aspects of treatment include the ease with which a drug can be swallowed, and its ability to be readily preserved or transported without requiring refrigeration or other special maintenance. Although the peritherapeutic advantages of a drug could not overcome the absence of direct therapeutic efficacy, the peritherapeutic distinctions would be valuable in choosing among drugs that have essentially similar ratings or only minor differences in direct therapeutic efficacy. Nevertheless, despite the importance to a patient of these peritherapeutic effects, they are seldom included in conventional assessments of *efficacy*.

Another important but generally neglected peritherapeutic issue is the difficulty of trying to maintain a schedule of diverse medications taken in diverse dosages. This issue is a patient-centered rather than drug-centered problem in therapy. With the aid of modern scientific technology, clinicians have managed to isolate the active ingredients of many drugs and to order these ingredients "scientifically" with the separate specifications of individual prescription. We have also, however, created a formidable burden for patients who must remember which drug to take and when to take it. A frequent sight in the outpatient department of modern medical centers is the pathetic bewilderment of an old man or woman, clutching six different bottles of medication, and trying to distinguish the one that must be taken four times daily before meals, from the ones that are taken twice daily after meals, every 8 hours, every 3 hours, at bedtime, and twice on weekdays but once on Saturday and Sunday. Although modern clinicians may look with disdain at the "polypharmacy" of the past, with its many different ingredients compounded into a single prescription, the patients were probably not confused by an array of medications. We have no data to indicate how faithfully those old multi-ingredient prescriptions were maintained, but several recent studies[4, 20, 28] have demonstrated the futility of expecting patients to adhere faithfully to our modern "polypharmacy" regimens, with many individual ingredients compounded into different drugs taken in different schedules.

In assessing the efficacy of drugs, all these "nuisance factors" in the patient's peritherapeutic convenience are regularly ignored because we do not know how to measure them. These factors could readily be identified, classified, and assessed, of course, if they were regarded as worthy of intellectual attention. But no one seems to think so, or at least no efforts seem to have been made. Moreover, such efforts will never be instituted as long as the demonstration of therapeutic "efficacy" is regarded merely as an exercise in the collection of randomized, double-blind, single-response, "statistically significant," hard data.

Aside from excluding the patient's convenience and comfort as an important constituent of pharmaceutical therapy, these constricted assessments of drugs also create bad science, because therapeutic regimens will be improperly evaluated if the patient's compliance is not suitably identified and analyzed. In many long-term trials involving the maintenance of oral drugs, the issue of compliance is ignored during analysis of the results. The posttherapeutic responses are attributed to the originally assigned regimens, regardless of whether the fidelity of adherence was good, bad, or nonexistent, and regardless of whether the patients, after developing difficulties in compliance or in other aspects of maintenance, had subsequently been transferred to other drugs. Such obdurate assessments of therapeutic efficacy may be accepted as statistically valid, but they will be regarded as neither scientific nor sensible by thoughtful clinicians and patients.

Although the peritherapeutic personal aspects of treatment cannot be ignored in any truly scientific methods of appraising the total efficacy of pharmaceutical preparations, the peritherapeutic issues are constantly neglected, particularly during the assessment of long-acting drugs and combinations of drugs, or when oral drugs are compared against injections. With the "soft" data of clinical symptoms omitted from analysis, and with the additional "soft" data of personal convenience also omitted, the results of treatment are often expressed exclusively in "hard" laboratory data. Since the variables contained in such data are seldom species-specific, a reader of the therapeutic reports might not be able to tell which species of animal was used in the investigation. Thus, the assessment of therapeutic efficacy may become deliberately dehumanized for the sake of scientific and statistical "validity."

5. The role of iatrotherapy. Although the diverse effects just cited may delineate the therapeutic action of a drug, they do not account for many other activities that occur during clinical treatment. The action of a drug on a patient is but one part of the total therapeutic environment. Another major part is played by the clinician who prescribes the drug.

Amid the general current attention to the pharmacologic and therapeutic efficacy of drugs, the therapeutic efficacy of a clinician seems to have been forgotten. Our statistical vocabulary does not include such terms as *concern, compassion, reassurance,* and *TLC* (tender loving care). Nevertheless, not only do these entities exist, but they also may have paramount importance in the treatment of patients. These iatric entities are often the only potent therapeutic agents at a clinician's disposal, and they are pre-requisite to the success of many pharmaceutical preparations.

The fundamental role of iatrotherapy in clinical practice is expressed in the old French admonition that is the guideline of every good practitioner:

> *Guerir quelquefois,*
> *Soulager souvent,*
> *Consoler toujours.*[*]

A drug may sometimes provide cure and may frequently provide relief, but only a clinician can consistently provide comfort, using the agents of human touch, gestures, and speech. In the many chronic distresses and self-limited acute illnesses that constitute the majority of situations for which people seek medical help, a dose of enthusiastic iatrotherapy given in conjunction with an ineffectual drug will usually make patients feel much better than a moderately effective drug delivered with little or no iatrotherapy.

Unlike a pharmaceutical preparation, however, iatrotherapy cannot be prescribed. It must be evoked. Not all doctors will spontaneously and constantly "give" of themselves, and even those who consciously try to do so may not maintain a persistently high level of "dosage". Consequently, an important and generally ignored action of therapeutic agents is their

effect in evoking iatrotherapy from the doctor. A clinician who believes he has no effective pharmaceutical agents to offer may also lose interest in offering himself as a therapeutic agent. Conversely, if he believes the drug is effective, he may prescribe it with an enthusiasm and confidence that is ultimately more forceful than the action of the drug itself. Thus, a drug that may intrinsically have little or no pharmacologic or therapeutic efficacy may nevertheless be used to produce good therapeutic effects.

The annals of unpublished clinical experience contain countless examples of this phenomenon, and many reports have appeared in the scientific literature.[3, 22, 30, 36] Among such examples are the major improvements noted in the abandoned patients of the "back wards" of many psychiatric institutions when psychiatrists began to do therapeutic trials of psychopharmacologic agents. The iatrotherapeutic attention and interest evoked by the trial itself produced substantial benefits for the "control" groups as well as for those who received the "active" agents. At nonpsychiatric academic institutions, iatrotherapy is often responsible for the improved morale that may occur when patients with "inoperable" cancer are transferred from the surgical to the medical service. The surgical house officer, believing he can do "nothing" for an inoperable patient, may tend to lose the personal interest that would evoke iatrotherapy. On the medical service, however, the patient may be buoyed up by attention from the chemotherapists, whose drugs may turn out to be ineffective, but whose concern and enthusiasm may transiently provide major therapeutic benefits.

The importance of iatrotherapy is, of course, one of the main reasons for performing double-blind investigations of drugs, and for insisting that active drugs be compared with a "dummy" or placebo agent rather than with no treatment. In order to determine the effectiveness of the drug itself, we deliberately try to exclude

---

[*]To cure occasionally; to relieve often; to comfort always.

the therapeutic action of the clinician. This exclusion provides important scientific data about the value of the drug when used in this isolated manner, but the data may not be applicable to the realities of ordinary clinical therapy, where a clinician participates without being "blind."

In particular, an overwhelming concern with proving the isolated effectiveness of drugs may be detrimental to the total treatment of patients in at least two important therapeutic situations:

1. For the various types of fatigue, depression, self-limited discomforts, and minor organic or major nonorganic symptoms that are regularly brought to family physicians, the doctor may give enthusiastic iatrotherapy as well as a drug in which he has had confidence for many years. If we perform a rigorous therapeutic trial and demonstrate that the drug is no better than placebo, we have illuminated the annals of science, but we may have also destroyed the doctor's confidence in the drug, and his motives for contributing himself to the therapy. Science may be advanced, but the doctor's patients may lose his action as an effective agent of treatment.

2. For many chronic organic maladies, a drug that has pharmacologic or short-term therapeutic efficacy may be ineffectual for long-term therapeutic goals. Thus the lowering of serum lipids may not prevent recurrent myocardial infarction, the cytotoxic destruction of neoplastic cells may not prolong survival in cancer, an anorexigenic drug may not enable the maintenance of weight loss, and the lowering of blood sugar by hypoglycemic agents may not prevent diabetic vascular complications. Nevertheless, the pharmacologic or short-term efficacy of the drugs, together with the absence of any alternative agents, may make a clinician prescribe the drugs for a longer period during which he simultaneously provides the comfort and aid of his own iatrotherapy to the patient. By determining that the drugs are "ineffectual" in long-term therapy and

by rejecting their usage in this manner, we may save patients from the costs and possible hazards of the drugs, but we may also deprive the patients of the iatrotherapeutic benefits induced by the doctor's faith in the drugs. Again, we may advance science while depriving patients of a good total therapeutic effect.

Acts of irrational faith have always played an important part in the treatment of human ailments, and are responsible for many of the therapeutic triumphs achieved, after failure of conventional "scientific" approaches, at religious shrines or by practitioners of diverse "unscientific" healing arts. To deny the personal role of the therapist and of other nonrational elements in the treatment of people is to deny the realities of nature, with which science is presumably concerned. To analyze only what is overtly rational while ignoring the nonrational constituents of natural events may lead to a pseudoscience based on irrational beliefs about the validity of inadequate methods and measurements.

This thorny problem is seldom subjected to public discussion, perhaps because it is not susceptible to scientific solution and because it involves an open recognition of the fact that doctors, like patients, may be "placebo reactors," and also that doctors often use pharmaceutical agents not for their inherent value, but as adjuncts or substitutes for iatrotherapy. It is easier for a doctor to prescribe a tranquillizer than to discuss a patient's lack of tranquillity; to prescribe an anorexigenic agent than to listen to the problems of maintaining caloric restriction; to prescribe a somnifacient agent than to explore the reasons for insomnia. Ideally, a doctor should always be ready and willing to give himself as an agent of treatment, but since the administration of iatrotherapy is often an arduous, time-consuming, and emotionally draining activity, and since doctors are human, they often minimize the activity or perform it only if suitably stimulated.

A doctor's awareness of the problem and his ability to cope with it have also been hampered by long-standing defects in medical education, which often emphasizes the pharmacologic action of drugs but not the totality of therapy, and which often allocates the role and contributions of iatrotherapy to the segregated pursuits of psychiatry. In addition to these difficulties, doctors also share with other people the urge to "do something," which has always been part of human nature, and which is particularly likely to develop or to be requested during the practice of clinical medicine. For these and other reasons, a spuriously effective drug often elicits in a doctor the "placebo reaction" that provides effective iatrotherapy.

Although the *safety* of a pharmaceutical agent must always be carefully checked to assure that it does no harm, the total issue of efficacy will often depend on the iatric as well as the intrinsically pharmaceutical elements of therapy. For the sake of pharmacologic science, however, we often deliberately exclude the iatric components of treatment, and restrict investigations to a comparison of active drug versus placebo, without studying a group of untreated patients. The result is often good as pharmacology but confusing as therapy. Suppose we find that 40 per cent of patients improve with a placebo and 50 per cent improve with drug *D*. If this difference is clinically meaningful and "statistically significant," we might conclude that *D* is an effective agent. On the other hand, suppose we had also tested an untreated group of patients and found but 5 per cent improvement. Our conclusion might now be somewhat different. We would realize that *D* is only a slightly effective agent and that iatrotherapy was the major source of the improvement, although the combination of drug *D* and iatrotherapy was more effective than placebo and iatrotherapy.

Suppose, however, that the improvement rates were 40 per cent with drug *D*, 40 per cent with placebo, and 5 per cent

with no treatment. We would decide that the drug is no better than placebo. If no other pharmaceutical agent had been shown to be effective for this clinical condition, a doctor might be unwilling to use a placebo as "active" treatment, and might conclude that patients should be left untreated. Instead of a 40 per cent improvement with the "ineffectual" drug *D*, the improvement rate might then be only 5 per cent. Thus, despite the absence of pharmaceutical efficacy for drug *D*, the physician's belief in the therapeutic agent had evoked a potent form of iatrotherapy so that the rate of improvement in the treated groups was 35 per cent higher than that in the untreated. If drug *D* had not been available to provoke the iatrotherapy, a major therapeutic benefit for patients would not have occurred.

These remarks are in no way intended to propose a return to the prescientific era when the contributions of iatrotherapy were elicited by a misplaced confidence in such ineffectual or dangerous agents as blood-letting, blistering, purging, and puking. But a transition from the old pre-science to a modern pseudoscience does not necessarily represent progress. The determination of a drug's pharmacologic efficacy, although obviously a basic necessity of any therapeutic investigation, is not the only necessity of therapeutic science. The complex therapeutic interplay of doctor, drug, and patient in clinical medicine can not be adequately investigated merely by studying the drug and the patient under "scientific" conditions that demonstrate the efficacy of the drug without clarifying the evaluation of therapy.

6. Identification of the patients. All of the foregoing discussion has been concerned with the problems of evaluating the events that occur after therapy begins. Assuming that these events can be thoroughly identified and properly evaluated, clinicians are then confronted with the additional problem of extrapolating the results. For this decision, clinicians must be able to correlate the results with the initial conditions of the patients under treatment. The performance of this correlation has also been greatly handicapped by the oversimplifications of current statistical designs for therapeutic trials.

Although the initial clinical features of patients are important harbingers of prognosis and determinants of therapy, these features are deliberately obliterated in therapeutic trials when all the patients are "lumped" together for randomization, and when suitable prognostic stratifications are not performed during the subsequent analyses. Among the clinical features that may need consideration for patients with the "same" diagnosis—particularly in chronic diseases—are the iatrotropy, cluster, severity, sequence, and timing of the diverse symptomatic manifestations.[9] Because the "soft data" that describe these clinical features are often omitted from statistical consideration, however, a clinician examining the results may be unable to determine which clinical type of patients had responded well or poorly to the therapeutic agents.

Another unfortunate custom in many statistical plans is to exclude all patients with major associated comorbid diseases.[10] For example, in trials of therapy for coronary artery disease, the population may be restricted to people who have only coronary disease, excluding those with diabetes mellitus, hypertension, gout, or other ailments. Such exclusions provide the statistical satisfaction of treating a "pure" population of patients with the "main" disease, but the results in these "pure" groups cannot readily be extrapolated to the impurities of clinical practice. An alternative and equally unfortunate statistical custom in the management of comorbidity is to include patients whose major comorbidity is inadequately classified. For example, in a trial of therapy to prevent vascular complications of diabetes mellitus,[33] patients with major comorbid diseases were admitted if judged to have a good prognosis, but the ingre-dients of the prognostic judgments were left unspecified and the comorbid ailments were not effectively identified.[13] When disputes arose about fatalities that occurred during the trial, the data could not be interpreted because of difficulties in ascribing the deaths to complications of diabetes, to the pre-existing comorbid ailments, or to the effects of treatment.

The final problem to be cited here is the difficulty of extrapolating results in a trial performed with a "compliance sample" of patients. Such a "sample" is created when ambulatory patients, before admission to a trial of long-term therapy, are first tested for their ability and willingness to comply with the planned diagnostic and therapeutic procedures. Patients who show inadequate compliance during the test period are then excluded from the trial. This type of preselection of patients seems reasonable because it avoids wasting the investigator's time treating patients who may later "drop out," and it reduces the difficulty of appraising results in patients who did not faithfully adhere to the prescribed regimens. Nevertheless, although the trial may demonstrate the efficacy of the drug, without data to indicate that the personalities and other clinical features of patients in a "compliance sample" are similar to the features of other patients with the same disease, we may be unable to draw conclusions about the way that the general population of diseased patients would respond to the drug.

B. Problems in safety

The estimation of safety is beset with many of the same types of problems just described for efficacy. No operational definition has been created for *safety;* no unequivocal standards have been established for the clinical and laboratory abnormalities that are acceptable as "safe" and those that are not; and the usual statistical approach to the problem of safety is to tabulate and compare the numbers of "side effects" or "adverse reactions" that occurred in patients treated with the tested drugs or placebo. Since no operational criteria are provided to identify these "side effects" and "adverse reactions," the results can often achieve "statistical significance" without having any scientific specificity or clinical applicability.

With respect to multiple responses, no criteria have been established to weigh the amount of "unsafety" that is acceptable in exchange for "efficacy." (For example, if major surgical operations were evaluated in the same manner as new drugs, the operations would probably never be allowed "on the market," because of the almost constant occurrence of postoperative pain and permanent cutaneous scarring.) In reference to the diverse goals of treatment, no delineations have been drawn for the differences between pharmacologic safety, and safety in short-term or long-term therapy. As for the distinctively personal reactions of patients and doctors, no standards have been created to distinguish between habituation, abuse, or other problems in the chronic maintenance of drugs.[8, 18] Thus, no pejorative terms are applied for the chronicity of therapy when a diabetic patient takes insulin at the start of each day to achieve normoglycemia or when a businessman takes whisky at the end of the day to achieve relaxation. But the term "habituation" would be applied if the same businessman took a barbiturate at bedtime to achieve sleep, and the term "abuse" would probably be applied if he took a long-acting amphetamine daily to maintain weight reduction.

To discuss the many principles of *safety* that have been neither clinically specified nor operationally defined would extend this essay to an inordinate length. Instead, I shall restrict the remaining discussion to just one of the available topics: the question of operationally identifying an "adverse reaction." There are many different types of undesirable reactions that can occur during pharmaceutical treatment. They have been given such names as *cumulation, tachyphylaxis, tolerance, intolerance, toxicity, overdosage, side effects, secondary effects, idiosyncrasy, hypersensitivity,* and *allergic reactions.* Although the definitions do not always agree, these terms are generally defined in most textbooks of pharmacology.

Unfortunately, however, the definitions are not satisfactory for clinical practice because they follow the wrong logical direction. In clinical practice, a physician examines a patient with certain clinical and laboratory manifestations and must then decide their cause. Are they due to the evolving course of the main disease, to the evolving course of an antecedent comorbid disease, to the superimposition of a new comorbid disease, or to the patient's anxiety and other psychic reactions? Or do they represent an "adverse reaction" to a drug? And, if so, what kind of reaction and to which drug, if more than one was being taken?

To make these decisions in a reproducible, consistent manner would require that suitable diagnostic-therapeutic algorithms be established by clinicians who are connoisseurs of human illness and of clinical therapy. Since such algorithms have been neither established nor planned, the statistical tabulation of "adverse reactions" and the creation of "guidelines" for interpreting those statistics in modern therapeutic practice can proceed unencumbered by any of the elemental principles of science.

• • •

These intellectual maladies of clinical therapy cannot be cured merely by the further application of inappropriate statistical theories, by "crash" programs and bureaucratic fiats, or by recommendations from scientists who have had little or no personal responsibility for the continuing care of patients. The problems arise in clinical activities, and can be best perceived and solved by connoisseurs of those activities.

Some of the work will require the intellectual "dissection" of existing patterns of clinical reasoning. To harden "soft" clinical data, to classify comorbidity and other taxonomically neglected clinical features of patients, and to differentiate diagnostically among the diverse causes of posttherapeutic reactions will require the formation of algorithmic criteria.[12] For these algorithms, the ingredients of clinical reasoning must be expressed in a manner that will delineate specific observations and decisional strategies whose constituents and logic are now relegated to the mystical realms of "clinical judgment."[9]

For other necessary activities, the main challenge is to establish standards and goals that do not now exist. Since no distinctive principles have been developed for defining meaningful differences in response, for evaluating patients' peritherapeutic responses, and for choosing and "weighting" constituents in composite indexes of multiple response, the principles must now be created *de novo* as a product of careful deliberation and consensual validation.

To appraise long-term therapeutic results, however, the work must go beyond intellectual activities at a conference table by suitable clinicians from academic and nonacademic sources. Massive clinical efforts will be needed for gathering appropriate data from practitioners, and for developing appropriate research activities at academic medical centers. At these centers, an abundant population of patients is available for the necessary scientific observations and investigations, but the opportunity has been generally neglected in favor of scientific challenges in the laboratory.[11] Although the demonstration of *pharmacologic* safety and efficacy is a legitimate responsibility of pharmaceutical manufacturers, the industry cannot be held liable for the larger and long-term issues of clinical therapy. The manufacturer of a surgical therapeutic instrument is obligated to show that the instrument works properly, but can not be asked to prove that surgeons will always use it wisely or that patients will always benefit from the operative procedure.

Neither science nor the public will be well served if the determination of safety and efficacy in drug treatment is assigned exclusively to the pharmaceutical industry and if the supervision of this assignment is delegated exclusively to federal regulatory agencies. Since the issues of pharmaceutical therapy, rather than pharmacology alone, comprise concepts and data unique to clinical practice, the issues cannot be properly contemplated, identified, analyzed, or regulated unless connoisseurs of clinical practice participate in a suitable manner. Without such participation, the assessment of safety and efficacy will continue to be based on ideas that are inadequate for clinical practice and on rules that may be calamitous to it.

The public will continue to demand regulations that assure the safety and efficacy of pharmaceutical therapy, and regulations will inevitably be created in response to this demand. Without modification of current procedures, however, the regulations will succeed in replacing "clinical experience" that is scientifically unspecified by "scientific" statistics that are clinically worthless. If academic and practicing clinicians want these regulations to be both scientifically meaningful and clinically sensible, the clinicians cannot continue to evade their own paramount responsibilities while complaining about the work done by the statisticians, pharmaceutical companies, and federal personnel to whom the responsibilities have become allocated by default.

References

1. Ad Hoc Committee to Revise the Jones Criteria (modified) of the Council on Rheumatic Fever and Congenital Heart Disease of the American Heart Association: Jones criteria (revised) for guidance in the diagnosis of rheumatic fever, Circulation 32:664-668, 1965.
2. Beckman, H.: Pharmacology. The nature, action and use of drugs, ed. 2, Philadelphia, 1961, The W. B. Saunders Company.
3. Beecher, H. K.: Measurement of subjective responses, New York, 1959, Oxford University Press.
4. Bonnar, J., Goldberg, A., and Smith, J. A.:

Do pregnant women take their iron? Lancet **1**:457-458, 1961.

5. Bowman, W. C., Rand, M. J., and West, G. B.: Textbook of pharmacology, Oxford, 1968, Blackwell Scientific Publications.

6. Burgen, A. S. V., and Mitchell, J. F.: Gaddum's pharmacology, ed. 6, New York, 1968, Oxford University Press.

7. DiPalma, J. R., editor: Drill's pharmacology in medicine, ed. 3, New York, 1965, McGraw-Hill Book Co., Inc.

8. Dunlop, D.: Abuse of drugs by the public and by doctors, Brit. Med. Bull. **26**:236-239, 1970.

9. Feinstein, A. R.: Clinical judgment, Baltimore, 1967, The Williams & Wilkins Company.

10. Feinstein, A. R.: Clinical biostatistics. IV. The architecture of clinical research (continued), CLIN. PHARMACOL. THER. **11**:595-610, 1970.

11. Feinstein, A. R.: What kind of basic science for clinical medicine? New Eng. J. Med. **283**: 847-852, 1970.

12. Feinstein, A. R.: Taxonorics. I. Formulation of criteria, Arch. Intern. Med. **126**:678-693, 1970.

13. Feinstein, A. R.: Commentary. Clinical biostatistics. VIII. An analytic appraisal of the university group diabetes program (UGDP) study, CLIN. PHARMACOL. THER. **12**:167-191, 1971.

14. Garb, S., Crim, B. J., and Thomas, G.: Pharmacology and patient care, ed. 3, New York, 1970, Springer Publishing Company, Inc.

15. Goldstein, A., Aronow, L., and Kalman, J. M.: Principles of drug action: the basis of pharmacology, New York, 1968, Harper and Row, Publishers.

16. Goodman, L. S., and Gilman, A.: The Pharmacological basis of therapeutics, ed. 4, New York, 1970, The Macmillan Company.

17. Goth, A.: Medical pharmacology. Principles and concepts, ed. 4, St. Louis, 1968, The C. V. Mosby Company.

18. Green, D. M.: Pre-existing conditions, placebo reactions, and "side effects," Ann. Intern. Med. **60**:255-265, 1964.

19. Grollman, A., and Grollman, E. F.: Pharmacology and therapeutics. A textbook for students and practitioners of medicine and its allied professions, ed. 7, Philadelphia, 1970, Lea and Febiger, Publishers.

20. Joyce, C. R. B.: Patient co-operation and the sensitivity of clinical trials, J. Chron. Dis. **15**: 1025-1036, 1962.

21. Krantz, J. C., Carr, C. J., and Ladu, B. N.: The pharmacologic principles of medical practice, ed. 7, Baltimore, 1969, The Williams & Wilkins Company.

22. Lasagna, L., Mosteller, F., vonFelsinger, J. M., and Beecher, H. K.: A study of the placebo response, Amer. J. Med. **16**:770-779, 1954.

23. Laurence, D. R., editor: Symposium on quantitative methods in human pharmacology and therapeutics, London, 1958, New York, 1959, Pergamon Press, Inc.

24. Mainland, D.: The estimation of inflammatory activity in rheumatoid arthritis. Role of composite indices, Arthritis Rheum. **10**:71-77, 1967.

25. Modell, W.: Relief of symptoms, ed. 2, St. Louis, 1961, The C. V. Mosby Company.

26. Meyers, F. H., Jawetz, E., and Goldfien, A.: Review of medical pharmacology, Los Altos, Calif., 1968, Lange Medical Publications.

27. Musser, R. D., and O'Neill, J. J.: Pharmacology and therapeutics, ed. 4, Toronto, 1969, The Macmillan Company, Collier-Macmillan Ltd.

28. Porter, A. M. W.: Drug defaulting in a general practice, Brit. Med. J. **1**:218-222, 1969.

29. Report of a WHO Scientific Group: Principles for pre-clinical testing of drug safety, Technical Report Series No. 341, Geneva, 1966, World Health Organization.

30. Rickels, K., editor: Non-specific factors in drug therapy, Springfield, Ill., 1968, Charles C Thomas, Publisher.

31. Ropes, M. W., Bennett, G. A., Cobb, S., Jacox, R., and Jessar, R.: 1958 Revision of diagnostic criteria for rheumatoid arthritis, Bull. Rheum. Dis. **9**:175-176, 1958.

32. Tedeschi, D. H., and Tedeschi, R. E., editors: Importance of fundamental principles in drug evaluation, New York, 1968, Raven Press.

33. University Group Diabetes Program: A study of the effects of hypoglycemic agents on vascular complications in patients with adult-onset diabetes. Part I: Design, methods, and baseline characteristics. Part II: Mortality results, Diabetes **19**: (Suppl. 2) 747-830, 1970.

34. Waife, S. O., and Shapiro, A. P., editors: The clinical evaluation of new drugs, New York, 1959, Paul B. Hoeber, Inc.

35. Wilks, S. S.: Some aspects of quantification in science, p. 5, *in* Woolf, H., editor: Quantification, Indianapolis, 1961, Bobbs-Merrill Company.

36. Wolf, S.: Placebos: Problems and pitfalls, CLIN. PHARMACOL. THER. **3**:254-257, 1962.

37. Wolstenholme, G., and Porter, R., editors: Drug responses in man (Ciba Foundation Volume), Boston, 1967, Little, Brown & Company.

38. Zaimis, E., editor: Evaluation of new drugs in man, *in* Proceedings Second International Pharmacological Meeting, vol. 8, Oxford, 1965, Pergamon Press.

CHAPTER 19

The difficulties of pharmaceutical surveillance

After being approved for the open market, a drug becomes used in a broader spectrum of clinical situations and durations than those for which its efficacy and safety were originally studied. The careful supervision of what happens in these new circumstances is often called *monitoring* or *surveillance*. Since *monitoring* has acquired many other connotations, such as the vigilant observation of patients in an intensive care unit or the scrutiny of investigators adhering to a research protocol, the word *surveillance* has fewer ambiguities than *monitoring* and seems preferable as a label for the process of "watching over" a drug in its expanded spectrum of applications.

The challenge of pharmaceutical surveillance has become a major problem for the public, for physicians, and for the pharmaceutical industry and its federal regulators. What mechanisms can be used to determine promptly when a drug is dangerous, so that we can be spared another thalidomide disaster, or when it has unforeseen benefits—such as the role of lidocaine in arrhythmias or methotrexate in psoriasis—that were not discovered during the pre-marketing investigations? In this essay, I should like to note some of the fundamental difficulties and to discuss some of the bio-

statistical methods that might be used to get scientific answers to these questions.

A. The basic phenomena

Although many discussions of *surveillance* begin with the idea of finding rates of adverse events associated with use of a drug, the basic phenomena under observation are much more profound and complex. Before any rates can be calculated, we must be able to decide what is an "adverse reaction," whether it is caused by a drug, and which drug has caused it. These decisions require an evaluation of the following sequence of three entities:

$$\text{PERSON} \xrightarrow{\text{DRUG}} \text{EVENT.}$$

To conclude that an "adverse drug reaction" has occurred requires a careful dissection of the intricate mixture of constituents contained in each of these three entities.

1. The event. The events that are noted after use of a drug can be classified as desirable, negligible (or innocuous), or undesirable. Certain undesirable events can be intended or anticipated, such as the pain associated with an injection. Other undesirable events, which are not anticipated, are the contenders for receiving the designation of "adverse drug reaction," Before any other planning can begin, a standardized, consistent mechanism must

This chapter originally appeared as "Clinical biostatistics—XXVIII. The biostatistical problems of pharmaceutical surveillance." In Clin. Pharmacol. Ther. 16:110, 1974.

be established for designating the desirability of the observed events and for deciding which ones are the adverse-reaction candidates. The current absence of such a mechanism, as noted later, is a fundamental obstacle to any clinical or biostatistical efforts aimed at designing an effective process of surveillance.

2. The drug. Another frequently oversimplified aspect of the surveillance process is the idea that the events occurring after the use of a drug can regularly be associated with that drug. Many concomitant phenomena that occur while or after the drug is taken can produce effects whose cause must be differentiated from the effects ascribed to the drug. Among those phenomena are the use of another drug or drugs, the superimposition of a separate ailment that was not present when the "index" drug was begun, and the patient's exposure to diagnostic procedures or nonpharmaceutical therapy that may be followed by untoward consequences.

To evaluate the concomitant phenomena that may cause an adverse reaction, intricate judgments are needed in diagnostic and therapeutic reasoning. As noted later, no standardized, consistent mechanisms exist for performing these judgments.

3. The person. The human use of drugs also does not take place in standardized situations. Even if people have the same diagnosed disease, they may differ in their basic clinical states. Thus, two patients may both have acute myocardial infarction, but one may have chest pain alone whereas the other may have chest pain, respiratory distress, and a major cardiac arrhythmia. Even if two people have identical diagnoses, such as acute myocardial infarction, and identical clinical states, such as chest pain and respiratory distress, the drugs may be given for different clinical indications. One patient may receive Drug X for the chest pain; the other patient may be given the same drug for the respiratory distress.

In addition to diseases, clinical states, and clinical indications, two other impor-

tant variables—co-morbidity and demography—may differentiate the people receiving the same drug. Co-morbidity refers to the associated diseases that are present in addition to the principal disease; a patient with myocardial infarction alone is different from a patient who also has hypertension, diabetes mellitus, and gout. Demography refers to such personal features as age, race, sex, occupation, and family status.

These underlying characteristics help distinguish the baseline state of the person who takes the drug. They may also be prognostic harbingers of future events, occurring after the drug is given, that must be included as possible sources of an undesirable reaction. Thus, when an arrhythmia develops in a patient receiving digitalis for the treatment of congestive heart failure, a possible cause of the arrhythmia is a worsening of the initial congestive heart failure rather than a reaction to the digitalis. Similarly, when dementia develops in an elderly patient receiving digitalis for cardiac disease, a possible cause of the dementia is cerebral arterial insufficiency rather than digitalis toxicity.

B. The statistical rate

After these different aspects of the data have been disentangled, we can contemplate a statistical rate as

$$\left(\begin{array}{c}\text{ADVERSE}\\\text{REACTIONS}\end{array}\right) \Big/ \left(\begin{array}{c}\text{USE OF}\\\text{DRUG}\end{array}\right).$$

The *numerator* of this rate must be carefully determined since it represents the identification, association, and causal evaluation of the events just cited. The *denominator* of the rate must also be carefully determined since it represents the association of the numerator events with the risk taken in the exposed patients. Another reason for precise identification of the denominator is to permit valid extrapolation of the results. Unless we know the particular types of patients in whom adverse reactions occurred, we cannot draw clinically useful conclusions about what to do in future prescription of the drug.

When we consider the process of surveillance, however, we are not talking about either the numerator or denominator of this rate. Surveillance is what happens in the virgule (the slash mark) that separates the numerator and denominator. The virgule represents the time interval, between use of a drug and occurrence of subsequent events, during which we can impose the process of observing, detecting, evaluating, and recording those events. Many discussions of surveillance are devoted mainly to these "virgule activities," with emphasis on the various investigators, administrative mechanisms, and computer systems used for the acquisition and storage of data. These activities in the process of surveillance constitute its technology—the arrangements of medical setting, personnel, and data-gathering tactics that allow the desired information to be acquired. The more basic scientific strategies of surveillance, however, depend on decisions about the numerators and denominators: what kind of data to gather, what kind of patients to observe, and what principles to use for evaluation.

C. The technology of surveillance

A major accomplishment in pharmaceutical research of the past decade has been the development of "surveillance systems" at several different medical institutions.[1, 6, 16-18, 20, 25, 28, 31, 35, 41] These systems, which are intended to provide a continuous scrutiny of the use and effects of pharmaceutical preparations, have obtained quantitative information that was hitherto unavailable about the frequency of institutional prescription of different drugs and the frequency of associated adverse reactions. In some instances, a surveillance system has also been employed as a mechanism for performing an analog of Phase III clinical trials[26]; and for noting demographic factors[4, 24] that may influence the action of drugs.

Despite some major shortcomings that will be noted later, these systems represent an enormous achievement in the technology of pharmaceutical surveillance. One valuable demonstration has been the contributions that can be made by nurses,[4] pharmacists,[17] and other non-physician personnel in collecting data. Another noteworthy feature has been the documented importance of making planned, continuous observations[28] rather than relying on ad hoc, sporadic reports. A third substantial contribution has been the creation of suitable data formats for coding and storing much of the necessary information, and the development of computerized or other analytic methods[1, 25] that can be used when the data are tabulated and interpreted. In addition, of course, the results obtained during the surveillance have served to provide warnings of possible toxicity and appraisals of possible efficacy for a variety of different drugs and drug-interactions.[2] Regardless of the ultimate role of these institution-based surveillance systems, they have led to the development of useful technologic tactics that will be invaluable background for any future work in surveillance activities.

An institution-based surveillance system, however, is institution-based. The investigators can observe only the kinds of patients who are referred or self-referred to the institution and can study only the kinds of pharmaceutical preparations that are authorized or ordered at the institution. For the surveillance systems that depend on a population of hospital in-patients, the duration of observation usually lasts only as long as the patient is in the hospital. These drawbacks would not affect a system's ability to draw conclusions about what is happening in the institutional setting, but they would create serious limitations in answering more general questions about the surveillance of a wide variety of people using a wide variety of drugs for a wide variety of durations.

The fundamental problem of contemporary surveillance, however, is not the restricted scope of the observed patients, drugs, and durations in institution-based surveillance systems. The fundamental problem is the absence of a standardized, consistent, reproducible procedure for making the decision that a particular event is an "adverse drug reaction."

D. The identification of adverse reactions

In all of the surveillance systems just mentioned and in all of the reports assembled at the various surveillance registries that will be mentioned later, each of the tabulated "adverse reactions" was diagnosed as an act of individual clinical judgment. No clearly delineated and overtly specified method of operational procedures has been developed for making the decisions.[10] The investigators may regularly supply definitions and classifications[33] of the "adverse reactions," but a defined classification is quite different from an operational identification.

We can define *blood sugar* as the amount of a monosaccharide, $C_6H_{12}O_6$, that is present in 100 ml of whole blood, but this definition does not provide an operational identification of blood sugar. For an operational identification, we would need a set of sequential instructions, such as those that might be found in a laboratory manual describing a chemical method of measuring blood sugar. The directions would tell us to add a certain volume of blood to certain volumes of designated reagents under certain physical conditions; to place the resultant mixture in a spectrophotometer; and to convert the reading using certain pre-determined numerical factors. The result would be the value of blood sugar, operationally identified.

The medical and pharmaceutical literature currently contains many definitions that classify adverse drug reactions according to mechanism, existence, and severity. Their presumptive mechanism is usually classified as pharmacologic, allergic, or idiosyncratic. The pharmacologic reactions are further subclassified as primary excess effects, due to overdosage or over-

effectiveness; and secondary effects on non-primary targets or at sites of injection. The causal relation of a drug to an adverse reaction is often classified as definite (or "causative"), probable, possible, or doubtful (or "coincidental"). The severity of an adverse reaction can be cited as fatal, severe nonfatal, moderate, or mild.

But none of these definitions and classifications provides an operational identification or diagnostic algorithm[13] for deciding whether a particular undesirable event was due to the accused drug, to some other drug, to an interaction of drugs, to the evolving course of the main clinical state, to the evolving course of a baseline co-morbid state, to a superimposed new co-morbid state, or to some intervening diagnostic or other therapeutic procedure. A report from a Registry of Tissue Reactions to Drugs[23] is the only reference I have been able to find in which deliberate formal attention has been given to the diagnostic reasoning used in this activity. Among the data that might be included to justify decisions in the flow chart or criteria for making an operational identification are the known characteristics of the main clinical state and co-morbid state, the known patterns of response to the index and associated other drugs, the laboratory evidence of the drug's concentration in the patient, the time relationships between the adverse event and the intake of drugs, and the results of such additional tests as cessation (or "de-challenge") of the drug and its resumption (or "re-challenge").

In the absence of stated methods of operational identification for adverse reactions, investigative work in surveillance will continue to lack a fundamental ingredient of scientific evidence. The "adverse reaction," as the basic element under investigation, is not identified with precise, distinctive, reproducible criteria. We have no idea of the amount of variability among the physicians whose nondescript judgment is used to decide whether an observed event is or is not an adverse drug reaction. There have been no procedures for standardization; no tests of consistency; and no assessments of reproducibility. After we work our way through all the majesty of the computer print-out and the glory of the statistics, we find that the decision-making mechanism for identifying adverse reactions—for making diagnoses such as whether an episode of vomiting is due to digitalis, underlying heart disease, psychic tension, or spoiled food—depends on the vagaries of clinical judgment of an array of unstandardized physicians.

The first main step towards developing a valid biostatistical science of pharmaceutical surveillance will not be in creating additional technologies of surveillance. The first step is to arrive at reproducible methods for identifying an adverse drug reaction.

E. Epidemiologic strategies of surveillance

Like other epidemiologic challenges in the discernment of cause-and-effect relationships, pharmaceutical surveillance requires a comparative assessment of rates. The possible epidemiologic strategies contain a complex, almost bewildering, array of different numerators and denominators, "control" groups, and methods of getting data. The reader is hereby warned that this section of the text, as befits the intricacies of the subject, is neither simple nor easy to follow.

1. Cohort procedures. The cohort approach is the most scientifically logical way of answering a question about cause and effect; and the incidence rates that emerge from a cohort study are direct and simple to understand. The denominator consists of the number of people exposed to the "cause," which is the drug under investigation. The numerator consists of the number of those people who developed the "effect," which is the cited adverse reaction(s). The ratio of this numerator and denominator is an incidence rate, denoting adverse reactions per people taking the drug. This rate is then compared with the incidence of similar adverse reactions in a group of people treated in some other

manner. Several different procedures can be used for acquiring data about incidence rates in a cohort.

a. Prolective cohort. In a prolective[11] study, the investigators begin the research before treatment is given and before any adverse reactions have occurred. Groups of people taking the investigated drug or being treated in some other way are assembled and followed to note the occurrence of the adverse reactions. This is the type of procedure used in the hospital surveillance systems mentioned earlier.

b. Retrolective cohort. In this approach, the numerators and denominators consist of the same type of data used for a cohort—the incidence of adverse reactions in a defined population of exposed or nonexposed people—but the data for the compared groups are assembled retrolectively,[11] after the adverse reactions have occurred. Having noted some events that are believed to be adverse drug reactions, the investigator begins the research by collecting existing data—usually from patients' medical records—for the clinical course of a group of people who have received the suspected drug. By inspecting the data for the post-drug course of those people, the investigator determines the rate at which the suspected adverse reactions occurred. For comparison, the investigator assembles the recorded data of a similar group of people, treated in some other manner, and notes the rates of the same reactions in this controlled group. The data for the control group can be "concurrent," derived from people treated in some other way during the same calendar time interval in which the suspected drug was taken; or "historical," derived from an earlier group of patients with the same medical condition.

A retrolective cohort with a "historical control" group was the procedure employed when the hazards of thalidomide were first pointed out in the English language literature by W. G. McBride.[32] Without any elaborate research grants or epidemiologic flamboyance, McBride described his work in a letter, written to the editor of *The Lancet,* that is a model of clear thinking and reporting:

Congenital abnormalities are present in approximately 1.5% of babies. In recent months I have observed that the incidence of multiple severe abnormalities in babies delivered of women who were given the drug thalidomide . . . during pregnancy . . . (was) almost 20%.

c. Estimated cohort. In this circumstance, a group of patients receiving the suspected drug is not actually assembed and counted as the denominator of a cohort. Instead, the number of people taking the drug is estimated from its sales figures, supplied by the manufacturer. The numerator for this denominator is the number of suspected adverse reactions that have been reported in the geographic region to which the estimated denominator pertains. The data about the adverse reactions can be collected in a registry (as described later) or directly by the manufacturer of the drug. The rate in a comparative group is determined from "historical controls" or from analogous data assembled for some other drug that has the same type of clinical usage.

2. Other procedures. For all of the three methods just described, the frequency of adverse reactions was calculated as an incidence rate, with appropriately exposed (or non-exposed) people in the denominators and the corresponding adverse reactions in the numerators. In all of the methods that follow, the logic of cohort data is altered. The number of people receiving the drug is not determined and cohort incidence rates are not calculated. Instead, the decisions rest on several other types of epidemiologic rates.

a. Secular mortality associations. In this procedure, the basic research data are issued by the Bureau of Vital Statistics (or some appropriate counterpart), when it publishes the annual rate of death attributed to a specific disease in the general population. The pattern noted in a calendar sequence of these annual mortality rates is called a *secular trend.* Observing an apparently inappropriate change in the trend, an investigator may suspect that the change is due to an alteration in treatment for the disease. After assembling data about the time when a suspected pharmaceutical agent was introduced, the investigator notes the secular trend for sales curves or other usage of the agent. The concomitant secular trends in both mortality and drug usage are then associated for a cause-effect conjecture. The inference drawn from such a secular mortality association was the basis for beliefs[21] that aerosol bronchodilators had led to an increase in deaths from asthma in England and Wales.

b. 'Event' trohoc. This approach consists of a modification of the classical trohoc[12] (or "case-control") study. The investigators begin by assembling a group of people (or "cases") who are known to have had the particular event that is suspected of being an adverse reaction to the drug. In this group of "cases," the investigators then determine the number of people who had previously taken the accused drug. For comparison, the investigators determine the previous usage of that drug in a "control" group of people selected because they have not had the event under scrutiny. The prevalence rates of the drug's usage in the "cases" and the "controls" are then compared directly or compressed into a "risk ratio." The "cases" are usually selected from in-patients at a hospital, and the "controls" can be chosen from other patients in the hospital or from suitable sources outside the hospital. The population studied in this approach is called an *event trohoc* (rather than a *disease trohoc*) because the cases and controls are chosen according to the presence or absence of the event that is suspected of being an adverse drug reaction.

An event trohoc was surveyed for the type of research used to suggest that oral contraceptive pills might lead to thrombophlebitis[22, 39, 42] and that the use of certain estrogens in pregnancy might lead to vaginal carcinoma in the offspring.[19] Although modern-day hospital surveillance systems were established for performing cohort studies of drug effects, the investigators can also use the collected data for trohoc research. Because of the positive relationship found in a trohoc study performed with data of a pharmaceutical surveillance system,[27] an interesting current controversy has arisen about the association between coffee-drinking and myocardial infarction. The relationship was denied in a cohort study performed by the Framingham epidemiologic team.[7]

c. Registry collections. All of the other epidemiologic procedures to be described here are based on the analysis of data assembled at the institutional,[43] municipal,[37] national,[8, 9] or international[38] registries that have been established to solicit, receive, and store the adverse-reaction case reports voluntarily submitted by physicians or by other qualified reporters. Because of the way the data are assembled, they contain numerators without denominators. The data can be used to count the frequency of the adverse reactions associated with specific drugs and to provide warnings based on changes in frequency,[44] but the registry data alone provide no indication of the total usage of the drugs or the number of users who were reaction-free.

An appealing tactic with registry data is to convert the frequency counts of drug reactions into crude incidence rates for an estimated cohort of drug users. The number of drug reactions is the numerator; the denominator is estimated as noted earlier; and the comparison is with historical or other suitable control groups. Other analyses of the registry data are based exclusively on information stored at the registries. From the many possible strategies, which have received thorough descriptions by Finney,[14, 15] only three will be mentioned here.

1. Secular trends. The investigator notes the frequency count of the number of reactions reported during successive calendar intervals. Suspicions are aroused by an unexplained increase in the secular trend of frequencies of the reports. (These secular "reaction" rates differ from the secular

mortality rates mentioned earlier. A mortality rate contains three ingredients: the number of deaths per specified population per specified time interval. A secular "reaction" rate contains only two ingredients: the number of reactions reported per specified time interval.)

2. Registry trohoc. A diverse group of clinical entities will have been reported in the registry as the adverse reactions for any drug, D. Suppose we are interested in a particular type of reaction, X. Using the trohoc principle, we can choose a "case" group to consist of all the reactions reported for D. We then note the prevalence of X among those reactions. For comparison, our "control" consists of the prevalence of X among the total number of reactions reported for some other drug or drugs.

3. Accrual rate. At any point in time, the registry will contain a certain number of reported adverse reactions for the drug. During an ensuing interval of time, new reports are acquired. The size of this increment, when divided by the previous number of reports, produces an accrual rate of new reactions for that drug during the cited time interval. This rate can be compared against the analogously calculated accrual rate for some other drug or for all drugs.

F. Cause signals, causes, rate signals, and rates

The different epidemiologic strategies that have just been described can be employed in at least four different ways. In one circumstance—the cause signal—we have no idea that a particular drug and a particular undesirable event are related. The purpose of the signal is to raise suspicions of this possibility. Once our suspicions have been alerted, we may then want to get additional evidence to decide whether the relationship between the drug and the event is actually causal, and whether the event should be regarded as an adverse reaction to that drug.

In a different circumstance, we begin with the belief that the event is an adverse reaction, and we want to know the frequency of its occurrence. We might also want to have a mechanism—the rate signal—to alert us to changes in frequency that might suggest the occurrence of new or unforeseen toxicity for the drug. The mechanism that produces a cause signal may not necessarily be the mechanism for proving cause; and the mechanism that produces a rate signal may not always indicate the true rates of the adverse reactions.

1. Cause signals. If an undesirable event is clinically unique, such as the sudden growth of feathers on a person's forearm, we may have no difficulty deciding that it is an extraordinary reaction and we may immediately suspect the associated drug. Our main quest will then be to decide the frequency rate of the reaction and its acceptability in exchange for the benefits of the drug. If the undesirable event is clinically rare, such as phocomelia or retrolental fibroplasia, a sudden increase in its usual frequency may suffice to trigger our suspicions that something unsatisfactory is happening.

If the undesirable event, however, is a relatively frequent clinical occurrence—such as cataracts, jaundice, peptic ulcer, or thrombophlebitis—doctors may not be ready at first to suspect that the event is an adverse drug reaction. The event may be initially ascribed to the main condition under treatment or to a co-morbid condition, rather than to a pharmaceutical reaction. Lasagna[29] has described a series of situations—including the bleeding associated with aspirin—in which adverse drug effects remained unrecognized for a long time.

Neither the trohoc nor the registry procedures can be used to generate such signals. Trohoc studies begin only after a suspicion exists; they are intended to explore the intensity of the possible causal relationship, not to signal a suspicion. Studies of registry data begin with data that were submitted by doctors whose suspicions have already been aroused and who have already made causal decisions.

Secular mortality associations can suggest that an undesirable event is happening, but can not *per se* signal that a particular drug (or class of drugs) is involved. Consequently, the principal method of generating cause signals for a particular drug is with cohort procedures that compare the events occurring in the drug-treated group and in a control group.

2. Causes. After a signal of suspicion has been raised, the next step may be to decide whether the drug can be held causally responsible for the associated event. If the indictment was based on cohort data, the available evidence may be suitable not only for suspecting an association but also for suggesting that the association is causal. Quite often, however, the cohort data may be both retrolective and unquantified, based on clinical hunches and recollections that are quite satisfactory for arousing suspicions, but inadequate for providing proof. The investigators may then look for more cogent evidence elsewhere.

Since conclusions about a causal relationship have been drawn before a registry report is submitted, the data of a registry cannot be used for assessing causal relationships. The epidemiologic pursuit of causal investigations must therefore depend on the use of cohorts, event trohocs, or secular mortality associations. The secular associations are the scientifically weakest[5] of these activities, containing many uncertain elements that may produce misleading or distorted results. Event-trohoc studies are also scientifically weak[12] but can be strengthened when special precautions (which are seldom employed) are taken to eliminate or adjust for major sources of potential bias. Prolective cohort studies, although the most powerful of the scientific approaches, are often difficult (or extremely expensive) to conduct in suitable populations.

A well designed project using a retrolective cohort is a potentially effective although often overlooked research strategy for these goals. For example, the many trohoc investigations performed to study association between oral contraceptive pills and thrombophlebitis could also have been done—with probably no more effort or cost—as studies on retrolective cohorts, appropriately chosen from practicing physicians' rosters of patients receiving different forms of contraception. The potential bias involved in the non-random assignment of therapy for the cohorts could probably be identified and adjusted more readily than the analogous and additional forms of bias that are present in trohoc research.[12]

Nevertheless, the epidemiologic data routinely collected by practicing physicians (inside or outside of academia) are usually rejected as potential sources of valuable research information. A retrolective cohort can yield data about the same kind of population, followed in the same clinical and chronologic direction, as a prolective cohort.[11] Because the data are not collected with the defined scientific standards that are possible in prolective research, however, the use of retrolective cohorts is usually spurned in favor of the standardized information available from the inverted logic of trohoc research.[12] The resolution of this issue depends on an important point in the philosophic orientation of science: do we want an imprecise answer to the right question or a precise answer to the wrong question?

3. Rate signals. If the "adverse reactions" have been thoroughly and reliably diagnosed, the techniques used with registry data—examining secular trends, drug trohocs, and accrual rates—can provide useful signals of changes in the incidence rate of reactions. The true rates, of course, cannot be determined from registry data, but could be approximated by the previously described technique of cohort estimation. (Another valuable source of rate signals is the adverse reaction case reports assembled by the manufacturers of the drug. These reports can be used in a manner analogous to that of registry data.) Event trohocs are used to explore cause, rather than rates of incidence; and secular mortality associations provide data about rates of death per disease, not rates of adverse reaction per drug. The prolective surveillance of a cohort would obviously provide signals about a change in rate; but retrolective cohort studies would usually not begin until a change in rate has been signalled by other sources of data.

4. Rates. Regardless of whether or not a rate signal has been received, the only way of determining the incidence rate of adverse drug reactions is to study a cohort of people receiving the drug. None of the registry procedures, secular associations, or trohoc investigations can provide an incidence rate. Even when the frequency of reactions is acquired from registry data or when a "risk ratio" has been calculated in trohoc research, the conversion of the results to an approximation of incidence has required an estimation of the size of the exposed cohort, using data from sales curves of the drugs or other suitable sources.

G. The goals of surveillance

After wading through the diverse terms, concepts, and tactics of the preceding two sections, the reader is probably ready to return to the main issue. Here, too, however, we encounter another scientific strategy that has been imprecisely specified. What is the purpose of pharmaceutical surveillance? Is it intended to provide an "early warning system" or a set of clinical guidelines for use of the drug?

1. Early warning system. Almost everyone would agree that a prime goal of surveillance is to provide early warning about a dangerous drug. In designing a system of surveillance, however, we would have to know what kind of danger. We would obviously want to be warned about clinical catastrophes, such as death, phocomelia, or retrolental fibroplasia. Do we also want to know, however, about less catastrophic events? What about clinical nuisances, such as transient skin rashes or reversible jaundice? And what about paraclinical abnormalities—such as elevations and depressions of white blood count, serum calcium, or blood urea nitrogen—that have no overt manifestations in clinical signs or symptoms?

To construct a system of surveillance, we would need to know whether it is supposed to detect the first, the first two, or all three of these dangers. The techniques of observation, the population to be observed, and the data to be acquired will obviously depend on what we want to accomplish. Nevertheless, these distinctions are seldom specified in discussions of surveillance. Several years ago, for example, when a federal agency asked for bids on a contract to provide "surveillance," the instructions to the potential bidders contained no statements about which goals, if any, were to be covered in the proposal.

Because the general methodologic problems are so enormous, a successful approach to surveillance might begin by detecting clinical catastrophes. If an effective system can be constructed for providing an early warning about catastrophes, the system might later be amplified to include clinical nuisances and paraclinical abnormalities.

2. Clinical guidance. A quite different approach to the surveillance issue is to view the process not as a warning system but as an evaluation system. The objective is to find out not merely what is bad but also what is good about a drug.

The clinical trials that were done before the drug was approved for marketing will have provided preliminary evidence about its usage and consequences. This information will pertain, however, only to the cohorts of patients and dosages of drug that were studied in the trials. When the drug enters the general market, it will be used in a greatly expanded spectrum of people, clinical states, and durations. The purpose of the surveillance would be to cover the new spectrum of anticipated or unanticipated benefits and the new spectrum of adverse effects. With this information available, we could compare the qualitative characteristics and quantitative frequencies of the events that occur in the spectrum of risks and benefits. This type of comparison would allow us to assess the "risk/benefit ratio" that is so frequently discussed but so seldom documented or quantified.

What emerges would presumably be a balanced evaluation of the drug, providing effective guidance for its future clinical usage. This is the kind of clinical guidance that has been informally (and often anecdotally) developed after many years of pragmatic experience with such drugs as aspirin, digitalis, and insulin. The purpose of a formal surveillance system for new (or old) drugs would be to attain the guidance information more promptly, effectively, and quantitatively than might be done if we waited for the appropriate "distillation" of clinical experience alone.

H. Evaluation of epidemiologic strategies

Having contemplated the available epidemiologic methods and having noted the desired goals, we can now begin to evaluate the respective merits of different methods for different goals.

One point about the methods should be noted immediately: in order for any method to work, it must be made to work. Whatever be the procedure used for surveillance, the procedure itself must receive surveillance (or monitoring) to ensure that its planned activities are being carried out. The supervisors of a cohort surveillance system must check that all appropriate members of the cohort are entered into it and that the necessary data are being collected. The supervisors of a registry of adverse reactions must encourage the submission of reports by any physician who observes a reportable reaction. Furthermore, with either a cohort or a registry system, none of the available "signals" will be detected unless the collected data are frequently analyzed in search of signals.

As we consider the two main goals of pharmaceutical surveillance, however, certain procedural methods may seem preferable to others.

1. Early warning system. In an early warning system for clinical catastrophes, we would want to be sure that all possible uses of the drug (and all of the possible reactions to it) have the opportunity to enter the system. This desideratum cannot be achieved with the restricted focus of an institution-based procedure. An institutional surveillance system is confined to the cohort of people treated at the institution. In technologic operation, the system may attain statistical magnificence by acquiring numerator and denominator data, coding standardized forms, and applying computerized analyses; but the institutional system can not be relied upon to observe the totality of drug usage and reactions that can provide early warnings about clinical catastrophes.

For example, ambulatory pregnant women taking thalidomide would not have been part of a hospitalized cohort and thalidomide might not have been part of the pharmacopoeia used in a large outpatient clinic. Consequently, the phocomelia that followed thalidomide might not have been detected by institution-based prolective procedures. (The thalidomide disaster was actually detected by analysis of retrolective and estimated cohorts.[30, 32, 36])

If we want to learn about any clinical catastrophe that may occur in a person using a drug, we cannot limit our surveillance to the enumerated group of people who are followed in a cohort. A catastrophic event can occur in anyone who receives the drug, and the event must have a good chance of being reported. For this reason, the best way of routinely getting warnings about catastrophes that can emerge from the entire group of drug users is to collect adverse reaction reports in a registry maintained either by the manufacturer or by some other governmental or medical organization. The registry technique becomes desirable here for the very reason that makes it epidemiologically unappealing: there are no defined populations to constrain the denominators. By placing no restrictions on the denominator, i.e., by not demarcating an observed cohort, the registry allows a "total sampling," because anyone receiving the drug has an opportunity to be included when an adverse

reaction occurs. With improvements in the thoroughness of reporting and with greater care in analyzing the cited adverse reactions, the case report procedure can provide a satisfactory and relatively inexpensive approach to the goal of an early warning system.

The fundamental problem in relying on case report data in a registry is the thoroughness of reporting. This problem can be solved or minimized if the act of reporting is made especially easy with such procedures as a toll-free telephone call to the collecting agency, by total reassurance to reporting physicians that the information will be kept suitably confidential, and by encouraging physicians to trust the motives of the collecting agency. Thus, if practicing physicians (for whatever reason) develop apathy, hostility, or distrust toward federal agencies, the likelihood of an agency's receiving case reports will be reduced, and its registry data may be too incomplete to be valuable.

An additional problem in relying on registry data is the vigilance with which the data are scrutinized and analyzed. For an early warning signal to be noted, someone must be constantly looking out for it. Certain aspects of this watchman role may be better fulfilled by a "commercial" registry, maintained by the manufacturer of the drug, than by a "non-commercial" registry maintained by a national or international health agency. For example, the first public warning about thalidomide in the U.K. was issued not by a "non-commercial" registry, but by the drug's manufacturer, who announced its withdrawal from the market two weeks *before* any adverse reactions had been reported in the English language literature.[32] Had the "commercial" registries been even more vigilant on the European continent and in the U.K., the thalidomide catastrophe might have been noted sooner and its magnitude reduced.

Since a drug's manufacturer can be (and has been) held financially liable for compensating the victims, the manufacturer would be expected to exert a concerned self-interest in maintaining registries that can promptly detect overtly dangerous drugs before the consequences become fiscally as well as clinically catastrophic. While supplementing the manufacturer's vigilance for clinical disasters, the non-commercial registries can also be expected to provide signals, of the type noted earlier, about less dramatic clinical reactions that a manufacturer might not avidly scrutinize.

Another way of getting warnings about major clinical nuisances is through an institutional surveillance system. The extensive data assembled and analyzed in such a system could provide cause signals and other evidence for detecting non-dramatic reactions that might otherwise be overlooked. The main difficulty in using current surveillance systems for this purpose is the clinical imprecision with which the drug recipients and reactions have been identified. In many analyses, the reactions and drugs have been associated without further subdivision according to the clinical distinctions of the patients and conditions.

For example, in surveillance studies suggesting adverse cardiac effects of amitriptyline,[3, 34] no analyses were done to indicate whether the amitriptyline-treated patients and the "controls" received the drug for the same clinical indication; and whether the compared groups were similar in the prognostic severity of their baseline cardiac condition. In order for causal indictments to be convincing, the patients receiving the compared treatments must be shown to have comparable clinical conditions at baseline. With improvements in clinical specification and comparison, the institutional surveillance systems can make invaluable contributions to the screening process that provides "early warning" of clinical nuisances and laboratory abnormalities.

An alternative to the case report system or the institutional cohort is the use of *representative* cohorts as described in the next section. Such a procedure is probably too expensive to be used only for delivering early warnings. Furthermore, the size of the followed cohorts would have to be enormous to allow surveillance of ample numbers of patients with each type of clinical condition, treated with each corresponding pharmaceutical agent.

2. Clinical guidance. An adequate early warning system could be attained with the methods that have just been described, but a clinical guidance system creates a quite different challenge. As noted earlier, we would want to learn all about the clinical usage of the drug—its good effects as well as its bad ones. For thorough evaluation of the total spectrum and frequencies of both risks and benefits, we would have to investigate a prolective cohort. We could not use registries, trohocs, or secular mortality tactics because they do not include the appropriate population or data. A retrolective cohort technique would be also unsatisfactory because the patients' original medical records may not contain all the information needed to document the diverse facets of risk and benefit. Since a prolective cohort study is the only method of getting scientifically precise data about clinical usage of a drug, the main issue in research architecture is the choice of the cohort. What people are to be examined and how are they to be chosen?

The most straightforward answer to this question is to take a random sample of users of the drug. The procedure can be arranged by following the fate of a randomly selected fraction of batches of the drug prepared by the manufacturer. Alternatively, a random sample of pharmacists can be enlisted as a collaborating research team. The cohort of patients can then be chosen as a random sample of the people to whom the pharmacists dispense the drug. This type of "drug-cohort" investigation would not be easy to perform. It would require the creation of new types of research teams, working outside of institutional settings and enlisting suitable cooperation from manufacturers, pharmacists, physicians, and patients. Despite the obvious problems, such research may not be too difficult to do if the participants are properly approached. Pharmacists, practicing physicians, and their patients may welcome the opportunity to contribute to research surveys that are neither experimental nor esoteric, and that can provide better therapeutic knowledge for everyone.

The main disadvantage of studying such a drug cohort is that we would lack a control group. No analogous information would be available for the outcome of people with similar clinical conditions that were treated in some other way. To complete the picture, therefore, we would need to perform a separate investigation. For this purpose, we would want to take a random sample of practicing physicians from whom we could get suitable data about the selected clinical conditions and their post-therapeutic outcomes. Here, too, the performance of the research would entail many logistic difficulties, but the difficulties may become minor if medical societies enthusiastically endorse the plans and if practicing physicians accept the opportunity to work in a new form of clinical investigation that arises not from isolated academic or federal cloisters, but from the real world of medical care.

With these two representative samples of drug users and patient conditions, we could cover the necessary spectrum of pharmaceutical and clinical phenomena. The methods of implementing the basic design are beyond the scope of this discussion. The main point is that if we want a surveillance system to provide effective clinical guidance about the use of drugs, the job will not be easy. We shall have to study what is valid rather than what is convenient, and we shall have to develop an appropriate coterie of investigative personnel rather than to rely merely on restricted applications of institutional technology. This new challenge in clinical epidemiology would allow the people who are most involved in the use of drugs—manufacturers, pharmacists, practicing physicians, and patients—to become collaborating investigators who help solve the problems that the drugs create. The questions that originate in the extensive world of medical care would be answered not from data assembled by armchair epidemiologists or institution-bound academicians, but

from accounts of the events that actually occur in that world, as witnessed by representative members of the people who live in it.

Regardless of whether pharmaceutical surveillance is intended to provide early warnings or clinical guidance, we shall have to give more attention to the patient who gets the drug than to the technology of the surveillance or the manipulation of the statistics. The technology and the statistics are already well developed. What still remains as undeveloped scientific territory is the basic identification of an adverse reaction and of the clinical complexity that surrounds it.

References

1. Borda, I., Jick, H., Stone, D., Dinan, B., Gilman, B., and Chalmers, T. C.: Studies of drug usage in five Boston hospitals, J. A. M. A. **202:**506-510, 1967.
2. Boston Collaborative Drug Surveillance Program: Interaction between chloral hydrate and warfarin, N. Engl. J. Med. **286:**53-55, 1972.
3. Boston Collaborative Drug Surveillance Program: Adverse reactions to the tricyclic-antidepressant drugs, Lancet **1:**529-531, 1972.
4. Boston Collaborative Drug Surveillance Program: Decreased clinical efficacy of propoxyphene in cigarette smokers, CLIN. PHARMACOL. THER. **14:**259-263, 1973.
5. Bradford Hill, A.: Principles of medical statistics, ed. 9, New York, 1971, Oxford University Press.
6. Cluff, L. E., Thornton, G. F., and Seidl, L. G.: Studies on the epidemiology of adverse drug reactions. I. Methods of surveillance, J. A. M. A. **188:**976-983, 1964.
7. Dawber, T. R., Kannel, W. B., and Gordon, T: Coffee and coronary heart disease, Am. J. Cardiol. **33:**133, 1974. (Abst.)
8. DeNosaquo, N.: The registry on adverse reactions of the American Medical Association, Methods Inf. Med. **4:**15-21, 1965.
9. Editorial: Reporting of adverse reactions to drugs, Can. Med. Assoc. J. **92:**476-477, 1965.
10. Feinstein, A. R.: Clinical biostatistics. IX. How do we measure "safety and efficacy"? CLIN. PHARMACOL. THER. **12:**544-558, 1971.
11. Feinstein, A. R.: Clinical biostatistics. XI. Sources of 'chronology bias' in cohort statistics, CLIN. PHARMACOL. THER. **12:**864-879, 1971.
12. Feinstein, A. R.: Clinical biostatistics. XX. The epidemiologic trohoc, the ablative risk

ratio, and 'retrospective' research, CLIN. PHAR-MACOL. THER. **14**:291-307, 1973.

13. Feinstein, A. R.: An analysis of diagnostic reasoning. III. The construction of clinical algorithms, Yale J. Biol. Med. **47**:5-32, 1974.

14. Finney, D. J.: The design and logic of a monitor of drug use, J. Chronic Dis. **18**:77-98, 1965.

15. Finney, D. J.: Systematic signalling of adverse reactions to drugs, Methods Inf. Med. **13**:1-10, 1974.

16. Friedman, G. D., Collen, M. F., Harris, L. E., Van Brunt, E. E., and Davis, L S.: Experience in monitoring drug reactions in outpatients. The Kaiser-Permanente Drug Monitoring System, J. A. M. A. **217**:567-572, 1971.

17. Gardner, P., and Watson, L. J.: Adverse drug reactions: A pharmacist-based monitoring system, CLIN. PHARMACOL. THER. **11**:802-807, 1970.

18. Gray, T. K., Adams, L. L., and Fallon, H. J.: Short-term intense surveillance of adverse drug reactions, J. Clin. Pharmacol. **13**:61-67, 1973.

19. Herbst, A. L., Ulfelder, H., and Poskanzer, D. C.: Adenocarcinoma of the vagina. Association of maternal stilbestrol therapy with tumor appearance in young women, N. Engl. J. Med. **284**:878-881, 1971.

20. Hurwitz, N., and Wade, O. L.: Intensive hospital monitoring of adverse reactions to drugs, Br. Med. J. **1**:531-536, 1969.

21. Inman, W. H. W., and Adelstein, A. M.: Rise and fall of asthma mortality in England and Wales in relation to use of pressurized aerosols, Lancet **2**:279-285, 1969.

22. Inman, W. H. W., and Vessey, M. P.: Investigation of deaths from pulmonary, coronary, and cerebral thrombosis, and embolism in women of child-bearing age, Br. Med. J. **2**:193-199, 1968.

23. Irey, N. S.: Diagnostic problems and methods in drug-induced diseases. Parts I, II, and III, Washington, D. C., 1966, 1967, and 1968, respectively, American Registry of Pathology, Armed Forces Institute of Pathology.

24. Jick, H., Slone, D., Borda, I. T., and Shapiro, S.: Efficacy and toxicity of heparin in relation to age and sex, N. Engl. J. Med. **279**:284-286, 1968.

25. Jick, H., Miettinen, O. S., Shapiro, S., Lewis, G. P., Siskind, V., and Slone, D.: Comprehensive drug surveillance, J. A. M. A. **213**:1455-1460, 1970.

26. Jick, H., Slone, D., Shapiro, S., Lewis, G. P., and Siskind, V.: A new method for assessing the clinical effects of oral analgesic drugs, CLIN. PHARMACOL. THER. **12**:456-463, 1971.

27. Jick, H., Miettinen, O. S., Neff, R. K., Shapiro, S., Heinonen, O. P., and Slone, D.: Coffee and myocardial infarction. A report from the Boston Collaborative Drug Surveillance Pro-

gram, Boston University Medical Center, N. Engl. J. Med. **289**:63-67, 1973.

28. Koch-Weser, J., Sidel, V. W., Sweet, R. H., Kanarek, P., and Eaton, A. E.: Factors determining physician reporting of adverse drug reactions, N. Engl. J. Med. **280**:20-26, 1969.

29. Lasagna, L.: The diseases drugs cause, Perspect. Biol. Med. **7**:457-470, 1964.

30. Lenz, W.: Thalidomide and congenital abnormalities, Lancet **1**:45, 1962.

31. McDonald, M. G., and MacKay, B. R.: Adverse drug reactions. Experience of Mary Fletcher hospital during 1962, J. A. M. A. **190**:1071-1074, 1964.

32. McBride, W. G.: Thalidomide and congenital abnormalities, Lancet **2**:1358, 1961.

33. Melmon, K. L.: Preventable drug reactions—causes and cures, N. Engl. J. Med. **284**:1361-1368, 1971.

34. Moir, D. C., Crooks, J., Cornwell, W. B., O'Malley, K., Dingwall-Fordyce, I., Turnbull, M. J., and Weir, R. D.: Cardiotoxicity of amitriptyline, Lancet **2**:561-564, 1972.

35. Ogilvie, R. I., and Ruedy, J.: Adverse drug reactions during hospitalization, Canad. Med. Assoc. J. **97**:1450-1457, 1967.

36. Pfeiffer, R. A., and Kosenow, W.: Thalidomide and congenital abnormalities, Lancet **1**:45-46, 1962.

37. Reidenberg, M. M.: Registry of adverse drug reactions, J. A. M. A. **203**:31-34, 1968.

38. Royall, B. W.: Monitoring adverse reactions to drugs. WHO Chronicle, **27**:469-475, 1973.

39. Sartwell, P. E., Masi, A. T., Arthes, F. G., Greene, G. R., and Smith, H. E.: Thromboembolism and oral contraceptives: An epidemiologic case-control study, Am. J. Epidemiol. **90**:365-380, 1969.

40. Slone, D., Jick, H., Borda, I., Chalmers, T. C., Feinleib, M., Muench, H., Lipworth, L., Bellotti, C., and Gilman, B.: Drug surveillance utilizing nurse monitors, Lancet **2**:901-903, 1966.

41. Smidt, N. A., and McQueen, E. G.: Adverse reactions to drugs: A comprehensive hospital inpatient survey, N. Z. Med. J. **76**:397-401, 1972.

42. Vessey, M. P., and Doll, R.: Investigation of relation between use of oral contraceptives and thromboembolic disease, Br. Med. J. **2**:199-205, 1968.

43. Weston, J. K.: The present status of adverse drug reaction reporting, J. A. M. A. **203**:35-37, 1968.

44. Wintrobe, M. M.: The therapeutic millennium and its price: Adverse reactions to drug, *in* Talalay, P.: Drugs in our society. Based on a conference sponsored by The Johns Hopkins University, Baltimore, 1964, The Johns Hopkins Press.

MATHEMATICAL MYSTIQUES AND STATISTICAL STRATEGIES

Mathematical theories often produce fears or fascinations that divert medical readers and investigators from the many scientific problems discussed in the previous three sections. Readers who get flustered by parametric estimators, pooled variances, α levels, standard errors, confidence intervals, regression coefficients, β errors, and logistic transformations may be too confused to look behind the statistical facades and scrutinize the quality of the scientific architecture and data. Alternatively, after becoming infatuated by the idea that statistical methods are panaceas for the intellectual ailments of research, investigators may neglect basic scientific challenges in structure, bias, or data and may assume that any problems will be solved by multiple regressions, discriminant functions, analysis of covariance, or partitionings of chi-square.

These inappropriate attitudes about the power of statistical techniques are often encouraged by the way the techniques are taught. They may be presented for investigators as a set of "cookbook" instructions to be followed obediently, even if the "cook" has no idea of what is being done or why. For statisticians, the presentation may receive so inherently mathematical a focus that the cook becomes a connoisseur of ovens, stoves, and kitchen maneuvers, while remaining oblivious to the fundamental culinary objectives in texture, flavor, and taste.

The four essays in this section are concerned with basic statistical ideas that have been confusing, distracting, or scientifically hazardous for both investigators and statisticians. The first set of ideas is concerned with the major scientific distinctions between estimating a parameter and contrasting a difference. In most tests of "statistical significance," the investigator evaluates the likelihood that chance is responsible for the difference found when *two groups* are contrasted. The t-test, chi-square, and other conventional procedures used for this purpose are derived from mathematical theories that were developed for a different purpose: to estimate a parameter for a *single group*. The conversion from a one-group estimation to a two-group contrast was desirable because it offered major advantages in computation, but it has made the statistical process indirect, convoluted, and hard to understand. With the ease of computation that is offered by modern electronics, investigators may prefer to use an alternative method: the permutation tests that are direct, straightforward, and easy to understand.

The second essay deals with problems in the mathematical duplexity of certain directions—the "one-way" dependence or "two-way" interdependence of a relationship—and the choice of a unilateral or bilateral zone of probability for "rejection" of the celebrated null hypothesis. The third essay is devoted to an issue that is seldom considered in conventional instruction. The decision that a difference is "statistically significant" is somewhat like making a positive diagnosis, and the P value or probability zone established as an α level denotes the possibility that the diagnosis is falsely positive. If the difference is regarded as *not* statistically significant, however, the investigator takes the chance of making a false negative diagnosis. This latter problem, which rarely receives adequate attention when investigators study statistics, involves the contemplation of β levels and a different type of P value. The α and β levels of probability are the bases for a statistically popular indoor sport: the calculation of sample size in a research project.

The fourth essay contains a catalog of defects in the way investigators employ statistical tactics to summarize or display the data reported in scientific literature. The standard error is regularly used improperly in two ways: either instead of a standard deviation to show the spread of data or instead of a confidence interval to show the estimated zone of location for the mean. A ± sign frequently appears between a mean and a standard something, but the *something* is not identified. The graphical portrait that is needed to illustrate the relationship of two variables is often omitted and, instead, the results are summarized inefficiently or misleadingly with correlation coefficients or regression coefficients. Finally, and perhaps worst of all, the only reported results may be the statistical calculations for P values or F values; and the actual data may be neither presented nor summarized.

CHAPTER 20

Permutation tests and 'statistical significance'

The previous paper[13] in this series was concerned with the advantages and pitfalls of using a randomization process in sampling from a parent population. By depending on chance alone, the randomized selection removes any element of human choice in the sample, and allows the results to be interpreted with inferences based on statistical probability. These statistical inferences are particularly useful when the parent population is being sampled to estimate the value of an unknown parameter, such as the mean of a selected variable. From the results found in the random sample, the investigator can demarcate a zone of values, called a "confidence interval," and can have a specified "confidence level" for the probability that the true value of the parameter lies within the demarcated zone. The main pitfall of random sampling is that it does not indicate the reliability of the particular sample that was selected in the research. The randomization process provides no safeguards against the 5% of chance occasions in which a 95% confidence interval will be erroneous because

the "luck of the draw" produced a substantially distorted sample.

An antidote for this hazard is stratification. If cogent subgroups (or strata) can be defined beforehand, the members of the sample are selected randomly from within each stratum. If this type of pre-stratification is not feasible, the sample is drawn with a non-specific randomization, the cogent strata are demarcated afterward, and the data are analyzed within strata. The results found in the individual strata can then, if desired, receive a "standardized adjustment" to create a single value that estimates the desired parameter appropriately for the entire parent population.

As noted previously,[9-11, 13] the selection of cogent strata and the analysis of potential bias are crucial scientific requirements that have seldom been adequately fulfilled in modern clinical and epidemiologic research. The requirement is particularly necessary in these forms of research because the groups of people under investigation have almost never been assembled by random sampling. Almost all of the existing surveys of the causes, occurrence, and treatment of disease, and all of the existing experimental trials of therapy, have been based on groups that were not

This chapter originally appeared as "Clinical biostatistics—XXIII. The role of randomization in sampling, testing, allocation, and credulous idolatry (Part 2)." In Clin. Pharmacol. Ther. 14:898, 1973.

chosen randomly. The groups have consisted of people conveniently available to the investigators at such locations as hospitals, industrial plants, physicians' registries, schools, etc.

A. The two main uses of statistical inference

The discovery that medical researchers seldom use random samples often comes as a surprising shock to investigators who work in other domains. With inanimate materials, chemists achieve random samples routinely and easily as an aliquot of a homogeneous mass. With general human populations, social and political scientists give careful attention to methods of sampling and getting random selections. With medical populations, however, the investigative samples are almost never random. Why are medical researchers so delinquent?

The answer to this question is based on the two different purposes of statistical inference. A socio-political scientist often wants to estimate a populational parameter, whereas a medical investigator usually wants to contrast a difference in two groups. A random sample is mandatory for estimating a parameter, but has not been regarded as equally imperative for contrasting a difference.

1. *Estimation of parameters.* In polling political beliefs, our main concern is to get an estimate of the quantitative partition of public opinion. There is no contrast of any imposed experimental or control maneuvers. We simply want to find out what the people think politically, and we want to know how accurately the sample reflects the views of the public at large. We therefore want to estimate the values and confidence intervals of populational parameters. A random sample being crucial for these activities, a political scientist pays close attention to getting a suitable collection of people for the survey.

2. *Numerical evaluation of an analytic contrast.* The estimation of a populational parameter is not a major goal of most forms of clinical and epidemiologic research. The investigator usually wants to compare the effects of different maneuvers in the groups under study—the results noted in the exposed vs. non-exposed people, or in "case-control" vs. diseased, or in "treated" vs. "untreated." He is seldom interested in populational parameters or their confidence intervals. He wants to know whether the magnitude of the difference observed in the results of a particular set of data is more than can readily be expected from numerical chance alone.

The contrast of the numerical difference associated with different maneuvers is a fundamental purpose in many research activities, and is the primary objective of most clinical and epidemiologic investigations. This goal does not appear to be well understood, however, by some of the leading statisticians of our era. For example, so excellent a statistician as G. W. Snedecor[30] has stated that "the purpose of an experiment is to produce a sample of observations which will furnish estimates of the parameters of the population together with measures of the uncertainty of these estimates." This misconception of medical research is relatively widespread among statisticians, and may be responsible for some of their many current problems as consultants in biomedical investigation.[5, 6, 21, 31, 39]

For analytic contrast, an investigator seldom cares about estimating the parameter of some unexamined theoretical parent population, and seldom wants to measure the uncertainties expressed with such calculations as "standard error of the mean." He has performed a single act of research on a single collection of people, who were divided into two groups. He has noted a difference in the numerical data for the contrasted groups, and he wants to know whether this numerical difference might arise by chance alone.

Suppose an investigator has reported success rates of 75% in a treated group and 25% in a control group. Before drawing any further conclusions, we immediately want to know whether enough people were included in the research. Is the striking difference of 50% in the two success rates likely to have arisen by chance? If each treated group contained only four patients, so that the 75% and 25% values were obtained from the numbers 3/4 and 1/4, we would immediately suspect that the 50% difference could be a fortuitous occurrence. With only four people in each group, the difference is not convincing. On the other hand, if each group contained 200 people, so that the comparison of 75% vs. 25% was based on the numbers 150/200 vs. 50/200, we would feel reasonably sure that the 50% difference was not a happenstance numerical event.

Regardless of whether or not the 50% difference is "statistically significant," the results could not be extrapolated or even regarded as valid until we had given paramount consideration to the scientific architecture of the research. Were the two groups prognostically comparable before treatment? Were the treatments allocated without bias? Were the two compared treatments carried out with equal skill by the physicians and with equal compliance by the patients? What were the criteria for "success," and was it observed and detected without bias? Unless we were assured of propriety in these aspects of scientific method, we might reject any further attention to the data. Assuming that the research was properly done, however, we can evaluate the numerical difference as a separate statistical question. For this decision, we are interested merely in the statistical aspects of the numbers. We want to know what role chance might have played in the numerical distinctions. The design of the research is a quite different issue, to be pondered with quite different analytic criteria. The statistical issue deals with fortuitous possibilities in the pattern of numerical alternatives.

For the two cited instances (3/4 vs. 1/4 and 150/200 vs. 50/200), each with a 50% difference in the contrasted rates, the pos-

sible numerical alternatives that chance might provide seemed quite obvious by what Mainland[22] has called the "eye test." We could draw a reasonable conclusion by just looking at the data. The decision would be more difficult if the 75% and 25% came from such numbers as 9/12 vs. 5/20, or 3/4 vs. 10/40. For these and for the many other contrasts whose numerical distinctions cannot be immediately judged with an "eye test," we want some cerebral mechanisms to supplement the ocular perceptions. One major purpose of statistical theory is to provide those cerebral mechanisms. The mechanisms consist of procedures for testing "statistical significance." The rest of this discussion is concerned with the role of randomization in those tests.

3. **The fundamental reasoning in a numerical contrast.** To contemplate a numerical difference between two groups, the investigator would reason as follows. Suppose the two modes of treatment have identical effects. (Statisticians call this supposition the "null hypothesis"). According to this hypothesis, there would be no difference in the treatments and the two groups of patients should have had similar responses, but certain differences could have arisen by chance simply from the way the patients were originally divided to form the two groups. The investigator would therefore consider what might have happened to the data if the patients had been divided by chance some other way, but if each patient still had the same result. How great a difference would have been noted in the two groups?

As the investigator begins to recognize alternative patterns of arrangement for his two groups of patients, he becomes ready to consider all the possible ways in which the two groups might have been formed from the available set of patients. He can then contemplate the difference in results that would occur with each arrangement, and the frequency with which the individual differences are "exceptional" —equaling or exceeding the difference that was actually observed in the research. If these theoretical "exceptions" occur often enough, the investigator would conclude that the observed difference may well be due to chance. If the exceptions are sufficiently infrequent, he would decide that the observed difference is unlikely to be a chance event, and he would reject the "null hypothesis," concluding that the two treatments gave "significantly" different results.

In order to pursue this strategy of reasoning, the investigator must make an arbitrary choice about how infrequently an event can occur to be regarded as *sufficiently infrequent*. The traditional decision is to set this infrequency at either 1 in 20 or 1 in 100. The selected value of 0.05 or 0.01 (or some other choice) is then called the α level of probability. With α chosen, the relative frequency of the exceptional results, which is called a P value, is noted. If P is equal to or smaller than α, the observed difference will be regarded as uncommon enough to be called "statistically significant."

We have now taken care of almost all the necessary reasoning and judgments, but one crucial decision still remains. How do we go about contemplating the pattern of all the possible arrangements of the observed data in the two groups? The answer to this question will determine the particular test that is chosen and the way the test is interpreted.

B. The statistical approach to "significance"

The most fashionable current statistical methods for examining the possible patterns of the data depend on an intellectual ritual that is more than 60 years old. In this ritual, the investigator does not actually examine the possible patterns of the data. Instead, he substitutes certain theoretical patterns and principles, described in the sections that follow.

1. *Statistical principles.* The most popular statistical tests of "significance" are the t test and chi-square. Despite the common application of these tests in scientific research, very few investigators are aware of the underlying doctrines with which the tests are constructed and used.

The basic concept is the idea of a sampling distribution for a test statistic. The *test statistic* is created from the results observed in the research. For the t test, the test statistic is calculated as $t = (\bar{x}_A - \bar{x}_B)/SE$. In this formula, $\bar{x}_A$ and $\bar{x}_B$ are the means of the two compared groups, A and B. SE is a quantity, discussed later, that estimates the "standard error" of the difference in these means. For the chi-square test, the test statistic is calculated as $X^2 = \Sigma[(o_i - e_i)^2/e_i]$. In this formula, o_i and e_i are, respectively, the observed and expected values of each distinct subgroup, i, whose attributes were counted.

The test statistic is interpreted according to the following theory. If we repeatedly drew random samples from a parent population (replacing each sample afterward), and if we calculated the value of the test statistic for each sample, the different values would appear with different frequencies. The proportionate occurrence of those frequencies, when plotted against the various individual values of the test statistic, would form a curve called a *sampling distribution*. For an infinite number of samplings, the curve would be a smooth "probability density" for the selected test statistic. (The familiar bell-shaped Gaussian curve is the pattern of one type of probability density.)

Each particular test statistic has its own pattern of sampling distribution. The curve need not be determined empirically from infinite sampling and can be constructed, instead, on the basis of a complex equation, derived from statistical theory. (If the test statistic requires a consideration of "degrees of freedom," the sampling distribution contains a family of curves—one for each value in the array of degrees of freedom.)

The sampling distribution for the t statistic is called a t distribution and was discovered by W. S. Gosset,[32] writing pseudonymously as "Student." The sampling distribution for the X^2 statistic is almost always related to a chi-square distribution, which was popularized by K. Pearson[27] but actually discovered much earlier.[20, 26] Because the X^2 statistic is almost never considered apart from the associated χ^2 distribution, most investigators omit the distinction between X^2 and χ^2, and refer to both the test statistic and its sampling distribution as χ^2. I shall continue that tradition here, and use χ^2 rather than X^2 in the rest of this discussion.

Once the curve of sampling distribution is available, it can be used to determine the probability of random occurrence for any noted value, v_o, of the test statistic. When an ordinate to the curve is erected at v_o, the area beneath the curve that lies beyond this ordinate will indicate the probability (P value) of randomly encountering a value of the test statistic that is "exceptional," i.e., as extreme or more extreme than v_o.

To avoid the nuisance of making graphic calculations of these areas, various tables have been constructed for each test statistic and its sampling distribution. These tables° show the P values associated with each value of the test statistic for different "degrees of freedom" (d.f.) in the sampling. Thus, at 29 d.f. and t = 0.854, the P value is 0.40; at 1 d.f. and χ^2 = 3.92, the P value is <0.05.

To test "significance" in a particular set of results, we would calculate the value of the test statistic for our observed data. We would find the associated P value in an appropriate table. We would then accept or reject the null hypothesis according to whether or not this P value exceeds the chosen level of α. If α was set at 0.05 and if P turns out to be < 0.05, we would reject the null hypothesis and proclaim the results to be "statistically significant."

2. Statistical assumptions. In order to use the principles of probability that un-

derlie this sampling-distribution approach, we must make several important assumptions about the two groups of people whose results we wanted to compare:

a. We assume that the two groups were selected as random samples from the same parent population.

b. We assume that the treatments (or other distinguishing maneuvers) were allocated randomly to the members of the groups.

c. We assume that the target variable (i.e., the result) occurs with a specific type of frequency distribution in the parent population.

d. We assume, for the t test and for most applications of chi-square, that this distribution is Gaussian (or "normal").

e. For the t test, we assume that the variance found in the two samples is essentially similar.

When the null hypothesis is added to all these other assumptions, we then can estimate the theoretical frequency, or P value, with which the "exceptional" differences would occur. In actual practice, of course, none of these assumptions in steps a-e may be correct:

a. The groups studied in modern clinical or epidemiologic research are seldom selected as random samples.

b. For the many clinical and epidemiologic research projects that are performed as surveys, the maneuver under investigation was not assigned randomly. A random allocation of the maneuver can occur only in experimental clinical trials.

c. We almost never know the exact distribution of the target variable in the parent population.

d. In many of the groups studied in medical research, we know that the target variable does *not* have a Gaussian distribution, and often departs from it dramatically.

e. In many of the groups contrasted with a t test, we know that the variance of the two samples is *not* similar.

Nevertheless, despite all these violations of the basic theory for the test procedures,

---

°All values cited in this paper are from the tables contained in Documenta Geigy.[7]

they are constantly employed and accepted. Let us now consider how they are done.

3. *Performance of the tests.*

a. The t test. Suppose an investigator has two groups, each containing four people, treated with agents A and B respectively. The target variable has values of 20, 15, 12, and 6 units for the four people in Group A. The corresponding values in Group B are 7, 3, 2, and 1. The mean in Group A, $\bar{x}_A = 13.25$ units, seems substantially higher than the corresponding mean in Group B, $\bar{x}_B = 3.25$ units, and so we want to test for "statistical significance."

To do so, we can employ the t concept in two different ways. The method that is most popular among investigators is to calculate the value of the t statistic directly from the data, using the formula, $t = (\bar{x}_A - \bar{x}_B)/SE$.

We are now temporarily stymied by the fact that we do not know the value of SE, which is the standard error of the difference in the parametric means of the parent population. To get out of this dilemma, we estimate SE by introducing another new concept, called *pooled variance*, and denoted as s^2. For the observed two groups A and B, having the respective variances $s_A{}^2$ and $s_B{}^2$, the pooled variance can be calculated according to the formula:

$$s^2 = \frac{(n_A - 1)\, s_A{}^2 + (n_B - 1)\, s_B{}^2}{(n_A - 1 + n_B - 1)}$$

Since $(n_A - 1)s_A{}^2 = \Sigma x_A{}^2 - (\Sigma x_A)^2/n$, we perform the required calculation in Group A to get $(n_A - 1)s_A{}^2 = 805.00 - 702.25 = 102.75$. By an analogous calculation, we get $(n_B - 1)s_B{}^2 = 63.00 - 42.25 = 20.75$. Substituting back in the formula for s^2 gives us

$$s^2 = \frac{102.75 + 20.75}{3 + 3} = 20.5833$$

Now that we have the pooled variance, we can find the "standard error" of the difference between the two means, $\bar{x}_A$ and $\bar{x}_B$. The formula for this is

$$SE = \sqrt{s^2\left(\frac{1}{n_A} + \frac{1}{n_B}\right)}$$

Substituting in this formula, we get

$$SE = \sqrt{20.5833\left(\frac{1}{4} + \frac{1}{4}\right)} = 3.208$$

We now can insert the value of SE into the previous formula to get

$$t = (\bar{x}_A - \bar{x}_B)/SE = 10/3.208 = 3.117$$

At this point, we are ready to use a table to find the value of P associated with this value of t, but first we choose the interesting entity called "degrees of freedom." The rationale for this name and choice are too elaborate[35] for further discussion here. Let us accept the statistical doctrine that the value for the "degrees of freedom" in this test of two groups is $n_A - 1 + n_B - 1 = 6$. Accordingly, we would now look for the P value associated with a t of 3.117 at 6 degrees of freedom.

We still have yet another judgment to make, however. Although usually expressed in statistical phrases, the judgment is really a scientific decision. Do we want one-sided (or "one-tailed") versus two-sided (or "two-tailed") probability values for t? The scientific rationale for this decision was outlined earlier in this series[12] and will not be further considered here. To allow the discussion to proceed, let us look up the results for both decisions. We find, with the cited values, that the two-sided P value for the numerical contrast in our two groups is between 0.025 (where t is 2.969) and 0.02 (where t is 3.143). For a one-sided interpretation, these values would be halved, and P would be between 0.0125 and 0.01.

We now would conclude that our results are "statistically significant," since P is below the customary boundary of 0.05, regardless of whether we interpret the result as one- or two-sided.

A different way of using the t concept is to calculate a confidence interval around the observed difference in means. In this approach, which is often recommended by statisticians[25] but seldom used by investigators, an additional set of theoretical statistical principles is introduced with the following reasoning:

If we repeatedly drew an infinite array of samples for A and B from the parent population, and if we calculated the difference of the means $(\bar{x}_A - \bar{x}_B)$ for each sample, we would expect to get a Gaussian distribution for those differences. With the assumption of the null hypothesis, the true parametric means $(\mu_A$ and $\mu_B)$ for Groups A and B are regarded as equal, and so $\mu_A - \mu_B = 0$. Therefore, working at an α level of 0.05, we would expect the 95% confidence interval for $\bar{x}_A - \bar{x}_B$ to include the value of 0. If the calculated results for this confidence interval in our sample do not include the value of 0, we would reject the null hypothesis at the 0.05 level.

The confidence interval is calculated as $(\bar{x}_A - \bar{x}_B) \pm (t \times SE)$. To determine its size, we would begin by consulting an appropriate table to find the proper value of t. At a 95% confidence level and at 6 degrees of freedom, the t value associated with a P of 0.05 is 2.447. We now multiply this value of t times the standard error of 3.208 to get 7.85. Since 10 is the value of $|\bar{x}_A - \bar{x}_B|$, we add and subtract 7.85 to get a confidence interval range of 2.15 to 17.85. Since this interval does not include 0, we reject the null hypothesis and conclude that the observed difference in means is "statistically significant."

b. The chi-square test. The chi-square test would be applied for the type of "categorical" data obtained in the following situation: Suppose valid criteria have been established for determining post-therapeutic "success" or "failure," and suppose an investigator observes a success rate of 7/8 (88%) in patients treated with Agent X and a corresponding rate of 2/7 (29%) in patients treated with Agent Y. The difference of 59% is impressive, but the groups are small, and the investigator is worried about the possible role of chance.

To apply the classical approach to determining χ^2 for these results, we express the data in the form of a 2×2 contingency table. This arrangement is often called a "fourfold" table because its basic "cells" contain four distinct subgroups:

	Successes	Failures	TOTAL
Group X	7	1	8
Group Y	2	5	7
TOTAL	9	6	15

To calculate χ^2, we proceed as follows:

With the null hypothesis, we assume that treatments X and Y give identical results. If so, the anticipated proportion of successes in each treatment group would be 9/15. We thus would expect $(9/15) \times 8 = 4.8$ successes in Group X, and $(9/15) \times 7 = 4.2$ in Group Y. With analogous reasoning, the expectation of failures would be $(6/15) \times 8 = 3.2$ in X, and $(6/15) \times 7 = 2.8$ in Y.

Note that we have now violated a basic principle of human life. People are integral units, rather than decimals or fractions, and we cannot realistically expect to find 2.8, 3.2, or any other fragmented number of human beings in a group. Such an insistence on realistic details would keep us from using the chi-square test, so we elect to ignore this issue and we accept the bizarre expectations as a minor aberration in the statistical theory.

With these assumptions and expectations, we are now ready to calculate chi-square as the sum of the values for "(observed-expected)^2/expected" in each of the four cells of the table.

These calculations for our data yield the following results:

$$\frac{(7\text{-}4.8)^2}{4.8} + \frac{(1\text{-}3.2)^2}{3.2} + \frac{(2\text{-}4.2)^2}{4.2} + \frac{(5\text{-}2.8)^2}{2.8} =$$
$$1.008 + 1.513 + 1.152 + 1.729 = 5.402.$$

An alternative and easier way of generally calculating χ^2 is to express our contingency table as follows:

	Successes	Failures	TOTAL
Group X	a	b	A
Group Y	c	d	B
TOTAL	S	F	N

The formula for χ^2 is then $(ad\text{-}bc)^2 N / (ABSF)$. Substituting our data in this formula, we get $(35 - 2)^2 \times 15 / (8 \times 7 \times 9 \times 6) = 5.402$.

Entering an appropriate table of probability at the one degree of freedom that pertains for a "fourfold" test, we find that the two-sided P is 0.025 for $\chi^2 = 5.024$ and 0.01 for $\chi^2 = 6.635$. We can therefore state that for a χ^2 of 5.402, the value of P is $0.01 < P < 0.025$. For a one-sided test, these probabilities would be halved. For either a one-sided or two sided interpretation, therefore, the result is "statistically significant" at the 0.05 level.

About 40 years ago, Frank Yates[38] introduced a "continuity correction" to be applied in the chi-square calculation when the expected values in the cells are small. For many years thereafter, investigators were troubled[3] about when to use the Yates correction, because the term "small" was not precisely defined. Different statisticians proposed different values of "small", ranging from 1 to 5 as expectations in the cells. In recent years, the entire use of the Yates correction has become controversial,[23, 33] and certain statisticians[16] have argued that it should be abandoned altogether. Nevertheless, because the numbers in the data we observed here certainly seem "small," let us apply the Yates correction. The formula is $\chi^2 = (|ad-bc| - \frac{N}{2})^2$ $N/(ABSF)$. Substituting our data in this formula gives $\chi^2 = (|35-2|-7.5)^2 \times 15/ (8 \times 7 \times 9 \times 6) = 3.225$.

We are now in trouble. If this chi-square value receives a two-sided interpretation, we find that $0.05 < P < 0.10$, and the result is *not* "statistically significant." If the interpretation is one-sided, however, the P values are halved, so that $0.025 < P < 0.05$ and "significance" has been found. We are thus left with considerable ambiguity. According to the way we calculate and interpret chi-square, the results either are or are not "statistically significant." For the moment, let us conclude that they "tend" toward "significance."

4. *The conceptual deviations.* We can now pause to review our original goal, and to note the amount of conceptual deviation and extraneous ideas that were produced by the statistical strategies. We originally wanted to know how often an "exceptional" difference would have been noted if our original groups had been rearranged in some other manner. The sampling-distribution tactic does *not* provide a direct answer to this question. Instead of looking at the distribution of potential differences in our observed data, we have looked at the theoretical sampling distribution of a contrived test statistic.

We originally wanted no mathematical ideas more complex than a count of the relative frequency for the exceptional differences. Instead, we have been forced to contemplate parametric values for an imaginary parent population, and we have become immersed in such extraneous concepts as *probability densities, expected values, degrees of freedom,* and *standard error of the difference in means.*

This indirect statistical approach to the problem, with all of the attendant digressions and impositions, has received widespread acceptance for more than half a century because most investigators do not know of any other methods for testing "statistical significance." Even today, many textbooks of statistics contain no mention of alternative procedures, and most statistical consultants do not inform their clients that any other options are available. To assess "statistical significance" for the numerical difference noted in two groups, most investigators devoutly believe in only two procedures: the t test if the data are dimensional, expressed in means; and the χ^2 test if the data are categorical attributes, expressed as proportions or percentages.

C. The investigator's quest for significance

Amid all of the elaborate mathematical reasoning needed for these two statistical tests, not a single thought was devoted to a scientist's primary purpose in contemplating "significance." The scientist's first concern is with the magnitude of the observed difference. It is big enough to be important?

1. *Clinical importance.* The judgment about the "material significance"[17] or practical importance of the difference found in an analytic contrast is often called "clinical significance." The judgment depends entirely on scientific rather than statistical

Table I. *Methods of citing a contrast*

	Original data cited in means	Original data cited in percentages
Group A	69 units	75% success
Group B	46 units	25% success
Absolute Difference |A-B|	23 units	50%
Ratio: A/B	3:2 or 1.5:1	3:1
Ratio: B/A	0.67:1	0.33:1
Percentage drop from A	$\frac{23}{69} = 33\%$	$\frac{50}{75} = 67\%$
Percentage rise from B	$\frac{23}{46} = 50\%$	$\frac{50}{25} = 200\%$

principles. A difference of 2 units in the mean values for two groups may seem important if the respective means are 1 and 3; and trivial if the respective means are 2951 and 2953.

There are several ways to express the contrast noted in two groups. The standard approach is to subtract one result from the other, which provides a value for the difference. Another approach is to form a ratio of the two results. A third approach is to express the difference as a percentage of one result or the other.

These diverse approaches for contrasting results are shown for two different types of data in Table I. An important point to note from Table I is that the investigator can enlarge or de-emphasize the magnitude of a contrast according to the way in which he chooses to express it. In particular, the percentage increment or decrement from one group to another could be noted, on the left side of Table I, as either 33% or 50% according to whether the percentage change was assessed as a drop from Group A or a rise from B. Similarly, on the right side of Table I, the corresponding increments or decrements would be either 67% if based on A or 200% if based on B. What appears to be a distinctive percentage drop of 67% for one investigator might appear, for another investigator, to be a very high "risk ratio" of 3:1.

Regardless of the particular contrast that is chosen and the way it is expressed, the investigator must make a decision about its apparent importance. A ratio of 3:1 or a difference of 50% clearly seems major.

A ratio of 87:86 or a difference of 1% does not seem particularly important, but might be quite pertinent in certain special circumstances (particularly for a rise in a bank's interest rate on loans). The evaluation of this distinction is entirely a matter of scientific judgment for which statistical procedures of testing significance, despite their intricate cerebral mechanisms, are totally "decerebrate." A difference of major scientific value might be not statistically significant if the numbers of persons in the groups are too small. Conversely, a minor difference—no matter how trivial—can become statistically significant if large enough numbers of people are included in the test.

An investigator is therefore interested in statistically testing a distinction that is clinically important. A clinically unimportant distinction might ordinarily not be tested, or, if tested, its "statistical significance" would be ignored. If the difference is clinically important, however, the investigator will worry about small numbers in his groups. This is the situation for which he wants to know whether significant odds exist against the difference arising by chance. If the numbers of people in the groups are large enough, the statistical distinction will usually be clearly evident by an "eye test," and a statistical procedure will serve merely to embellish the values for P. If the results are appraised exclusively in P values, the test may sometimes be inadvertently misleading. Thus, with data of *20/25 (80%)* vs. *18/25 (72%)*, the 8% difference in results does not seem impressive clinically. It is also not "statistically significant," since $\chi^2 = 0.439$ and $P > 0.5$. If the group were ten times larger, so that the results were *200/250 (80%)* vs. *180/250 (72%)*, the 8% difference would still not seem particularly impressive clinically. The value of chi-square would now be ten times larger, however, and for $\chi^2 = 4.39$, the result is "statistically significant" at $P < 0.05$.

Having considered the primacy of judging clinical importance, we may now proceed to what an investigator seeks in a statistical test of "significance."

2. Random probability. If the cited statistical tests had not been developed, the issue of "statistical significance" could be approached with a direct implementation of the fundamental reasoning noted at the end of Section A. The investigator would think as follows:

a. My research project contains a total of N people, divided so that n_A are in Group A and n_B in Group B.

b. Suppose there is no real difference in the effects of the two maneuvers used in Groups A and B. Then the results observed in the individual people would be the same regardless of whether they were allocated to Group A or B.

c. Let me now consider all the possible ways in which a group of N people can be divided into two groups, each containing n_A and n_B members. For each of those divisions—using the data for the people I have actually observed—let me calculate the mean (or percentage) for each group, and the difference between the means (or percentages).

d. Let me now see, among that array of differences, how often I encounter an "exceptional" value that equals or exceeds the one observed in my research.

e. The relative frequency of the "exceptional" occurrences will denote the probability that the observed difference might have arisen fortuitously if the patients had been divided into any other one of the possible arrangements.

f. If this P value does not exceed my chosen level of α, I shall reject the null hypothesis and decide that the observed difference is "statistically significant."

a. Data expressed in means. To illustrate this procedure, let us consider the same data that we examined earlier to perform the t test. The results in Group A are 20, 15, 12, and 6 units, with a mean of 13.25. The results in Group B are 7, 3, 2, and 1 units, with a mean of 3.25.

If these eight people were arbitrarily divided into two pairs of quartets, how many diverse pairs of quartets could be formed? Assuming that each person maintains the same individual results, what difference would have been noted in the means for each of those pairs of quartets? How often would those differences equal or exceed the 10 units we have noted? These questions can be answered by resorting to another type of mathemetical procedure: the arrangement of permutations and combinations.

If N different objects are divided into two groups, one containing R objects and the other containing N-R objects, there is a mathematical formula for expressing the number of distinctly different combinations. It is[*]

$$\frac{N!}{R! \; (N\text{-}R)!}.$$

For the data of the 8 people here, we would therefore have

$$\frac{8 \times 7 \times 6 \times 5 \times 4 \times 3 \times 2 \times 1}{(4 \times 3 \times 2 \times 1) \times (4 \times 3 \times 2 \times 1)} = 70$$

different combinations of two groups, each containing four people.

A more intuitive way of understanding this result is as follows. Let the eight objects be called *s, t, u, v, w, x, y, z*. For Group A, the first member can be chosen in 8 different ways, the second member in 7 ways, the third in 6 ways, and the fourth in 5. Once these members are chosen, the membership of Group B is fixed, since the remaining four members go into B. Of the 1680 ways (= 8 × 7 × 6 × 5) in which the members can be arranged for Group A, each individual quartet will repeatedly appear in a series of permutations. Thus, the quartet *w, x, y, z* can be permuted as *w, y, z, x; x, y, z, w; z, y, x, w;* and so on. The number of different permutations for a group of four different objects is 24 (= 4 × 3 × 2 × 1). Thus, each distinctive quartet will appear in 24 ways among the 1680 arrangements. We therefore divide 1680 by 24 and get 70 as the number of distinctive quartets that could be formed by dividing eight objects into two groups of four each.

Half of these 70 arrangements are similar but opposite. Thus, the quartet *w,x,y,z*

---

[*]The exclamation point in the formula refers to the "factorial" of a number. Thus $5! = 5 \times 4 \times 3 \times 2 \times 1$. By convention, $0! = 1$.

Table II. *Means and differences in means for 35 arrangements of eight observations divided into two groups*

Group A	Group B	Mean, Group A	Mean, Group B	Difference in means, A-B
20, 15, 12, 7	6, 3, 2, 1	13.5	3.0	10.5
20, 15, 12, 6	7, 3, 2, 1	13.25	3.25	10.0
20, 15, 12, 3	7, 6, 2, 1	12.5	4.0	8.5
20, 15, 12, 2	7, 6, 3, 1	12.25	4.25	8.0
20, 15, 12, 1	7, 6, 3, 2	12.0	4.5	7.5
20, 15, 7, 6	12, 3, 2, 1	12.0	4.5	7.5
20, 15, 7, 3	12, 6, 2, 1	11.25	5.25	6.0
20, 15, 7, 2	12, 6, 3, 1	11.0	5.5	5.5
20, 15, 7, 1	12, 6, 3, 2	10.75	5.75	5.0
20, 15, 6, 3	12, 7, 2, 1	11.0	5.5	5.5
20, 15, 6, 2	12, 7, 3, 1	10.75	5.75	5.0
20, 15, 6, 1	12, 7, 3, 2	10.5	6.0	4.5
20, 15, 3, 2	12, 7, 6, 1	10.0	6.5	3.5
20, 15, 3, 1	12, 7, 6, 2	9.75	6.75	3.0
20, 15, 2, 1	12, 7, 6, 3	9.5	7.0	2.5
20, 12, 7, 6	15, 3, 2, 1	11.25	5.25	6.0
20, 12, 7, 3	15, 6, 2, 1	10.5	6.0	4.5
20, 12, 7, 2	15, 6, 3, 1	10.25	6.25	4.0
20, 12, 7, 1	15, 6, 3, 2	10.0	6.5	3.5
20, 12, 6, 3	15, 7, 2, 1	10.25	6.25	4.0
20, 12, 6, 2	15, 7, 3, 1	10.0	6.5	3.5
20, 12, 6, 1	15, 7, 3, 2	9.75	6.75	3.0
20, 12, 3, 2	15, 7, 6, 1	9.25	7.25	2.0
20, 12, 3, 1	15, 7, 6, 2	9.0	7.5	1.5
20, 12, 2, 1	15, 7, 6, 3	8.75	7.75	1.0
20, 7, 6, 3	15, 12, 2, 1	9.0	7.5	1.5
20, 7, 6, 2	15, 12, 3, 1	8.75	7.75	1.0
20, 7, 6, 1	15, 12, 3, 2	8.5	8.0	0.5
20, 7, 3, 2	15, 12, 6, 1	8.0	8.5	−0.5
20, 7, 3, 1	15, 12, 6, 2	7.75	8.75	−1.0
20, 7, 2, 1	15, 12, 6, 3	7.5	9.0	−1.5
20, 6, 3, 2	15, 12, 7, 1	7.75	8.75	−1.0
20, 6, 3, 1	15, 12, 7, 2	7.5	9.0	−1.5
20, 6, 2, 1	15, 12, 7, 3	7.25	9.25	−2.0
20, 3, 2, 1	15, 12, 7, 6	6.5	10.0	−3.5

might be in Group A and the quartet *s,t,u,v* might be in Group B; or vice versa. Consequently, there are really 35 distinctively different pairs of quartets to be considered. Those arrangements for the numbers 20,15, 12,7,6,3,2 and 1 are shown in Table II, together with the means and difference in means for each of the 35 arrangements. Exchanging the contents of Groups A and B, and reversing signs for the differences in means, we could obtain the remaining 35 arrangements that complete the 70 possibilities for those eight numbers.

By inspecting the results of Table II, we can get the answers to the questions asked earlier. An "exceptional" difference in means of 10 units or more in favor of Group A occurs twice in the 35 arrangements shown in Table I. If we completed the rest of the table to form 70 arrangements, we would find that a difference of means of 10 units or more in favor of B would also occur twice. Thus, at a two-sided level of interpretation, for any difference of 10 units or more, the probability is 4/70 = 0.05714. At a one-sided level of interpretation, for the difference of 10 units in favor of A, the probability is 2/70 = 0.02857.

These results are different from what we found earlier with the t test. At a two-sided level of interpretation, P was between 0.025 and 0.02 with the t test, but it was 0.057 with the exact random permutation test. Thus, if we were adhering to a strict α level of below 0.05 for "statistical significance," we would draw different conclusions from the two tests. At a one-sided level of interpretation, however, both results would be "significant." P was below 0.0125 with the t test and was 0.029 with the random permutation test.

From Table II, we can also note the fallacy of the 95% confidence interval calculated earlier. According to the calculated confidence interval, the differences in means for 95% of the samples in the observed distribution should lie between 2.15 and 17.85. As noted empirically in Table II, however, none of the differences exceeded 10.5, and 12 of the 35 pairs of samples had absolute differences that were smaller than 2.16. If our research had been done to estimate parametrically the difference in means of the two parent populations, and if we had used the conventional statistical wisdom, we would have had a quite different set of results.

b. Data expressed in percentages. If we wanted to perform an analogous procedure with the earlier data on which we did a chi-square test, the reasoning would be as follows: We have a total of 15 people, divided so that 8 are in one group and 7 in the other. Of those 15 people, 9 were successes and 6 were failures. Assuming that treatments X and Y yield the same results, so that the patients would be successes or failures no matter how they were divided, let us consider all the possible ways in which these 15 people— containing 9 successes and 6 failures— can be divided into two groups of 8 and 7. In how many of those arrangements would we find a difference in success percentages that is at least as large as the 59% encountered in the actual results we observed?

To answer this question, we could con-

struct a table similar to Table II, showing all possible arrangements of the 15 people, and we could then note the frequency of the difference in percentages for the two groups in each arrangement. The table would be quite long because of the many different arrangements to be considered. [The number of possible arrangements is $15!/(8! \times 7!) = 6435$.]

Fortunately, an easier way of determining the desired information was developed by R. A. Fisher.[15] If the table has the construction shown earlier with the letters a,b, . . . ,F,N, Fisher showed that the proportion of the permutations that would give rise to this particular arrangement is

$$P = \frac{A! \; B! \; S! \; F!}{N! \; a! \; b! \; c! \; d!}$$

For the particular table we observed, this value would be

$$P = \frac{8! \; 7! \; 9! \; 6!}{15! \; 7! \; 1! \; 2! \; 5!}$$

This formidable looking fraction can be calculated using a table of factorial logarithms. Alternatively, with appropriate cancellations of numbers in numerator and denominator, the fraction reduces to $24/(13 \times 11 \times 5) = 0.03357$. This value tells us the proportion of times that our arrangement of the 15 people would yield the particular table under consideration.

Another way of reaching this same result is to recognize that the 9 successes in this table can be arranged in $9!/(7! \times 2!) = 36$ ways. The 6 failures can be arranged in $6!/(5! \times 1!) = 6$ ways. The number of possible ways of forming the table is thus $36 \times 6 = 216$. Since there are a total of 6435 possible arrangements, the P for this particular table is $216/6435 = 0.03357$.

For purposes of illustration, we can work out similar values for each of the 7 possible tables that can be formed with the cited constraints of the four marginal totals for the 15 people: 9 successes and 6 failures; 8 people in Group X and 7 in Group Y. These 7 arrangements are shown here in Table III, containing individual probabilities (= 0.00140 + 0.03357 + ... +

Table III. *Arrangements for 8 people in Group X and 7 people in Group Y, having a total of 9 successes and 6 failures*

Arrangements of $\begin{Bmatrix} a & b \\ c & d \end{Bmatrix}$	[Group X-Group Y] Difference in percentage of successes	Probability value
$\begin{Bmatrix} 8 & 0 \\ 1 & 6 \end{Bmatrix}$	100%- 14% = 86%	0.00140
$\begin{Bmatrix} 7 & 1 \\ 2 & 5 \end{Bmatrix}$	88%- 29% = 59%	0.03357
$\begin{Bmatrix} 6 & 2 \\ 3 & 4 \end{Bmatrix}$	75%- 43% = 32%	0.19580
$\begin{Bmatrix} 5 & 3 \\ 4 & 3 \end{Bmatrix}$	63%- 57% = 6%	0.39161
$\begin{Bmatrix} 4 & 4 \\ 5 & 2 \end{Bmatrix}$	50%- 71% = -21%	0.29371
$\begin{Bmatrix} 3 & 5 \\ 6 & 1 \end{Bmatrix}$	38%- 86% = -48%	0.07832
$\begin{Bmatrix} 2 & 6 \\ 7 & 0 \end{Bmatrix}$	25%-100% = -75%	0.00559

0.07832 + 0.00559) that can be added to form a sum of 1.

By examining Table III, we can get an immediate answer to our original question. A difference in percentages of 86% occurs with a P of 0.00140; 59% with a P of 0.03357; and (at the other "tail") – 75% with a P of 0.00559. These are the only percentage differences that are as large as or larger than the one we observed. Therefore, the two-sided random probability of the result we observed is the sum of these three probabilities, or 0.04056. The one-sided probability is 0.03497. Expressed in fewer digits, the two-sided P is 0.04 and the one-sided P is 0.03.

This is the exact answer to our original question. The answer is precise, unambiguous, unencumbered by any peculiar expectations about fractional people, and unembroiled in any controversy about the Yates correction. (We might also note that this particular case supports the people who oppose the Yates correction. At a two-sided interpretation and a 0.05 level of α, the exact probability test and the uncorrected χ^2 value would have led us to declare "significance"; the corrected χ^2 value would not.)

D. The use of permutation tests

The types of test performed in the foregoing section are called *randomization tests* or *permutation tests*. To avoid another confusing usage of the word *randomization,* I shall call them *permutation tests.* They are based on forming all possible distinctively different permutations of the actual data observed by the investigator. We then determine the relative frequency with which our observed result or a more "exceptional" one is found among those permutations. This relative frequency is the P value we seek.

1. *Advantages of permutation tests.* These tests have many obvious attractions for investigators engaged in real-world scientific research:

a. The result of each permutation test is a direct, exact probability value for the random likelihood of the observed difference in results (or of a more exceptional one). In contrast, the t test and chi-square test are indirect procedures, yielding a result that is not a probability value but a "score" for the test statistic, t or χ^2. This score must then be converted into a probability statement after a search in an appropriate table. Furthermore, because of constraints in the tables, the probability statement is usually an approximation (such as "0.025 < P < 0.05"), rather than an exact value.

b. The permutation tests do not require any unwanted inferential estimations of means, variances, pooled variances, or other parameters of an unobserved, hypothetical parent population. The tests are based only on the evidence that was actually obtained.

c. The investigator is not forced into making any erroneous assumptions either that the contrasted groups were chosen as random samples from the parent population, or that the maneuvers under study were randomly allocated to the two groups. A permutation test tells what would happen if the actual people under observation had been randomly distributed into the two groups, but it requires no conceptual ideology about random choices from a parent population or random allocations of treatment.

d. The investigator is not forced into making any erroneous or unconfirmable assumptions about a Gaussian (or any other) distribution for the parent population or about equal variances in the contrasted groups.

e. A permutation test can be applied to groups of any size, no matter how large or small. There are no "degrees of freedom" to be considered or calculated. For categorical data in a contingency table, there is no need to worry about the magnitude of the "expected" value, no need to calculate expectations based on fractions of people, and no need to keep abreast of the latest state of the controversy over whether or not to apply Yates correction.

Permutation tests have existed for a long time. The procedure used as a counterpart of the χ^2 test for contrasting percentages in a 2×2 contingency table is moderately well known and is called the *Fisher exact probability test*. The procedures that can be used as permutation counterparts of the t test for contrasting the means of dimensional data are not eponymically labelled, but have been discussed by Fisher[15] and by such other prominent statisticians as Pitman,[28] Welch,[36] and Wald and Wolfowitz.[34] Although no specific examples have been cited here, permutation tests also exist for ordinal data. Some of the best known tests for ranked ordinal data were created by Wilcoxon[37] and are associated with his name. Because permutation tests require no assumptions about distributions or parameters of a parent population, they are sometimes called *distribution-free*[2] or *non-parametric*[29] tests.

Although permutation tests offer major advantages to clinical and epidemiologic investigators, the tests are relatively unknown and untaught. Most courses in biostatistics for medical students contain little or no mention of non-parametric procedures. When mentioned, the procedures are usually confined to various types of

ranks tests for ordinal data. The Fisher exact probability test is omitted from most biomedical instruction, and also from most textbooks of biostatistics or elementary statistics. The use of a permutation test to supplant the t test is mentioned almost nowhere in the textbooks. The only place I could find such a test cited among the many texts devoted to biostatistics or biologic applications of statistics is in an excellent new paperback book by Colquhoun.[4]

2. *Disadvantages of permutation tests.* After discovering the advantages of these tests, an investigator usually wants to know why he was not told about them before.

At least three features—of inertia, ideology, and information—make minor contributions to the existing state of statistical desuetude:

a. It is easier for many teachers to continue the inertia of teaching what they were taught years ago than to revise the contents of the curriculum.

b. Investigators or consultants who ideologically believe that the goal of science is to estimate parameters and variances will have no enthusiasm for tests that do not include or rely on these estimations.

c. Many statisticians have a deep-seated horror of doing anything that may entail "losing information." This type of "loss" would occur if dimensional data were converted into ordinal ranks for the sake of a non-parametric test that uses the ranks rather than the observed values. Since ranks are used in almost all of the tests popularly known as *non-parametric,* and since all of these tests depend on the principle of random permutations, a statistician may erroneously conclude that all non-parametric tests create a loss of information. The conclusion is wrong because the non-parametric permutation tests illustrated here make use of the original values of the data, not the ranks.

The three features just cited are of minor importance, however. The main reason for the neglect of permutation tests is the difficulty of calculating the results. The diverse products and quotients for arrays of factorial numbers create formidable problems in calculation. The calculations cannot readily be done on a desk calculator, even with sophisticated modern capabilities. For the Fisher exact probability test of a 2×2 contingency grouping, a statistician can avoid doing many of the calculations, because tables[7, 14, 22] have been prepared to cite the decisive P values of this test for all possible 2 × 2 arrays in which the total value of N is no larger than 70. These tables extend over many pages, however, and are more cumbersome to use than the simpler one-page tables for χ^2. Besides, whenever N exceeds 70, the Fisher test result must be individually calculated. For the permutation equivalent of a t test on the means of two groups, no routine tables can be prepared. Each such test must be separately computed from the individual values of the observed data. As Bradley[2] has pointed out,

> Despite their excellent properties, . . . (these randomization) tests . . . are little more than statistical curiosities. The fact that the distribution of the test statistic is conditional upon the obtained set of observation values makes each separate application a unique test and prevents the compilation of tables that can be used repeatedly.

The permutation procedures that an investigator would regard as optimal statistical tests have therefore been generally unpublicized and unused not for intellectual reasons, but for ease of computation. They have been a nuisance to calculate. During the past 50 years, the magnitude of this nuisance was great enough to make statisticians prefer what was computationally attractive rather than what was scientifically desirable. In the era of the digital computer, however, these calculational difficulties will ultimately disappear. When the costs of computation have become cheap and desk terminals ubiquitous, an investigator will be able to turn to his terminal as readily as he now turns to his desk calculator, and will be able to get the results of an appropriate permutation test with no more time or effort than it now takes to do a t test or a χ^2 test.

Furthermore, in situations where the sample sizes are relatively large, requiring an inordinate amount of computer time to form and examine the entire array of distinctive permutations, the complete permutation test can be truncated into a "Monte Carlo" type of "randomization test." For this procedure, a program can be written for the computer to generate random numbers successively; to use these numbers for preparing 1000 appropriate randomizations of the observed data; to calculate the value of the difference in results noted for each such randomization; and to note the frequency with which "exceptional" values occur for the differences. This frequency, divided by 10, would yield the desired P value.

3. The acceptance of conventional tests. At this point in the discussion, the reader may be wondering how the t and χ^2 tests have been able to survive so well. If the tests are so unsatisfactory, why have they received such widespread acceptance?

The answer to this question is that the tests are not unsatisfactory. Despite their cited disadvantages, they generally work well enough to yield reasonably reliable approximations of the more exact results provided by permutation procedures. In both theoretical contemplations and empirical comparisons,[1, 8, 24] the probabilities calculated with the traditional tests have often closely agreed with what is obtained by permutation tests. Particularly when the sample sizes are large, the chi-square tests and t tests produce P values that are generally similar to those derived by the counterpart permutation procedures.

For this reason, investigators have generally had little reason to challenge the conventional techniques. Concerned with scientific principles of designing and conducting research, an investigator often pays little attention to the statistical theories used for testing numerical differences. Besides, a good investigator generally relies on an "eye test" to tell whether or not the results are significant. He may regard the use of the statistical tests either as the last refuge of the investigatively destitute, or as a quantitative frippery that is needed to satisfy the demands of reviewers, editors, and granting agencies. In these circumstances, as long as the statistical test produces the P value required for numerical "significance," the investigator may not care about how the test operates or whether its theoretical principles are constantly violated during the operations.

The main difficulty with this intellectual complacency is that the conventional tests may be unreliable in small-sized groups, which are the particular situations in which an investigator is most concerned about the role of chance. In the two examples that were shown earlier, the conventional t and χ^2 tests might have caused the investigator to draw false conclusions if α were set at the 0.05 level. When the sample sizes are small, the statistical tests become particularly important, and the use of an accurate test becomes crucial. When sample sizes are large, the statistical tests are less important and a good approximation is quite acceptable.

Thus, a statistician defending the general use of t and chi-square tests in modern research could point to their frequent accuracy. With the same argument, an old school clinician might point out that diabetes mellitus can usually be diagnosed by tasting the urine or applying Benedict's reagent. With the availability of better and equally easy ways to diagnose diabetes, however, these old procedures were gradually replaced by techniques that are more reliable. Similarly, when the aid of computers allows permutation or randomization tests to be performed easily, the t test and χ^2 test will probably begin to disappear as routine procedures. Even without computers, however, the permutation tests are the preferable and perhaps mandatory procedures to be used with small-sized groups.

For more than 60 years, clinical investigators have used statistical tests that are computationally feasible rather than tests that are intellectually desirable. In the age of the computer, this aspect of the "substitution game" need not be continued in scientific research. As Kempthorne has stated: "Making . . . assumptions of normality and then applying the battery of mathematical tests is not a satisfactory basis for experimental inference. . . . Tests of significance . . . have frequently been presented by way of normal law theory, whereas their validity stems from randomization theory.[18] . . . The proper way to make tests of significance . . . is by way of the randomization (or permutation) test."[19]

4. *The ultimate value of permutation tests.* A more substantive disadvantage of the traditional statistical tests has been their adverse effect on the reasoning used for "hypothesis testing." In scientific investigation, the hypothesis is a strictly scientific phenomenon. As the basis for the research, the hypothesis comprises all of the scientific nuances in reasoning, planning, and evaluating. In statistical inference, however, the hypothesis is converted into a strictly algebraic phenomenon. It is a pair of symbols joined by an equals sign, usually expressed in the form of "$H_0: \mu_1 = \mu_2$."

In forming this algebraic "hypothesis," a statistician is almost required to suspend attention to the realities of research. To use the associated tests, the statistician must assume that the research was ideally conducted—that there is no bias in observation, no bias in selection, no bias in allocation, no bias in chronologic grouping, and no bias in target detection. These assumptions may liberate a statistician from any inhibitions about using the t test or χ^2 test, but they may also distract him from an imperative concern with the validity of the assumptions themselves.

A good investigator, on the other hand, would accept the algebraic phrasing of the *null hypothesis,* but would give it no serious attention. The scientific contents of a hypothesis usually bear no relation to any mathematical probabilities, and the contents are neither confirmed nor refuted by the probabilities. A scientific hypothesis is evaluated according to the way the research was designed and executed, not according to mathematical theories. Recognizing that his groups were not drawn randomly, that the investigated maneuvers were not allocated randomly, and that the data may fulfill none of the other conventional statistical assumptions, a knowledgeable investigator will use the statistical test purely for its numerical appraisals. He expects the test to describe the arithmetic of chance, not the validity of science. For the latter goal in scientific design, he will contemplate profound issues for which the question of whether $\mu_1 = \mu_2$ is either trivial or irrelevant. Unfortunately, however, because the statistical tests have become so over-emphasized, because the investigator may be awed by their mathematical intricacy, and because the term "significance" has become so seductive, many investigators will suspend their own sensibility and will credulously conclude that the scientific hypothesis was confirmed by an appropriate result in a computed test of the statistical "hypothesis."

The ultimate value of the permutation tests, therefore, is that their intellectual directness, precision, and simplicity will free both the investigator and the statistician from a deleterious pre-occupation with sampling distributions, pooled variances, and other mathematical distractions. An investigator who comprehends the principles of his statistical tests will be less inclined to give idolatrous worship to a numerical "significance" that has no scientific connotation. A statistician who need not rely on stochastic abstractions as his main stock in trade can improve his work as a consultant by devoting greater attention to fundamental issues in the scientific design and conduct of research. The investigator and the statistician can then begin to understand each other more effectively and to collaborate more productively in pursuing the many significant scientific challenges that are not contained or expressed in the esoteric mathematics of current approaches to "statistical significance."

• • •

With or without this new utopia, a third major problem in randomization still awaits consideration. The next paper in this series will be concerned with randomized allocations in clinical trials.

References

1. Baker, F. B., and Collier, R. O., Jr.: Some empirical results on variance ratios under permutation in the completely randomized design, J. Am. Stat. Assn. **61**:814-820, 1966.
2. Bradley, J. V.: Distribution-free statistical tests, Englewood Cliffs, N. J., 1968, Prentice-Hall, Inc.
3. Cochran, W. G.: Some methods for strengthening the common χ^2 tests, Biometrics **10**: 417-451, 1954.
4. Colquhoun, D.: Lectures on biostatistics, Oxford, 1971, Oxford University Press.
5. Cox, C. P.: Some observations on the teaching of statistical consulting, Biometrics **24**: 789-801, 1968.
6. Daniel, C.: Some general remarks on consulting in statistics, Biometrics **24**:1029, 1968. (Abst.) (Complete report, Technometrics **11**:241-245, 1969.)
7. Documenta Geigy. *In* Diem, K., editor: Scientific tables, ed. 6, Ardsley, N. Y., 1962, Geigy Chemical Company.
8. Edgington, E. S.: Statistical inference and non-random samples, Psychol. Bull. **66**:485-487, 1966.
9. Feinstein, A. R.: Clinical biostatistics. VII. The rancid sample, the tilted target, and the medical poll-bearer, Clin. Pharmacol. Ther. **12**:134-150, 1971.
10. Feinstein, A. R.: Clinical biostatistics. X. Sources of 'transition bias' in cohort statistics, Clin. Pharmacol. Ther. **12**:704-721, 1971.
11. Feinstein, A. R.: Clinical biostatistics. XI. Sources of 'chronology bias' in cohort statistics, Clin. Pharmacol. Ther. **12**:864-879, 1971.
12. Feinstein, A. R.: Clinical biostatistics. XVII. Synchronous partition and bivariate evaluation in predictive stratification, Clin. Pharmacol. Ther. **13**:755-768, 1972.
13. Feinstein, A. R.: Clinical biostatistics. XXII. The role of randomization in sampling, testing, allocation, and credulous idolatry (Part 1), Clin. Pharmacol. Ther. **14**:601-615, 1973.
14. Finney, D. J., Latscha, R., Bennett, B. M., and Hsu, P.: Tables for testing significance in a 2×2 contingency table, Cambridge, 1963, Cambridge University Press.
15. Fisher, R. A.: The design of experiments, ed. 6, New York, 1951, Hafner Publishing Company.
16. Grizzle, J. E.: Continuity correction in the

χ^2 test for 2×2 tables, Am. Stat. **21**:28-32, 1967.

17. Hodges, J. L., Jr., and Lehman, E. L.: Testing the approximate validity of statistical hypotheses. J. Roy. Stat. Soc. (Series B) **16**:261-268, 1954.

18. Kempthorne, O.: The randomization theory of experimental inference, J. Am. Stat. Assn. **50**:946-967, 1955.

19. Kempthorne, O.: Some aspects of experimental inference, J. Am. Stat. Assn. **61**:11-34, 1966.

20. Kendall, M. G., and Buckland, W. R.: A dictionary of statistical terms, ed. 3, Edinburgh, 1971, Oliver & Boyd, Ltd.

21. Kimball, A. W.: Errors of third kind in statistical consulting, J. Am. Stat. Assn. **52**: 133-142, 1957.

22. Mainland, D.: Elementary medical statistics, ed. 2, Philadelphia, 1963, W. B. Saunders Co.

23. Mantel, N., and Greenhouse, S. W.: What is the continuity correction?, Am. Stat. **22**:27-30, 1968.

24. McHugh, R. B.: Comment on "Scales and statistics: Parametric and non-parametric," Psychol. Bull. **60**:350-355, 1963.

25. Natrella, M. G.: The relation between confidence intervals and tests of significance, Am. Stat. **14**:20-22, 33, 1960.

26. Pearson, E. S.: Some reflexions on continuity in the development of mathematical statistics, 1885-1920; pp. 339-353, *in* Studies in the history of statistics and probability, Darien, Conn., 1970, Hafner Publishing Company.

27. Pearson, K.: On the criterion that a given system of deviations from the probable in the case of a correlated system of variables is such that it can reasonably be supposed to have arisen from random sampling, Philosophical Mag. **50**:157-175, 1900.

28. Pitman, E. J. G.: Significance tests which may be applied to samples from any populations, J. Roy. Stat. Soc. (Series B) **4**:119-130, 1937.

29. Siegel, S.: Nonparametric statistics for the behavioral sciences, New York, 1956, McGraw-Hill Book Company, Inc.

30. Snedecor, G. W.: The statistical part of the scientific method, Ann. N. Y. Acad. Sci. **52**:792-799, 1950.

31. Sprent, P.: Some problems of statistical consultancy, J. Roy. Stat. Soc. (Series A) **133** (Part 2): 139-164, 1970.

32. Student (W. S. Gosset): The probable error of a mean, Biometrika **6**:1-25, 1908.

33. Veldman, D. J., and McNemar, Q.: In defense of the chi-square continuity correction, Proc. Am. Psychol. Assn., pp. 69-70, 1972.

34. Wald, A., and Wolfowitz, J.: Statistical tests based on permutations of the observations, Ann. Math. Stat. **15**:358-372, 1944.

35. Walker, H. M.: Degrees of freedom, J. Educ. Psychol. **31**:253-269, 1940.

36. Welch, B. L.: On the z test in randomized blocks and Latin Squares, Biometrika **29**: 21-52, 1937.

37. Wilcoxon, F., and Wilcox, R. A.: Some rapid approximate statistical procedures, Pearl River, N. Y., 1964, Lederle Laboratories.

38. Yates, F.: Contingency tables involving small numbers and the χ^2 test, Supplement, J. Roy. Stat. Soc. **1**:217-235, 1934.

39. Zelen, M.: The education of biometricians, Am. Stat. **23**:14-15, 1969.

CHAPTER 21

The direction of relationships, hypotheses, and probabilities

A statistician who begins to work in the real world of science and who gives suitable attention, as R. A. Fisher[13] advised, to "the duty of getting his head clear on the principles of scientific inference", may also find, as E. A. Cornish[5] has noted, "that the traditional machinery inculcated by the biometrical school was wholly unsuited to the needs of practical research".

One of the major problems in the current machinery is the ambiguous concept of *control*. As discussed earlier[8] in this series, the word *control* can have at least twelve different uses in clinical science, but statisticians are seldom taught about the differences. Consequently, when asked to give advice or guidance, a consultant statistician may sometimes confuse himself, the investigator, or the research by making inappropriate or erroneous assumptions about "controls" and "controlled experiments"[8].

In this essay, I should like to consider another important type of confusion created by the disparity between the theories of academic biometry and the realities of scientific research. The difficulties arise as a series of issues in *direction*. The direction may be expressed with such phrases as *forward* or *backward, before* or *after, affected* or *inter-related, greater than* or *less than,* and *one-sided* or *two-sided.*

This chapter originally appeared as "Clinical biostatistics—XXXII. Biologic dependency, 'hypothesis testing', unilateral probabilities, and other issues in scientific direction vs. statistical duplexity." In Clin. Pharmacol. Ther. 17:499, 1975.

Many scientific activities involve a single direction of planning, observing, or analyzing. Most statistical strategies, however, are deliberately intended to be bidirectional. After spending years of academic training in the duplexity of these bidirectional theoretical principles, the statistician may later have difficulty in recognizing or coping with the challenges that occur when real-world research has a specific unidirectional orientation.

I have already discussed some of these directional difficulties in earlier installments[7, 9] of this series. I shall here briefly review the previous discussion and then proceed to the newer topics, which involve the use of direction in analyzing statistical "associations", in formulating statistical "hypotheses", and in using tables or graphs of statistical probability.

A. Directional pursuit of a population

This issue refers to the difference between *cohort* research, in which the investigator follows a population forward from cause towards effect; and *trohoc* research[9], in which the population is studied backwards from effect towards cause. Because of the differences in chronologic direction, the results of trohoc research are particularly likely to be distorted by diverse forms of bias[6, 7] that are difficult to discover, adjust, or remove.

The statistician (or epidemiologist) who neglects the logical perils of a backward scientific direction may blithely assume that cohort and trohoc research should yield essentially the same data, which can be analyzed with essentially the same mathematics. Oblivious to the need for carefully examining bias rather than avidly manipulating numbers, the data analyst may then focus on the statistical rather than the scientific contents. After the numbers are agglomerated into an "odds ratio" that ablates the true values of the "risks" under assessment[9], the investigator may delude himself and his readers into believing that a "significant" value for this ratio confers credibility upon whatever conjecture is being tested.

B. Time of data collection

The second problem to be noted is really an issue of before-or-after timing rather than cause-effect direction. In many forms of investigation, the research data are obtained from an existing compendium of recorded information. The compendia of data may include such sources as patients' birth certificates, medical records, and death certificates. In other circumstances, the investigator gets the data directly from the patients, using pre-planned forms, standardized interviewing procedures, etc. The first method of assembling research data "afterward" from existing records can be called *retrolective,* and the second or "beforehand" method can be called *prolective*[7, 9]. Regardless of the timing with which the data are collected, the investigated population can be followed backward from effect toward cause as a *trohoc;* or forward from cause toward effect as a *cohort.*

These distinctions between the directional pursuit of a population and the timing used for assembly of research data have been confused by the application of the same words, *retrospective* and *prospective,* to both types of activity. Probably the best solution to this epidemiologic ambiguity is to remove the words *retrospective* and *prospective* from circulation. The terms *cohort* and *trohoc* can be applied to the pursuit of populations; and *prolective* and *retrolective* can be used for the collection of data. Neither the scientific nor the statistical confusion can be resolved if *prospective* and *retrospective* continue to receive a duplex duty. The duplexity becomes especially confusing

when the term "retrospective prospective" is used for a retrolective cohort study; and when "prospective retrospective" is used for a prolective trohoc study.

C. The direction of a relationship

In looking at the association of two variables, we can consider them as being dependently or interdependently related. For example, in a scattergraph of points for a group of infants and children, showing age along one axis and weight along the other, we can contemplate the interdependent relationship between age and weight, as expressed statistically in a *correlation coefficient*. The basic idea contained in a correlation coefficient is not that age affects weight, or vice versa; the coefficient is simply an index of the way that the two variables are inter-related.

In most scientific circumstances, however, an investigator would approach this relationship with a definite direction in mind. Believing that weight is affected by age, the investigator would analyze the data looking for an index to express this biologic dependency. The usual statistical expression would be a *regression coefficient,* indicating the slope of the line showing weight's regression on age.

The idea of a regression for two variables, x and y, is that one is mathematically dependent on the other. The mathematics can go in either direction. We can find the way that y regresses on (i.e., is dependent upon) x; or we can find the way that x regresses on y. Although the mathematics is flexible enough to calculate a regression coefficient for both directions, a biologic judgment must be employed to decide which coefficient we want to use. The decision here is based on a biologic rather than mathematical concept of dependency.

On the other hand, if we want a correlation coefficient, there is no need for thinking about a biologic direction. Besides, even if an investigator had such thoughts, the statistical duplexity of the correlation coefficient would destroy all mathematical traces of a biologic direction. The way in which a correlation coefficient performs this feat can be noted if we inspect the algebra of the calculation. Suppose we have an array of paired values x_i, y_i for each of a series of n patients. The respective means are $\bar{x}$ and $\bar{y}$. From the array of paired data, we can calculate the variance of the x values as $s_{xx} = \sum(x_i - \bar{x})^2/(n - 1)$ and the variance of the y values as $s_{yy} = \sum(y_i - \bar{y})^2/(n - 1)$. We can also calculate the covariance between x and y as $s_{xy} = \sum(x_i - \bar{x})(y_i - \bar{y})/(n - 1)$.

Now suppose that the x_i values represent age and that the y_i values represent the weight of the children. The question an investigator might want to ask is: "How does age affect weight"? In statistical terms, this question is: "What is the regression of weight on age"? The answer is provided by calculating a regression equation, which has the form $\hat{y}_i = a + bx_i$. (The ^ mark is placed over the $\hat{y}_i$ value to distinguish y_i, the actually observed value at each point of x_i, from the $\hat{y}_i$ value that is being estimated from the regression equation.) The main answer to the investigator's question is computed by using a least-squares procedure (demonstrated in any standard statistical text) to obtain the value of b, the regression coefficient that shows the slope of the line. With the variance symbols and values noted in the preceding paragraph, the regression coefficient is calculated as $b = s_{xy}/s_{xx}$.

A statistician might not be content, however, with this unidirectional approach to the data. We can also get the statistical answer to another question: "What is the regression of age on weight"? It is not a question that the investigator wants answered, since he probably has no interest in exploring the idea that weight affects age. Nevertheless, an alternative regression equation is there statistically. Its form is $\hat{x}_i = a' + b'y_i$; and its regression coefficient is $b' = s_{xy}/s_{yy}$.

The next step in the statistical reasoning is easy. Since we have two possible regression coefficients, since we don't want to be unkind to either one, and since statisticians like to arrive at a simple single index for expressing complex relationships, let us achieve that simple index by multiplying the two regression coefficients together. The product, in another splendid bit of statistical jargon, is called the *coefficient of determination* and can be expressed as $r^2 = bb' = (s_{xy}/s_{xx})(s_{xy}/s_{yy})$. If we take the square root of this product, we have

r, the correlation coefficient. The correlation coefficient is thus obtained as the geometric mean of the two opposing regression coefficients, and we have carefully destroyed any scientific direction that might have been used in the research or in the investigator's thought processes.

With this technique, if we contemplated the correlation of weight and age for a group of infants and children, we would act as though we didn't know whether weight depended on age or whether age depended on weight. We would get the coefficient for the regression of weight on age; we would get the coefficient for the alternative regression of age on weight; we would ablate the direction of these coefficients by multiplying them together; and we would get the correlation coefficient by taking the square root of the product. The result eliminates any statistical necessity for thinking about a scientific direction. The correlation coefficient is a remarkable duplex value: it goes in both directions at once.

After being calculated in this duplex manner, the correlation coefficient is also regularly abused and misinterpreted. Many investigators will perform a test of "significance" on the result and report the associated P value, without ever citing the actual value of r. In this way the reader is kept from knowing whether the correlation of the two variables is quite close (such as r = .94) or almost non-existent (such as r = .06). All we can tell is whether the P value is below or above .05.

Another important issue in interpreting an r value arises from the role of r^2, rather than r. The reason r^2 is called the coefficient of "determination" is that it denotes (or determines) the proportionate amount of variance that has been reduced by fitting a straight line to the data.

This distinction is based on the following reasoning and mathematics. Suppose we have worked with the regression of y on x. The original variance in the y values around their mean, before we fitted the regression equation, was s_{yy}. With algebraic calculations that are shown in most statistical textbooks, it can be demonstrated that s_r, the variance of the y values around the regression line, is $s_r = s_{yy} - bs_{xy}$. The amount of variance that has been reduced by fitting the regression line is therefore s_{yy}

$-s_r$, which is bs_{xy}. The proportion of the original variance that has been eliminated (or "explained") by the regression is bs_{xy}/s_{yy}. Since $b = s_{xy}/s_{xx}$, this expression becomes $(s_{xy})^2/(s_{xx})(s_{yy})$, which is the formula for r^2.

Consequently, if we want a reasonable idea of whether the regression line has done much for the general variance of the system, we should really look at the value of r^2 rather than r. The act of squaring r creates a reversal in size that may surprise many investigators who ordinarily expect the square of a number to be larger than the original number. Because the value of r must lie between -1 and $+1$, the value of r^2 is inevitably smaller than the value of r, except on the rare occasions when r is exactly -1, 0, or $+1$. Thus a correlation coefficient of 0.5 may sometimes seem impressive until we recognize that $r^2 = 0.25$ and that only about a fourth of the total variance has been affected by the "correlation".

The continued popularity of the correlation coefficient is surprising in view of the many authoritative statisticians who have actively denounced it. R. A. Fisher[14] said, "It is seldom . . . desired to express our conclusion in the form of a correlation coefficient". In more modern writing, Armitage[1] states that although "the correlation coefficient has played an important part in the history of statistical methods, it is now of considerably less value than the regression coefficients". Donald Mainland's opinion[19] was that "of all the statistical expressions commonly used in medicine", Pearson's coefficient of correlation was "perhaps the most mysterious, misunderstood and misleading. . . . If it were abolished in medicine we would lose very little, because the valuable information it contains can be found by . . . regression analysis".

In view of all these remarks about the undesirability of correlation coefficients, why have they remained so popular? One principal reason is that the correlation coefficient is "standardized" for units, always being between 0 and $|1|$, whereas the size of a regression coefficient will depend on the magnitude of the units used for expressing the x and y variables. Thus, in examining the relationship of weight to age in children, if we decide to express age in months rather than years, there will be a 12-fold change in the magnitude of the regression coefficient. After a regression coefficient, b, has been noted, the correlation coefficient is therefore an excellent device for "checking" that the size of b has not been made unduly large or small because of a capricious choice of units for expressing the x (or y) variables.

Probably the main reason for the popularity of correlation coefficients, however, is that they eliminate the need for having a sense of direction in the research. They allow the investigator, as well as the statistical consultant, to avoid making any decisions about whether y depends on x or vice versa. The investigator is liberated from having to do any difficult scientific thinking and can concentrate on the mathematics. This aspect of the correlation procedure may account for its frequent use in certain research domains where the investigator hopes that statistical procedures, such as factor analysis (a multivariate correlation technique), will generate hypotheses and decisions from the data. With factor analysis or with its multivariate cousin, principal component analysis, the variables are all analyzed as an interdependent mélange.[10] No dependent (or target) variable is established and none need be contemplated. The conclusions can emerge not from scientific thought, but from the statistical analysis.

Despite these disadvantages, the correlation coefficient continues to be the single most common index of association that appears in general medical literature. In the survey of usage of statistical procedures that was reported a year ago[12], correlation coefficients were found to have been employed almost twice as often as regression coefficients. (The ratio of usage was 52 to 30.) When I cited the results of that survey, I pointed out some of the poor or inappropriate statistical practices (such as unlabelled $\pm$ signs and inadequate descriptions of dispersion) that were being encouraged by medical editors and their statistical consultants. To that list of malefactions can now be added the excessive use of a directionless scientific wanderer—the duplex correlation coefficient.

D. The direction of a statistical "hypothesis"

Most discussions of "statistical hypotheses" and "tests of significance" contain no attention to perhaps the most important fundamental point: the reason for doing the test. These tests are not sought for casual, haphazard, or random purposes. In order to decide to do the test, the investigator must have received a stimulus. This crucial stimulus, to which we shall return later on, is usually an impressive difference in the results of two groups.

When such a difference has been found, the investigator will want to do a statistical "test of significance". The purpose of the test is to confirm the adequacy of the numbers by indicating that the two groups contain enough people (or objects) so that the difference is unlikely to arise by chance. For example, if patients treated with Agent A have a 25% improvement rate and patients treated with Agent B have a 75% improvement rate, the 50% difference between the groups is obviously impressive. Our confidence in this initial impression might disappear immediately, however, if we learned that each group contained only 4 patients, so that the 25% vs. 75% was based on the numbers 1/4 vs. 3/4.

The possibly fortuitous aspects of these small numbers are intuitively evident by an "eye test", but if we wanted to be more statistically precise about the judgment, we could proceed as follows. If the two treatments A and B are identical, what we have observed is a total group of 8 people of whom 4 later had a successful outcome. When these 8 people were divided into two groups, each containing 4 members, what was the likelihood that, by sheer chance, one group would contain 3 successful patients and the other group would contain 1 successful patient?

This question can be answered with several forms of statistical calculation. Perhaps the simplest is to determine the exact probability for the random likelihood of the occurrence[11]. There are 70 different ways $[= 8!/(4!)(4!)]$ in which a group of 8 people can be divided into two groups, each containing 4 people. There is only one way of getting a

split as extreme as 0/4 vs. 4/4. [The calculation is $\{4!/(4!)(0!)\} \times \{4!/(0!)(4!)\} = 1$.] There is also one way of getting the split that is 4/4 vs. 0/4. There are 16 ways of getting the split of 1/4 vs. 3/4. [The calculation is $\{4!/(3!)(1!)\} \times \{4!/(1!)(3!)\} = 4 \times 4 = 16$.] There are also 16 ways of getting the split 3/4 vs. 1/4. Finally, with an analogous set of calculations based on $(4!)/(2!)(2!)$, we would find that there are 36 ways of getting the split of 2/4 vs. 2/4.

Of the 70 possible ways in which these 8 people could be divided by chance alone, we would therefore find on 17 occasions that the split is at least as large as the observed result of 1/4 vs. 3/4. This relative frequency of 17/70 has a P value of .24. If we did not care about whether A or B was the superior agent, the result we observed would occur by chance on 34 of the 70 occasions, with a P value of .48. Thus, in the 8 patients we have been considering, an unequal split in the success rates was almost as likely to occur by chance as the equal split of 2/4 vs. 2/4.

The investigator who did an "eye test" and concluded that 1/4 vs. 3/4 was not "statistically significant" probably did not go through all of this computation. He may be gratified, however, to know that the statistical results agree with his intuition. Another circumstance in which an investigator could draw a conclusion by "eye test" would occur if the 25% vs. 75% difference was based on the numbers 100/400 vs. 300/400. Here the investigator's scientific intuition would indicate that the numbers are surely large enough to be "statistically significant". (An investigator who trusts neither his eyes nor his intuition about these data can do a chi-square test, which yields $\chi^2 = 200$, $P < .000001$; so that there is less than one chance in a million that the difference arose fortuitously.)

The two circumstances that have just been described (1/4 vs. 3/4 and 100/400 vs. 300/400) are extreme instances in which a statistical conclusion about "significance" could be drawn by any sensible investigator who merely looked at the data. In most other circumstances, however, the size of the numbers is not immediately convincing in either direction. An example of such a situation for 25% vs. 75% would occur with the numbers 3/12 vs. 9/12. For these and many other numerical contrasts that create an impressive difference, the investigator wants statistical help to convince himself and his audience that the difference is not merely a fortuitous act of numerical chance.

The statistical strategy that provides this help begins with the invocation of a "null hypothesis". As shown in the preceding example, we make the assumption that the two treatments are equivalent and that therefore they should produce the same results. With this assumption, we then determine how often, by chance alone, we would encounter a difference that is as large as, or larger than, the one we actually observed. If this chance encounter is sufficiently uncommon—for example, having a relative frequency of less than one time in twenty, so that $P < .05$—we would reject the null hypothesis and declare the difference to be "statistically significant".

The statistical reasoning seems convoluted, but it works quite well and it is actually analogous to certain aspects of clinical diagnostic reasoning. In many acts of diagnosis, a clinician contemplates an array of alternative possibilities that he then rejects (or "rules out"), leaving the actual diagnosis as the possibility that was not rejected. Thus, we diagnose a patient as having a *common cold* by excluding such alternatives as *pneumonia, hay fever, septicemia,* etc. In null-hypothesis reasoning, we use a reverse kind of exclusion. We assume that the two treatments are equivalent and we find the likelihood that chance alone would produce the observed difference between them. If this likelihood is too small, we reject the null hypothesis and conclude that the treatments are different.

What the foregoing discussion should have served to make clear is that the idea of a "hypothesis" is quite different for statisticians and scientists. For a scientist, a hypothesis is a complex array of concepts that outline the architecture and goals of the research, indicating the phenomenon that is to be examined and either demonstrated or refuted. Is coronary

bypass surgery worth its risks in patients with angina pectoris? In mothers who smoke cigarettes, is the lower average birth weight of infants caused by the smoking or by features intrinsic to the smoker? Does DNA have a double-helical structure? To formulate a hypothesis, the scientist must choose what to explore, how to explore it, what to consider as a contrasting counter-hypothesis, and how to explore the counter-hypothesis. The diverse scientific decisions involve intensive thought about a large variety of issues in choices of the initial state, the comparative maneuvers, and the subsequent state of the material or people examined in the research.

For a statistician, however, the hypothesis is a simple algebraic equation that can be cited in the same rote way for almost every research project, regardless of the investigator's methods, materials, or goals. Thus, to examine the "statistical significance" of a set of research data, the statistician need not think about any of the scientific complexities that entered the design and conduct of the research. Instead, to formulate the null hypothesis, the statistician can convert everything into a single line of eight symbols that are usually put together as:

$$H_0: \mu_1 = \mu_2$$

In this array of symbols, the "H_0:" indicates that what follows is the statement of the statistician's null hypothesis. The symbols μ_1 and μ_2 refer to the means for a selected variable in the populations exposed to the contrasted maneuvers, designated as 1 and 2. This algebraic statement allows the complexity of the research to be neatly dissected, removed, and repackaged so that it need no longer be considered. From the many types of events and data observed in the research, a single variable is chosen. We calculate the means from the values of this variable that were observed in the members of groups 1 and 2; and we then assume, with the null hypothesis, that the two means are identical in the parent population from which these groups came.

At this point, a thoughtful scientist may immediately raise some objections. Why express the results as a mean? Why can't we use a median or a percentage, or some other summary value? The answer to this objection is that some other citation could be used. The null hypothesis can be expressed with whatever measurement we wanted to employ. For a percentage, the null hypothesis might be cited as H_0: $\pi_1 = \pi_2$.

The scientist might now want to know why the statistician expresses the hypothesis by using Greek symbols that represent the parameters of a parent population. Why not use the actual values found in the "samples" that constituted groups 1 and 2? Why not say, for the mean, H_0 : $\bar{x}_1 = \bar{x}_2$ (rather than $\mu_1 = \mu_2$); or for a proportion, H_0: $p_1 = p_2$ (rather than $\pi_1 = \pi_2$)? The answer to this question is that a classically trained statistician always thinks about a great imaginary parent population out there somewhere in the sky, consorting with its Greek parameters. The statistician may never observe the members of that population, get its data, or determine its parameters, but he must create the imaginary population in order to do the infinitely repetitive imaginary samplings that will allow him to work with sampling distributions, confidence intervals, and the other intellectual paraphernalia that occupy classical parametric tests of "statistical significance".

Besides, the results obtained with the parametric tactics are usually not too different from what can be found with the modern permutation tests that are more directly suitable for scientific research[11]. (The permutation procedures develop their "parent" distributions, relative frequency counts, and probability values not from any theoretical models but from the actual data encountered in the investigation.) Furthermore, even when the data are analyzed with permutation procedures, the null hypothesis is still invoked as a starting point by assuming that treatment-1 (or maneuver-1) is equivalent to treatment-2 (or maneuver-2). So if the scientist doesn't like $\mu_1 = \mu_2$, he can re-write things as $T_1 \backsimeq T_2$ or $M_1 \backsimeq M_2$.

Finally, the scientist may say, isn't it silly to use the results for only one variable during an evaluation of what has happened in a complex experiment containing observations for multiple variables and multiple outcomes? The statistician's answer would be that a null hypothesis can be formulated and a test of

"significance" performed for each of those variables. Instead of doing one "test of significance", we could do two, or five, or a hundred—one test at a time for each of the pertinent variables. Alternatively, the statistician might offer to perform a multivariate test of significance[10], incorporating all of the different outcome phenomena into a single test result such as Hotelling's T^2 or Mahalanobis' D^2.

At this point, the scientist might wonder about what interpretation can be used for those multiple individual tests; or whether the single all-encompassing multivariate test contains suitable values and judgments for the relative importance of the different individual variables that are all bunched together. But the scientist wants to get back to the basic issues and so he is willing to feel placated enough to proceed to the next act of statistical reasoning.

Like a scientist, a statistician recognizes that the mere statement of a hypothesis is not enough. There should also be an alternative or counter-hypothesis, which can be symbolized as H_A. If the null hypothesis is H_0: $\mu_1 = \mu_2$, what should be the counter-hypothesis? In order to answer this question, we must contemplate yet another aspect of direction in research. To a statistician, this question is answered with H_A: $\mu_1 \neq \mu_2$. By using the $\neq$ sign and saying merely that μ_1 does not equal μ_2, we can cover the entire array of alternative possibilities while requiring no knowledge or scientific perception about any of them. There is no need to contemplate whether μ_1 is larger than μ_2 or smaller; or how much larger or smaller the difference may be. The scientist may be thinking about $\mu_1 > \mu_2$ or $\mu_1 >>> \mu_2$, or vice versa; but the statistician will automatically assume merely that $\mu_1 \neq \mu_2$, unless the scientist deliberately specifies otherwise.

This type of "otherwise" thinking actually occurs so often that in many acts of scientific reasoning, the statistical null hypothesis is an erroneous statement. The expression for many null hypotheses should *not* be H_0: $\mu_1 = \mu_2$; it should be H_0: $\mu_1 \leq \mu_2$. The alternative should not be H_A: $\mu_1 \neq \mu_2$; it should be H_A: $\mu_1 > \mu_2$. For example, when we test a new treatment against a placebo, we anticipate that

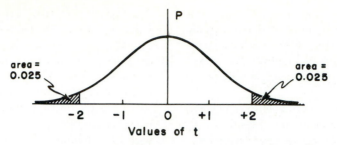

Fig. 1. Demarcation of area under the curve at P = .05 for a two-sided distribution of t, at 100 degrees of freedom. (The vertical axis here and in Fig. 2 is marked "P" but is really a probability "density" at each point. The P value is the area under the curve beyond a specific ordinate.)

the treatment will be *better* than placebo. If we thought that the treatment might be worse, we wouldn't be testing it. Consequently, we are interested in a directional null hypothesis, which is that the treatment is either no better than placebo or is worse.

At this point, a classically trained statistician, reluctant to abandon the rigidity of his traditional duplex thinking, might respond by pointing out that in the sagacities of statistical plans, we must anticipate the possibility that the new treatment may be worse than placebo. The scientist could then immediately respond that he is quite aware of that possibility and quite interested in it, but it is not part of his *scientific* hypothesis. If the research results show that the new treatment is worse than placebo, the scientist will usually have no desire to confirm the "statistical significance" of the inferiority. The scientist's next step will be either to start looking for a newer and better treatment; or to try to determine what went wrong in either the treatment or the investigation that produced results so contrary to the scientific hypothesis.

There are circumstances, of course, in which a scientist really does want to examine both of the alternative directions. One example is a comparison of two treatments in which there is no reason to suspect that one is better than the other. Another example is in an efficacy trial of a new drug vs. placebo, where we might be looking at an outcome such as side effects, for which we might want to test the superiority (or inferiority) that is found in either direction.

For all these reasons, the formulation of an alternative statistical hypothesis should not be a reflex act of writing $\mu_2 \neq \mu_2$. Since the investigator, not the statistician, knows (or should know) the scientific hypothesis of the research, the investigator must make certain that the alternative algebraic hypothesis is established on the basis of specified scientific direction, rather than rote statistical duplexity.

E. Unilateral vs. bilateral directions of probability

The main reason for giving so much attention to the algebraic formulation of these hypotheses is that they determine how the subsequent P values will be calculated or interpreted.

When we compute the relative frequencies that become P values in a permutation test[11], we have to decide whether to look in one direction or both. If the observed probabilities are 2/7 vs. 6/8, the array of unilateral possibilities to be considered under the null hypothesis are the permutations that would produce the results of 2/7 vs. 6/8, 1/7 vs. 7/8, and 0/7 vs. 8/8. These are the arrangements that would yield a difference that is just as large or larger—in the same direction—as the difference we actually observed. Using the Fisher exact probability test[11, 14], we would find that the random relative frequencies (or probabilities) for these arrangements respectively are .0914, .0087, and .0002, so that their sum, which is .1003, would be the unidirectional P value. If the size of the difference was our main concern, regardless of the direction from which the difference emerged, we would have to contemplate some additional arrangements of the same data. These arrangements, coming from the opposite direction, would be 7/7 vs. 1/8 and 6/7 vs.

2/8. The relative frequencies of these two arrangements, respectively, are .0012 and .0305, with a sum of .0317 as the probability on the other side. For a bilateral probability value in the exact test, therefore, the answer would be .1003 + .0317 = .1320.

The reasoning and the decisions are quite straightforward when we use a permutation test, such as the Fisher exact probability test, because it gives us the actual probability values for random rearrangements of the results that were observed in our data. In classical statistical tests of significance, however, everything becomes more complicated. First we calculate a "test statistic", such as t or chi-square, from the data that were actually observed. This is the last thing we do that involves real data. Everything else takes us into the world of mathematical conjecture. First, we conjure up a grand theoretical parent population in the sky. Then we find the "sampling distribution" of the "test statistic" by conjuring up an infinite number of random samples taken from that parent population, with each sample having the same number of "degrees of freedom" as the groups we actually observed in our research. For each of those individual imaginary samples, we calculate the value of t or chi-square. From each of those individual calculated values of t or chi-square, we prepare a graph showing their relative frequencies of occurrence. This curve of relative frequencies becomes the basis for the probability values we seek. At the value of t or chi-square that was observed in our data, we erect a perpendicular line to the curve. The area under the curve that lies outside this perpendicular line is the P value that we want.

An example of what this all looks like is contained in Fig. 1, which shows the curve of the sampling distribution at 100 degrees of freedom for the test statistic that is called *t*. The curve is symmetrical, with one probability area of .025 lying beyond the value of t = +2, and a similar probability area lying beyond t = −2. If we want to know the random chance of finding a t value whose absolute magnitude is 2 or greater, we would add the sum of those two areas, which is P = 0.05. If our hypothesis goes in a single direction, so that we want to know the random chance of t being greater than

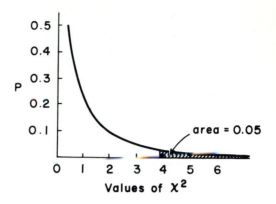

Fig. 2. Demarcation of area under the curve at P = .05 for the distribution of χ^2 at 1 degree of freedom.

+2, we would contemplate only the right hand "tail" of this distribution. For the one-sided hypothesis, P is 0.025.

Fig. 2 gives an example of the sampling distribution of chi-square for 1 degree of freedom. This is the particular chi-square curve that is pertinent for the 2 × 2 "contingency" tables to which the chi-square test is commonly applied. This curve is not symmetrical because χ^2 never takes on any negative values. In the calculation of χ^2, we square the observed difference in the two proportions, p_1 and p_2. Regardless of whether we are interested in $p_1 - p_2$ or in $p_2 - p_1$, χ^2 depends on $(p_1 - p_2)^2$, which is the same as $(p_2 - p_1)^2$. Consequently, the values of χ^2 are always positive, and the associated probabilities in the χ^2 distribution are always bilateral. They include both the possibility that $p_2 > p_1$ and the possibility that $p_2 < p_1$.

To determine the sampling distribution for each test statistic at each degree of freedom, to draw the curves of each array of relative frequencies, and to calculate the areas that lie under the curve beyond each value of the test statistic would be a formidable chore. Fortunately, we can be spared all this work because our statistical colleagues have already done it for us. They have worked out the complete details of each theoretical sampling distribution for each test statistic at each "degree of freedom". The details have been organized so that we need not even look at the distribution curve to erect a perpendicular line and measure an "external" area of probability. This area has already been measured for us. It becomes the P values that are listed in the familiar tripartite tables that show a confluence of three items: the value of t (or whatever test statistic is being used); the associated number of degrees of freedom; and the associated value for P.

In using these tables, however, we still have to decide whether the P value we seek is unilateral ("one-sided") or bilateral ("two-sided"). If the alternative hypothesis is $\mu_1 \neq \mu_2$, the test is bilateral, since we want to know the possibility that μ_1 is either greater than or less than μ_2. If the alternative hypothesis is unidirectional, such as $\mu_1 < \mu_2$, the probability should correspondingly have only one direction.

To illustrate this point, suppose we have found a mean value of 11.3 in Group A and a mean of 14.4 in Group B. According to the null hypothesis, we want to know the likelihood of finding a difference of 3.1 units by chance. Suppose each group contains 51 members, with the standard error estimated as 1.7 units for the population. The associated value of t would be $3.1/1.7 = 1.82$. If our test is two-sided, we are really asking for the probabilities that are found on both sides of the symmetrical t-distribution—the probability of getting a value of t greater than 1.82 and the probability of getting a value of t less than -1.82. The sum of those two probabilities is what emerges in the conventional bilateral test. When we look in a table of two-sided probabilities for t at 100 degrees of freedom, we see that $P = 0.1$ for $t = 1.661$ and $P = .05$ for $t = 1.982$. Consequently, for our observed t of 1.82, we find that $.05 < P < .1$, so that the result is not "statistically significant".

On the other hand, if we expected Group B to have a larger value than Group A, so that our null hypothesis was $\mu_A \leq \mu_B$, the subsequent test would be one-sided. We would want to know only the probability of encountering a value of t greater than 1.82. To find this information, we can either go to a set of tables that show the one-sided probabilities or we can take half the probability values listed in a table of two-sided results. For the situation just described, we would get $.025 < P < .05$, and the result would now be "statistically significant". Thus, according to the way we formulate the null hypothesis and use the t-tables, the same set of data may or may not be "statistically significant".

When the procedure is a chi-square test, rather than a t-test, the situation is somewhat trickier. On seeing the asymmetrical "one-tail" curve of the chi-square distribution, users of the test may become confused and may conclude erroneously that the associated P value refers to a unilateral probability. The fact is, however, that the idea of two-sidedness is built into the calculation of chi-square itself. In a t-test for $x_A = 10$ vs. $\bar{x}_B = 12$, the t value is opposite to what we would get if $\bar{x}_A = 12$ and $\bar{x}_B = 10$. If $p_A = .10$ and $p_B = .12$, however, the chi-square value is identical to what we would get for $p_A = .12$ and $p_B = .10$. Because the probabilities associated with the asymmetrical chi-square curves are always two-sided, we cannot find a one-sided result by looking for a value on the "other side" of the curve. We simply take half the associated value of probability. For example, in the customary table of chi-square values at one degree of freedom, P is 0.10 when χ^2 is 2.706 and P is 0.05 when χ^2 is 3.841. Consequently, a χ^2 value of 3.12 would not be "significant" in a two-sided test because $0.05 < P < 0.1$. If the test were one-sided, however, this same value of χ^2 would become "significant" at $P < .05$ because the associated probability values would be halved.

These illustrations of both the permutation and the "test statistic" methods of getting a P value have shown why an investigator will usually prefer the unilateral tests of probability. They are more consistent with the unidirectional design of a scientific hypothesis and they also offer a "better" P value for the same investment in research data. The results are always more likely to be "statistically significant" if the probabilities are evaluated in a one-sided manner.

Many statisticians, however, are reluctant to accept the idea of allowing a directional scientific decision to affect the operation of a duplex statistical procedure. One of the most vigorous statements of the statistical ideology was provided by Langley[17] as follows:

> There is a lot of muddled thinking about this particular aspect of statistical inference, even in high places. . . . The whole aim of statistical tests is to eliminate guesswork and to put inductive logic on a mathematical footing, and this means that these tests must remain completely objective. This impartiality, this freedom from human foible, is only possible if we stick to two-sided probabilities. . . . (The problem) is solved simply by using two-sided probabilities as a routine for all significance tests.

This adamant opposition to the use of one-sided probabilities is particularly likely to arise among statisticians who have consulted extensively for research in education, psychology, and the social sciences. In these domains, the investigator is seldom able to study the effects of interventional maneuvers and may have difficulty specifying a dependent relationship or a directional hypothesis. Consequently, certain investigators sometimes try to generate their scientific hypotheses after the data have been analyzed rather than beforehand, and the investigators may often want to juggle the statistical hypothesis into a unilateral direction in order to get the P values down below the magic marker level of 0.05. These research strategies have been thoroughly debated in an extensive series of publications of which many statisticians seem lamentably unaware. Anthologies of the controversy over hypothesis testing and number of "sides" for probability are presented in references 21 and 23.

In the domain of biologic and clinical science, the ability to study interventional maneuvers (with either experiments or surveys) often allows the investigator to formulate a unidirectional scientific hypothesis. Accordingly, one might expect contemporary biometricians to be reasonably flexible about whether the statistical test should be one-sided or two-sided. To check this expectation, I went through my collection of 18 books that are devoted to medical or biologic statistics. I found, to my surprise, that two of the most famous books—by Fisher[14] and by Bradford Hill[3]—contained no mention (or at least none that I could find) of the distinction between a unilateral or bilateral direction for probability. A medical reader who relied on these two books might never discover that such decisions have to be made whenever he uses a table of probability values.

The remaining textbooks could be divided into three categories. The describe-but-don't-prescribe books contain an account of the two kinds of decisions, but do not seem to provide any instructions on how to make the decision. The even-handed-approach books, as exemplified by Schor[22] and by Huntsberger and Leaverton[15], describe the two different kinds of hypotheses and indicate the circumstances in which each hypothesis should be applied. Mainland[19], who must have met a trauma of investigators who wanted to alter their hypotheses after the data were analyzed, prefers two-sided tests because "we should beware of the temptation to lower our standards by giving ourselves a better chance of obtaining a 'positive' result". The other books containing a two-sides-are-almost-always-better-than-one argument range from Campbell's view[4] that "one-sided tests are justified only rarely but . . . we ought always to consider their possible relevance" to Armitage's assertion[1] that "it will be safe to assume that significance tests should almost always be two-sided".

My own view is in accord with the even-handed school. Since the decision should always be based on scientific rather than statistical considerations, there is no reason for a statistician to approach the decision with any mathematically authoritative pontifications or preconceptions. The investigator should be obligated to state, before the analysis, whether his scientific hypothesis is unidirectional or bidirectional; the statistical hypothesis should then be appropriately one-sided or two-sided; and the unilateral or bilateral aspects of probability should follow accordingly. From time to time, a statistical consultant will encounter an investigator who cannot state any form of direction. This difficulty usually arises not in deciding whether to go one way or two ways in the statistical null hypothesis, but because the scientific hypothesis itself is either malformed or amorphous. The research is directionless because it is aimless. In this situation, the statistical consultant can do everyone a service not by conservatively applying the "objective" two-sided tests of "significance", but by advising the investigator to re-think the goals and aims of the research itself.

F. The size of the rejection zone

We can now turn our attention to a magnitude, rather than a direction, that is an integral part of statistical hypothesis testing.

At the end of either a one-sided or two-sided test is a statistically blessed region called the *rejection zone*. It is the place where the investigator can happily set aside the null hypothesis and proclaim those magical words—sacred to reviewers, editors, and granting agencies— "statistical significance". The rejection zone is demarcated by the choice of a fixed probability level, called α, which is usually taken to be either .05, .01, or .001. If the P value in the research data is below the chosen level of α, we reject the null hypothesis, state that the results are "statistically significant", and conclude that the observed difference is real.

This is the "positive" conclusion that an investigator usually wants to attain in doing a test of "significance". The level of α establishes the proportionate risk that the conclusion will be falsely positive—that a correct null hypothesis has been erroneously rejected. If the null hypothesis is true, we would want to accept it and draw the "negative" conclusion that the results are "not significant". The likelihood of being correct in this decision will be $1 - \alpha$. Consequently, if $\alpha = .05$, and if we make decisions for 100 instances in which the null hypothesis is true, we will be right 95 times and wrong 5 times. The value of $1 - \alpha$, which is thus equivalent to the specificity of a diagnostic test, is also the source of statistical concepts of "confidence". If $\alpha = .05$, our confidence level is $1 - \alpha$, or 95%, that we will be right when we accept the null hypothesis and conclude that a difference is "not significant". As α gets smaller, our "confidence" rises in the specificity of the negative decision.

The smaller the magnitude of α, the greater is the exuberance with which "significance" is proclaimed when the P value falls below α. For some investigators, if P is respectively below

.05, .01, or .001, the upward verbal declension of significance ascends from "statistically significant" to "highly statistically significant" to "very highly statistically significant". For others, the sequence is *significant, decisive,* and *conclusive*[20]; or it may be *significant, highly significant,* and *determinant.*[2] I have sometimes heard the sequence or *super, wow,* and *eureka.* In computer print-outs, the machine's grandiloquence is restrained to a symbolic Guide-Michelin expression of *, **, or ***.

A sober scientist, encountering all this verbal or symbolic jubilation about a P value, may wonder how these sacred boundaries were ordained and why the sanctification should arise from the test of a *statistical* hypothesis, in contrast to the analysis of a *scientific* hypothesis and its associated results. In a later essay in this series, I shall give detailed discussion to the perversion of the word "significance" as one of the many intellectual pollutants that an inappropriate use of statistical theory has brought to modern medical science. For the moment, however, we can focus on the choice of the magic level of $\alpha = .05$.

The role of this number in demarcating "significance" has become so widely accepted and worshipped that one might expect to find a record of the time and place when the apotheosis occurred. No such record, however, seems to exist. I have looked through a series of books devoted to the history of probability, statistics, and science, but the historians do not seem to have taken note of an event so prominent in the development of a statistical hegemony over scientific decisions.

According to Donald Mainland[18], the statistical use of the term "significance", although usually ascribed to R. A. Fisher, was probably introduced in 1896 by Karl Pearson. Pearson's boundary for dividing "significance" from "non-significance" was an entity called the *probable error,* an idea that has since become archaic. Fisher was probably the person who moved the boundary to .05. This choice seems to have arisen from a mathematical phenomenon that could be easily converted into a mnemonically convenient statistical tool. In a Gaussian distribution of data, 95% of the values are in a zone spanned by the mean plus or minus

1.96 standard deviations. Because 1.96 was so close to 2, the number 2 could be easily remembered and the expression $\mu \pm 2\sigma$ (or $\bar{x} \pm 2s$) became a quick, simple shorthand for denoting the zone in which the "common" values of a distribution would be encountered. The 5% of values that lay outside this zone would be regarded as uncommon or "rare".

The next step in the reasoning was easy to take. An event that occurred in the outside 5% zone could be regarded as different enough from the other 95% of events to be called "significant", and to be deemed unlikely to have happened by chance. The fact was, of course, that such events *could* regularly occur by chance, with an occurrence rate of about 1 in every 20 chance occasions. Nevertheless, a boundary was needed for making individual decisions and .05 seemed as good a boundary as any other, particularly since it had the pleasant relationship with 2σ.

Some of Fisher's language is elsewhere quoted by Mainland[19] as follows:

If P is between .1 and .9, there is certainly no reason to suspect the hypothesis tested. If it is below .02 it is strongly indicated that the hypothesis fails to account for the whole   the facts We shall not often be astray if we draw a conventional line at .05 and consider that . . . (lower) values . . . indicate a real discrepancy. . . . It is convenient to take this (.05) point as a limit in judging whether a deviation is to be considered significant or not.

Fisher did not succeed in getting these concepts universally accepted by the statistical establishment. In what is generally accepted today as the "bible" of theoretical statistics, Kendall and Stuart[16] make no mention of .05, .01, or any other specific number as the boundary between what they call the *critical region* and the *acceptance region*. Furthermore, the idea of "statistical significance" does not appear anywhere in the three volumes of the Kendall and Stuart text. In a footnote, the authors explain that they "shall not use" the term because it "can be misleading".

For the world of psychologic and social science research, however, and for many biometric priests and their clinical acolytes, Fisher's words and boundaries have now become sacred writ. Research publications are accepted or rejected; clinical trials are maintained or abruptly terminated; pharmaceutical agents are allowed on the market or withdrawn; and scientific reputations are made or lost—all on the basis of the magisterial phrase and number: *statistical significance at $P \leq .05$*.

G. The size of the substantive difference

The historians who ultimately review the course of twentieth century clinical science will probably not be surprised that an act of critical scientific judgment was converted into an arbitrary numerical shrine. So many judgmental procedures have been obliterated during the twentieth century worship of technology, so many crucial human attributes have been neglected or deliberately omitted during the collection of "hard" data, so many inadequately designed and inadequately analyzed statistical enumerations have become established as the standards of epidemiologic research, and so much effort has been made to arrive at objectivity even at the sacrifice of sensibility—that the conversion of scientific hypotheses to P values will probably be regarded as merely a minor note in the dominant intellectual cacophony of the era.

It is also not surprising that scientists confronted with complex decision-making would have searched for a reliable and effective guideline. Anyone confronted with difficult decisions would seek whatever good advice might be available. What the historians will probably regard as astonishing, however, is that the "enlightened" scientists of the twentieth century would have been so obsequious in accepting a guideline that was neither reliable nor effective.

The P values that arise from statistical "tests of significance" are unreliable guidelines to scientific decisions because P values are totally dependent on the size of the groups under investigation. No matter how trivial or foolish the scientific hypothesis and no matter how petty or inconsequential the difference that is being analyzed, the results will be "statistically significant" if the size of the sample is large enough.

For example, in a test of the difference in means between two groups each of size n, having means x_1 and $\bar{x}_2$ and variances $s_1{}^2$ and $s_2{}^2$, the value of t is $(\sqrt{n})(\bar{x}_1 - \bar{x}_2) \div (\sqrt{s_1{}^2 + s_2{}^2})$. Because of the multiplication by $\sqrt{n}$, if $\bar{x}_1$, $\bar{x}_2$, s_1, and s_2 remain the same, the value of t will rise or fall (and the P value will get correspondingly smaller or larger) merely with changes in the size of n. Analogously, in a test of the difference in percentages p_1 and p_2, between two groups each of size n, the value of chi-square is

$$2n\,(p_1 - p_2)^2 \div [(p_1 + p_2)(2 - p_1 - p_2)]$$

Chi-square thus equals 2n times a particular "function" of p_1 and p_2. Regardless of the individual values found for p_1 and p_2, or their difference, chi-square will rise or fall and the P value will change correspondingly, entirely according to the size of n.

For this reason, an investigator who observes an impressive difference in $\bar{x}_1 - \bar{x}_2$ or in $p_1 - p_2$ is entirely justified in performing a t-test or a chi-square test to determine whether n is large enough to indicate that the result is unlikely to arise by chance. Beyond that probabilistic assessment, however, the investigator engages in a weird distortion of scientific reasoning if he makes decisions that depend on degrees of "significance" in the value of P itself, or if he allows trivial differences to become magnified into "statistical significance" merely because the size of n was large enough to make anything become "significant". The use of P values in this manner has been an especially unfortunate aspect of modern "biostatistics", and the trap has been particularly treacherous for analysts of the huge numbers that sometimes appear in epidemiologic data.

In addition to being unreliable, P values are not an effective guideline to scientific decisions. The magnitude of P has nothing to do with the quantity that should ordinarily concern a scientist: the size of the difference. In the days before investigators became infatuated with statistical tests, a scientist was obligated to establish more than a hypothesis and more than a direction for the hypothesis. The scientist also had to decide about an increment. This increment—the difference in the results of the contrasted groups, as expressed by $\bar{x}_1 - \bar{x}_2$ or by $p_1 - p_2$—was what might be called *substantive significance* or *clinical importance*.

An investigator who observed a 28% improvement rate in the treated group, and 26% in the controls, might have no interest whatsoever in testing the null hypothesis that $p_1 = p_2$ or even that $p_1 < p_2$. To decide that the observed difference was important, the investigator would want p_1 (the value in the treated group) to exceed p_2 by a substantial increment such as 10%. The scientific hypothesis in the research would then be $(p_1 - p_2) \geq .10$, or $p_1 \geq (p_2 + .10)$. For this purpose, the opposite (or null) hypothesis would be that $p_1 < (p_2 + .10)$.

With this statement of a scientifically important increment, the simple algebra of the statistical hypotheses has been invaded by another symbol. It is Δ, the magnitude of the increment that is substantively significant. This increment seldom receives any major attention in statistical textbooks or discussions, possibly because the size of Δ cannot be determined with any act of statistical conjecture or computational prestidigitation. To pay attention to Δ, the statistician must acknowledge the primacy of scientific judgment.

Despite the neglect by statisticians, the size of Δ is usually what makes an investigator decide to use tests of statistical significance. If the observed difference, d, exceeds the size of a chosen increment, Δ, an astute investigator will want assurance that the result is "statistically significant". If d is too small, the investigator may not bother with any probabilistic calculations.

Once we recognize that traditional scientific inference depends on Δ, whereas traditional statistical inference depends on α, we are ready to contemplate yet another aspect of direction in the differences between scientific and statistical reasoning. This new directional activity is usually labelled with the Greek letter β. In statistical terms, $1-\beta$ refers to the "power" of a significance test. In scientific terms, β refers to the directional aspect of being right or wrong when conclusions are drawn about α. Expressed in diagnostic terms, β is the rate of false negative decisions about accepting the null hypothesis, and $1-\beta$ is the "sensitivity" of a positive decision.

These conclusions are regularly discussed (seldom with any real attention to Δ) in statistical textbooks, but the associated reasoning now appears most frequently in another one of the twentieth century's favorite applications of statistical numerology: "the estimation of sample size" for a clinical trial. The strategy, tactics, and abuse of this procedure will be deferred for separate discussion in a future installment of this series.

References

1. Armitage, P.: Statistical methods in medical research, New York, 1971, John Wiley & Sons, Inc., pp. 159 and 104.
2. Atkins, H.: Conduct of a controlled clinical trial, Br. Med. J. **2:**377-379, 1966.
3. Bradford Hill, A.: Principles of medical statistics, ed. 9, New York, 1971, Oxford University Press.
4. Campbell, R. C.: Statistics for biologists, Cambridge, 1967, Cambridge University Press, p. 61.
5. Cornish, E. A.: Preface to Reference 14.
6. Feinstein, A. R.: Clinical biostatistics. X. Sources of 'transition bias' in cohort statistics, CLIN. PHARMACOL. THER. **12:**704-721, 1971.
7. Feinstein, A. R.: Clinical biostatistics. XI. Sources of 'chronology bias' in cohort statistics, CLIN. PHARMACOL. THER. **12:**864-879, 1971.
8. Feinstein, A. R.: Clinical biostatistics. XIX. Ambiguity and abuse in the twelve different concepts of 'control', CLIN. PHARMACOL. THER. **14:**112-122, 1973.
9. Feinstein, A. R.: Clinical biostatistics. XX. The epidemiologic trohoc, the ablative risk ratio, and 'retrospective' research, CLIN. PHARMACOL. THER. **14:**291-307, 1973.
10. Feinstein, A. R.: Clinical biostatistics. XXI. A primer of concepts, phrases, and procedures in the statistical analysis of multiple variables, CLIN. PHARMACOL. THER. **14:**462-477, 1973.
11. Feinstein, A. R.: Clinical biostatistics. XXIII. The role of randomization in sampling, testing, allocation, and credulous idolatry (Part 2), CLIN. PHARMACOL. THER. **14:**898-915, 1973.
12. Feinstein, A. R.: Clinical biostatistics. XXV. A survey of the statistical procedures in general medical journals, CLIN. PHARMACOL. THER. **15:**97-107, 1974.
13. Fisher, R. A.: Design of experiments, ed. 8, New York, 1966, Hafner Publishing Co., p. 2.
14. Fisher, R. A.: Statistical methods for research workers, ed. 14, Edinburgh, 1970, Oliver & Boyd, Ltd., p. 177.
15. Huntsberger, D. V., and Leaverton, P. E.: Statistical inference in the biomedical sciences, Boston, 1970, Allyn & Bacon, Inc., pp. 150-151.
16. Kendall, M. G., and Stuart, A.: The advanced theory of statistics (in three volumes), Longon, 1963, Charles Griffin & Co.
17. Langley, R.: Practical statistics (paperback), London, 1968, Pan Books Ltd., pp. 143 and 146.
18. Mainland, D.: The significance of "nonsignificance", CLIN. PHARMACOL. THER. **4:**580-586, 1963.
19. Mainland, D.: Elementary medical statistics, ed. 2, Philadelphia, 1964, W. B. Saunders Co., pp. 222 and 330.
20. Miller, D. A.: Significant and highly significant, Nature **210:**1190, 1966.
21. Morrison, D. E., and Henkel, R. E., editors: The significance test controversy—a reader, Chicago, 1970, Aldine Publishing Co.
22. Schor, S. Fundamentals of biostatistics, New York, 1968, G. P. Putnam's Sons, Inc., p. 157.
23. Steger, J. A., editor: Readings in statistics for the behavioral scientist, New York, 1971, Holt, Rinehart and Winston, Inc.

CHAPTER 22

Sample size and the other side of statistical significance

'Statistical significance' is commonly tested in biologic research when the investigator has found an impressive difference in two groups of animals or people. If the groups are relatively small, the investigator (or a critical reviewer) becomes worried about a statistical problem. Although the observed difference in the means or percentages is large enough to be biologically (or clinically) significant, do the groups contain enough members for the numerical differences to be 'statistically significant'?

For example, if Group A has a mean of 9.8 units and Group B has a mean of 17.3 units, the difference may be biologically impressive because the second mean is almost twice as large as the first. On the other hand, if the two groups each contain only a few members, or if the data are widely dispersed around the mean values, our biologic impression may not be sustained numerically. The statistical assessments may show that the observed difference could quite easily have arisen by chance alone.

The statistical procedures used to test the numerical 'significance' of an observed difference between two groups have been discussed in several previous installments[4, 6] of this series. The calculations used for the procedures depend on the kind of basic data in which the results were expressed. For dimensional data, the results would be cited as means and the usual statistical procedure would be a t test. For nominal or existential data, the results are expressed as fre-

quency counts that are converted to proportions, percentages, or rates; and the usual statistical procedure would be a chi-square test. (To avoid making unproved assumptions about the distribution of a hypothetical parent population, we can replace the t test by a Pitman permutation test and the chi-square test by a Fisher exact probability test.) If the data are expressed in ranked ordinal values, the usual statistical procedure would be the Wilcoxon rank sum test or the Mann-Whitney U test.

Although each of these tests is chosen according to the type of data under examination, the underlying statistical strategy is identical. It follows the same principle that was used to prove theorems in elementary school geometry. We assume that a particular conjecture is true. We then determine the consequences of that conjecture. If the consequences produce an obvious absurdity or impossibility, we conclude that the original conjecture cannot be true, and we reject it as false.

When this reasoning is used for the statistical strategy that is called "hypothesis testing", the argument proceeds as follows. We have observed a difference, called δ (delta), between Groups A and B. To test its 'statistical significance', we assume, as a conjecture, that Groups A and B are actually not different. This conjecture is called the *null hypothesis*. With this assumption, we then determine how often a difference as large as δ, or even larger, would arise by chance from data for two groups having the same number of members as A and B. The result of this determination is the *P value* that emerges from the statistical test procedure.

This chapter originally appeared as "Clinical biostatistics—XXXIV. The other side of 'statistical significance': alpha, beta, delta, and the calculation of sample size." In Clin. Pharmacol. Ther. 18:491, 1975.

At this point in the reasoning, the statistical strategy departs from what was used to prove theorems in grade school geometry. In geometry, there were no problems in deciding whether or not to reject the assumed conjecture, because the geometrical logic regularly brought us to a situation that was impossible, i.e., the P value was zero. In such a circumstance, the original conjecture could not be maintained. It had to be wrong because it could not possibly be right. With statistical inference, however, the results can seldom, if ever, be so conclusive. The P value that emerges from the calculations in the statistical test may be as small as .000001, or even smaller, but it never becomes zero. There is always a possibility, however infinitesimal, that the observed difference arose by chance alone. Accordingly, unlike the situation in geometry, we cannot use a statistical test to prove with total certainty that the original conjecture is wrong. There is always a chance of 1 in 20, or 1 in 50, or whatever the P value is, that the original conjecture (i.e., the null hypothesis) is right.

To draw statistical conclusions, therefore, we must establish a concept that was not necessary for the inferential reasoning of grade school geometry. This concept is called an α (alpha) *level* of 'significance'. It is used to demarcate the *rejection zone*. If the P value that emerges from the statistical test is equal to or smaller than α, we decide that we shall reject the null hypothesis. In doing so, we demarcate α as the risk of being wrong in this conclusion—but it is a risk we must take in order to have a statistical mechanism for drawing conclusions. In geometrical inference, α was always zero. In statistical inference, α is customarily chosen to be .05, i.e., 1 in 20, although some investigators (or editors) may select other boundaries such as .1 or .01.

A previous paper[6] of this series contained a discussion of the arbitrary way in which .05 became designated as the customary level of α. The designation came, not as a pronouncement of the Deity or from the deliberations of an international committee, but from a habit of R. A. Fisher. Noting that a conclusion had to be drawn after a statistical test was performed, and knowing that an α level was necessary to draw the

conclusion, Fisher chose α to be .05. The rest of the statistical world followed.

A. Statistical reasoning and diagnostic analogies

This reasoning is regularly applied in a way that makes the statistical appraisal of 'significance' resemble a clinical diagnostic test.

1. α level and 'diagnostic specificity'. In using .05 or whatever other α level is selected as boundary for the rejection zone, an investigator specifies the deliberate chance that he wants to allow of being wrong when he decides that the observed difference in his two groups is real. There will exist a probability of magnitude P, however, that the null hypothesis is correct— that the observed difference in the groups has arisen simply by chance, and that the conclusion is wrong.

The α level is thus analogous to the risk of getting a *false positive* result in a diagnostic test[5]. Suppose we make a diagnosis of lung cancer after finding a positive result in the Pap smear of a patient's sputum. If the patient does in fact have lung cancer, the diagnostic decision is correct—a true positive. If the patient does not have lung cancer, the diagnosis is wrong—a false positive conclusion. In the customary situation of hypothesis testing, we want to make a positive decision, rejecting the null hypothesis and concluding that the observed difference is real. The α level indicates the statistical risk that this decision may be wrong and that there is actually no difference between the groups. The value 1-α can therefore be likened to the *specificity* of a diagnostic test, which is the likelihood that the test will have a negative result when the disease is absent. The value of 1-α denotes the likelihood of being correct when we do not reject the null hypothesis and thereby conclude that the observed difference is not 'statistically significant'.

The kind of reasoning used in forming a 'null hypothesis' and in establishing levels of α and 1-α is based on the idea that the 'disease' we are looking for, i.e., a real difference between the groups, is absent. The chance of a false positive diagnosis is α; and the chance of a true negative diagnosis is 1-α. Consequently, if we set α at .05, we take a 5% chance of being wrong if we reject the null hypothesis (i.e., draw a positive conclusion) and a 95% chance of being right if we concede the null hypothesis (i.e., fail to draw a positive conclusion).

This analogy to a false positive result and to the specificity of a diagnostic test can make the α and $1-\alpha$ concepts particularly easy for clinicians to understand, since the idea of a diagnostic test does not appear in the general statistical phrase by which α level is usually called *Type I error*. Probably the main reason for the statistical nomenclature is the difference in the way investigators and statisticians use the inverted logic that customarily goes into hypothesis testing. To an investigator, the test is usually done for a positive reason—to demonstrate that a biologically impressive difference is also statistically impressive. The investigator thus regards a doubly negative phenomenon (rejection of the null hypothesis) as a *positive* event, analogous to getting a positive result in a diagnostic test. In general statistical usage, however, the acceptance or rejection of the null hypothesis is seldom associated with any negative or positive intellectual virtues. Thus, for statistical definitions, a Type I error consists of rejecting the null hypothesis when it is actually true.

2. The calculation of P_A. To apply these principles requires the calculation of a P value for the observed data and the observed difference, δ. This particular P value, which is the conventional one usually cited in medical literature, will be designated here as P_A to distinguish it from other P values that will be discussed later. The procedures used for calculating P_A are presented in detail in textbooks of statistics and will be summarized as follows:

a. The simplest and most generally applicable statistical strategy rests on the idea of a "critical ratio" or "z-score". For any single value randomly chosen from a Gaussian distribution whose constituent values are x_1, x_2, x_3, etc., a critical ratio can be calculated as $z = (x_i - \mu)/\sigma$. In this formula, μ is the mean of the parent distribution; σ is its standard deviation; and x_i is the single value with which we are concerned. If the data under consideration consist of a series of means of samples, each of which has n members randomly drawn from the same par-

ent population, these means also have a Gaussian distribution. Their mean is also μ, but their standard deviation is $\sigma/\sqrt{n}$. This standard deviation of a series of means is called SE, the 'standard error' of the mean. The corresponding critical ratio for any of these means, $\bar{x}$, is $z = (\bar{x} - \mu)/(\sigma/\sqrt{n})$.

b. If we want to analyze a difference in the means, $\bar{x}$ and $\bar{y}$, of two samples, we seek the distribution of a new variable, $w = \bar{x} - \bar{y}$. This variable, which has its own mean, will have a "common" standard deviation that can be calculated in one of two ways. If we assume, by the null hypothesis, that the population variances of $\bar{x}$ and $\bar{y}$ are equal, we can create a "pooled variance" for w. If we do not assume equality of population variances for $\bar{x}$ and $\bar{y}$, then the common variance of w equals the sum of the variance of $\bar{x}$ and the variance of $\bar{y}$. In particular, if the mean values, $\bar{x}$ and $\bar{y}$, happen to be proportions, p_1 and p_2, we can calculate the common variance as follows:

1. If we assume that the population values for $p_1 = p_2$, the common mean for both samples is $\bar{p} = (np_1 + np_2)/2n = (p_1 + p_2)/2$. The common variance of the difference in proportions is $2\bar{p}(1 - \bar{p})/n$.

2. If we do not assume that the population values for $p_1 = p_2$, the common variance is calculated as $[p_1(1 - p_1) + p_2(1 - p_2)]/n$.

The corresponding z values for these two cases would be $(p_1 - p_2)/\sqrt{2\bar{p}(1 - \bar{p})/n}$ in the first instance, and $(p_1 - p_2)/\sqrt{[p_1(1 - p_1) + p_2(1 - p_2)]/n}$ in the second. In general, the formula for calculating the z value of a difference in means is

$$z = \frac{\text{difference in means}}{\text{"standard error" of the difference}}$$

c. Regardless of whether a particular critical ratio of z is calculated for a single mean or for a difference in means, the z values have some distinctive, important properties. If we drew a large series of samples, consisting of single means or differences in means, and if the sample sizes were themselves large, and if a z score were calculated for each sampling, the array of z values would approximate a 'standard normal' distribution, having a mean of 0 and a standard deviation of 1. Furthermore, each positive (or nega-

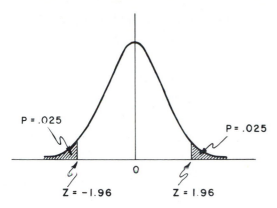

Fig. 1. Standard Gaussian distribution showing values of z for two-sided P = .05.

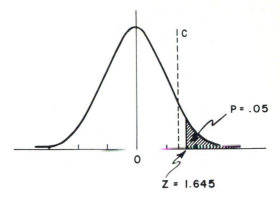

Fig. 2. Standard Gaussian distribution showing value of z for one-sided P = .05. Line drawn at c represents an observed value.

tive) value of z will be associated with a value of P, which represents the amount of 'exterior' probability as the area that lies beneath the standard Gaussian curve to the left (or right) of an ordinate erected at z. Because the entire area below the curve has a probability value of 1, the value of P for the area beyond z will be .5 when z = 0 (since half of the curve lies to the right—or left—of the corresponding ordinate). Some other pertinent results, which can be found in the tables of most statistical textbooks, are as follows:

z value	0	1.28	1.645	1.96	2.58
P value	.5	.1	.05	.025	.005

d. For any selected exterior level of probability, α, there will correspond a value of z_α, denoting the point on the abscissa at which an area of α is cut off under the probability curve. Thus, if α is set at .005, $z_{.005} = 2.58$. The choice of the associated z values for an α level depends on whether the area of exterior probability is being considered in a one-sided or two-sided direction. For a two-sided test, the exterior probability area is divided symmetrically at the extremes of the curve. Thus, if $\alpha = .05$ for a two-sided test, we would seek the value of z for $\alpha/2$, which is $z_{.025} = 1.96$. This distinction is shown in Fig. 1. For a one-sided test, however, all of the exterior probability is placed on one side of the curve, as shown in Fig. 2. Thus, if $\alpha = .05$ but if the test is one-sided, we would seek the value of $z_{.05}$, which is 1.645. This shift

from a two-sided to a one-sided test therefore reduces the value of z from 1.96 to 1.645. The line drawn at *c* in Fig. 2 shows the location of an observed difference, $p_2 - p_1$, and the associated z value. (The actual z value is determined as $z_c = (p_2 - p_1)/SE$.) Since c does not lie within the shaded boundary, the observed $p_2 - p_1$ difference would be regarded statistically as 'not significant' in a one-sided test at the selected level of α.

e. With an appropriate statistical table showing z and P values, we can thus readily move back and forth from an observed difference in two proportions (or means), to a value of z, to an associated value of P. When the calculations are performed after the data have been obtained, this P value is the P_A mentioned at the beginning of this section.

3. *The calculation of sample size for α and Δ levels.* The Type-I or α-error approach that has just been described has often been used to determine—before the research is performed—the sample size required to attain 'statistical significance' in a contrast of two groups. For this process, the formula that was used to get the value of z is algebraically manipulated so that we solve for n instead.

a. *Information needed for calculations.* Four items of information must be assigned, estimated, known, or assumed in order to do the calculations.

1. We must assign a value of *delta* that

will be regarded as a biologically impressive difference between the means (or rates) found in the control group and in the treated (or 'experimental') group. Because this value of delta is assigned before the research, it will be designated here as Δ, to distinguish it from the δ value observed after the data are obtained.

2. We must estimate the standard error of the difference in the means or rates of the two groups. For rates or percentages, we will know from previous research the particular value, p_1, that is to be expected in the control group. The experimental group will then be required to have a value p_2 which is higher or lower than p_1 by the amount, Δ. We can then calculate the standard error of the assigned difference, $p_2 - p_1$, by using the formula described in the previous section. [For dimensional data, we take Δ to be the difference in means, and we assume that the experimental group will have the same variance (or standard deviation) that is expected in the control group.]

3. We assign a level of α (thereby indicating z_α) as the chosen level of 'significance.' [This level of α actually represents P_α.]

4. We assume that the two groups will each be of size n, and that the total sample size will be $N = 2n$.

b. Example of calculations. To illustrate this process, suppose we will regard a new treatment as 'useful' if it raises the percentage of success by 10% from its customary level of 50% in the control group. For a one-sided result, statistically significant at the level of $\alpha = .05$, how large a sample do we need if this difference actually occurs?

We have assigned $\Delta = .1$ and $\alpha = .05$. Since the test is one-sided, we find from the table that $z_{.05} = 1.645$. Since we know that $p_1 = .50$, we estimate $p_2 = p_1 + \Delta = .60$. We quickly determine $\bar{p}$ as $(p_1 + p_2)/2 = .55$. Assuming the null hypothesis, the common variance of the difference in p_1 and p_2 is $2\bar{p}(1 - \bar{p})/n$, which is $(2)(.55)(.45)/n = (.495)/n$. We now have all the information we need to solve for n in the formula

$$z = \frac{\Delta}{\sqrt{2\bar{p}(1 - \bar{p})/n}}.$$

Squaring both sides and isolating n, we get

$$n = \frac{z^2[2\bar{p}(1 - \bar{p})]}{\Delta^2}.$$

Substituting appropriately, we find

$$n = \frac{(1.645)^2(.495)}{(.1)^2} = 133.9 \simeq 134.$$

Since n is the size of one sample, the total group needed for the proposed research would be 2n, or 268 patients. Had we decided to use a two-sided test of probability (just in case the treatment was 10% *worse* than the controls) the value of z would have been $z_{.025} = 1.96$ and n would have been calculated to be $(1.96)^2(.495)/(.1)^2 = 190.2 \simeq 191$ patients. The total required sample size would have been 382 patients.

Readers who feel more comfortable with the chi-square test of 'significance' than with the z procedure might like to see how this same result can be attained using the chi-square formula. As shown elsewhere[3], the formula for calculating chi-square for frequency data expressed as two proportions, each from a group of size n, is

$$\chi^2 = \left[\frac{(n)\,(n)}{2n}\right]\left[\frac{\Delta^2}{\bar{p}\bar{q}}\right]$$

where $\bar{q} = 1 - \bar{p}$. This formula can be solved for n to yield $n = 2\bar{p}(1 - \bar{p})\chi^2/\Delta^2$. For $\alpha = .05$ in a two-sided chi-square test at 1 degree of freedom (as befits a test of two proportions), the critical value of χ^2 is 3.84. Substituting this value of χ^2 into the formula gives us exactly the same result that was obtained with the z procedure.

The reason for using the relatively unfamiliar z procedure, rather than our old friend chi-square, is that the z procedure can be applied for dimensional data as well as for proportions. More importantly, the z procedure is especially useful for illustrating the additional concepts that are to appear shortly.

4. The role of β and 'false negatives'. All of the strategies and tactics that have just been discussed constitute a long-standing, well established statistical procedure that is still used by many investigators as the 'natural' way to calculate sample size. In 1928, however, Jerzy Neyman and Egon S. Pearson[10] pointed out that the reasoning was incomplete. According to the Neyman-Pearson argument, a statistical test of 'significance', like a medical test of

Table I. *Analogies of conclusions in diagnostic and statistical reasoning*

	Diagnostic reasoning	
	Disease is really:	
Result of diagnostic test	*Present*	*Absent*
Positive	True positive diagnosis	False positive diagnosis
Negative	False negative diagnosis	True negative diagnosis

	Statistical reasoning	
	Significant difference is really:	
Result of statistical test	*Present, i.e., null hypothesis not true*	*Absent, i.e., null hypothesis true*
Reject null hypothesis	No error; probability: $1-\beta$	Type I error: Probability: α
Concede, i.e., do not reject null hypothesis	Type II error; probability: β	No error; probability: $1-\alpha$

diagnosis, has another side to it. In diagnosis, when thinking about the situation where the disease is absent, we recognize that a diagnostic test will yield either a *false positive* diagnosis or a *true negative* diagnosis, but what about the situation where the disease is present? We have thus far ignored this other side of diagnostic reasoning. What about the *false negative* or *true positive* diagnoses that will occur if the disease actually exists? In statistical reasoning, the counterpart to a false negative diagnosis is the error we would make if we conceded the null hypothesis and concluded that the observed difference was not statistically significant when, in fact, an important difference really existed.

In Fig. 2, for example, the value of c that was converted to a z score for the observed difference, $p_2 - p_1$, would have been declared 'not significant' statistically. How can we be sure of this decision? Perhaps the value of z_c is compatible with some other curve drawn farther to the right, in which the true difference of $p_2 - p_1$ is larger and more biologically significant than what was observed? If the true difference is biologically important and if we

failed to draw that conclusion, we would have made an erroneous decision. This type of false negative conclusion is what statisticians call a *Type II error*, and a new array of reasoning was created to work out its mathematical relationships.

The first step in the proceedings is to get a mathematical name for the likelihood of this type of error. If α was the boundary of probability demarcated for a false positive error, we can use the symbol β as the boundary for false negative error. Furthermore, if $1-\alpha$ corresponds to the *specificity* of a diagnostic test, $1-\beta$ will correspond to its *sensitivity*—the likelihood of making a positive diagnosis when the disease is present. Consequently, working at selected levels of α and β, we would have a $1-\beta$ chance of being right when we reject the null hypothesis (if it is false), and a $1-\alpha$ chance of being right when we concede it (if it is true). The associated analogies of the "diagnostic" and statistical reasoning are shown in Table I.

The terms *sensitivity* and *specificity* provide an idea of the diagnostic power of a test and help indicate the confidence that can be placed in the test. These same concepts are used (although somewhat differently) for the statistical nomenclature. As shown in Table I, the level of $1-\beta$, corresponding to the sensitivity of the test in correctly making a positive diagnosis, is often called the statistical *power* of the test. The level of $1-\alpha$, corresponding to the specificity of the test in correctly making a negative diagnosis, does not have a particular statistical word, such as *power*, attached to it. Its level is sometimes cited, however, as the *confidence* with which a null hypothesis is conceded. With this set of vocabulary and concepts, we can characterize a statistical test of significance by citing the α level and the power (or $1-\beta$ level) at which the test is employed for a difference, Δ. We might thus want to talk about a particular test as having a 95% chance (= $1-\beta$) of correctly rejecting the null hypothesis at the 5% level (= α) if the true difference is Δ.

The value of Δ is what allows us to specify just what is happening during the tests of statistical hypothesis that are under scrutiny. In ordinary statistical testing, the hypothesis we really wanted to accept is called the *alternative hypothesis*. It is expressed as H_A and is written (for a two-sided test) as H_A: $\text{mean}_1 \neq \text{mean}_2$. For a one-sided test, H_A could be written as $\text{mean}_1 < \text{mean}_2$ or as $\text{mean}_1 > \text{mean}_2$. To accept this alternative hypothesis, we engaged in a pattern of reasoning that called for rejection of the null hypothesis, which is written as H_0: $\text{mean}_1 = \text{mean}_2$.

When we add a β-type of reasoning to this previous form of α reasoning, we become interested in testing two separate hypotheses. One of these is the conventional null hypothesis, H_0, which says $\text{mean}_1 = \text{mean}_2$. The other is the alternative hypothesis, H_A, which is expressed in the form of $\text{mean}_2 - \text{mean}_1 = \Delta$ or (if two-sided probabilities are used) as $|\text{mean}_2 - \text{mean}_1| = \Delta$. The realities, decisions, and corresponding probabilities of error are shown in Table II. The most important point to be noted here is that a Type II (or beta) error can occur when we accept the null hypothesis. Since this is equivalent to the error of falsely rejecting H_A, we can determine the magnitude of probabilities for a Type II error by considering the consequence of a rejection of H_A.

An illustration of this situation is shown in Fig. 3. On the left of this figure is the Gaussian distribution of z values under the assumption that H_0 is true. To the right of the vertical line drawn at c, we have a zone in which H_0 will be falsely rejected at an alpha level that corresponds to c. The curve at the right of the figure shows the distribution of z values under the assumption that H_A is true. To the left of the vertical line drawn at c, we have a zone in which the acceptance of H_0 will be associated with a false rejection of H_A.

B. Strategies in β statistics

We can now contemplate two new kinds of statistical procedures: a new kind of P value and an additional way of determining sample size.

1. The calculation of β-error. In an ordinary *post hoc* test of 'statistical significance', the P_A value that we determined (from the z value of the observed results) told us about the possibility of a Type I or α error. In calculating

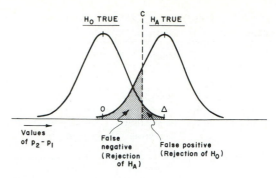

Fig. 3. Distributions for null hypothesis, H_0, and for alternative hypothesis, H_A. For further details, see text.

Table II. *Hypotheses, conclusions, and types of statistical error*

Reality	Decision*	Type of error	Probability
H_0 true; H_A false	Accept H_0	None	$1-\alpha$
	Reject H_0	False positive	α
H_0 false; H_A true	Accept H_0	False negative	β
	Reject H_0	None	$1-\beta$

*If H_0 is accepted, H_A is rejected; and vice versa.

sample size, we chose a specific level for this error and called it α or P_α. If we assign a Δ value, however, and contemplate just how large the true difference might really be for the two contrasted groups, we can determine the 'other side' of statistical significance. We can calculate a P_B value for the possibility of a Type II or β error.

The procedure used for this determination can be illustrated in reference to the curves of Fig. 3.

a. The left hand curve in Fig. 3 has its mean at 0, and represents the distribution of values for $p_2 - p_1$ under the null hypothesis, with H_0 assumed to be true.

b. The right hand curve in Fig. 3 has its mean at Δ, and represents the analogous distribution of $p_2 - p_1$ under the alternative hypothesis, H_A.

c. The line drawn at c represents an observed value of $p_2 - p_1$. [Alternatively, as we shall see later, it can represent an assigned value for α or for β.]

d. A z-value can be determined for any of these points by appropriate reference to a standard error. Thus, for an observed value of $p_2 - p_1 = \delta$, under the null hypothesis,

$$z_c = \frac{\delta}{\sqrt{[2\bar{p}(1 - \bar{p})]/n}}$$

and

$$z_\Delta = \frac{\Delta}{\sqrt{[2\bar{p}(1 - \bar{p})]/n}} .$$

The value of z_c, as shown in the hatched area of Fig. 3, will indicate the probability of a false positive rejection of H_0.

e. Under the alternative hypothesis, H_A, the stippled area to the left of c will indicate the likelihood of a false positive rejection for H_A. If c represents the observed value of δ, this point is located at $\Delta - \delta$, and the associated negative value for z_B is

$$z_B = \frac{\Delta - \delta}{\sqrt{[p_2(1 - p_2) + p_1(1 - p_1)]/n}}$$

f. For most practical purposes, we can assume that the two standard errors are equal, i.e., that $2\bar{p}(1 - \bar{p}) = p_2(1 - p_2) + p_1(1 - p_1)$. For example, if $p_1 = .50$ and $p_2 = .70$, the respective values for these terms are 0.48 and 0.46. Consequently, if we let $v = 2\bar{p}(1 - \bar{p}) \simeq p_2(1 - p_2) + p_1(1 - p_1)$, the formulas we have been considering become

$$z_c = \delta\sqrt{n/v}$$
$$z_\Delta = \Delta\sqrt{n/v}$$

and

$$z_B = (\Delta - \delta)\sqrt{n/v} = z_\Delta - z_c.$$

g. By referring this z_B value to the associated one-sided P value, we obtain P_B, which is the probability of falsely rejecting the alternative hypothesis.

2. *Illustration of calculation for P*$_B$

a. *Equal sample sizes.* Suppose an investigator, comparing the rates of patient satisfaction with medical care at two hospitals finds that the rate of satisfaction was 70% (16/23) at Hospital A and 84% (19/23) at Hospital B. The investigator concludes that the difference is not statistically 'significant' because chi-

square $= 1.08$ and P is too large $(> .1)$ to be 'significant'. [Doing the statistical test by the z procedure, we would choose $\bar{p} = (16 + 19)/(23 + 23) = 76\%$. We then get $z_c = (.83 - .70) (\sqrt{23})/\sqrt{(2)} (.76) (.24) = (.13) (4.8)/\sqrt{.36} = 1.04$; and the associated P value is .15.] After drawing this conclusion, the investigator claims that the care at the two hospitals produces the same degree of satisfaction.

Contrary to his claim, however, we suspect that Hospital B does give better care, that its real level of patient satisfaction is actually 20% higher than in Hospital A, and that 'statistical significance' was absent in this study as an act of chance, possibly because the sample sizes were too small. What we would like to know, therefore, is the likelihood that the investigator may have been wrong in his conclusion. We use the formula $z_B = (\Delta - \delta)\sqrt{n/v} = (.20 - .13)\sqrt{23/.36} = (.07) (7.99) = 0.56$. The associated one-sided value for P_B is .288 or 29%. Thus, there is a good chance (of about 29%) that the investigator falsely accepted the null hypothesis if the true difference in rate of satisfaction at the hospitals is as high as 20%.

b. *Unequal sample sizes.* All of the foregoing calculations were based on the assumption that the observed proportions, p_1 and p_2, came from groups of equal sizes. If the sample sizes, n_1 and n_2, are unequal, then $p = (n_1p_1 + n_2p_2)/N$, where $N = n_1 + n_2$. Under the null hypothesis, the standard error of $p_1 - p_2$ is $\sqrt{\bar{p}\bar{q}\left(\frac{1}{n_1} + \frac{1}{n_2}\right)}$, where $\bar{q} = 1 - \bar{p}$. This expression becomes $\sqrt{N\bar{p}\bar{q}/n_1n_2}$. Under the alternative hypothesis, the standard error of $p_1 - p_2$ is $\sqrt{\frac{p_1q_1}{n_1} + \frac{p_2q_2}{n_2}} = \sqrt{(n_2p_1q_1 + n_1p_2q_2)/(n_1n_2)}$. For most practical purposes, we can assume that $\sqrt{N\bar{p}\bar{q}} = \sqrt{n_2p_1q_1 + n_1p_2q_2}$. The formula for finding beta error would then be $z_B = (\Delta - \delta)\sqrt{n_1n_2/N\bar{p}\bar{q}}$.

3. *The 'power curve' of a statistical test.* If we want to operate a statistical test at a fixed level of α for making decisions, we can readily determine the values of β that will be associated for any choice of α. In this case, the chosen level of α will determine an assigned value of

z_α, which will be the location of z_c in Fig. 3. Since we previously developed the formula that $z_B = z_\Delta - z_c$, we can substitute the assigned value of z_α for z_c and get $z_\Delta = z_\alpha + z_B$. Since z_Δ has a fixed value that depends on the magnitudes of $_\Delta$, n_1, n_2, N, $\bar{p}$, and $\bar{q}$, the values of z_α and z_B must sum to a constant. Consequently, if higher values are assigned to z_α, the values of z_B must decrease; and vice versa. This reciprocal relationship is analogous to what we have noted in a previous discussion[5] of sensitivity and specificity for a diagnostic test. If one increases, the other decreases.

This reciprocal aspect of the equation allows various statistical tests to be illustrated with "power" curves, which show the values of $1 - P_\beta$ that will occur with different choices of α. For example, consider the situation where the true values of the compared rates are $p_1 = 27\%$ and $p_2 = 45\%$, so that $\Delta = p_2 - p_1 = .18$ and $v = 2\bar{p}(1 - \bar{p}) = 0.46$. If we take a sample size of 80 for each group in a comparison, we will have $z_\Delta = \Delta\sqrt{n/v} = (.18)\sqrt{80/.46} = 2.37$. If we decide to reject the null hypothesis at a two-sided α level of .05, we would have $z_B = 2.37 - 1.96 = 0.41$. The associated P_B value would be .341 and the 'power' of the test would be 65.9%. If the null hypothesis were to be rejected at a two-sided α level of .1, $z_B = 2.37 - 1.645 = 0.73$, and the associated P_B value would be .233, giving the test the higher 'power' of 76.7%.

C. The calculation of a 'doubly significant' sample size

In the foregoing discussion, we worked on the assumption that the research was complete. We had our data; we had determined or assigned the level of P_A or P_α; and we wanted to know what P_B might be. A different application of these concepts occurs for the modern calculation of a 'doubly significant' sample size, which means that we want a sample large enough to be significant at the levels of both α and β. In the previous calculations, we began with known data for everything except z_B, and we solved for z_B. Now we begin by knowing (or assuming) all the necessary information except n, and we solve the equation for n.

1. Simplified procedure. The simplest approach for these calculations is to take the previously developed formula and to substitute the assigned values of z_α and z_β for their respective counterparts z_c and z_B. We then would have

$$z_\Delta = \Delta\sqrt{\frac{n}{v}} = z_\alpha + z_\beta.$$

If we square both sides and solve for n, we get $n = v(z_\alpha + z_\beta)^2/\Delta^2$. For example, suppose we expect that $p_2 = .70$ and $p_1 = .50$ and we want to attain statistical significance for a 2-sided α level of .05 and a one-sided β level of .05. What size should our sample be? We have assigned $\Delta = .20$, $z_\alpha = 1.96$ and $z_\beta = 1.645$. From previous calculations, we know that v is either 0.48 or 0.46. Let us call it 0.47. Substituting directly into the cited equation, we get $n = (0.47)(1.96 + 1.645)^2/(.20)^2$, and $n = 152.7$. We would thus need 153 patients in each group, for a total sample size of 306 patients.

2. Stricter procedure. In a mathematically stricter set of calculations, we make provision for the fact that the value of z_α is determined using the null hypothesis, whereas the value of z_β depends on the alternative hypothesis. Thus, the point c in Fig. 3 will define an α level of

$$z_\alpha = \frac{c}{\sqrt{2\bar{p}(1 - \bar{p})/n}}.$$

At this same point c,

$$z_\beta = \frac{\Delta - c}{\sqrt{[p_2(1 - p_2) + p_1(1 - p_1)]/n}}.$$

If we solve the first of these two equations for c, and substitute the results into the second, we get

$$z_\beta = \frac{\Delta - (\sqrt{2\bar{p}(1 - \bar{p})/n})(z_\alpha)}{\sqrt{[p_2(1 - p_2) + p_1(1 - p_1)]/n}}.$$

This equation becomes

$$\frac{1}{\sqrt{n}}\left\{z_\beta\left[\sqrt{p_2(1 - p_2) + p_1(1 - p_1)}\right] + z_\alpha[\sqrt{2p(1 - \bar{p})}]\right\} = \Delta.$$

Squaring both sides and solving for n, we get

$$n = \left(\frac{1}{\Delta^2}\right)\left\{z_\alpha[2\bar{p}(1 - \bar{p})]^{\frac{1}{2}} + z_\beta[p_2(1 - p_2) + p_1(1 - p_1)]^{\frac{1}{2}}\right\}^2.$$

This formula, which is less formidable than it looks, is the one that regularly appears in many statistical discussions[8, 11, 13] of sample size. In the numerical example just cited, the actual values are

$$n = \frac{1}{(.20)^2}\left\{1.96[2(.60)(.40)]^{\frac{1}{2}} + 1.645[(.70)(.30) + (.50)(.50)]^{\frac{1}{2}}\right\}^2$$

$$= \frac{1}{.04}\left\{1.96[.69] + 1.645[.68]\right\}^2$$

$$= \frac{1}{.04}\left\{1.35 + 1.12\right\}^2 = \frac{1}{.04}\left\{2.47\right\}^2 = 153.$$

The result is identical to what we obtained with the previous set of simplified calculations.

3. *Use of statistical tables.* These computations can be avoided if we make use of appropriate sets of prepared tables. A particularly good collection of tables, showing sample sizes for different values of α, β, Δ, and p_1, is contained in Table A-3 (pages 176-194) of the excellent textbook by Fleiss[7]. For example, if Δ is 5%, if α (two-sided) is .05, and if β (one-sided) is .05, Fleiss' Table A-3 shows that the size of n will range from 796 if p_1 = 5%, to 2669 if p_1 = 50%. If Δ is 20%, under the same conditions of α and β, the size of n will range from 99 if p_1 = 5% to 172 if p_1 = 50%. The values of n in Fleiss' tables are higher than those calculated in the preceding illustrations here because Fleiss' computations include a 'correction for continuity', analogous to that of the Yates' 'correction' in chi-square tests. Using a formula derived by Kramer and Greenhouse[9], the n values in our calculations can be converted to the n' values cited by Fleiss. The formula is

$$n' = \frac{n}{4}\left[1 + \sqrt{1 + (8/n\Delta)}\right]^2.$$

4. *Differences in sample-size methods.* We can now note the difference between calculating a 'singly' and a 'doubly significant' sample size. In the classical old formula for a 'singly significant' sample

$$n = \frac{z_\alpha^2 v}{\Delta^2}.$$

For the 'doubly significant' sample,

$$n = \frac{(z_\alpha + z_\beta)^2 v}{\Delta^2}.$$

The change to 'double significance' thus increases the sample size by a ratio of $[(z_\alpha + z_\beta)/z_\alpha]^2$, which is $\left[1 + \frac{z_\beta}{z_\alpha}\right]^2$. If we choose equal

values for our levels of α and β, the right hand ratio of z values will be 1, and the 'doubly significant' sample will be $(1 + 1)^2 = 4$ times as large as the first.

To illustrate this point, suppose we want to achieve a one-sided significance level of .05 in a clinical trial where the expected rates of success are 10% in the control group and 20% in the treated group. From these data, p_2 = .20, p_1 = .10, Δ = .10, and v is estimated as $(.20)(.80) + (.10)(.90) = 0.25$. [The alternative estimation for v would be $(2)(.15)(.85) = 0.26$.]

For the 'one-sided' calculations of sample size for α level significance, we would have

$$n = \frac{z^2 v}{\Delta^2} = \frac{(1.645)^2(.25)}{(.10)^2} = 67.65$$

and we would need $2 \times 68 = 136$ patients altogether.

To calculate sample size for both α and β levels of significance, we would have

$$n = \frac{(z_\alpha + z_\beta)^2 v}{\Delta^2} = \frac{(1.645 + 1.645)^2(.25)}{(.10)^2} = 270.6.$$

We would therefore need $2 \times 271 = 542$ patients, an amount that is about four times larger than before.

Two other important features to be noted about these formulas are the crucial roles of Δ and v. Since Δ is always a value between 0 and 1, the value of Δ^2 is always smaller than Δ. (For example, if Δ = .3, Δ^2 = .09.) Furthermore, the smaller the value of Δ, the smaller will be the value of Δ^2 and the larger will be the corresponding value of $(1/\Delta^2)$ which is used as a factor in determining n. Thus, the smaller the difference for which we want to show 'statistical significance', the larger is the sample size that is required. In fact, if we want to prove the null hypothesis exactly, and to show that p_1 and p_2 are absolutely identical, we would need a sample of infinite size because $\Delta = 0$.

Since v appears in the numerator of the factors that are multiplied to calculate n, the size of n will decrease as v decreases. The value of v, being dependent on $2\bar{p}(1 - \bar{p})$, will be at a maximum when p = 50% and will take minimum values near the polar extremes of 0% or 100%. Thus, if $\bar{p}$ is close to 0% or to 100%, v will be small and n will be correspondingly small. On the other hand, when $\bar{p}$ is very close to a polar extreme, a large value for Δ may be extremely difficult or unfeasible to obtain. The advantage of a very high or very low value for $\bar{p}$ may thus be completely obliterated by the associated disadvantages of a very small value for Δ.

D. The importance of β error

Because scientific research is usually directed at showing that two entities are different, most investigators depend on statistical tests that provide values only for P_A. The values of P_B are generally omitted, either because the investigator is unaware of their existence or because he is not concerned about them. The absence of attention to the possibility of β error is equivalent to setting the value of $z_\beta = 0$. For this value of z_β, the one-sided $P_B = .5$; and the 'power' of the test is $1 - P_B$ or 50%. In other words, the investigator takes a 50-50 chance of committing the false negative error of incorrectly rejecting the alternative hypothesis.

Most investigators accept this risk with equanimity, since their main concern in the customary situation of 'significance' testing is with α error—with a false positive conclusion. There are at least two major scientific circumstances, however, in which the role of β error becomes particularly important.

The first of these circumstances is a clinical trial in which we want to be sure of having a satisfactory chance of detecting a substantial Δ when it exists. If we fail to find 'statistical significance' at the α level, we might like to be reasonably confident about accepting the null hypothesis. This strategy is responsible for sample-size calculations that culminate in such phrases as "a 90% chance of finding a 20% difference at the .05 level". In this phrase, the associated statistical values are $\Delta = .20$, $\alpha = .05$ and (one-sided) $\beta = .1$.

The second (and perhaps more important) role of β error is in the situation where we want to show that two groups are similar rather than different. An example of such a situation is a clinical trial[12, 15] whose conclusion was that the quality of primary care provided by nurse practitioners is essentially equal to what is offered by physicians. Another example, which is an increasingly common situation in clinical pharma-

cology, occurs for tests of the bioequivalence of two pharmaceutical preparations. In such circumstances, we assign a value of Δ as the maximum permissible difference between the groups. If the observed difference is smaller than Δ, we shall conclude that the groups are essentially equivalent. As noted earlier, the value that is chosen for Δ and the magnitude of p_1 will be as important as the choices of α and β in determining sample size.

The high values of n that can emerge from these calculations will be a major problem in routine studies of bioavailability. In an example cited earlier, for α and β both equal to .05 and for $\Delta = 29\%$, the size of n could range from 84 to 143, according to the values of p_1. Since sample sizes of this magnitude will usually be unfeasible, the values of α and β may have to be made quite liberal. Thus, if α (two-sided) is increased to 0.2 and if β (one-sided) is increased to 0.15, the size of n will vary as follows:

Δ	5%	5%	20%	20%
p_1	5%	50%	5%	50%
n	254	728	38	57

These sample sizes, although smaller than before, are still substantially larger than the 6 to 10 patients whose data have been customarily examined for studies of bioavailability. If the bioavailability research is conducted in a "crossover" manner, in one group of patients rather than two groups, the paired arrangement of data will permit a further reduction in sample size. Nevertheless, if strict statistical standards become demanded for studies of bioequivalence, the problems of obtaining ample numbers of people for the tests may be so formidable that the studies will be impossible to conduct. Just as the old calculations of P_A for α error alone made no provision for β error, the new calculations of sample size of β error alone may have to be done without consideration of α error.

E. Caveats and abuses

A knowledge of β reasoning and the 'other side' of 'significance' can lead to prompt detection of a classical abuse in the way that statistical tests are often reported in medical literature. The β reasoning has also been applied to create new problems in the calculation of sample size

1. Conclusions when the null hypothesis is conceded.

In a routine statistical test of 'significance', what conclusion do we draw if the P_A value is higher than α? The correct answer to this question is that such a high P value makes us concede, i.e., fail to reject, the null hypothesis. With this concession, we conclude that the observed difference is statistically not significant. The wrong answer to the question is that we accept the null hypothesis and conclude that the difference is insignificant.

The distinctions between *concede* and *accept* and between *not significant* and *insignificant* can be clinically illustrated by recalling the purpose of the sputum Pap smear as a diagnostic test. We order the test in search of a positive diagnosis of lung cancer. If the test is negative, however, we cannot conclude that lung cancer has been ruled out. We would merely concede that we have failed to show its presence. To accept the negative diagnosis that lung cancer is absent, i.e., to rule it out, we would want to check results from additional tests, such as the chest X-ray.

Consequently, in a simple test of 'statistical significance', a high P value is like the Scottish verdict of *not proved*. When P_A exceeds α, we neither reject nor accept the null hypothesis. We concede it, or fail to reject it. Our conclusion must therefore be that the observed difference is *not significant,* rather than *insignificant.* To conclude that it is insignificant, we would have to accept the null hypothesis—a decision that would require additional evidence for the possibility of β error.

The previous example of satisfaction with care at two hospitals provided an illustration of the erroneous conclusions that can occur when $P_A > \alpha$. The investigator wanted to claim that the satisfaction was similar at the two hospitals, but we would not accept his claim because it had a 'power' of only 71%. In fact, if our original sample size was quadrupled, and if the proportion of successes remained the same, the resulting numbers would be 64/92 vs. 76/92 and the difference would be statistically significant at $P < .05$ even though the observed δ was only 13%.

Even when the two contrasted results seem quite similar, we still cannot conclude that their difference is *insignificant*. For example, suppose we have found a success rate of 3/7 (43%) for treatment A and 4/9 (44%) for treatment B. This result seems unimpressive, but it could readily arise by chance if the true success values for treatments A and B were, respectively, 29% and 56%. Thus, if we exchanged one success and one failure in the patients comprising groups A and B, we would get success rates of 2/7 (29%) for A and 5/9 (56%) for B. This difference is impressive although not statistically significant.

One of the main abuses of tests of statistical significance occurs, therefore, when an investigator who gets a high P value, i.e., $P_A > \alpha$, concludes that the observed difference between two groups is 'insignificant' and that the groups should be regarded as similar. If this type of reasoning were correct, we could always 'prove' that two treatments were identical, merely by using a small sample size for the study. Thus, if we put 3 patients in each group, a result as extreme as 0/3 (0%) successes for treatment *A* vs. 3/3 (100%) for treatment *B* could still not achieve 'statistical significance'. (The two-sided P value is .1.) From this failure to attain 'statistical significance', it would be absurd to conclude that the observed difference is insignificant and that the two treatments are equivalent. Nevertheless, such errors regularly appear in medical literature.

An analogous problem occurs when statistical tests are done to determine whether the act of randomization provided an equitable distribution of the patient groups before treatment began in a clinical trial. When good grounds exist for suspecting baseline inequalities, a high P_A value cannot alone be accepted as confirmation of their absence. The analysis is incomplete unless attention is also given to P_B. (A memorable example of such omissions occurred in analyses[1, 17] of the celebrated UGDP study of diabetes. When statistically significant differences were *not* found in certain analyses of baseline distinctions, the data analysts concluded that the baseline differences were insignificant, although no levels of β-error were cited.)

The point to be borne in mind is that an ordinary test of 'statistical significance' can be used only to reject the null hypothesis, not to accept it. The test either shows or does not show a 'significant' difference. It cannot show an 'insignificant' difference. To draw the latter conclusion, we would need to know the other kind of P value for the possibility of β error.

2. Problems in calculating sample size. With the increasing performance of controlled clinical trials, many alternative strategies have been proposed for determining sample size. So many different proposals have been made, in fact, that contriving new ways to gauge sample size seems to have become a favorite indoor sport of statistical theoreticians. The alternative strategies include schemata based on sequential analysis, Bayesian conjectures, and various 'play-the-winner' techniques. Schneiderman[14] has provided a well-written summary of the state of the art in some of the statistical ideologies. For practical purposes, the material presented here has been based on the currently accepted "conventional wisdom".*

Like many other statistical activities, a preoccupation with the mathematical tactics of determining sample size may often distract both statisticians and investigators from basic challenges that are the really fundamental issues in scientific research. In order to calculate a sample size, we often ignore these issues and assume that they have been taken care of. After the Neyman-Pearsonian, Bayesian, or other strategies have yielded a number in the sample size calculations, the clinical investigator may become awed by the precision of the number ('you will need exactly 984 patients') or flustered by its magnitude ('how the devil can I possibly get so many?'). As this number and negotiations about its reduction become the focus of attention, the clinician and statistician may forget that the basic scientific problems remain unresolved. Among them are the following:

a. The univariate choice of an endpoint. To determine p_1, p_2, and Δ, we must choose a single variable whose outcome will be the "endpoint" in the research. This concentration on only one kind of outcome is contrary to every tenet of good clinical investigation, which calls for an appraisal of the multitude of variables that are involved in a patient's responses to treatment. Nevertheless, there currently exist no satisfactory biostatistical procedures for either choosing sample size in a multivariate manner or preparing a clinically effective composite of important multiple variables into a single univariate index.

b. The focus on 'hard data'. Since everything in the sample size calculations depends on the endpoint noted in a single variable, statisticians usually want to be sure that this endpoint is an item of 'hard data', such as *death*. Since changes in death rates are usually smaller than the changes that can occur in important 'soft data' variables, the result of the focus on hard data is to create a relatively small value of Δ, which may lead to excessively large values for the calculated sample size. A more important consequence of the hard-data focus is that an important soft-data variable, such as vascular complications or quality of life, may become ignored in the early stages of biostatistical planning for the trial and may remain ignored (or poorly managed) thereafter. Because of this inattention to 'soft data', the most important clinical and human aspects of therapy—the associated risks, benefits, costs, joys, and sorrows of treatment—often become grossly neglected in the research[16].

c. The current uninformed choice of p_1. Because good data are seldom available for 'historical controls', the choice of p_1 (as an estimate of the outcome rate for the control group) becomes an act of guesswork that often turns out to be erroneous. If the error leads to a huge overestimate of sample size, the trial becomes excessively expensive.

d. The future uninformed choice of p_1. The estimate of a single value of p_1 has no real clinical precision. What is usually needed, instead, is a series of p_1 values—one for each of the cogent clinical strata[2] of patients subjected to therapy. If the data of large-scale randomized therapeutic trials are not analyzed with a cogent

*For my education in these concepts and for other helpful comments on this text, I am indebted to several clinical and statistical colleagues: Donald Archibald, Robert Deupree, Michael Gent, Walter Spitzer, and Carolyn Wells. Their aid is gratefully acknowledged here, while they are also absolved of responsibility for the contents.

clinical stratification, however, the results of a current trial cannot provide a good estimate of p_1 values for use in future trials. Today's expensive, unproductive therapeutic trial may thus be followed by tomorrow's.

e. The arbitrary choices of α and β. Despite the elaborate reasoning that has been discussed for choosing α and β, their values are seldom selected in the abstract intellectual manner described here. What often happens is that the statistician and investigator decide on the size of Δ. The magnitude of the sample is then chosen to fit the two requirements (1) that the selected number of patients can actually be obtained for the trial and (2) that their recruitment and investigation can be funded. The values of α and β are then adjusted to fit this number and a suitable mathematical rationale is then developed for presentation to the granting agency.

f. The arbitrary choice of Δ. As the difference that indicates 'clinical significance', the magnitude of Δ is often the most crucial issue in planning and evaluating the research. Despite this importance, the scope of Δ is not only constrained by the univariate restrictions noted earlier, but it also gets chosen arbitrarily. Judgments about the proper size of Δ have received almost no concentrated attention via symposia, workshops, or other conclaves of experts assembled to adjudicate matters of clinical importance. In the absence of established standards, the clinical investigator, on being badgered by the statistician to choose a Δ so that sample size can be calculated, picks what seems like a reasonable value. This value is tossed into the formula, using z_α, z_β, etc. If the sample size that emerges is unfeasible, Δ gets adjusted accordingly, and so do α and β, until n comes out right.

In some brave new world of the future, when clinicians begin to insist that large-scale therapeutic trials be truly clinical investigations as well as elaborate exercises in mathematics, better solutions may be developed for these clinical and scientific problems. In the meantime, clinical investigators can take comfort in knowing about the panacea-like marvels offered by modern statistical methods for determining α-error, β-error, and sample size. Even if we don't know what we're doing and even if we can't specify it, repeat it, or make good clinical sense out of it, we can still calculate the required populational numbers and determine the probabilistic uncertainties going in both logical directions. Not since the days of alchemy have scientists been able to rely on such dazzling transmutations.

References

1. Cornfield, J.: The University Group Diabetes Program. A further statistical analysis of the mortality findings, J. A. M. A. **217:**1676-1687, 1971.
2. Feinstein, A. R.: Clinical biostatistics. The purposes of prognostic stratification, CLIN. PHARMACOL. THER. **13:**285-297, 1972.
3. Feinstein, A. R., and Ramshaw, W. A.: A procedure for rapid mental calculation of the fourfold chi-square test, J. Chron. Dis. **25:**551-553, 1972.
4. Feinstein, A. R.: Clinical biostatistics. XXIII. The role of randomization in sampling, testing, allocation, and credulous idolatry (Part 2), CLIN. PHARMACOL. THER. **14:**898-915, 1973.
5. Feinstein, A. R.: Clinical biostatistics. XXXI. On the sensitivity, specificity, and discrimination of diagnostic tests, CLIN. PHARMACOL. THER. **17:**104-116, 1975.
6. Feinstein, A. R.: Clinical biostatistics. XXXII. Biologic dependency, 'hypothesis testing', unilateral probabilities, and other issues in scientific direction vs. statistical duplexity, CLIN. PHARMACOL. THER. **17:**499-513, 1975.
7. Fleiss, J. L.: Statistical methods for rates and proportions, New York, 1973, John Wiley & Sons, Inc.
8. Halperin, M., Rogot, E., Gurian, J., and Ederer, F.: Sample sizes for medical trials with special reference to long-term therapy, J. Chron. Dis. **21:**13-24, 1968.
9. Kramer, M., and Greenhouse, S. W.: Determination of sample size and selection of cases, *in* Cole, J. O., and Gerard, R. W., editors: Psychopharmacology: Problems in evaluation, National Academy of Sciences, National Research Council, 1959, pp. 356-371.
10. Neyman, J., and Pearson, E. S.: On the use and interpretation of certain test criteria for the purposes of statistical inference, Biometrika **20A:**175 and 263, 1928.
11. Pasternack, B. S.: Sample sizes for clinical trials designed for patient accrual by cohorts, J. Chron. Dis. **25:**673-681, 1972.
12. Sackett, D. L., Spitzer, W. O., Gent, M., and Roberts, R. S.: The Burlington randomized trial of the nurse practitioner: Health outcomes

of patients, Ann. Intern. Med. **80:**137-142, 1974.

13. Schlesselman, J. J.: Planning a longitudinal study. I. Sample size determination, J. Chron. Dis. **26:**535-560, 1973.

14. Schneiderman, M. A.: The proper size of a clinical trial: "Grandma's strudel" method, J. New Drugs **4:**3-11, 1964.

15. Spitzer, W. O., Sackett, D. L., Sibley, J. C., Roberts, R. S., Gent, M., Kergin, D. J., Hackett, B. C., and Olynich, A.: The Burlington randomized trial of the nurse practitioner, N. Engl. J. Med. **290:**251-256, 1974.

16. Spitzer, W. O., Feinstein, A. R., and Sackett, D. L.: What is a health care trial? J. A. M. A. **233:**161-163, 1975.

17. University Group Diabetes Program. A study of the effects of hypoglycemic agents on vascular complications in patients with adult-onset diabetes. I. Design, methods and baseline results; and II. Mortality results, Diabetes **19** (Suppl. 2):747-830, 1970.

CHAPTER 23

Problems in the summary and display of statistical data

After completing a research project, an investigator encounters several different challenges in the management of data. One of these challenges is in organizing and analyzing the information; another is in drawing conclusions; a third is in communicating the results.

The organizational activities consist of choosing the variables to be analyzed; preparing suitable arrangements of the data for each variable; and summarizing the data in a way that allows appropriate discernment of relations and contrasts. The formation of conclusions occurs in two different steps. From knowledge of the scientific background and architecture of the research, the investigator notes the magnitude of the observed relations and contrasts, and first uses scientific judgment to make decisions about their substantive importance. From the observed magnitudes and from the size of the examined groups, the investigator then uses mathematical inference to make decisions about "statistical significance".

Thus, an investigator might find, in one study, a difference of 30% in comparing the percentage improvement with two treatments in 10 people; or, in another study, a correlation coefficient of .05 for the relationship of two variables in 5,000 people. Using both scientific and mathematical methods of decision-making, the investigator might conclude that the ther-

apeutic difference was clinically important although statistically "not significant", whereas the cited correlation was statistically "significant" but clinically trivial.

The communication of results is a challenge that occurs after the others have been completed. To meet this challenge, the investigator must provide scientific colleagues with a clear account of what was done, what was found, and what was concluded. Unless this last challenge is suitably managed, the previous activities will have an unsatisfactory outcome. The research will not be reported in a manner that makes it comprehensible, appraisable, and usable by the scientific community.

The tools of statistics play diverse roles in these activities. The basic architecture[7] of the research and the choice of important variables depend on scientific rather than statistical decisions, but all the other procedures involve statistical methods. The techniques of *descriptive statistics* provide expressions for the numbers that are used to summarize data, to show relationships, and to indicate contrasts. To summarize data for individual variables, descriptive statistics offers such numerical expressions as means, medians, proportions, standard deviations, ranges, and percentiles. To show the relationships among variables, the descriptive statistical methods include two-way tables and graphs, correlation coefficients, and regression equations. To indicate contrasts, descriptive statistics supplies such expressions as increments, decrements, ratios, and proportionate

This chapter originally appeared as "Clinical biostatistics—XXXVII. Demeaned errors, confidence games, nonplussed minuses, inefficient coefficients, and other statistical disruptions of scientific communication." In Clin. Pharmacol. Ther. 20:617, 1976.

differences. The techniques of *inferential statistics* provide the mathematical methods for drawing probabilistic conclusions about the results cited in the descriptive expressions. The mathematics of inferential statistics produces such probabilistic statements as standard errors, confidence intervals, and the various tests that yield P values for correlation or regression coefficients and for the differences found in contrasts of means, proportions, or other descriptive summaries.

The descriptive statistical procedures are obviously basic necessities for communicating the results of scientific research. None of the inferential maneuvers can be applied until the descriptive processes are completed, and none of the inferential maneuvers have any substantive meaning or scientific acceptability unless the descriptive data are available for evaluation. Nevertheless, in the literature of modern biomedical science, many investigators and editors have become so infatuated with inferential or analytic statistics that the fundamental role of descriptive statistics has become neglected or perverted. The neglect occurs when investigators and editors make important decisions solely on the basis of P values or other inferential calculations, ignoring the magnitude of the contrasts and relationships from which the statistical calculations are derived. The perversion occurs when descriptive expressions for the contrasts and relationships are eliminated and replaced by the inferential statistical statements.

1. The demeaned error

The "standard error" has become a popular method of reporting results, although most of the investigators using this term do not know its definition, source, or connotations. If you doubt the foregoing remark, I invite you to take the following test. Choose an intelligent, reasonably critical "layperson" who knows nothing about statistics, but who understands the idea of an arithmetic average or mean, and who has enough common sense to question any statements you make that seem inconsistent or foolish. Now try to explain to that person exactly what is meant by the *standard error of the mean* and why you, as an investigator, use it

in your work. If the explanation is satisfactory to you, the other person should be looking baffled and seeking a clearer account. If the explanation is satisfactory to that other person, you should now be feeling quite uncomfortable. Your friend will be asking you why realistic scientists are engaging in abstract fantasies and why the flights of fantasy are described in such peculiar words as *standard error*.

A standard error has nothing to do with standards, with errors, or with the communication of scientific data. The concept is an abstract idea, spawned by the imaginary world of statistical inference and pertinent only when certain operations of that imaginary world are met in scientific reality.

a. The idea of 'error'. If you decide that you want to explain the phrase *standard error of the mean,* the first word with which to begin is the idea of *error.* This idea happens to have a realistic origin. It arose in reference to a practical problem that today would be called "observer variability". Suppose the same entity or substance has been measured several times and suppose the different measurements do not agree. For example, if the chemistry laboratory at your institution is particularly fastidious and conducts all its tests in quadruplicate, the lab may get such values as 249, 250, 247, and 258 mg/dl as measurements of cholesterol concentration in the same specimen of serum. Which one of these measurements should be issued by the lab as the formal, correct value?

The answer to this question involves some fundamental philosophic issues in the statistics of mensuration. Should we average all the values together and take the mean? If so, the "correct" result is 251. Should we take the average of the three values that remain after discarding the value of 258 because it seems to be an outlier, far away from the others? If so, the correct result is 248.7. Should we take an average based only on the two closest values? If so, the correct result is 249.5. The decision about which and how many values to include is beyond the scope of this discussion. For the moment, the point to be noted is that regardless of how the candidate values are chosen for inclusion, each of the "correct" results emerged from calculating the mean of the candidates.

The idea of using the mean as the *right* result is an old statistical tradition. The tradition is justified by its reasonableness—since there seems to be no better routine way of solving the problem—and is sanctified by more than a century of scientific usage.

Once we have chosen a mean, we can note the differences between the mean and the actual values that are observed in the measurements. If we call these differences *deviations,* the name is straightforward and non-pejorative. If the mean, however, has been endowed with the sublime virtues of truth, correctness, and propriety, the deviations can be suitably castigated for their failings. They can be called *errors.*

This use of the word *error,* of course, is itself untrue, incorrect, and improper. To call a deviation an *error* implies that there is something wrong with the measurement, that the equipment or the observer (or both) may not have been functioning accurately. In fact, however, if we had some unequivocal method for determining the accurate value of the measurement, we might have found that it was any one of the ''deviant'' results. The deviation may thus have had nothing wrong with it and its designation as an *error* made it a victim of a scientifically bizarre ''morality'' in nomenclature. Nevertheless, this demeaning use of *error* has persisted in statistical vocabulary, being embellished in such additional maledictions as *error variance* or *residual error* for the sum of the squared deviations around a fitted mean or for the deviations of observed measurements from a fitted line.

For many other statistical circumstances, however, the word *error* has been displaced from this unsatisfactory usage; and deviations from the mean are actually called *deviations.* At least two reasons can account for the displacement. The first reason is that the word *error* is obviously foolish when it is applied to deviations from the mean, not in different measurements of a single specimen, but in single measurements of different specimens. After all, if we determined the serum cholesterol of each member of a group of people, calculated the mean cholesterol for the group, and then found each person's deviation from the mean, we would be unacceptably silly if we referred to

those deviations as *errors*. This approach may seem silly today, but it was a basic principle of the reasoning used by Quetelet a century ago to lay the foundations of populational statistics. In transferring *deviations* and *variance* from being a property of individual measurements to being a property of individual people, Quetelet adopted the idea that the *mean* was also the *ideal.* The statistical glorification of mediocrity in people was perpetuated when Galton, Pearson, and other founders of the British school of biometry accepted both the conceptual transfer of *variance* and the associated nomenclature of *error*.

Although modern recognition of this folly should have been the main reason for evicting the word *error* from its former role in describing deviations, the second reason is probably more cogent. The word *error* was needed (as we shall see later) for a different job, describing a different type of deviation, occurring in a different type of modern world—the abstract imagery of statistical inference.

b. The idea of 'standard'. Once we have decided to use the mean as either the correct result or the focal point of a series of n measurements, we want to get an idea of the dispersion of values around that mean. The most obvious approach is to find the average dispersion or average deviation of the values. To take the sum of the deviations is a futile task, however, since they will always add up to zero, by virtue of the way they were defined. [If you wonder about this statement, recall that the mean is defined as $\bar{x} = \sum x_i / n$, where x_i is any one of the n measurements. The sum of the deviations is then $\sum(x_i - \bar{x})$, which becomes algebraically expanded to $\sum x_i - \sum \bar{x}$, which is $n\bar{x} - n\bar{x} = 0$.]

To get around this problem, we could take the sum of the absolute magnitudes of the deviations, regardless of whether they are positive or negative. This sum, when divided by n, would give the average absolute deviation—a value that is clear and reasonable. Unfortunately, because absolute values are a nuisance to calculate and work with, they are mathematically unappealing.

The next option is the one that has swept the field. To avoid the negative signs, we can square all the deviations. Preparing for getting an average, we now add those squared deviations together, as classically symbolized by $\sum(x_i - \bar{x})^2$. This expression, which is the sum of the squared deviations, happens to be very useful for other statistical manipulations and so it often gets a nickname, *sum of the squares,* and a special symbol, S_{xx}. (My own preference is to call this expression the *group variance,* but I shall adhere to the conventional nomenclature in this essay.)

If we now divide the sum of the squared deviations by n, which is the number of deviations (or observations), we get the mean squared deviation,

$$\frac{S_{xx}}{n} \text{ or } \frac{\sum(x_i - \bar{x})^2}{n},$$

which is also called the *variance.* By taking the square root of the variance, we get what is accurately called a *root mean squared deviation.* To shorten the phrase, the term might be called the *average square deviation.* The phrase that is actually used, however, is *standard deviation.*

I have been unable to find an answer for the question of why a distinctive scientific word like *standard* was pressed into this peculiar mathematical service. (According to F. N. David, the phrase *standard deviation* was first used by Karl Pearson.) Many other two-word alternatives were available, including *adjusted deviation* and *adapted deviation.* By suitable re-definition of the word *dispersion,* the root mean squared deviation could have been called the *dispersion* or the *mean dispersion.* The word *variance* might even have been reserved for this purpose, so that what is now called the *variance* or the *squared standard deviation* could have been called the *squared variance.*

With complete disregard for the important scientific roles of the words *standards* and *standardized,* however, the idea of *standard* was seized and joined to *deviation,* where it has remained in its status as a statistically fused, scientifically malformed neologism. What has made the malformation so acceptable and the phrase *standard deviation* so popular, of course, is that the idea (not the name) is an excellent way of communicating results. If the data have a Gaussian distribution, the standard deviation serves as a splendid summary of the dispersion of data around the mean. We can also describe the dispersion in a single expression by dividing the standard deviation by the mean to get the *coefficient of variation.* Furthermore, in Gaussian circumstances, we know that 95% of the data will be contained in a zone spanned on either side of the mean by two (actually 1.96) standard deviations. Thus, for many years, the most popular way of communicating a summary for a set of univariate data has been to cite the results in the form of mean ± standard deviation, usually symbolized as $\bar{x} \pm s$. [There are good reasons—as discussed earlier in this series[10]—for rejecting this fashion, replacing it with medians and percentile ranges; but this essay is concerned with the sins of the standard error, not the standard deviation.]

c. The entrance and emergence of indirect inference. The events just noted were routine procedures of the descriptive statistics that evolved in the days when scientific investigators were concerned with demonstrating what they had found. These statistical activities required no knowledge of mathematics (beyond the ability to do arithmetic) and no mental flights to any probabilistic aeries. When investigators performed comparisons, however, a role became available for statistical inference. The investigator's comparison might involve a direct contrast of two means or two proportions; or an indirect contrast of a greater-than-zero value for a correlation coefficient or regression coefficient against an assumed null value of 0. After deciding, from scientific judgment, that the contrasted results were substantively impressive, the investigator would then want to determine whether the observed groups were large enough for the results to be more than a chance occurrence.

The need to make this probabilistic decision brought statistical inference into scientific research. The two different mathematical ways to do the probabilistic analysis were described[9] previously in this series. One way was simple, straightforward, and easily comprehensible. It relied on permutations of the observed data to provide a specific distribution of alternative possibilities for arranging the results, showing exact P values for each alternative. The other way was complex, convoluted, and hard to understand. It relied on a gerrymandered transformation of the parametric theories developed for inferential estimation from single samples; an acceptance of numerous assumptions that could never be verified; and a willingness to think in the abstract domains of hypothetical populations, mathematically perfect distributions, infinite acts of sampling, pooled variances, and approximate P values. The first way was what scientists wanted; the second was what statisticians offered. The first way, in the era before computers, required difficult and sometimes formidable calculations; the second way, once one learned the rules of the game, was easily carried out with a desk (or handheld) calculator. Not because of any logical or scientific desirability, but merely because of calculational convenience, the second way has thus far been triumphant.

In the forseeable future, when digital computers have become cheap and easy to use and when hand-held, battery-powered computer terminals have become ubiquitous, the scientifically desirable, direct methods of statistical inference may become the conventional procedure for performing probabilistic contrasts. For the immediately foreseeable future, however, investigators must deal with the indirect forms of probabilistic reasoning, with statistical consultants who prefer that form of reasoning (because of its comfort, its familiarity, and perhaps its mystery), and with the adverse consequences that the indirect forms of statistical inference have had on scientific communication.

d. The confusion between estimations and contrasts. To be applied for evaluating comparisons, the indirect methods of statistical inference had to be altered from their original purposes. The original goal of the indirect inferential strategy was parametric estimation, not probabilistic contrast. The inferential tactics were initially intended for political poll-takers, market research analysts, and other people who attempt to estimate the "parameters" of a population by inferences drawn from the values found in a single random sample of that population. Thus, if we take a random sample of 150 potential voters in Connecticut, find that 81 of them say they will vote Republican, and thereby conclude that the Connecticut vote in favor of Republicans will be 54% in the next election, we perform a parametric estimation. If we find that the Republican preference is 44% among 150 clinical epidemiologists and 56% among 150 molecular biologists and if we thereby conclude that molecular biologists are more statistically significantly Republican than clinical epidemiologists, we perform a probabilistic contrast.

For parametric estimation, indirect statistical inference is a necessity, not a calculational luxury. In an estimation procedure, the investigator has only one sample. There is no second group available with which to form the permutations and other arrangements used in direct statistical inference for contrasts. With only one sample available, however, the estimating investigator must engage in educated guesswork (called *assumptions*) about the distribution and other characteristics of a hypothetical parent population; and must accept the other theoretical components of the process that leads from observed values in a sample to estimated values for its frame (or population).

The distinction between a parametric estimation from a single random sample and a probabilistic contrast for the results of two groups does not appear to be clearly understood by many statisticians and scientists. The consequent confusion may well be responsible for many of the major problems in communication that statistical analysis has brought to scientific research. An investigator performing a probabilistic contrast of two groups has no interest in parametric estimation, and uses indirect parametric principles of statistical inference only because he doesn't know anything else to do, or because he is computationally constrained, or because he has received misleading advice. Conversely, an investigator performing a parametric estimation from a random sample cannot apply direct principles of inference and uses the indirect methods because they are the best (and the only) tactics at his disposal.

The confusion among scientists is widespread and can readily be seen from the frequency with which indirect parametric techniques are applied to contrast the results of groups that were not selected as random samples and that therefore permit no parametric estimations. The confusion among statisticians is also widespread and can readily be seen from the frequency with which statisticians improperly use the word *samples* for groups that were not samples, the members of the group having entered the research because of their convenience and availability to the investigator. Perhaps the most dramatic example of statisticians' confusion was provided by the late G. W. Snedecor, one of America's leading statisticians and the principal instructor for a generation of contemporary statistical consultants. In the minds of scientific investigators, experiments are intended to allow comparisons of results that will provide valid answers to research questions. According to Snedecor[18], however, "the purpose of an experiment is to produce a sample of observations which will furnish estimates of the parameters of the population together with measures of the uncertainty of these estimates"

e. Estimating a mean and its standard error. In the rare circumstances in which a clinical or epidemiologic investigator has obtained a random sample for estimating a populational parameter such as a mean, the indirect statistical reasoning would go as follows.

In the available sample, we can calculate a mean and a standard deviation. From this information, how likely are we to be right or wrong in estimating the true mean of the parent population? To answer this question, we begin a long chain of abstract reasoning. Suppose we drew another sample and calculated its mean and standard deviation. Now suppose we obtained yet another sample and found its mean and standard deviation. Now suppose we repeated this process over and over, restoring each sample, if necessary, back into the original frame (or population) before the next sample was drawn.

As the process of repeated sampling continued, we would obtain a series of means, one for each sample. Let us now concentrate on that set of sample means and think of them as though they were the individual values in a collection of data. In fact, let us calculate the mean of the set of means and the standard deviation of those means. The value for the standard deviation of the means would need a name. We could call it the *standard deviation of the means,* but this term can be rejected either because it is too clear to be used in statistical nomenclature or because it might be confused with the other kind of standard deviation, calculated for individual single samples, not for the means of a series of samples. Besides, our old friend *error* has been hanging around, awaiting a call to active duty. To avoid letting this old soldier fade away, the standard deviation of the means (plural) will be christened the *standard error of the mean* (singular).

The philologic restoration of *error* and the transition from the plural to the singular of *mean* was accompanied by some basic acts of mathematical faith. It is this faith that enables you, as a realistic scientist, to forget that you have only one sample and that a repetitive sampling process never occurred. With this faith, you assume that such a process took place and you can then draw conclusions about its results. The conclusions, which represent the fundamental tenets of statistical inference for parametric estimation, can be stated as follows:

1. As the theoretical sampling process continues over and over, the mean of the means will approach the true value of the populational mean. Lacking the reality of repeated samples to tell us this true value, we must take a guess about it. There are convincing mathematical proofs to show that the best guess, i.e., the best estimate, for the populational mean will be the mean of our single available sample.

2. Although the mean of that single sample provides the best estimate of the populational mean, the variance of the single sample, calculated as S_{xx}/n, is not the best estimator of the populational variance. With a mathematical proof that is too complex to be shown here, it can be demonstrated that the populational variance is best estimated as $S_{xx}/(n-1)$. [This aspect of statistical inference is the reason that so many statistical textbooks and programmed calculators determine the standard deviation as $s = \sqrt{\sum (x_i - \bar{x})^2/(n-1)}$, rather than using the more intuitively "logical" value of n in the denominator. The commonly cited explanation—that $n-1$ is the "degrees of

freedom'' in the data—is another source of statistogenic confusion. It is an explanation that doesn't explain. The real reason is that the $n - 1$ calculation for the data in the sample offers a better estimate of the value in the population.]

3. With another mathematical proof that you will be spared here, it can be shown that this inferential value for the standard deviation in the single sample can be used to estimate the value for the standard error of the means assembled in all those hypothetical samples. With s calculated as $\sqrt{S_{xx}/(n - 1)}$, the standard error is calculated as $s/\sqrt{n}$.

The appearance of the square root of n in the denominator for the standard error indicates why a sampling process can be so expensive if we want highly accurate estimations. In order to halve the standard error, we must quadruple the sample size. For example, let us consider the standard error of the earlier illustration in which a random sample of 150 Connecticut voters indicated a 54% preference for the Republican party. The formula for getting the standard error of a proportion is $\sqrt{pq/n}$ where n is the sample size, p is the proportion, and $q = 1 - p$. The standard error of the proportion found in our political poll would therefore be $\sqrt{(.54)(.46)/150} = .04$, or 4%. If we wanted to reduce this standard error by one half, we could not merely double the sample size, since $\sqrt{(.54)(.46)/300} = .028$ or 2.8%. We would have to raise the sample size to 600, for which the standard error would be .02, or 2%.

f. Confidence interval around the mean. At this point, the friend whom you invited earlier to serve as a judge of your explanatory prowess should be asking some more questions: Why in the world have you bothered with all this mathematical explanation? What good is the standard error of the mean? What can you do with it? You may now smile happily because, at long last, you can provide a logical, easily understood answer that you hope will also deliver your *coup de grace*.

You can point out that the purpose of parametric estimation is not just to get an estimate of the mean, but also to indicate its ''uncertainty'', i.e., how close or far off the estimate may be from the true value. If we think about a series of repeated samples, yielding a series of means and a standard deviation— oops, standard error—for those means, we can

now invoke the old principle of Gaussian distributions. According to this principle, if we take the mean of our series of means, a range spanned by twice (or 1.96 times) the standard error on either side of that mean will contain 95% of the means found in all of the repeated samples. Re-phrased in a more easily understood manner, this statement says there is a 95% chance that the true populational mean lies in the zone $\bar{x} + 2s_{\bar{x}}$, where $s_{\bar{x}}$ represents the standard error of the mean and where $\bar{x}$, our sample mean, is used to estimate the populational mean. Thus, for the previously cited political poll, with a Republican preference of 54%, having a standard error of 4%, there is a 95% chance that the true Republican preference for the population is 54% ± (2)(4%), which is a zone between 46% and 62%. If the standard error is reduced to 2%, the true result has a 95% probability of being somewhere between 50% and 58%.

What we have just done is to construct what is called a *confidence interval around the mean.* The procedure is based on several theoretical principles and practical requirements.

1. From the mathematical structure of a Gaussian distribution, we know that specified zones of probability (or relative frequency) occur at specified standard deviations on either side of the mean of the collection of data. Thus, an interval that spans 1.96 standard deviations bilaterally around the mean will encompass 95% of the data in the distribution. A corresponding interval, based on 1.645 standard deviations, will encompass 90%; and 2.58 deviations will encompass 99%.

2. Reversing this process, if we decide how much of the probability (90%, 95%, 99%, or some other number) we want to cover in a distribution, we can use appropriate mathematical tables to find the associated number for multiplying the standard deviation. (This number is often called z and it takes such values as 1.645, 1.96, or 2.58.)

3. The results of the technique just cited pertain to the actual data for any Gaussian distribution. These principles are the reason for the conventional descriptive statement that approximately 95% of the data are spanned by the interval x ± 2s. In the particular world of statistical inference that now is under considera-

tion, however, we deal with a hypothetical distribution of the means of a hypothetical set of repeated samples. The standard deviation for that hypothetical distribution is the standard error of the mean. According to the Gaussian principles, we would therefore expect 95% of those hypothetical means to be located in an interval spanned by $x \pm 2 \ s/\sqrt{n}$. Since we have used $\bar{x}$, the sample mean, to estimate μ, the populational mean, we would thus be 95% confident that the true mean of the sampled population lies within that interval.

4. This "confidence" requires sustenance from several additional principles or requirements. First, to allow the use of Gaussian principles, the hypothetical distribution of the means must be Gaussian. This reassurance is provided by an extraordinary, crucial mathematical demonstration, called the *Central Limit Theorem,* which shows that the collection of means of repeated samples from a parent population has a Gaussian distribution, regardless of the way in which the parent population is itself distributed. Secondly, to allow principles of random probability to be applied, the single sample with which we actually work must be drawn randomly. Third, the z-values in the probability table are applicable only to large samples. If the sample we work from has a small size, the z values should be replaced by t values, taken from an appropriate table of probabilities associated with the t-distribution described by W. S. Gossett, writing under the pseudonym, "Student". Fourth, we must be prepared for the occasional fickleness of chance. Although we can be 95% confident that the true population mean will be located in our 95% confidence interval, there is always that one time in 20 when it will not, when our confidence will be a delusion, and when the inferential estimation, based on a confidence interval using a standard error, has led us to a wrong result.

2. Confidence games

The confidence interval technique has been an effective tool for investigators in social science, political science, and marketing research. These investigators, confronted with the challenge of estimating a population parameter from a single random sample, have found confidence intervals to be a valuable and probably irreplaceable procedure for indicating the zone in which the true value of a mean is likely to occur. The confidence interval helps show the uncertainty of the estimate made from a random sample and helps in calculating the size of the group needed in future acts of random sampling.

In clinical and epidemiologic research, however, the groups under investigation are almost never selected as random samples; and the investigator's main interest is in contrasting results for two or more groups, not in estimating parameters for a single sample. In these forms of research, neither the standard error nor the confidence interval can supply suitable answers to the fundamental challenges of communication and probabilistic contrast.

For communicating the data, the investigator should show or summarize what he found. The summaries are provided by indications of the data's central tendency (expressed in such terms as means, medians, and proportions) and dispersion (expressed in such terms as range, percentile ranges, and standard deviation). The standard error and confidence interval are not summaries of evidence; they are acts of inference. They do not describe the data. They provide, at most, a guess about the location of the mean of a mythical population in which the investigator may have no interest; and to which, even if interested, he cannot relate his results because the investigated group was not randomly sampled from that population.

(As long as statistical consultants maintain the belief that any selected groups can be arbitrarily regarded as random samples, the consultants will persist in giving unsuitable advice. It is true that parametric techniques of inference can be, and are, regularly applied for probabilistic contrasts of groups that were not selected randomly. The reason the parametric techniques are effective, however, is not because the contrasted groups can arbitrarily be regarded as random samples, but because the P values that emerge from the indirect parametric calculations are often quite similar to those accurately obtained by direct permutation methods. The persistence of the arbitrary fiction about random sampling during a probabilistic contrast of groups allows the attention of the consultants and their clients to be diverted into thinking about abstract statistical inference, rather than searching for realistic sources of bias in the selection of the groups. The pervasive neglect of this problem is probably the single greatest cause of malpractice[8] in academic biostatistical consultation today.)

For drawing probabilistic contrasts, an investigator wants to know the likelihood that the observed difference arose by chance. He can determine this probability either directly, using permutation techniques, or indirectly, using parametric inference. In the latter situation, the standard error is not a communicative entity; it is merely a component of the parametric calculations that are performed en route to a P value.

In fact, the standard error of the individual groups does not appear in probabilistic tests where the means or proportions of two groups are contrasted. Such procedures as the t test or chi-square test for two groups depend on a pooled standard error, not on the standard errors in each group. Thus, in two groups containing n_1 and n_2 members and standard deviations of s_1 and s_2 respectively, the t test for the standard error of the difference in means relies on a "pooled variance", which is calculated as $[(n_1 - 1)s_1^2 + (n_2 - 1)s_2^2]/(n_1 + n_2 - 2)$. The individual standard errors, which would be $s_1/\sqrt{n_1}$ and $s_2/\sqrt{n_2}$, do not appear in the formula for the calculations. Similarly, in the chi-square test, the standard error of the difference in two proportions, p_1 and p_2, relies on a "pooled variance", which is calculated as PQ, where $P = (n_1 p_1 + n_2 p_2)/N$, and $Q = 1 - P$. Again, the individual standard errors, which would be derived from $p_1 q_1/n_1$ and $p_2 q_2/n_2$, do not appear in the calculations.

If the individual standard errors appeared in either the t-test or chi-square test formulas, there would be something unusual about the test procedure. We would be using the test for a purpose that is different from an ordinary probabilistic contrast. When the null hypothesis is invoked for the customary contrasts, the assumption is made that each of the two groups is a random sample from the same parent population. In seeking the hypothetical distribution of

the differences in the means (or proportions) of two concomitant samples from the same population, we use the pooled variance to estimate the standard error of the means of the population of differences.

There are at least two unconventional circumstances in which the individual standard errors of each group actually appear in the calculations. One of these situations is a probabilistic procedure where we do *not* invoke the null hypothesis. Thus, in the kinds of statistical tests done to examine "beta errors" on the "other side of statistical significance"[12], we would use the standard error values in each group for our estimations—but we would then be doing a probabilistic contrast that has different goals and procedures from those customarily used to test statistical significance. Henrik Wulff[19] has described another such situation—occurring after the primary (or null hypothesis) test of "statistical significance" is found to be positive, so that the null hypothesis is rejected. Accepting the idea that the two groups are different and wanting to get an idea of the true magnitude of this difference, we can calculate a confidence interval around the difference, using each group's standard error in the calculation. This procedure would be valid for a difference in the two groups created by the randomized allocation of treatment in a clinical trial, but the results cannot be extrapolated beyond those two groups, unless the combined groups were originally sampled randomly from patients eligible for inclusion in the trial.

Why, then, you may now be asked by your common-sensical friend, have investigators and editors so often been playing the confidence game of reporting results in terms of standard errors or confidence intervals? The act might be justified, although not wholly proper, if the reported results are immediately subjected to inferential testing; but if no inferential tests are done, the only role of the standard errors and confidence intervals is to distort and conceal the data. The reader wants to know the actual span of the data; but the investigator displays an estimated zone for the mean.

This substitution gives the data a much more compact appearance, particularly in graphical displays where lines are drawn on both sides of the mean at a distance of either one standard deviation or one standard error. The data will look "tighter" if this distance is demarcated by using the standard error, as an inferential estimate around the mean, rather than the standard deviation, as a summary of dispersion. The demarcated zone will thereby be reduced in size because the standard error, being calculated as $s/\sqrt{n}$, is always smaller than the standard deviation; and because a 95% confidence interval based on twice the standard error is always smaller than a 95% data interval based on the standard deviation. The viewer of the "tighter" graph may then think that the data have much less variability than is actually present. After all, results shown as ⊢•⊣ seem much less disperse than ⊢——•——⊣, even though the two drawings are derived from exactly the same set of data, with the first showing the mean ± standard error and the second showing the mean ± standard deviation.

Although this kind of substitution gives a misleading idea of the dispersion of the data, and although the distortion has become ubiquitous in medical literature, statistical textbooks contain few if any admonitions against the activity. The procedure is also unmentioned among the many other communicative distortions cited in Darrel Huff's splendid book, *How to Lie with Statistics*[15]. For statistical and scientific analysts who are concerned with evidence rather than inference, a major crusade may be necessary to evict the standard error from the pretentious deception it creates in the communication and graphical display of scientific data.

Some investigators might want to argue that a drawing of the magnitude of the standard errors is helpful in gauging the statistical significance of differences in groups. This argument is based on mathematical misunderstandings. If the investigator really does want to illustrate "statistical significance", a well marked set of 95% confidence intervals would be a better demonstration than standard errors. If the 95% confidence intervals do not overlap around the two means or two proportions, the difference between them is significant at $P < .05$. If this approach is to be used, however, each confidence interval on the graph should have exactly the same width, since, according to the null hypothesis, it should be calculated from the pooled standard error for the groups.

An investigator who draws a graph with two or more points, each point having a different sized band for the standard error around it, may

believe he is offering an excellent illustration of statistical significance in the data. In fact, however, he is deluding himself and misleading his readers. If he wants to show the dispersion of the data, the bands should be based on standard deviations, not standard errors; and if he wants to show inferential "statistical significance" for differences in the means, the bands should represent confidence intervals, not standard errors. To show "statistical significance", the confidence bands should be of similar width for each group, having been calculated from the common standard error of the means, according to the pooling principle used in testing the null hypothesis.

3. The nonplussed minus

Perhaps the worst abuse of statistical symbolism in communicating data is the nonplussed minus sign: a "±" that appears in the form of $a \pm b$ without any indication of what is meant by b. The a almost always refers to the value of a mean; but the b, unless clearly identified, can refer to many things. It usually denotes either the standard deviation of the data or the standard error of the mean. If marked *s.d., s.e.,* or *s.e.m.,* the expression for b can be understood by the reader. If the reporting investigator also indicates the group size, *n,* the reader can quickly do the calculations needed to go from either the standard deviation to the standard error, or vice versa. If there is no indication of what term is reported after the "±" sign, however, the reader has no idea of whether it refers to standard deviation, standard error, or something else entirely. Although a reader might expect the editors of scientific journals to guard against this malefaction, it frequently appears in many places, even in such highly prestigious general journals as *Lancet* and the *New England Journal of Medicine*.

About eight years ago, the problem received open airing in a commentary, published in *Science,* by Churchill Eisenhart[5], who urged that "the shorthand form $a \pm b$ should be avoided in abstracts and summaries; and never used without explicit explanation of its connotation". In response to subsequent letters, Eisenhart[6] quoted Ku's remark[16] about the "loss of information through oversimplification", Branscomb's survey[1] of the "useless literature explosion", and added the following new indictment:

My colleagues in the National Bureau of Standards Office of Standard Reference Data find that an appalling fraction of the literature in any specific field contains data not worthy of critical evaluation. Estimates of the faulty fraction range from 50 to over 90 percent. The three principal reasons for failure appear to be: the experimental work was done incorrectly; the sources of uncertainty were not analyzed; or the work was not reported in sufficient detail to permit evaluation.

In the field of medical literature, this estimate probably is closer to 90 percent (or higher) than to 50 percent; and a fourth principal reason might be added to the three other reasons for the failures: the research was poorly designed, because the investigator (or the investigator's consultant) was trained to think only about simple issues in the design of *experiments,* not about the many complexities of architecture that occur in planning the non-random *surveys* that constitute most medical research.

As the editors of scientific journals recall that their major purpose is the communication of evidence and not merely computations of tests of "statistical significance", greater efforts may be taken to avoid the nonplussed minus phenomenon. One effective mode of prophylaxis might be to include warnings against the orphan "±" sign in the journal's stylebook. If the investigators, reviewers, and editors do not guard against this problem, the manuscript redactor might be asked to serve as the last line of defense. While simultaneously fixing any dangling participles, removing periods from abbreviations such as *e.g.* and *mg.* and changing the spelling of *technique* to *technic,* the redactor can check that the right hand side of each "±" sign is identified. Redactors might also be given the job of expunging such confusing expressions[2] as "variances are ±1 SD".

In customary scientific usage, of course, the *b* of an *a* ± *b* expression refers to the accuracy of the measurement. Thus, if someone reports that a specimen weighs 27 ± 2 mg, the idea is that its weight can be anywhere from 25 to 29 mgm. In statistical usage, the ± sign has this same meaning if it refers to a confidence inter-

val around a mean. A statement such as "the 95% confidence interval was 250 ± 10" implies that in a series of random samples taken from this same parent population, 95% of the means would lie between 240 and 260. But what is the value of the ± sign when it is applied to the standard deviation or standard error? A reader who wants to use the information cannot do so directly. To form a 95% interval of either dispersion or inference, the reader would have to multiply the s.d. or s.e. by 2 (or 1.96) and then add and subtract the result from the mean. If the purpose is to communicate the spread of the data or the estimation of the true mean, why not cite the interval directly for the reader? And if the idea is to show spread of the data, why not calculate the 95% zone around the mean by using the percentile technique, rather than the standard deviation, which is so often inapplicable because the data are not Gaussian?

Probably the only valid answer to these questions, aside from intellectual inertia, is the saving of space. To cite the boundaries of a 95% zone of dispersion would require two numbers rather than one and some indication of how the zone was determined. Thus, instead of an expression such as "mean ± s.d. = 27 ± 13", an investigator using a 95% inner percentile range would say "mean; 95% i.p.r. = 27; 2 − 57". Alternatively, an investigator using Gaussian range statistics could say "mean; 95% G.r. = 27; 1 − 53". The extra few spaces needed for the latter expressions would be more than compensated by the enormous increase they would offer in communicative clarity. The journal's editor could readily regain the space needed for these statements of evidence by throwing out some unnecessary P values and a few other excessive, noncommunicative items of inferential statistical baggage.

4. The inefficient coefficient

To summarize the distribution of data for a single variable, we use at least two indexes: one for central tendency and the other for dispersion. To summarize the relationship of two variables, the usual index is a single coefficient: either a correlation coefficient, for the nondirectional interdependency of the two varia-

Table I. *Hypothetical data showing results of three new methods vs. old method of measurement*

| Results of old method, X (x_i) | Results of new methods | | |
	Method Y (y_i)	Method Z (z_i)	Method W (w_i)
1.0	3.6	−8.0	0.0
2.0	3.6	−2.0	3.0
3.0	3.7	1.0	2.0
4.0	4.0	4.0	5.0
5.0	5.0	5.0	4.0
6.0	6.0	6.0	7.0
7.0	7.0	7.0	6.0
8.0	7.3	10.0	9.0
9.0	7.4	13.0	8.0
10.0	7.4	19.0	11.0
Mean	5.5	5.5	5.5
Correlation coefficient with x_i	.96	.97	.95
Regression coefficient with x_i	.54	2.44	1.06
Coefficient of determination (r^2)	.92	.94	.91

bles; or a regression coefficient, for the directional dependency of one variable on the other. In a previous essay in this series[11], I discussed the relative merits of these two coefficients, emphasizing the duplicity and defects of the correlation coefficient for situations in which the relationship clearly had a specific direction. The main point to be noted now is the gross inefficiency of both of these coefficients for communicating scientific data. We can also lament the sad irony that allows the relatively simple data for one variable to be summarized with two indexes, whereas the greater complexity of two variables gets summarized with only one.

The main flaws of the correlation coefficient and the regression coefficient can be paraphrased from a remark once made to me by a newspaper reader who said she preferred the tabloid *New York Daily News* to the august *New York Times*. ''The Times'', she said, ''gives me all the news that's fit to print, but it doesn't tell me what's happening''. Similarly, correlation or regression coefficients provide a statistically suitable summary of bivariate relationships, but do not show some of the most important features that a scientific reader would like to know.

For example, consider the kind of a challenge that often confronts clinical chemists. Suppose we have three new different methods for measuring a chemical substance and we want to compare the results of the new methods against those of the established old method. A popular approach for this analysis is to note the correlation coefficient between the value obtained for each specimen by the old method and the corresponding values obtained with the new. When these coefficients are calculated for each of the three new methods, we find apparently excellent agreement. The respective correlation coefficients against the old method X, are .96 for method Y, .97 for method Z, and .95 for method W.

A clinical chemist who relied only on correlation coefficients might therefore conclude that all three of these new methods are excellent and that they are essentially equivalent. A scientific clinical chemist would insist on examining the data. In Table I, the values of x_i show the results obtained with the old method in 10 specimens; and the values of y_i, z_i, and w_i show the results obtained when the same specimens were measured respectively, by methods Y, Z, and W. For all three methods, as indicated in Table I, the correlation coefficients against the old method are excellent and almost identical, ranging from r = .95 to r = .97.

Neither the coefficients nor the tabulated data will clearly show, however, what becomes promptly apparent if we look at a graph of the actual relationships, as portrayed in Fig. 1. The graphs show that Method Y achieves its excellent correlation by virtue of its identical values in the middle of the spectrum. At either end of the spectrum, however, Method Y has terrible results, producing flattened results that make the total data resemble an S-curve. On the other hand, Method Z also gives identical values in the middle of the spectrum, but turns sharply downward and upward at the extremes. Method W, in contrast to the other two, does not give identical values anywhere, but successively vacillates 1 unit above and 1 unit below the old values.

We might have gotten a clue to these major disparities in the three methods by noting the

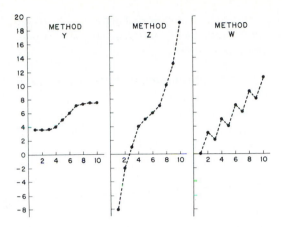

Fig. 1. Results of Methods Y, Z, and W (on ordinates) vs. Method X (on abscissa). Lines drawn by eye-fit of points.

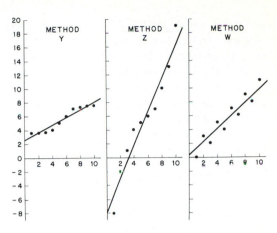

Fig. 2. Results of Methods Y, Z, and W (on ordinates) vs. Method X (on abscissa). Lines drawn by mathematical calculation of regressions.

substantial differences, listed in Table I, for the three regression coefficients, which are respectively about 0.5, 1.0, and 2.4 for methods Y, W, and Z. These regression coefficients merely tell us, however, that the fitted lines have different slopes. They do not tell us whether the lines are appropriate (i.e., that the data may be non-linear); and the coefficients do not indicate where and how the lines may fit badly. In fact, because the excellence of fit is supposed to be indicated by the *coefficient of determination,* which is r^2, and because the r^2 values of .92, .94, and .91 suggest excellent fits, a purely statistical analyst might conclude that all the linear correlations are splendid, although the graphical portraits obviously contradict this conclusion. The straight lines drawn from the mathematical calculations, in fact, do provide good fits, as shown in Fig. 2; but the direct visual portraits shown in Fig. 1 might make a clinical chemist reluctant to accept any of these three new methods as being satisfactory replacements for Method X.

The example just cited is but one of the many different types that could have been used. Good textbooks of statistics will provide many other illustrations; and a particularly useful account of the diverse problems is provided in Mainland's text[17] and in an intriguing new book[4] by Ehrenberg. Because the problems can occur in so many different ways, there is no simple, easy procedure that will get rid of the difficulties

caused by the inefficiency of correlation and regression coefficients for summarizing relationships of two variables. Perhaps the most useful approach is to insist that no bivariate relationship can be properly communicated merely with a coefficiented summary. To get a more effective indication of what is happening, some other things are necessary. Among those other things are the following:

a. Insist on examining the graphical portrait of the data. Looking at the tabulated results alone will not show the relationships as clearly as the scatter-graph.

b. Insist on seeing the calculated regression line for the points on the graph. (If the two variables cannot be biologically designated as dependent and independent, look at the two regression lines that are obtained when each variable is placed in the dependent role.)

c. Always look at the values for both the correlation and the regression coefficients. See whether their computed values are consistent with the results you would anticipate by *visually* fitting a line to the data.

d. Badger, cajole, and prod your friendly journal editor to get him (or her) to maintain the foregoing three standards for communicating reports of scientific data, even if the journal's statistical reviewers fail to ask for compliance with the standards.

e. When the raw data are available, try breaking the data up into at least three parts—for low, intermediate, and high values of the independent variable that serves as x or its equivalent. Determine the correlation and regression coefficients for each of these three parts. If the corresponding coefficients are similar for each part and also for the complete data, then the overall summary coefficients are reasonably reliable. If major differences occur in coefficients for the parts vs. coefficients for the whole, beware. Something funny is going on, requiring further exploration and interpretation.

The procedures just cited can be helpful when the correlation and regression coefficients deal with a relationship between two variables. In a multivariate situation, everything is much more complicated. There is no easy way to draw graphical portraits of the relationship between the dependent variable, y, and the multiple independent variables to which it is related in such tactics as multiple linear regression or multiple logistic regression. These multivariate relationships cannot be visualized in any realistic manner, since the mathematical model calls for "additive effects", taking place in an "n-dimensional space" that is too imaginary to be portrayed.

The problems of trying to conduct scientific communication amidst these complex mathematical models are enormous and will be saved for discussion in a future installment of this series. Only two points will be noted now. The first is a distressing feature of modern statistical life: the frequency with which careful investigators abandon their common sense and scientific skepticism when credulously accepting the results of multiple regression analyses whose models, mechanisms, and machinations the investigators do not understand. The second point is the communicative deception that occurs when investigators report the results of multiple regression procedures by citing the *b* (or beta) regression coefficients alone, without reporting the coefficient of multiple determination, R^2, that would give the reader an idea of how well (or how badly) the data are fitted by the imaginary regression surface. Regardless of whether this deception is deliberate or inadvertent, good editors should not permit it to occur. The results of multiple regression maneuvers should not be accepted for publication unless accompanied by

a coefficient of multiple determination, which would cite the regression model's overall "goodness of fit".

5. The substitution of inference for evidence

In all of the problems that have just been listed, the scientific communication was incomplete. The data were summarized with expressions that were inadequate or inefficient for reporting all the distinctions needed in scientific appraisals—but the investigator had at least tried to communicate. With increasing frequency in modern biomedical journals, alas, no such effort is made.

The observed evidence is often not reported or summarized at all. It may not be even cited in confidence intervals. Instead, the only thing that gets listed is an array of P values (or F values) to show the inferential results of the "tests of significance" (or the "variance ratios"). Nothing is published to show the observed evidence—in either raw or summary form—from which the inferential calculations were derived.

A separate but related problem occurs when the investigator reports the results of inferential calculations without indicating what statistical test was used for the calculations. This form of defective communication has become particularly prevalent as computers have become increasingly used for the data analyses. One of many available striking examples is the following statement[3], appearing in a respected, usually well-edited medical journal: "Statistical analyses were carried out with a Hewlett Packard computer and program". The authors made no further comment—and the editors apparently requested no more—about what kind of "program" or even which type of "Hewlett Packard computer"

These perversions of scientific communication have become so commonplace that even statisticians have been writing warnings[13, 14] about the problem. Like some of the other problems, this one can be easily solved by a re-orientation of just a few people: the editors of medical journals. We cannot hope to re-orient a generation of statisticians who have been systemically trained to focus on inference while ignoring evidence; nor can we hope to re-orient a generation of investigators who have been systematically trained to honor statistical advice without questioning it, particularly if compliance leads to getting grants funded and papers approved for publication. The number of contemporary editors is much smaller, however, and, besides, editors are ordinarily open-minded people. Having been spared any systematic education that would directly prepare them for being editors, they usually approach the job without any allegiance to entrenched academic paradigms. The editors should therefore be readily amenable to education and re-orientation.

And the best person to help re-orient the editors is you, dear reader, you. Make yourself into a one-person vigilante committee. Whenever a journal that you read publishes the results of anonymous statistical tests; when the tests are identified but the data are absent; or when any other of the foregoing list of defects appears—call it to the editor's attention. Remind the editor about the evils of producing statistical guns without scientific butter; about the obvious necessity for publishing scientific evidence, not just analytic statistical inference. If necessary, wave some sort of flag, composed of quotations and illustrations from suitable references. In this bicentennial year, we cannot expect a major revolution that will totally liberate the communication of evidence from all of its statistical oppression, but a small band of suitably oriented medical editors can easily institute reforms that will restore many of the fundamental liberties needed for the pursuit of science.

References

1. Branscomb, L. M.: Quoted by Eisenhart, Ref. 5.
2. Cowan, D., Bowman, S., Fratianne, R. B., and Ahmed, F.: Platelet aggregation as a sign of septicemia in thermal injury, J. A. M. A. **235**:1230-1234, 1976.
3. Dawborn, J. K., Page, J. D., and Schiavonne, D. J.: Use of 5-fluorocytosine in patients with impaired renal function, Br. Med. J. **2**:382-384, 1973.
4. Ehrenberg, A. S. C.: Data reduction, London, New York, 1975, John Wiley & Sons, Inc.
5. Eisenhart, C.: Expression of the uncertainties of final results, Science **160**:1201-1204, 1968.
6. Eisenhart, C.: Statistical uncertainties, Science **162**:1332-1333, 1968. (Response to letter-to-editor.)
7. Feinstein, A. R.: Clinical biostatistics. III-V. The architecture of clinical research, CLIN. PHARMACOL. THER. **11**:432-441, 595-610, and 755-771, 1970.
8. Feinstein, A. R.: Clinical biostatistics. VI. Statistical "malpractice"—and the responsibility of a consultant, CLIN. PHARMACOL. THER. **11**:898-914, 1970.
9. Feinstein, A. R.: Clinical biostatistics. XXIII. The role of randomization in sampling, testing, allocation, and credulous idolatry (Part 2), CLIN. PHARMACOL. THER. **14**:898-915, 1973.
10. Feinstein, A. R.: Clinical biostatistics. XXVII. The derangements of the "range of normal," CLIN. PHARMACOL. THER. **15**:528-540, 1974.
11. Feinstein, A. R.: Clinical biostatistics. XXXII. Biologic dependency, 'hypothesis testing', unilateral probabilities, and other issues in scientific direction vs. statistical duplexity, CLIN. PHARMACOL. THER. **17**:499-513, 1975.
12. Feinstein, A. R.: Clinical biostatistics. XXXIV. The other side of 'statistical significance': Alpha, beta, delta, and the calculation of sample size, CLIN. PHARMACOL. THER. **18**:491-505, 1975.
13. Goldstein, H.: Notes on the presentation of statistics in medical papers, Dev. Med. Child Neurol. **13**:674-675, 1961.
14. Hoaglin, D. C., and Andrews, D. F.: The reporting of computation based results in statistics, Amer. Statist. **29**:122-126, 1975.
15. Huff, D.: How to lie with statistics, New York, 1954, W. W. Norton & Co., Inc.
16. Ku, H. H.: Expressions of imprecision, systematic error, and uncertainty associated with a reported value, Meas. Data **2**: 72, 1968.
17. Mainland, D.: Elementary medical statistics, ed. 2, Philadelphia, 1963, W. B. Saunders Co.
18. Snedecor, G. W.: The statistical part of the scientific method, Ann. N. Y. Acad. Sci. **52**:702-700, 1950.
19. Wulff, H. R.: Confidence limits in evaluating controlled therapeutic trials. Lancet **2**:969-970, 1973. (Letter-to-editor.)

THE ANALYSIS OF MULTIPLE VARIABLES

Some of the greatest challenges for creative biostatistical research today are in developing improved methods to analyze the data of multiple variables simultaneously. Every medical investigation provides data for multiple variables, which include demographic, clinical, paraclinical, therapeutic, etiologic, or other information. In analyzing results, however, the investigator usually examines the variables one at a time for means, dispersions, and distributions; or two at a time for correlations, simple regressions, or the contrasts tested with such techniques as t-test and chi-square. When more than two variables are examined simultaneously, the process becomes multivariate and the intricate complexity begins.

Although the plethora of available statistical techniques for multivariate analysis is an indication that none is satisfactory, the constant proliferation of new methods (most of which are minor variations on old methods) has served to obscure both the major flaws of the existing procedures and the basic challenges of what needs to be done. A multivariate analysis is a type of classification procedure. The data expressing the states of a set of multiple variables are arranged to produce a numerical entity that expresses (or classifies) the state of something else. The basic character of the statistical analysis and the result is determined by this *something else*. It can be the specific focus of a dependent target event (or variable); or it can be a nonspecific denominational name, such as a *factor* or *cluster,* which serves to summarize, rather than focus, the interdependency of the multiple variables.

Medical investigators encounter problems in both the denominational and the targeted forms of classification. Denominational problems occur during the challenges of creating suitable demarcations and names for living organisms or for diseases, particularly in the diagnostic categories of psychiatry. Targeted challenges involve either prognostic predictions about a patient's outcome or etiologic correlations with causes of disease. The targeted decisions, as discussed in the first essay in this section, have the major advantage of allowing an external validation. Any targeted mathematical construction can be validated by determining how accurately the results indicate the state of the external target variable. By contrast, a purely denominational system cannot be validated. It can be graded for its quantitative effects on the system's internal variance, covariance, or other mathematical indexes, but it cannot be tested for the frequency with which it is right or wrong.

The second essay in this section contains a relatively simple description and brief evaluation of the various statistical maneuvers that are currently available for multivariate analysis. The interdependent maneuvers, such as factor analysis and cluster analysis, have the handicap of not being aimed at a target variable; the targeted maneuvers, such as multiple regression and discriminant function analysis, depend on additive linear models that may be biologically inappropriate; and all of the existing systems—targeted or untargeted—have the major disadvantage of excluding clinical judgment from their construction and of obfuscating clinical meaning in their results.

In contrast to the purely mathematical processes, clinical investigators have developed an effective, comprehensible set of principles for a clinically oriented model of multivariate analysis. The clinical model is illustrated by staging systems for cancer. The stages are demarcated as multivariate clusters (or strata) that are prognostically targeted, clinically meaningful, and easily understood. Although staging systems for cancer have received worldwide dissemination and application, the underlying principles have generally been ignored. Confronted by challenges in other aspects of multivariate analysis, investigators usually rely exclusively on mathematical strategies and seldom attempt to create the analog of a clinical staging system.

The merits of the clinical model have probably been neglected because it involves hitherto nondescript judgmental decisions, because its principles have not been clearly stipulated, and because no methods have been established for evaluating the results. In the last four essays, I have tried to describe the judgments, stipulate the principles, and establish methods of evaluation. The objective of these activities in "prognostic stratification" (which seems to be a better name than "staging") is to preserve the basic intellectual and scientific advantages of the clinical model, while increasing its statistical precision and power. The optional forms of multivariate analysis, like all other issues in clinical biostatistics, should contain a suitably balanced combination of clinical coherence and statistical quantification.

CHAPTER 24

On homogeneity, taxonomy, and nosography

An ancient but persistent problem in biologic science is the ascertainment of homogeneity for compared substances. When the effects of two or more different maneuvers are investigated in the usual scientific sequence of INITIAL STATE → MANEUVER → SUBSEQUENT STATE, the entities that receive the compared maneuvers must be appropriately similar. If these entities have important initial differences, a pre-maneuveral bias will be introduced into the research and may invalidate its results.[15, 16]

The entities compared in research can easily be made similar if they can be physically divided into equal parts or aliquots. For this type of simple partitioning to be satisfactory, however, the entity must consist of homogeneous material. If the material contains several distinctly different ingredients, the separated parts might be equal in size or weight but unequal in the proportionate content of those different ingredients. To avoid such disproportions, the material to be studied is usually made homogeneous—by mixing, grinding, or other mechanical techniques—before the homogenate is physically partitioned into the aliquots that become subjected to the maneuvers under investigation. This type of physical homogenization and partition is readily achieved for the inanimate substances that are studied in physics, chemistry, and geology, and for the animate fragments (slices of organs, sections of tissues, suspensions of cells) that are studied in reductionist biology.

In organismal biology, however, the basic entity cannot be physically divided because it is an intact organism or animal. Although symmetrical regions of a single animal can sometimes be contrasted, the usual "material" of organismal research consists of two or more animals or groups of animals. In such circumstances, an investigator cannot prepare and divide a homogenate to achieve initial similarity for his compared substances. Consequently, organismal biologists are confronted by a major scientific problem that requires relatively little attention in the natural sciences or in reductionist biology. As a

Under the same name, this chapter originally appeared as "Clinical biostatistics—XIII." In Clin. Pharmacol. Ther. 13:114, 1972.

prerequisite to scientific investigation, the organismal biologist must develop methods of establishing and ascertaining homogeneity for individual animals or groups of animals.

One common procedure is the use of litter-mates. If a group of animals consists of litter-mates that were born, grown, and maintained under identical conditions, an investigator can feel reasonably assured that the members are individually similar. This litter-mate tactic is seldom possible, however, for biologic groups composed of people. An investigator performing clinical or epidemiologic research cannot rely on a common uterine origin for his human "material," and must use some other approach to distinguish homogeneity in people.

In making these distinctions, an investigator must differentiate between similarity in two individuals and in two groups. The two letters *A* and *A* are similar, as are the two letters *B* and *B,* or *C* and *C.* The two groups of letters *AAA* and *AAA* are similar, as are the two groups *ABC* and *ABC,* but the former group is homogeneous and the latter is heterogeneous. Since statistical comparisons are based on groups, our main concern here will be the homogeneity rather than mere similarity in groups. For example, an investigator can form two similar groups of four animals by assigning to each group one member from a litter of frogs, chicks, dogs, and porpoises. In these two groups, however, the membership will be so heterogeneous that any data based on the group, rather than on individual members, may be meaningless. To allow statistical techniques to be applied to the groups studied in scientific research, a biologic investigator must therefore ensure not merely that his groups are alike, but particularly that the individual members are similar enough to warrant their combination into a group.

The determination of a satisfactory similarity for people and of a satisfactory homogeneity for human groups is another basic aspect of scientific "architecture" that has been generally neglected in modern biostatistics. By what methods do we decide that a group is homogeneous? If it is heterogeneous, how do we divide it into homogeneous subgroups? How do we decide that a particular subgroup, although heterogeneous, is homogeneous enough to be maintained as a group? If heterogeneous people can be divided several ways into different kinds of homogeneous subgroups, which type of partition is most desirable?

All of these questions are fundamental to the architectural design of clinical or epidemiologic research, but neither the questions nor the answers appear in most textbooks devoted to statistics, biostatistics, or statistical concepts of "experimental design." Statisticians have been concerned with homogeneity of variance in measurements for a group of objects, not with homogeneity in the objects themselves. As discussed previously,[17] a group of objects that has suitably small variance around the measured mean might statistically be regarded as homogeneous even though the objects consist of small dogs, large cats, huge birds, and infant children. Statistical reasoning begins with the assumption that the objects in the "sample" are themselves homogeneous; the variance found in the sample is then ascribed to such features as inconsistencies in measurement, the vicissitudes of sampling, or the effects of the investigated maneuver. With this reasoning, statisticians have developed various "adjustments" that can be used when heteroscedasticity (i.e., inequality in variance) is found in compared "samples," but the adjustments themselves can not be used to demonstrate whether the samples consist of dogs, cats, birds, or children.

The absence of statistical methods for dealing with this problem is occasionally acknowledged in textbooks of statistics. In 1956, Snedecor[31] said:

What shall be done with samples that are not homogeneous? If there is no uniform probability of occurrence . . . any conclusions are based on flimsy evidence. There is no assurance that, if the experiment were repeated, the same set of probabilities would be existent. If one doesn't know why the probabilities change or in what manner, he can set up no experimental controls. The first step must be toward improved knowledge of the techniques of selecting and handling the experimental material. Only after the sources of variation are discovered may valid comparisons be made.

Since statistical techniques are applied only after the assumption that the samples are homogeneous, the problem of making them homogeneous is a challenging responsibility of biologists, clinicians, and other investigators familiar with the realities of scientific research.

A. The role of taxonomy

Since no two people are exactly alike, the attainment of total similarity for a group of people, or even for two people, is impossible. A pair of identical twins might be indistinguishable in physical appearance and in chromosomal patterns, although one of the twins is a good cook but a poor baseball player, whereas the other plays baseball well but cooks poorly. Although the twins might look identical, we would certainly differentiate between them if we were hiring a cook or choosing a baseball teammate.

Similarly, we might assemble two groups of people who are individually identical in age, race, height, weight, skinfold thickness, and many other discernible characteristics. If these identities are satisfactory for whatever purpose we plan to use the groups, we might then regard the groups as homogeneous. If our purpose, however, is to perform a test of efficacy for oral contraceptive agents, the identities just cited would be inadequate. We would certainly want the two groups to be similar in sex, and, in fact, we would exclude men from admission to membership. We would also exclude women whose potential for conception is compromised by age, by previous surgery, or by the absence of suitable opportunity.

The decision about similarity thus depends on the purpose of the classification. People who are homogeneous for one purpose might be heterogeneous for another, and vice versa. A team of baseball players all wearing the same uniform will be homogeneous in outer garments, despite major differences in individual age, height, nationality, and athletic skills. Another team of players, wearing different individual uniforms, might be homogeneous in these other characteristics, despite their sartorial diversity.

1. The two meanings of 'classification.' The term *classification* can refer to two different procedures. In one case, a suitable set of terms or categories already exists, and we "classify" an object by choosing the appropriate term from the titles listed in this set. In the second case, a suitable set of categories does not exist, and a classification is performed to establish a new set of terms for future usage. The first of these procedures depends on the successful accomplishment of the second. The diagnostic act of identification requires the availability of a taxonomic array of diagnostic categories.

Thus, if we want to establish a diagnosis for a patient's chest pain, we must first create (or be given) a series of diagnostic titles—such as *myocardial infarction, dissecting aortic aneurysm,* and *acute pericarditis*—from which to choose the appropriate term. If we want to indicate the severity of chronic renal disease, we look for some suitable array of categories—such as *mild, moderate, severe* or *Grade 1, Grade 2, Grade 3,* etc.—in which to express the severity.

In the activities of medical practice, a clinician is often concerned with classification as an act of diagnostic identification. In the biostatistical literature, the word *classification* is also employed mainly in this diagnostic sense. The more fundamental scientific usage of *classification,* however, is taxonomic—the creation of the categories later employed for diagnoses or for other identifications. This paper and the two that follow it will be concerned with taxonomy as a basic scientific process that produces categories and systems of classification.

2. The contribution of taxonorics. The scientific discipline of *taxonorics*[13] is a branch of taxonomy. Taxonomy is concerned with the choice of topics to be classified and the strategy to be used in the classification; taxonorics is concerned with the details of categories used in the classification. Thus, the decision to classify library books according to subject matter (or content), rather than color or size, is an act of taxonomy; the Dewey Decimal System and the Library of Congress System are two different taxonoric methods for performing the classification. The decision to classify patients with breast cancer according to anatomic features of the cancer (rather than the patient's age, occupation, symptoms, or birthplace) is an act of taxonomy. The Columbia, Manchester, and International TNM staging systems are three different taxonoric procedures used in this taxonomy. Similarly, we could taxonomically decide that the property, age, warranted a system of classification. We could then taxonorically create at least three different systems: the broad categories of *young, middle-aged*, or *old;* the decade categories of *0-9, 10-19, 20-29, 30-39*, etc.; or the annual unit categories of *0, 1, 2, 3, . . ., 99, 100*, etc.

The taxonomic decisions and taxonoric categories established in a system of classification are of paramount scientific importance. They become the basis not only for identifying what is under investigation, but particularly for subsequent conclusions about similarity, since two entities are regarded as similar for a particular property (or "variate") if they are identified in the same category of the classification established for that variate. Thus, if age is classified according to annual units, a person who is 78 and another person who is 85 years old would not be similar, but they would become similar (identified as *old*) if age were classified only in the three broad categories cited in the previous paragraph. Since the available categories of classification are the basis for decisions about similarity, taxonomy and taxonorics are fundamental to the study of homogeneity. The taxonomist and taxonorist establish the topics and categories that will be used for expressing the decisions.

3. The functions of taxonomy. A system of classification can be created for at least three different functions: denomination, qualification, and prediction. In denomination, a group of entities is assigned a common name or category. In qualification, a group of terms is created to describe or qualify additional features of a named entity. In prediction, the qualifying terms refer to some anticipated future outcome for the named entity.

For the environment of a particular sports event, we might denominate the main participants as *horses*. We might further describe (or qualify) the horses with such terms as *yearling, filly, good mudder*, and *front-runner*. We might then predict which horses are most likely to win or lose a forthcoming race. These predictions might be expressed in such categories as *favorite* and *longshot*. In clinical medicine, we would denominate a particular biologic entity as a *patient* and the patient's disease entity might be called *myocardial infarction*. We might then qualify that diseased patient according to such descriptive features as age, sex, symptoms, and electrocardiographic data. In prediction, we would prognosticate for the patient by using such terms as *good risk, bad risk*, or *moribund*.

Each of these three functions of taxonomy has a different goal in clinical medicine, and presents different scientific challenges and problems. In the taxonomy of qualification, we deal with such issues as the formation of indexes to describe gradation (e.g., *small, medium, large*), transition (e.g., *smaller, same, larger*), desirability (e.g., *better, worse*) and other important characteristics of clinical phenomena. In the taxonomy of prediction, we deal with issues in prognostic stratification and other methods of anticipating the future. In the taxonomy of denomination, we decide what kinds of entities should be associated together under a common name.

Since we must give something a name

before we describe it further or anticipate what will happen to it, the classification of denomination takes precedence in any general consideration of taxonomy. The rest of this discussion is therefore devoted to denomination. The taxonomy of prediction will be the topic of the next two papers in this series, and the taxonomy of qualification will be discussed at a later date.

B. The taxonomy of denomination

The central act of classification in clinical medicine is the denomination of disease. All our activities in public health, in epidemiology, and in clinical practice depend on the way that we classify, recognize, and identify diseases. Despite its fundamental importance, however, the taxonomy of disease has received little or no attention in the modern world of "basic science." Many physicians today are unfamiliar with the word *nosology*, which refers to the concepts and nomenclature of disease, and with *nosography*, which refers to the particular terms used as nomenclature.[10, 11] Medical students, particularly during courses in pathology, are taught an array of diagnostic terms for disease entities, but the educational process seldom includes consideration of how and why the entities and terms were chosen. In the universe of human ailments and anomalies, how do we decide which ones should be stipulated as *diseases*?

A generation ago, the attempt to answer this question might have seemed like an exercise in scholasticism, but the issue has now become vital to scientific progress in clinical medicine:

1. The increasing development of paraclinical technology has led to the detection of many new entities that require classification. Clinicians can now recognize and must decide about appropriate nomenclature (and connotations) for such "new" ailments as *cytomegalic inclusion disease, heavy chain disease, 21-trisomy,* and the *empty sella syndrome*.

2. The dissemination of new technology via multiphasic screening programs and other periodic examinations has led to the discovery of diverse unexpected abnormalities in people who are otherwise in good health. How greatly "diseased" are these people?

3. The usual mechanism for classifying new diseases formerly depended on advances in scientific knowledge. As new evidence was obtained and new concepts developed, new "diseases" were recognized and old "diseases" altered. This intellectual mechanism of science can now be replaced by statistical and computer procedures that do not provide new evidence, and that rely, instead, on new methods for processing the data of existing evidence. For example, the statistical technique of *factor analysis* has been used to demarcate diagnostic categories for certain psychologic ailments, and the computer procedures of *numerical taxonomy* have been employed to delineate "diagnostic" subgroups in the spectrum of several chronic diseases that will be discussed later.

The last of these three points is the main reason for attention to taxonomy in a paper dealing with biostatistics. If statistical theory and computer calculations can be used in the future to create or classify the denominations of disease, the basic ideas behind the taxonomic strategies warrant careful consideration.

1. The principles and problems of denomination. A denomination provides a name that is a "summary" of the entity represented by the name. Thus, by summarizing certain qualities of the observed entities, such denominations as *person, book,* or *chair* will promptly convey an idea of the object that they represent. The rapid transmission of this idea is obviously the greatest power of a summary, but the summary itself will also create many problems. What characteristics of the entity serve as the focus for the summary? How many characteristics are included? How do we choose and combine them? What are the effects of the exclusions?

a. The focal "essence." The denominational nomenclature of science has depended for years on the Aristotelian concept of an "essence." The "essence" is a conclusion about the basic nature of an entity; it is the crucial distinction that makes the entity what it is. To denominate the elements of chemistry, for example, the taxonomy of the Periodic Table depends on an essence of atomic weight and valence. An alternative essence (such as physical state, viscosity, or color) could have been chosen, but weight and valence were regarded as the most important distinctions with which to differentiate one chemical element from another. In the system used for classifying books at most public libraries, the main essence is content, rather than author, size, or typography. For other taxonomic purposes, the essence is chosen to be the ancestry, cause, or "genesis" of the observed entity. This type of classification is performed when a patient's sore throat is diagnosed as a streptococcal infection.

In the essence approach to taxonomy, a specific focus is selected as the orientation of the classification. A different approach is based on the concept of overall similarity rather than focal essence. In the similarity approach, we would regard a group of entities as similar if they resemble one another in a large array of different characteristics that are not specifically directed toward a distinct focus. Thus a group of people with the same age, race, sex, and symptom of sore throat might be regarded as similar, even though they have different etiologic agents for the sore throat.

b. The type of reasoning. The reasoning used for denomination is empirical, if it depends on classifying the observed evidence; and inferential, if it depends on deductions or inferences about the observed evidence. We perform an empirical classification when we say that a patient's chest pain represents *angina pectoris,* and an inferential classification when we call it *coronary artery disease.*

When a classification is based on overall similarity, the observed evidence is classified empirically. When the classification depends on a focal essence, the reasoning will be empirical or inferential according to whether or not the essence was observed among the available evidence. Thus, if we diagnose coronary artery disease exclusively on the basis of a patient's history, chemical tests, and electrocardiograms, a diseased coronary artery has not been demonstrated. The diagnosis is inferential. If coronary disease has been demonstrated via arteriography, surgery, or necropsy, the diagnosis is empirical. In the previously cited examples of taxonomy for chemical elements and library books, the reasoning was empirical because the focal essence (weight and valence, or content of text) was present among the evidence used for the classification.

Because of the difficulties of confirming the accuracy of an inference or achieving standardization in the way diagnostic inferences are performed, an empirical rather than inferential taxonomy seems more likely to enhance scientific consistency during the subsequent use of the system.[11]

c. The scope of inclusion. Regardless of whether a summary is oriented toward a focus, and toward evidence or inference, how many details should it include? Should all properties of an entity, or just a few, be represented in the scope of the summary? This distinction can be cited as the difference between *encompassing inclusion* and *selective exclusion.*

For example, when we contemplate the differences that distinguish such entities as *people, books,* and *chairs,* we generally ignore the height, weight, and age of the entities. The names and concepts that differentiate people, books, and chairs were based on selective rather than encompassing summaries, and furthermore, height, weight, and age were "excluded," i.e., not regarded as crucial properties, when the selections were made.

In traditional scientific approaches to

taxonomy, the denominational summary has been based on selective exclusion rather than encompassing inclusion. Thus, a disease name such as *myocardial infarction* conveys some carefully selected ideas about the abnormal condition of a heart, but excludes any information about concomitant abnormalities in the brain or liver. From the name *myocardial infarction*, moreover, we would not know whether the heart is a person's or an animal's, and we would know nothing of the age or sex of the body from which the heart came.

d. The method of aggregation. Regardless of which and how many properties are included, they must be combined or aggregated to form the summary. How is this aggregation to be performed? One method is to assign a weight or score to each element, and to add these scores together to form the summary value. This technique has not been generally used for denomination in clinical medicine, but it has been employed in qualitative taxonomy for such composite indexes as the Apgar score and the Lansbury index of activity in rheumatoid arthritis. A modified "addition" technique is employed in the current diagnostic criteria[1] for rheumatic fever, where the diagnosis requires the presence of two "major" and one "minor" manifestations or vice versa. The other type of taxonomic aggregation depends on conjoining elements, rather than adding scores. Thus, the entity *boy* is a conjunction of the elements *male* and *child*; the entity *myocardial infarction* is a conjunction of the elements *myocardium* and *infarction*.

The difference in these two types of aggregation can be described as *additive scores* vs. *conjoined elements*. The conjunction technique has been the more traditional procedure in scientific taxonomy.

e. The assignment of weights. The conjunctive technique of classification creates no graded weights or scores for the elements it contains. Since each element is either present or absent, the assignment of a weighted score consists only of the decision to include or exclude that element. In the additive technique, however, each element is either assigned a specific score, or is associated with a coefficient that affects the "weight" or "value" of the element. Regardless of whether the rating is done by inclusion-exclusion, by specific score, or by associated co-efficients, the "weights" can be assigned according to arbitrary judgment or statistical calculation.

The difference in these two methods of assigning weights—judgmental vs. statistical—will be illustrated later.

f. The consequences of exclusion. No matter how each of these techniques is used in preparing the summary, the result is an incomplete description of the observed entity. Certain details that are inevitably condensed or omitted during the summary procedures may be important for other identifications of the entity. Consequently, after a main denominational taxonomy has been established on the basis of a reduced summary of details, a supplemental taxonomy may be necessary to preserve and classify some of the excluded information. For example, the books at most public libraries are listed and stored according to a denominational taxonomy that "summarizes" the book according to its content. Nevertheless, additional taxonomies are usually maintained as catalogs for such details as the titles of the books and the names of the authors. The medical periodical literature is "summarized" in the *Index Medicus* according to content and authors of the published papers, but additional aspects of content ("key words") are catalogued in a reference system called *Medlars*, and the interrelationship of bibliographic listings is catalogued in a system called the *Citation Index*.

2. The controversies of biologic taxonomy. The diverse methods of creating denominations will obviously lead to disputes about which methods are best. These disputes have not yet become prominent in medical taxonomy, probably because the newer techniques have not yet received widespread usage or enthusiastic support. In non-medical biology, however, a major controversy about taxonomy has flourished for more than a decade. The biologic debates are worth our attention here because they help illustrate the basic issues, and because they are germane both to certain problems that have already become evident in medical taxonomy, and to other problems that will become more prominent in the future with increasing use of statistics and computers in medical activities.

The biologic controversy is not easy to understand or explain, partly because many concepts have not been well defined, and partly because so much unfamiliar jargon has been employed in the verbal battles.[30] Among the different words or phrases that abound in the debates are: *phyletic, phylogenetic, phenetic, patristic, cladistic, taximetry, taxometry, taxon, typology,* and *neo-Adansonian.* I shall here attempt to describe only those aspects of the controversy that seem most cogent for the subsequent medical discussion.

The traditional system of classification for biologic organisms was developed empirically by Linnaeus two centuries ago, according to an "essence" based mainly on observed methods of locomotion and reproduction. The classification formed by Linnaeus provided most of the basic *phyla, orders, genera,* and *species* that are found in biologic taxonomy today. The Linnaean system was later modified to incorporate the inferential ideas of evolution developed by Darwin. With this modification, the "essence" of the taxonomic focus became transferred to concepts about cause (in this case, phylogenetic ancestry) that have always dominated the scientific quest for explanation. The now-classical biologic taxonomy, which can be called *phyletic,* is thus based on the particular attributes of an organism that are regarded as most important for biologic meaningfulness in a

scientific explanation of the organism's evolutionary origin. The taxonomy depends on a "causal" or phylogenetic essence, on inferences about phylogeny, and on the judgmental selection of key properties that are combined conjunctively.

The phyletic system has been subjected to severe criticism[23, 32, 33] during the past decade. The system has not been satisfactory for classifying certain "lower" biologic organisms—such as bacteria[4] and worms[29]—that are not readily analyzed with concepts of phylogeny and evolution. The phyletic categories also do not include consideration of many types of biochemical and other modern technologic data that were not available to Linnaeus and Darwin. Furthermore, according to the critics, the particular characteristics judged to be the "essence" of an organism are selected arbitrarily and are validated only by the inferences of the Darwinian theory of evolution.

As a replacement for classical phyletic taxonomy, the critics have proposed a system that is entirely empirical, with no inferences about "genesis" of the classified entities. The system is also encompassing, rather than selective, because the decisions about classification are based on all the observed characteristics of an entity, rather than an exclusive few. The new system replaces the focal essence of evolutionary ancestry with a summary of overall similarity (or "affinity") among entities. The summary is prepared additively rather than conjunctively, and the "weights" are determined with an elaborate series of statistical calculations rather than with arbitrary human judgment. Because the focal concept of phylogeny has been rejected in favor of the overall similarity of "phenotype" relations, the new system is usually called *phenetic.*

In the phenetic system, all the characteristics of a group of entities are examined, and a series of similarities (or affinities) are determined (as described later) for each characteristic of each entity. The values of affinity for the individual characteristics are then additively combined into a single value that represents the summated "co-efficient" for that entity. A specific category (or *taxon*) is created for entities whose co-efficients have values that are sufficiently close to one another. Higher-order groupings can be created by combining "adjacent" taxons.[32]

A crucial issue in this system of classification is the strategy for defining affinity or similarity. The similarity between characteristics is determined statistically by calculating certain correlations or "distances" between the numerical unit values assigned to the characteristics.

As a simplified example of the "distance" calculation, consider three entities, X, Y, and Z, and their "unit" values for two characteristics (or variables), A and B. For entity X, the unit values for A and B are 4 and 8, respectively; for entity Y, the corresponding values are 5 and 3; and for entity Z, the values are 9 and 4. In "distance" for variable A, entities X and Y are closest to each other; and in "distance" for variable B, the two closest entities are Y and Z.

For each pair of complete entities, however, we would like to know not the distance among individual variables, but the distance among all variables. This distance can be calculated by using the Pythagorean theorem of analytic geometry. If we consider variables A and B simultaneously, the distance between entities X and Y is $\sqrt{(4-5)^2 + (8-3)^2} = \sqrt{26}$. The distance between Y and Z is $\sqrt{(5-9)^2 + (3-4)^2} = \sqrt{17}$, and the distance between X and Z is $\sqrt{(4-9)^2 + (8-4)^2} = \sqrt{41}$. Consequently, if only variables A and B were being considered, Y and Z would have the greatest "affinity" of these three entities, since they have the shortest inter-variable "distance."

When more than two variables are involved in characterizing the observed entities, the calculation of similarity by using distance (or other statistical concepts) becomes mathematically formidable. For this reason, computers have played a prominent and crucial role in the development of a phenetic *numerical* taxonomy.[32] The performance of such a classification proceeds as follows: (1) choose a group of objects to be classified; (2) select the variates that differ among the objects; (3) subdivide the variates that are composite (e.g., con-vert *complexion* into *color of eyes, color of hair,* etc.); (4) eliminate variates that are redundant or highly interdependent (e.g., *color of shoes* and *color of shoelaces*); (5) standardize the units in which the remaining variates are expressed; (6) determine the mutual affinities for each variate of each object; (7) compute an affinity co-efficient for each object by combining its affinity values for each variate; (8) create groups by joining the objects with similar affinity co-efficients.

The "affinity co-efficients" can be computed from an n-dimensional generalization (by Mahalanobis) of the "distance" tactic just described. Alternatively, a numerical taxonomist can use other statistical procedures bearing such majestic titles as cluster analysis, discriminant function, principal components, centroid factors, and canonical relationships. The phenetic approach is thus antipodal to the phyletic approach in each of five main principles noted earlier. The phenetic procedures are non-focal, empirical, encompassing, additive, and statistical.

In the counter-attack[5, 24, 25, 28, 30, 34] against a phenetic taxonomy for biology, one of the most prominent of the cited defects is the apparent absence of a scientific goal. The traditional goals of science are to explain and to predict, but the phenetic classification is not oriented toward either "causal" explanation or prognostic prediction. Another prominent defect is that the new system remains highly arbitrary. It has replaced the arbitrary human judgments about biologic "meaning" by arbitrary statistical judgments about "affinity," and by arbitrary calculations that emerge during the computer's manipulation of the data. The statistical strategies themselves also have certain fundamental flaws that have been particularly well discussed by Fleiss and Zubin.[19]

Aside from these problems and from the question of validity for the basic statistical techniques, a major objection to phenetic numerical taxonomy is that the denominations it creates are not recognizable "names." It produces a series of "similarity clusters" whose "similarity" is entirely numerical, emerging from statistical calculations but not from biologic reasoning. The computed clusters can be named in a straightforward alphabetical or numerical fashion, but the denominated entities are unfamiliar and provide no immediate biologic recognition. As an outrageous example, suppose we used numerical taxonomy to classify newborn babies according to all of the observable clinical and paraclinical data. Immediately after a child is delivered, the baby's parent will ask, "what is it?" Instead of *boy* or *girl,* the reply might be *Taxon D* or *Taxon Q.*

The absence of familiar names and concepts would be particularly distressing in circumstances where the replaced term is classical and well-established. Many modern biologists have been appalled at the idea of supplanting traditional titles with an index number produced by a computer, just as many clinicians (as noted later) were fiercely resistant during the 19th century when new names were being introduced for old "diseases." On the other hand, for the entities revealed by new data or by new concepts, a new nomenclature is obviously necessary, and the terms need not conflict with any previous titles. Thus, modern clinical biologists have not balked at the application of such contemporary neologisms as *episomes, ribosomes, genomes, epimers, codons, cistrons, pheromones,* and *emperipolesis* for some of the entities discerned with modern technology, nor has there been major objection to such "numerical" nomenclature as *Stage I, Stage II,* and *Stage III* for the clusters of entities that are used to classify the dissemination of cancer. Provided that the new name is meaningful, its unfamiliarity or its expression in numerical, alphabetical, or other terms should not create an important scientific problem. A *rose* would presumably still be recognized by some other name, as long as appearance and sweetness of smell were accepted as the "essence" of the characteristics to be denoted.

Since both the phyletic and phenetic taxonomies are used for the general purpose of biologic denomination, neither form of taxonomy can readily be validated. We can determine whether a prediction is right or wrong by observing the outcome of events, but no standard of accuracy can be established for a denomination. The main validation for both phyletic and phenetic taxonomy is based on the same conceptual beliefs that produced them. Phyletic taxonomy is chosen and accepted because it seems to make "sense"

biologically. Phenetic taxonomy is chosen and accepted because it produces a "similarity" that is quantified statistically.

C. The current state of nosography

Many of the problems just cited for biologic taxonomy have analogous counterparts in nosography: the medical taxonomy of disease. The essence of the classification for disease has always been focal, but the focus has shifted in different medical eras and with different scientific advances. For many centuries, the focus was the most prominent clinical manifestation of the ailment, and the taxonomy was purely observational. *Fever, cyanosis, asthma,* and *consumption* were the names of diseases. With the advent of frequent necropsy in the 19th century, the focus was changed from observed manifestation to morphologic explanation, and the taxonomy became inferential.[10] Such diagnostic names as *infarction, inflammation,* and *carcinoma* were deduced during the patient's lifetime as causal explanations for the observed clinical phenomena. Since these explanations could usually not be verified until the patient's death, the taxonomy was inferential when applied to living patients. A protracted controversy raged during the 19th century and early 20th century as many clinicians expressed resistance to the new morphologic "diseases" that were replacing the old clinical "diseases."[11]

With the later development and application of new paraclinical technology in microbiology, chemistry, radiography, endoscopy, biopsy, and catheterization, new forms of evidence became available to allow new concepts of etiology, and to provide direct empirical data that could be obtained in living patients to substantiate the etiologic diagnoses.

1. Comparison with biologic taxonomy. As a result of the cited technologic changes, modern nosography resembles classical biologic taxonomy in having a generally "phyletic" orientation, but nosography also has certain major differences:

1. Unlike the rigorous logical standard-

ization and relative stability brought to biologic taxonomy by the work of Linnaeus and Darwin, medical taxonomy has been eclectic and unstable. Whenever a clinical name of disease could be suitably supplanted by an etiologic term, the transfer was performed; otherwise, the old diagnostic name remained. Thus, the old *angina pectoris* became the new *coronary artery disease* and the old *familial hemolytic jaundice* became the new *spherocytosis*, but the ancient *gout, rheumatic fever, diabetes mellitus,* and *measles* are still in service as venerable veterans of medical nomenclature. Because the new terms were incorporated into nosography without regard to any established criteria or standards of logic, the current taxonomy of disease is a polyglot of diverse ideas and names. The available diagnostic terms for disease include different categories of topography, morphology, physiology, biochemistry, microbiology, genetics, "clinical states," syndromes, symptoms, signs, and habits.[11]

At least two different taxonoric catalogues have been developed for citing the names of current "diseases." The Standard Nomenclature of Diseases and Operations[2] (SNDO) was popular for many years in the United States but has recently become increasingly supplanted here, as well as internationally, by the International Classification of Diseases, Adapted[38] (ICDA). The ICDA, like the SNDO, contains no criteria for diagnostic decision or identification, but provides coding numbers for individual diseases and for certain arbitrarily formed rubrics. The rubrics and codes are revised every ten years by an international committee.

The problems produced by inconsistencies in the logic of diagnostic taxonomy and in the arbitrariness of the nosographic coding systems have been discussed elsewhere.[11, 12] In the absence of operational criteria for applying the taxonomy, the same clinical entity may receive different diagnostic names in different countries; the diagnoses may be applied non-reproducibly in the same country; and major changes in the occurrence rates of "disease" may be caused by alterations in diagnostic technology and in the rubrics chosen as master categories in the coding system.

2. Although both biologic and medical taxonomy are phyletically oriented toward "causal" explanations, the availability of paraclinical tests often provides empirical evidence of the proposed medical causes. Thus, the diagnosis of streptococcal infection can be converted from inference to evidence with the results of an appropriate paraclinical procedure. The diagnosis of tuberculous pneumonia in a living patient was a deductive speculation a century ago, but the diagnosis today can readily be demonstrated with the paraclinical technology of roentgenography (which "shows" the pneumonia) and microbiology (which shows the tubercle bacillus). Similarly, the idea of disease due to endocrinopathy—the old concept of "deranged humors"—was formerly a matter of conjectural inference. Today, via experimental evidence obtained from ablation or manipulation of glands in both animals and man, the idea is thoroughly documented.

Furthermore, many other medical diagnoses have remained observational, rather than etiologic, because suitable etiologic explanations do not exist. The names of such "organic" diseases as *essential hypertension* and *systemic lupus erythematosus,* and most of the diagnostic nomenclature of mental and psychic illness (*schizophrenic, passive-aggressive, manic-depressive*) have been based on direct observation, rather than etiologic explanation.

In pursuing this eclectically etiologic but pragmatically empiric approach to diagnostic nomenclature, medical nosography has maintained the other characteristics of phyletic taxonomy. The diagnostic terms are generally based on the exclusion of apparently extraneous information, the conjunction of the selected "cogent" data, and the use of human judgment for the conjunctions.

2. Outstanding defects in current nosography. The preservation of a phyletic approach in diagnostic nomenclature has currently remained unchallenged, because an etiologic orientation appeals to a scientist's search for meaning and for suitable explanations to account for observed phenomena. In addition, medical nosography has been able to avoid two of the three main pitfalls noted for phyletic biologic taxonomy. Because many etiologic diagnoses can be demonstrated empirically, nosography does not rely on inference alone. Because the taxonomic categories have regularly been augmented and altered as the result of new technologic evidence, nosography is not confined to traditional data and concepts.

A third pitfall of phyletic biologic taxonomy is its unsatisfactory application to certain organisms that cannot be classified with phylogenetic concepts. Although this problem has its counterpart in medical taxonomy, the outstanding current defects of nosography arise from its omissions, not its contents. These defects are not encountered in biologic taxonomy, because biologists do not regularly attempt to change the denominated organisms, whereas the main job of clinicians is to treat or prevent disease.

a. Etiologic inadequacies. For diseases whose cause is not known or not readily demonstrable, an etiologically oriented nomenclature creates many practical problems. The nomenclature itself may become inconsistent, with arbitrarily chosen terms of either individual description (such as *hypertension*) or the clustered descriptions that are represented in the many syndromes and eponyms of medical diagnosis. The application of the nomenclature may be inconsistent in circumstances where the inference cannot be conveniently confirmed. Thus, the clinician can observe and clearly describe a *stroke,* but formal nosography in living patients regularly forces him into the unproved inferential diagnosis of *thrombosis, hemorrhage,* or *embolism.*

For ailments that are psychic rather than "organic," an empiric validation of cause is seldom available, even after necropsy. In the absence of such validation, psychologists and psychiatrists have had much less enthusiasm than their "organic" colleagues for an etiologic approach to medical taxonomy. In the search for a suitable

nosography for psychic illness, psychologists have been attracted by the phenetic approach offered in such statistical procedures as *factor analysis.* The validity of the procedures is uncertain,[20, 27] but they have exerted great appeal and have achieved considerable popularity.

b. The restrictions of summation. The fundamental current defect of medical nosography, however, arises not from the principle of etiology, but from the principle of summation. When the diverse aspects of a sick patient are compressed into the name of a disease, neither the sickness nor the patient is adequately described.

(1). PROBLEMS IN CO-MORBIDITY. The mortality data assembled by the Bureau of Vital Statistics are currently reported for a single disease that is chosen to be the "cause of death," regardless of how many other diseases occurred in each patient, and regardless of how many of those co-morbid diseases might have been equally good choices for lethal primacy.[12, 14] The results of therapy are also commonly reported for a group of people with a "main" disease, regardless of how those results may have been affected or distorted by the presence of co-morbid ailments.[14]

One approach to this problem has been for "vital statistics" to list all the diseases that were present at death, instead of confining the patient to a single diagnostic category. The approach has obvious merits,[21] but it does not resolve the various inter-relations of co-morbidity that must be classified when a patient is identified for the statistical analysis of either epidemiologic or therapeutic data.[14] Another approach that has been used in many therapeutic trials is to exclude all people with co-morbid diseases and to restrict the cohort to a "pure" group of patients with only the "main" disease. The statistical merits of this approach are vitiated by the inapplicability of the results to the "impurities" constantly encountered in clinical practice.

(2). PROBLEMS IN THE SPECTRUM OF A DISEASE. Many major chronic diseases have a diverse clinical spectrum of manifestations that can range from the asymptomatic to the moribund, and from the *forme fruste* to the typical presentation to the esoteric complication.[11] None of these important distinctions in the "clinical type" of a disease is indicated by its name alone. A patient with *pulmonary emphysema* can be jogging pleasantly in a park or gasping for air in a respirator. A patient with *cerebral arteriosclerosis* can be functioning in a normal manner or can be devastatingly incapacitated.

To classify these additional facets of the spectrum of disease has required the development of new forms of taxonomy. A phyletic form of "clinical taxonomy" has been proposed to indicate the existence (or absence) of iatrotropic complaints, "primary" manifestations, and "secondary" manifestations for each disease.[11] In the taxonomy proposed in the Standardized Nomenclature of Pathology[7] (SNOP), the denomination for a single ailment is expanded into four principal components of topography, morphology, etiology, and function. A somewhat similar multi-component system of classification[8] was developed for heart disease in 1923, and the published classification is now in its 6th edition.[9] The augmented contents of SNOP offer a more complete description for individual human ailments than is otherwise attainable, but the SNOP is based mainly on pathology, not on clinical phenomena, and no taxonomy is provided for the diverse symptomatic and co-morbid clinical events that must be considered in therapy.

An interesting new approach in classifying the clinical spectrum of a disease has been to abandon a phyletic orientation, and to employ the computerized phenetic tactics of numerical taxonomy.[3, 26, 37] The procedures have been used to demarcate subgroups of patients within the spectrum of such ailments as anemia,[26] goiter,[6] leukemia,[22] and hepatic cirrhosis.[36]

In one recently published study,[36] 400 patients with cirrhosis received a numerical taxonomic classification based on 56 different clinical and paraclinical variates that were each registered as present or absent. A dissimilarity co-efficient (*dico*) was calculated for each pair of patients. The *dico* value was $(n-x)/n$, where n was the number of variates observed in both patients, and x was the number of variates in which both patients had the same data. Thus, two patients with identical data for each variate would have a *dico* of zero. If all the data were different, the *dico* would be one. On the basis of the *dico* levels noted in the diverse pairs of patients, the investigators were able to isolate two different groups of patients with distinctly different *dico* values and with somewhat different clinical characteristics. A group of 26 patients contained more women, a more frequent history of hepatitis, and more abnormal liver function tests than a larger group of 104 patients in whom men and a history of alcoholism predominated.

Since the numerical taxonomic procedures were not directed at a specific target in either etiology or prognosis, it is not surprising that the taxonomic results were disappointing. The authors concluded the investigation by wondering "whether the relatively poor grouping of the present material is due to inclusion of 'noise data' or is a biologic fact."

(3). PROBLEMS IN THERAPY. The taxonomy of clinical medicine must serve a much greater range of functions than the taxonomy of biology. A clinician does more than identify; he intervenes. His medical taxonomy must therefore be suited not just for diagnosis of disease, but for identifying the people and the phenomena of clinical management encountered in prophylactic treatment, in remedial treatment, and in caring for patients. The current nosography of disease is not satisfactory for this challenge.

The use of a summation nomenclature, particularly in an era when chronic diseases are a prime medical problem, has served not to create homogeneity but to ensure heterogeneity in any group of patients with the same "main" disease. This heterogeneity is especially important in planning and evaluating treatment, because the choice of many of the targets of treatment will depend on the patient's clinical state, not on the name of the disease; and because a patient's prognostic expectation for achieving those targets will also depend on the symptoms and associated co-morbidity of the clinical state, not on the name of the disease.[11] The diverse phenomena of human illness that are so crucial for the therapeutic management of a sick person are obliterated when the patient's condition is summarized in a single title called a *diagnosis*.

Some of the defects in classifying the clinical spectrum and co-morbidity of a "main" disease have already been discussed. Other defects arise from the absence of a suitable "qualification taxonomy" to describe the targets of treatment, the initial degrees of severity, and the degrees of improvement or accomplishment.

A new approach to the targets of treatment is contained in Weed's "problem-oriented medical record,"[35] where the traditional nomenclature of diagnosis is replaced by a list of the names of "problems." The patient's physician chooses the problems that will be cited on this list, and chooses the names with which the problems will be labeled. The problems can be denoted with the titles of such entities as clinical symptoms, morphologic disorders, biochemical derangements, conventional diseases, psychic disturbances, and socio-economic difficulties. The Weed system provides a flexible nomenclature for identifying the different targets that receive clinical attention, but the system is not intended to deal with the unsolved taxonomic problems in classification of clinical spectrum, co-morbidity, and gradations of initial severity and of therapeutic accomplishment.

D. Taxonomic challenges in prediction

All of the activities just described for biologic, clinical, or other forms of denomination were concerned with classifying a state at a single point in time. No matter how the diagnostic taxonomy was formed —empirically or inferentially; phenetically or phyletically; with or without the aid of computers; with or without additional classifications of spectrum and co-morbidity—each title represented the contemporary state of the observed entity. Some of the systems of diagnostic taxonomy may be better than others, but each diagnostic category (irrespective of the taxonomic

system) has acted as a focus of uni-temporal homogeneity. If the diagnostic terms were standardized and applied correctly, we could be assured that the people who received a particular diagnostic identification were "homogeneous" in having the cited condition, at the cited point in time.

This type of uni-temporal taxonomy, if otherwise satisfactory, would be quite adequate for any medical needs that were restricted to denomination alone. In those situations where the main target under investigation is the occurrence or non-occurrence of a disease, the various categories of uni-temporal denomination would provide an array of names satisfactory for diagnostic citation. For example, in a study of the prevalence of rheumatic fever in a general population, the main taxonomic issue is the diagnosis of rheumatic fever. As long as a patient fulfills the denominational criteria[1] for this diagnosis, he will enter the statistics as a "unit" of rheumatic fever, regardless of its particular clinical type, regardless of the severity of the manifestations, regardless of co-morbidity, and regardless of the outcome.

In many other forms of clinical epidemiologic research, however, the main target under investigation is a transition, rather than a single state in time. The purpose is to discern a change between two states, or to note whether the first state makes a person more or less susceptible to developing the second state. In this type of cohort research, the investigator usually wants to determine whether the change or the susceptibility is affected by a particular maneuver. The maneuver under study may be exposure to an etiologic cause of disease, or treatment with an agent intended to remedy an existing disease or keep it from getting worse. To evaluate the statistical results of such maneuvers, which are constantly studied in the cause-cohorts of epidemiologic research and in the intervention-cohorts of clinical therapy, an investigator has two sets of problems in homogeneity: the homogeneity of initial state diagnosis *and* the homogeneity of prognostic anticipation for the target event in the subsequent state.

The attainment of initial state homogeneity is relatively easy, since it is an arbitrary act. The investigator uses whatever diagnostic terminology he wishes to specify the "admission criteria" or "eligibility criteria" for entrance into the cohort, and he is assured of homogeneity for these standards as long as they are observed. Despite the homogeneity created by fulfillment of the eligibility criteria, however, the members of a cohort may be markedly disparate in properties that determine susceptibility to the target event.[15]

For example, to study the treatment of well-differentiated epidermoid carcinoma of the right lower lobe of the lung in white men aged 50 to 55 years, we would assemble a cohort of people who are homogeneous in the stated features of race, sex, age, histology, and primary topography. With all of the cited homogeneity, this cohort is still prognostically heterogeneous. The men whose cancer is localized, who are asymptomatic, and who have no co-morbidity will have a much higher survival rate than those with metastatic lesions, with substantial loss of weight, and with major co-morbidity.[18] If survival is the target event used to assess treatment, we would have to subclassify the patients further according to anatomic localization of the cancer and the other clinical features that determine the likelihood of survival. An entirely new taxonomy, based on prediction rather than denomination, would be needed to provide the categories for this classification. The objective of the new taxonomy is to provide homogeneity not in diagnosis, but in prognosis.

This kind of predictive subclassification (or prognostic stratification) is necessary to avoid the 'transition bias'[15] that can arise when compared cohorts contain disproportionate amounts of patients who are prognostically disparate. The stratification is also necessary for other crucial aspects of efficient design and valid analysis in cohort statistics. The process of prognostic stratification is thus fundamental to the scientific performance of cohort research. The strategy and tactics of this process will be the topic for discussion at our next two meetings.

References

1. Ad Hoc Committee to revise the Jones criteria (modified) of the Council on Rheumatic Fever and Congenital Heart Disease of the American Heart Association: Jones criteria (revised) for guidance in the diagnosis of rheumatic fever, Circulation **32**:664-668, 1965.
2. American Medical Association. Standard nomenclature of diseases and operations. ed. 5. Thompson, E. T., and Hayden, A. C., editors, New York, 1961, Blakiston Division, McGraw-Hill Book Co., Inc.
3. Baron, D. N., and Fraser, P. M.: Medical applications of taxonomic methods. Br. Med. Bull. **24**:236-240, 1968.
4. Beers, R. J., and Lockhart, W. R.: Experimental methods in computer taxonomy, J. Gen. Microbiol. **28**:633-640, 1962.
5. Blackwelder, R. E.: A critique of numerical taxonomy, Syst. Zool. **16**:64-72, 1967.
6. Bouckaert, A.: Computer diagnosis of goiters. I. Classification and differential diagnosis; II. Syndrome recognition and diagnosis; III. Optimal subsymptomatologies, J. Chron. Dis. **24**:299-310; 311-320; 321-327; 1971.
7. Committee on Nomenclature and Classification of Disease of the College of American Pathologists. Systematized nomenclature of pathology, College of American Pathologists, Chicago, 1965.
8. Committee on Cardiac Clinics of the New York Heart Association for the Prevention and Relief of Heart Disease. Requirements for an ideal cardiac clinic and a system of nomenclature, Boston Med. Surg. J. **189**:762-768, 1923.
9. Criteria Committee of the New York Heart Association. Diseases of the heart and blood vessels. Nomenclature and criteria for diagnosis, ed. 6, Boston, 1964, Little, Brown & Company.
10. Faber, K.: Nosography in modern internal medicine, New York, 1923, Paul B. Hoeber, Inc.
11. Feinstein, A. R.: Clinical judgment, Baltimore, 1967, The Williams & Wilkins Co.
12. Feinstein, A. R.: Clinical epidemiology. II. The identification rates of disease, Ann. Intern. Med. **69**:1037-1061, 1968.
13. Feinstein, A. R.: Taxonorics. I. Formulation

of criteria, Arch. Intern. Med. **126**:679-693, 1970.

14. Feinstein, A. R.: The pre-therapeutic classification of co-morbidity in chronic disease, J. Chron. Dis. **23**:455-469, 1970.

15. Feinstein, A. R.: Clinical biostatistics. X. Sources of 'transition bias' in cohort statistics, CLIN. PHARMACOL. THER. **12**:704-721, 1971.

16. Feinstein, A. R.: Clinical biostatistics. XI. Sources of 'chronology bias' in cohort statistics, CLIN. PHARMACOL. THER. **12**:864-879, 1971.

17. Feinstein, A. R.: Clinical biostatistics. XII. On exorcising the ghost of Gauss and the curse of Kelvin, CLIN. PHARMACOL. THER. **12**:1003-1016, 1971.

18. Feinstein, A. R.: Scientific defects in the staging of lung cancer, *in* Carbone, P. P., moderator: Transcription of NCI Combined Clinical Staff Conference. Lung cancer: Perspectives and prospects, pp. 1005-1011, Ann. Intern. Med. **73**:1003-1024, 1970.

19. Fleiss, J. L., and Zubin, J.: On the methods and theory of clustering, Multivariate Behavioral Res. **4**:235-250, 1969.

20. Gower, J. C.: Some distance properties of latent root and vector methods used in multivariate analysis, Biometrika **53**:325-338, 1966.

21. Guralnick, L.: Some problems in the use of multiple causes of death, J. Chron. Dis. **19**:979-990, 1966.

22. Hayhoe, F. G. J., Quaglino, D., and Doll, R.: The cytology and cytochemistry of acute leukemias: A study of 140 cases, London, 1964, Med. Res. Council Special Report Series 304.

23. Heywood, V. H., and McNeill, J., editors: Phenetic and phylogenetic classification, London, 1964, Systematics Association.

24. Inglis, W. G.: The purpose and judgments of biological classifications, Syst. Zool. **19**:240-250, 1970.

25. Johnson, L. A. S.: Rainbow's end: The quest for an optimal taxonomy, Proc. Linnean Soc. New South Wales **93**:8-45, 1968.

26. Lipkin, M., Engle, R. L., Davis, B. J., Zworykin, V. K., Ebald, R., Sendrow, M., and Berkley, C.: Digital computer as aid to differential diagnosis: Use in hematologic diseases, Arch. Intern. Med. **108**:56-72, 1961.

27. Mainland, D.: A medical experimenter looks at factor analysis, *in* Notes on Biometry in Medical Research, Note 27, pp. 39-60, VA Monograph 10-1, Supplement 4, August, 1968. Veterans Administration, Washington, D. C. 20420.

28. Mayr, E.: The role of systematics in biology, Science **159**:595-599, 1968.

29. Moss, W. W., and Webster, W. A.: Phenetics and numerical taxonomy applied to systematic nematology, J. Nematol. **2**:16-25, 1970.

30. Simpson, G. G.: Current issues in taxonomic theory, Science **148**:1078, 1965.

31. Snedecor, G. W.: Statistical methods, ed. 5, Ames, Iowa, 1956, Iowa State University Press, p. 482.

32. Sokal, R. R., and Sneath, P. H. A.: Principles of numerical taxonomy, San Francisco, 1963, W. H. Freeman & Co.

33. Symposium on numerical taxonomy, *in* Cole, A. M., editor: Proceedings of a colloquium held in the University of St. Andrew's, September, 1968, London, 1969, Academic Press, Inc.

34. Warburton, F. E.: The purposes of classifications, Syst. Zool. **16**:241-245, 1967.

35. Weed, L. L.: Medical records, medical education, and patient care, Chicago, 1969, Year Book Medical Publishers, Inc.

36. Winkel, P., Paldam, M., Tygstrup, N., and The Copenhagen Study Group for Liver Diseases: A numerical taxonomic analysis of symptoms and signs in 400 patients with cirrhosis of the liver, Comput. Biomed. Res. **3**:657-665, 1970.

37. Wishart, D.: The use of cluster analysis in the classification of diseases, Scottish Med. J. **14**:96, 1969. (Abst.)

38. World Health Organization: Manual of the International Statistical Classification of Diseases, Injuries, and Causes of Death, vols. I and II, Geneva, 1957. (A revision of this publication was issued in two volumes in 1962 by the United States Department of Health, Education, and Welfare under the title, *International Classification of Diseases, Adapted.*)

CHAPTER 25

A primer of multivariate analysis

The analysis of multiple variables probably received little or no attention when contemporary clinicians were taught about statistical methods. The topic is either absent from most textbooks of elementary statistics and biostatistics; or, if present, it is saved for advanced instruction in which a medical student seldom participates. Multivariate analysis has nevertheless become a frequent event in the literature that now confronts a clinical reader. Such multivariate procedures as discriminant functions, multiple regression, factor analysis, and cluster analysis regularly occur among the methods used in reports that appear not only in specialty medical journals, but also in journals intended for a general clinical audience.

During the past year, while on leave at the new McMaster University School of Medicine in Canada, I joined with biostatistical colleagues and other interested investigators in a series of seminars, called the "Multivariate Forum." Our goal was to exchange information and mutual education about these relatively new or esoteric tools in the armamentarium of statistical analysis. The discussions were in-

tended to clarify some of the confusion that currently exists about nomenclature, operating principles, and applications of multivariate statistical procedures. Among the other contributing participants in the sessions were: G. D. Anderson, M. Gent, C. H. Goldsmith, G. B. Hill, A. S. Macpherson, M. A. Rahim, R. S. Roberts, D. L. Sackett, W. O. Spitzer, D. L. Streiner, and E. Vayda. One of my "homework" assignments was to prepare a summary of what had been learned (at least by me) during the "course." In this paper, I shall share that summary with the readers of this series.

A. Problems in concepts and purposes

An immediate problem associated with the term *multivariate analysis* is the scope of topics to which it refers. Topics that are included in one textbook may be omitted or deliberately excluded from another. A second problem is that the textbooks do not contain a clear outline of the functional purposes to which multivariate techniques can be applied. Such outlines—a boon to the user of statistical procedures—are sometimes presented in standard texts,[6, 19, 36] but are not included among the statistical principles, matrix manipulations, and computer calculations that are discussed in books on multivariate

This chapter originally appeared as "Clinical biostatistics—XXI. A primer of concepts, phrases, and procedures in the statistical analysis of multiple variables." In Clin. Pharmacol. Ther. 14:462. 1973.

analysis. Rather than following the conventional statistical taxonomy, I prefer to arrange the topics in this essay according to the types of analytic situations for which multivariate procedures can be used. As background for that arrangement, I shall first cite the different kinds of multiplicity that can be called *multivariate*, and the different purposes for which univariate or multivariate procedures can be employed.

1. Features of possible multiplicity.

a. Number of groups. The number of groups under statistical analysis can be one, two, or many. Thus, we might refer to the mean weight of men (one group); of doctors and lawyers (two groups); or of people treated with agents W, X, Y, or Z (many groups).

b. Number of temporal occasions. The data for the members of a group can be obtained on one, two, or many occasions. Thus, we might talk about the mean blood glucose found in a cross-sectional survey of men (one occasion); the change noted in patients' blood glucose values before and after a particular treatment (two occasions); or the pattern of values found in the "curve" for the diverse time points of a glucose tolerance test (many occasions).

c. Number of classes in a variable. The term *variable* will be used here to refer to a class of data. Thus, *sex* is a variable expressed with a nominal scale that has the values of **male** or **female**. *Serum cholesterol* is a variable expressed in such dimensional scalar values as . . . , **250, 251, 252,** . . . mg/100 ml.

A single variable can contain elements from one, two, or many classes of data. *Height* is a variable that includes one class of information. *Ponderal index,* calculated as a specified ratio of height and weight, is a single variable that includes two classes of data. The *Apgar score,* a single variable that is used to describe the condition of newborn babies, is obtained as the sum of additive values for five classes of data. Each of the three vari-

ables just cited is univariate, because it is expressed in a single scale of values, but the variables were constructed to include contributions, respectively, from one, two, or five variables.

The terms *composite* or *multidimensional* are often used to describe a single variable that contains elements from two or more separate variables; and the mixture is often cited with such names as *index, score, factor,* or *stage.* Familiar examples of such composite variables in daily life are the *wind-chill factor* and *temperature-humidity index.* Probably the most familiar medical example of a composite variable is the classification of patients with cancer according to anatomic, topographic, and other elements that are expressed as **Stage I, Stage II,** etc. For the discussion that follows, the term *variable* refers to a class of data expressed in a single scale of values, regardless of whether or not the variable is composite.

d. Relationship of variables. The relationships that exist among the individual variables are particularly important in multivariate analysis. According to the analytic purposes, these relationships can be regarded mathematically as independent, interdependent, or dependent.

The variables are all *independent* if they are analyzed without regard to any direct relationship that may exist among them. Thus, if we report the individual results for cholesterol, age, and hematocrit for a group of patients, making no effort to associate any of these variables, they have been dealt with in a wholly independent way.

The variables are *interdependent* if we examine the general relationship among all of them without specifying any particular variable(s) as a focus or target of the relationship. Thus, when we obtain the traditional correlation coefficient (Pearson's r) between cholesterol and hematocrit for a group of patients, we note the interdependence of these two variables. We do not mean to imply that cholesterol depends on hematocrit, or vice versa. The type of interdependence noted with Pearson's r is a bivariate correlation, because only two variables are involved. In the multivariate situation, we might want to correlate the interdependence of a series of variables, such as cholesterol, hematocrit, glucose, weight, and age.

The relationship is *dependent* if one or more variables has been chosen as a target that can be affected by one or more of the other variables. The term *dependent* is used for the target variable(s), and *independent* for the affector variable(s). Thus, if we want to know the way that cholesterol varies with (i.e., is affected by) hematocrit, we regard cholesterol as the dependent, and hematocrit as the independent variable. A more familiar medical relationship is that of *survival rate* as a dependent variable, and *stage of cancer*, as the independent variable.

These mathematical concepts of independence, dependence, etc. are often confusing to scientists who reserve the idea of "dependence" for circumstances in which one phenomenon has had a demonstrated influence on another. In mathematical usage, the concept of dependence refers only to the way the variables have been arranged for analysis. A real "dependence" need not be present. Thus, we could choose the baseline *stage of cancer* as a target variable, and analyze its dependence on the subsequent *survival rate* as the independent variable. The results might be silly, but the analysis is mathematically legitimate.

In many analytic circumstances, there are one dependent variable and multiple independent variables. For example, we might look for development of coronary artery disease, as a univariate (dependent) target, in relation to the multiple baseline (independent) variables of sex, age, weight, smoking habits, blood pressure, and cholesterol. Occasionally, the dependent variables may also be multiple. Thus, in relation to the array of independent variables just cited, we might contemplate the dependent variables simultaneously as development of coronary artery disease, change in work capacity, and cost of medical care.

2. The scope of multivariate analysis.

The relationship among variables is the key issue in certain statistical decisions about the topics that can be called *multivariate*. Many statisticians restrict the term *multivariate analysis* to two types of situation: (1) for relationships among three or more interdependent variables; or (2) for dependent relationships in which the target consists of two or more variables, rather than a single variable. Multiple regression would thus be regarded as a univariate technique because a single variable is the dependent target, despite the multiple variables that occur in the independent role.

This restricted scope of the word *multivariate* can be a useful way of indicating the particular circumstances to which the corresponding statistical theory will be applied, but the restriction has two major disadvantages. The first is that the restriction is not uniformly maintained. Many statistical discussions of multivariate analysis include such "univariate" but "multivariabled" techniques as multiple regression and discriminant function analysis. The second, and more important, disadvantage is that the word *multivariate* is too valuable a general descriptive adjective to be limited to only a small subset of its legitimate domain. In the title of this essay, for example, I was forced to use the phrase *analysis of multiple variables*. The preferable term, *multivariate analysis*, is shorter, clearer, and etymologically correct, but is excluded by the current arbitrary boundaries. The essay includes several "multivariable" topics for which the name "multivariate" has been proscribed.

Since many intellectual restrictions are often altered to comply with scientific necessities, the term *multivariate analysis* should be allowed to assume its proper role as a name for circumstances in which multiple variables are under analysis, regardless of whether they are independent, interdependent, or dependent. I shall therefore use *multivariate analysis* here in its unrestricted sense, with apologies to anyone who may protest that the purity of statistical nomenclature has been violated. The vigor of the protest can be mitigated by reminder of the many other terms—such as *significance, normal, precision, error,* and even *regression*—that have had their original medical or scientific meaning altered in current statistical usage.

3. The purposes of the analysis. Multivariate techniques can be employed for each of the three major general purposes of statistical analysis—reduction, association, and inference. Those purposes will be briefly reviewed here, with illustrations from univariate and bivariate procedures extended to their multivariate counterparts.

a. Reduction. There are at least four different ways in which statistical analysis is used to "reduce" data.

(1). FOR OBSERVATIONS. The most familiar and commonly used reduction of data consists of two tactics for summarizing the observations in a single variable. One such summary indicates a *central location,* such as a mean or median. The other summary indicates *dispersion,* and is often expressed as a variance (or standard deviation), or as a quantile range.

In the multivariate situation, no new concept is needed to cite the means of each variable; they are noted individually. A new concept does arise, however, for multivariate dispersion. We can talk about the variance for each individual variable, but the availability of several variables allows us also to consider the covariance of each variable with every other variable. The values for these variances and covariances are usually expressed in an arrangement called, appropriately enough, a *variance–co-variance matrix.*

(2). FOR CATEGORIES. The categories of a single variable are often reduced by combination of two or more adjacent entries. Thus, if serum cholesterol were expressed as **below 210, 210-250, 251-275, 276-300,** and **above 300,** we might reduce these five categories to three as follows: **below 251, 251-275,** and **above 275.** Multivariate combinations of categories are represented by such composite terms as **tall old men,**

containing elements joined from the variables of height, age, and sex. Another type of multivariate reduction is achieved by assigning numerical values to the individual categories, and by adding the values for several categories together to form a multidimensional single index, such as the *Apgar score.*

(3). FOR VARIABLES. The reduction of variables has no counterpart in univariate data, since more than one variable is required for the process. In multivariate situations, the objective is to arrange the variables in a manner that emphasizes their relative statistical importance. This objective can be achieved in at least two different ways. In one method, the variables that seem unimportant are directly eliminated from analysis. (This is the basic tactic employed in stepwise regression techniques, as noted later.) A second method is to create a new set of variables, based upon combinations of the old ones. For example, if we have three variables, x, y, and z, we might create three new variables

$$w_1 = a_1x + b_1y + c_1z,$$
$$w_2 = a_2x + b_2y + c_2z, \text{ and}$$
$$w_3 = a_3x + b_3y + c_3z.$$

The coefficients for the different values of a, b, and c are selected in such a way as to make w_1 the most important of the new variables, and w_3 the least important. (The criteria for assessing "importance" usually depend on maximizing or minimizing certain features of variance and covariance). If w_3 is sufficiently unimportant, it might then be eliminated from consideration, so that our original three variables (x, y, and z) would be reduced into two new ones: w_1 and w_2. This is the basic tactic employed, as noted later, in principal component analysis and factor analysis.

(4). FOR INDIVIDUAL PEOPLE. The individual people under analysis are commonly "reduced" in the univariate situation by using one of the variables, such as *sex,* to divide (and combine) the people into groups, such as male and female. A single target variable is then reported for each group. Thus, we can list the individual values of cholesterol for every one of our observed people, or we can summarize the results indiscriminately by giving a single mean for all of them. The summary is more refined, however, if we divide (or reduce) the people into groups and cite the mean cholesterol separately for men and women.

In the multivariate situation, the groups of people are demarcated by the composite categories, such as tall old men, that were mentioned earlier. The tactic of forming groups of individual people is used for the procedures, noted later, that are called *cluster analysis* and *multivariate stratification*.

b. Association. The association between two variables is familiar to most users of analytic statistical techniques. For dimensional variables, the association can easily be illustrated on a graph, and is usually expressed by the correlation coefficient, r. If the two variables are not dimensional, the association is often shown with a two-way contingency table. The chi-square test often applied to such tables is a measurement of the "significance" of the association, rather than the association itself. When pertinent, the association in non-dimensional data can be calculated with such eponym-laden statistics as Guttman's lambda, Yule's Q, Goodman and Kruskal's G, Kendall's tau, Spearman's rho, or Cicchetti's C.

In the multivariate situation, the association between variables can be either dependent or interdependent. In the *dependent* relationship, when several independent variables are being "predictively" associated with the target variable(s), the result can be expressed as a multiple regression equation in the form

$$y = b_0 + b_1x_1 + b_2x_2 + b_3x_3 + \ldots + b_nx_n.$$

In this equation, y is a target variable, such as death due to coronary disease; and $x_1, x_2, \ldots, x_n$ are variables such as age,

race, blood pressure, etc. Except for the constant, b_0, each of the b_i coefficients represents a type of correlation between each of the corresponding independent variables, x_i, and the dependent variable, y. In simple regression between two variables, the equation is expressed in the form, $y = b_0 + b_1x$. The value for b_1 in the simple equation is directly related to the correlation coefficient, r, in that $b_1^2 = (r^2)$ (variance of y)/(variance of x). In multiple regression, the b_i coefficients are much more complex to calculate, but the basic idea of correlation with the target variable is maintained.

In the multivariate *interdependent* situation, things become confused because there is no target variable to which each of the many variables can be related. They are supposed to be associated with one another, but, in the absence of a dependent variable, there is no target available to indicate the particular direction in which the association should be aimed. One obvious approach is to see how the variables correlate with one another by noting their covariance relationships, but this type of multiple correlation may not be the desired goal when multivariate interdependent associations are analyzed. The goal may be to determine the "resemblance" or "affinity" that exists among the individual objects described by the different variables. The problem is then to create a particular statistical index that can best denote the resemblance or affinity. A plethora of different indexes has been proposed for this purpose. I shall mention some of their names here merely for readers to savor the nomenclature: Euclidean distance, Mahalanobis D^2, Jaccard's S_J, Sokal-Michener's S_{SM}, Cain-Harrison's R_{jk}, and Canberra metric. A detailed account of these and many other measures of multivariate "affinity" is provided by Cormack[9] and by Sokal and Sneath.[37]

When so many alternatives exist for a particular procedure, it is obvious that none of them is wholly satisfactory, and all of them are fraught with the difficulties described in an excellent, lucid critique by Fleiss and Zubin.[18]

c. Contrast. A third principal purpose of statistical techniques is to allow inference about a contrast. This is what happens when we engage in "hypothesis testing" to calculate "statistical significance" for the differences observed when two or more entities are contrasted. The available statistical tests could have been created (like the t-test or chi-square) to evaluate the contrast directly. Alternatively, an inferential test can be performed by applying certain formulas to the results found in a measurement of association. Such tactics allow us to determine "statistical significance" for the bivariate correlation coefficient, r, or for the various b_i coefficients that are found in multivariate analysis of dependent relationships.

4. The problems of computation. The existence of multiple variables for multiple people will provide large amounts of different types of information. Merely to express the arrangement of data is a complicated procedure. The average clinician who feels uncomfortable with such symbols as Σ and $\bar{x}$, and who tries to hide when faced with dy/dt, will probably go into exile at first view of the matrix algebra[35] used for multivariate data. Beyond its inherent awesomeness, the algebra requires an amount of calculation so formidable that multivariate analysis seems relatively novel today not because it is new, but because its arithmetic drudgery made it unfeasible for frequent use until the advent of digital computers that could do the calculations quickly and accurately. Kendall,[25] for example, mentions that

In 1945 I did some calculations on a set of time series that took me three weeks on a desk machine. A short while ago I had a similar set done and the work took three seconds.

With computers available to do the "number crunching," multivariate techniques have now become popular because they can be easily applied, but two new hazards have been introduced. The first is that the techniques may be too popular and too readily available. An investigator today can "plug" his data into a "canned program" and get a series of results without ever understanding what they mean, without recognizing what was done to his data inside the "black box," and without determining whether the computer program did in fact provide a correct translation of the basic mathematical strategy. For example, many investigators who currently use multivariate "canned programs" do not know how the program deals with information that is absent or unknown for a particular variable in a particular person, and are not aware of the strikingly different results that can sometimes be obtained if certain arbitrarily chosen "operational parameters" are altered.[5]

A second hazard is that computers will be used merely to automate rather than to improve the *status quo* of statistical theory. The energy that has gone into constructing many computer programs for multivariate analysis has often been expended merely in arranging the automated application of existing statistical doctrines. Since these doctrines are not always well suited to the problems of analyzing multivariate clinical or epidemiologic data, investigators who become addicted to the existing programs may lose the opportunity to use the computer for creating new and potentially better approaches to the problems.

Clinical and epidemiologic investigators thus have a double incentive to become familiar with multivariate techniques: to avoid the intellectual serfdom of being ignorant and overly credulous when receiving the computer's print-out; and to learn enough about the problems to be able to evaluate and sometimes inspire proposals for better solutions.

B. Techniques of analysis

With these concepts of multiplicity and purpose, we can now proceed to consider a taxonomy of multivariate procedures, classified according to the types of data analyses for which they can be applied. Whenever possible, I have noted the counterpart procedures that might be used for the simple univariate or bivariate analyses with which many readers may already be familiar. To enliven the discussion, I have added some personal appraisals to indicate the particular procedures that, in my own experience, appear to have little value for clinical or epidemiologic analyses. I hope readers who have had experiences that either confirm or refute these comments will write to enlighten me.

I shall not attempt to explain the diverse mathematical principles that are the basis for the multivariate strategies. Some of these principles involve complex matrix algebra that I do not yet fully understand myself. An investigator who plans to use any of the multivariate procedures can find details of their theory and operation in appropriate publications. Unfortunately, most of the textbooks[2, 4, 24, 31-34] on this subject are difficult to understand (even by card-carrying statisticians), and at least one of the books would be a leading candidate for my own personal award for maximum communicative inscrutability. The clearest brief account I have found is in a paperback British text by Hope.[22] The texts by Tatsuoka[40] and by Cooley and Lohnes[8] provide moderately clear expositions, and many details of the corresponding computer programs. A clearly organized but mainly theoretical discussion of certain procedures is provided by Kendall and Stuart.[26]

1. Temporal occasions. We here assume one group of people and observations on one variable. If the observations are obtained on one occasion, the main statistical goal would be to reduce the data, using expressions such as the mean and standard deviation. If the observations are obtained on two occasions, the goal would usually be to contrast the individual pairs

of results for each person. The paired t-test is the classic example of a customary procedure for this contrast. If the observations are obtained on multiple occasions, time becomes an additional variable, and we get into an apparent analog of multivariate analysis. The analog is more apparent than real, however, because such multitemporal data can often be expressed in the form of a simple regression equation, with time as the independent variable.

The difficulty with this simple expression is that many forms of multitemporal data cannot be fitted with the linear model assumed in the usual regression equation. To fit the diverse patterns that can occur in multitemporal data requires a special form of statistical analysis concerned with *time series.* This type of analysis is complex not because of multiple variables, but because of multiple patterns of curves in the single variable whose response to time is being depicted by the statistical formulation. I know of no circumstances in clinical epidemiologic investigation where time-series analysis has provided really important or useful results, and the topic will not be further discussed here.

2. Contrast of groups. When the results of two or more groups are being contrasted, the names of the groups become the independent variable, and the particular type of observation under assessment becomes the dependent or target variable. Thus, if we perform a t-test on the mean survival times noted with Treatment X and Treatment Y, the treatments are the independent variable, and survival time is dependent. If we want to contrast the results in two groups for several dependent variables simultaneously (such as survival time, relief of symptoms, occurrence of side effects, and cost of treatment), the multivariate analog of the t-test is called *Hotelling's* T^2. Another multivariate test used for this purpose is Mahalanobis' D^2.

If the number of groups under contrast is three or more, and the target is univariate, the standard procedure is the F-test in the analysis of variance. An important point to note here is that the analysis of variance indicates only whether a "significant" difference exists when all the groups are considered simultaneously. In many instances, investigators may want to select pairs of groups for direct comparison by t-test. In this situation, the usual concepts of "statistical significance" do not hold. For example, if we have 7 groups, we could perform 21 ($=7\times6/2$) pairwise t-tests among them. At the 0.05 level, one of these 21 tests might turn out to be "significant" by chance alone. Consequently, the t-test analyses must be modified according to certain statistical principles used for "multiple comparisons."[39]

If three or more groups are being simultaneously contrasted for more than one target variable, the multivariate procedure is the *multivariate analysis of variance*. In many places in the literature, this procedure is acronymically abbreviated as MANOVA, and the univariate technique is called ANOVA.

3. Measures of association for variables. In these situations we deal with multiple variables for a single group of people. The results might then be applied to the individual members of that group, or tested for "prediction" on members from some other group.

a. Interdependent. We have already discussed the measures of association used when the variables are interdependent. For two variables, the statistical procedure is Pearson's r for dimensional data, or one of its diverse analogs when the data are nominal or ordinal rather than dimensional. For more than two variables, the multivariate association is assessed with one of the many available indexes of multiple correlation or "affinity."

b. Independent. A technique called *profile analysis* has been proposed for assessing the contrived spatial relationship of a series of independent variables. Consider a graph in which a series of variables, such as serum cholesterol, blood sugar, weight, hematocrit, and serum bilirubin, are marked separately but successively as individual locations on the x-axis. At each location, the value found for that variable in a particular patient is plotted as a point in the y-direction. We now connect the points for that patient to form a polygonal pattern on the graph. This pattern is called a *profile*. If we plot the points for a series of patients, we get a series of polygonal profiles.

The relationships of these lines to one another are studied in profile analysis. I have referred to the associations as *independent* because there is no specific target variable, and because the multiple variables are not assessed interdependently. What we analyze is a group of different linear shapes.

The exact value of profile analysis is obscure, and I know of no clinical circumstance in which it has provided valuable results. Furthermore, because the variables are placed in a completely arbitrary arrangement on the x-axis, the shape of profiles can be greatly altered by changing the location of the variables. Thus, in the foregoing example, we might get a quite different set of shapes if our succession of variables was changed from the previously cited order into the following: hematocrit, weight, serum cholesterol, serum bilirubin, and blood sugar.

c. Dependent.

(1). ONE TARGET VARIABLE; RANKED. For a relationship between one dependent and one independent variable, the standard procedure is simple linear regression. For a single dependent variable and more than one independent variable, the standard procedure is multiple linear regression.[10] In most situations the procedure is used with each of the variables expressed alone in its first order or "power." The regression equation can be augmented to include quadratic terms, such as x_1^2, or combinations of "interacting" terms, such as

$x_1 x_2$. An illustration of a multiple linear* regression equation with such additional variables is

$$y = b_0 + b_1 x_1 + b_2 x_2 + b_3 x_3 + b_4 x_1{}^2 + b_5 x_2 x_3 + b_6 x_1 x_2 x_3.$$

The investigator must decide, usually as an act of arbitrary judgment, to insert such quadratic or interaction terms into the regression equation.

The dependent variable in the regression technique must be expressed as a number that can be ranked, but the number can come from an ordinal as well as a dimensional scale. In particular, the dependent variable in multiple linear regression is often expressed dichotomously for the occurrence or non-occurrence of an event, such as death or the development of coronary artery disease. The absence of the event is then ranked as *0*, and its presence as *1*.

After the data for a group of people are analyzed to provide coefficients of a multiple regression equation for a dichotomous target event, the equation can be applied to "predict" results for individual people. The predictions are stated as the calculated probability for the likelihood that the target event will occur in that person. In some individual situations, however, the results of this calculation may yield impossible probability values that are either below 0 or greater than 1. To avoid these statistical unpleasantries, the format of the regression procedure can be modified so that the results of the calculation always emerge in values between 0 and 1. The algebraic tactic used for the modification is called the *logistic function*.[42] It leaves the basic regression principle intact but expresses it in slightly different terms. This procedure has recently become popular among epidemiologists, who often refer to it as *multiple logistic regression*.

(2). ONE TARGET VARIABLE; UNRANKED. When the dependent variable is expressed in one of several possible *nominal* categories, such as an occupation or a disease diagnosis, its relationship to the multiple independent variables cannot be determined with the regression procedure, which requires ranked values for the target variable. The alternative multivariate tactic used for this type of nominal association is called discriminant function analysis. If the target variable can be expressed in only two dichotomous categories, the results of discriminant function analysis are identical to those of multiple regression.

If the target variable contains nominal groups listed in three or more polytomous categories, the analysis usually produces two or more discriminant functions. Each function, expressed as a weighted combination of the multiple independent variables, forms a type of "line" that divides the "space" of data into the "sectors" where members of the different target categories are most likely to be encountered. When a particular person's data are entered into the discriminant function equations, the calculated results are then used to predict his membership in one of the groups. The discriminant function procedure thus seems particularly applicable for mathematical strategies of diagnosis, where it has sometimes been employed. Since prognosis is usually directed at a target variable expressed in ranked categories, the discriminant and regression procedures can be used interchangeably for this purpose.

---

*The word *linegr* has been a source of confusion for many investigators, including myself. The basic equation, $y = b_0 + b_1 x_1$, is for a line with y-intercept, b_0, and with slope, b_1. When the equation includes multiple variables, such as $b_2 x_2 + \ldots + b_n x_n$, we can imagine it to be a "line" or "hyperplane" in n-dimensional space.

The idea of linearity would thus imply that the x_i variables are all expressed in their first order (or "power"). For the mathematics of estimation, however, the b_i coefficients, not the x_i variables, are regarded as arranged in a linear manner.[9] Thus, an equation of the form

$$y = \frac{b_2 - b_1}{b_1} x_1 + e^{b_1 b_2} x_2$$

would come from nonlinear regression, although it describes a plane.

Clinical investigators have been wrong in complaining about the clinically unreal "linearity" assumed in the many regression equations that omit combinations (or "interaction") of variables. The proper focus of the complaint is the restriction to first-order terms of single variables only.

(3). MORE THAN ONE TARGET VARIABLE. When the dependent as well as the independent variables are multiple, the relationship between them is expressed in a statistical technique called *canonical correlation.* The equation takes the form

$$a_1y_1 + a_2y_2 + a_3y_3 =$$
$$b_0 + b_1x_1 + b_2x_2 + b_3x_3 + \ldots + b_nx_n$$

I do not know of any examples in clinical investigation where this technique has had demonstrated value.

4. **Procedures for associative reduction.** The association of multiple variables can also be performed with techniques of reduction that are intended either to demonstrate important variables (or combinations of variables); or to create clusters of categories that demarcate groups of people. The process of associative reduction uses different techniques for interdependent and dependent relationships of variables.

a. Interdependent variables.

(1). REDUCTION OF VARIABLES. Two multivariate procedures are available for this activity. One is called *principal component analysis;* the other, *factor analysis;* and both are difficult to understand. True comprehension requires a familiarity with the arcane world of determinants, eigenvectors, latent roots, characteristic equations, adjugate matrixes, axis rotations, and factor loadings. Every investigator I have met who uses these techniques either does not fully comprehend the complicated mathematics or has been unable to provide a succinct explanation. Even Hope,[22] whose description of the procedures is the clearest I could find, confesses at the end that the reader may have been left "bewildered" by the succession of arithmetic and algebraic relations.

In both the factor and the component techniques, the original variables are recombined in diverse ways to form new variables. These new combinations are made up of *components* or *factors* that are regarded as important in reducing, summmarizing, or weighting the number of original variables. The main difference between the two techniques, according to Kendall,[24] is

. . . in component analysis we begin with the observations and look for components, . . . (working) from the data toward a hypothetical model. In factor analysis we work the other way round; that is to say, we begin with a model and require to see whether it agrees with the data . . .

Another basic difference, according to Lawley and Maxwell,[29] is that ". . . whereas a principal component analysis is *variance-*orientated, a factor analysis is *covariance-*orientated."

Although component analysis seldom appears in medical literature, factor analysis has become well accepted and often used in psychologic research. At many university computer centers today, more computing time is probably consumed by factor analyses than by any other type of multivariate calculations. The psychologists' preference and enthusiasm for this technique may be attributable to its original formulation by psychologists rather than by statisticians, and to the hope that the results, in a somewhat dubious analogy from the many vectors of the associated matrix algebra, might reveal the "vectors of the mind."

I am reluctant to disparage the factor analytic technique because I have had so little direct experience with it and because many capable psychologists seem to think it is important. Nevertheless, it has been used frequently for many years without having produced any major, enduring, or generally accepted scientific contributions. In the few applications with which I am familiar, the results were either scientifically meaningless, or, if apparently worthwhile, could have been anticipated and effectively arranged through an incisive judgmental examination of the basic data, together with some simple statistical procedures.

The best appraisal I have seen of factor analysis was presented by Donald Mainland[30] in a biometric "note" that should be mandatory reading for any investigator who contemplates using the procedure. Another thoughtful assessment, contained in a general critique of multivariate procedures, was recently published by Kowalski.[23] For readers who are willing to struggle with the mathematics, a well organized description of the principles and computations of factor analysis has been provided by Cattell.[7] Amid the generally favorable evaluation, Cattell mentions the hazards of certain maneuvers that may create "meretricious neatness," "perpetrate a hoax," "inflate specious, incorrect common factors," or act by "contaminating the form of the important factors."

(2). FORMATION OF GROUPS OR "CLUSTERS". The statistical process of forming groups from interdependent multivariate data, without regard to a target variable, is called *cluster analysis*. It is currently a particularly fashionable multivariate activity, because computers can now be used to do certain numerical manipulations that formerly were unsuitable even for desk calculators. A subset of cluster analysis is a diverse array of techniques included in a domain called *numerical taxonomy*,[37] which refers to the use of computer-aided cluster analysis for challenges in the taxonomic classification of biologic organisms.

A cluster analysis requires two arbitrary decisions: (1) choice of an index of similarity or affinity between every pair of units in the population under analysis, and (2) choice of a method for sorting the indexes to form the clusters of units. The problems in making the first decision were discussed earlier. The second decision creates its own problems for choosing one of several available strategies for aggregation. The aggregates can be formed as demarcated clumps or hierarchial "nests," and they can either be all delineated at once, or created in a stepwise sequence in which certain units are first paired together as a "root" that is then augmented by other units to form small clusters that are ulti-

mately united into larger clusters. Some of the current controversies associated with numerical taxonomy and cluster analysis were discussed in a previous paper[12] in this series.

When the interdependent variables are not expressed dimensionally, the data may be cited as frequency counts in a multiple-variable contingency table. The condensation[20] of categories in these tables is an activity analogous to cluster analysis.

b. Dependent variables. In this circumstance, we have a series of multiple independent variables that are to be predictively associated with a single target variable, but we want the result to be "economical," either with a reduced number of variables or with a reduction of the population into groups.

(1). REDUCTION OF VARIABLES. To reduce the number of variables, techniques of multiple regression or discriminant function analysis are applied in a "stepwise" manner.[11] The equations are formed by successively selecting the particular variables that appear to be most important, and by entering only those variables that make a substantial contribution to the prediction. The criteria for "importance" and "substantial contribution" are usually based on reducing the "unexplained" variance in the target variable.

There has been considerable debate[3, 10] about the merits of these stepwise techniques, which can be performed in diverse ways, including stepping up, stepping down, etc. In theory, the predictions should be more accurate when all the available variables are included in the procedure. In practice (and in some recent expositions of theory), however, the results seem to be better when stepwise techniques are used to reduce the number of variables to the few that are most important.

(2). MULTIVARIATE STRATIFICATION (TARGETTED CLUSTERS). These techniques are new (some of the details not yet having been formally reported) and have not yet begun to receive discussion in statistical

textbooks of multivariate analysis. All of the techniques have been mentioned in previous papers [13-16] of this series. The techniques are used to identify targetted clusters of multivariate strata. In contrast to regression or discriminant function analyses, which produce coefficients for variables, the stratification procedures demarcate groups of people with combinations of characteristics that have been chosen for their effect on the target variable.

In three of the techniques, the groups are created with the use of a formal algorithmic strategy in a computer program that makes the process of selection take place in the same type of "automated" manner that would occur with a series of mathematical equations. The best known of these procedures, the "AID" program devised by Sonquist and Morgan,[38] is based on reduction of variance in the rate of the target event. Another technique, developed by Klein[27] and his colleagues,[21] depends on the principle of "congruent fit." The third technique, now reported only in a preliminary abstract,[17] depends on a successive polarization of target rates.

In the fourth technique, which was described in earlier papers[14-16] devoted to multivariate prognostic stratification, the groups are formed by a succession of judgments based on both clinical and statistical desiderata. This is the only one of the predictive multivariate techniques that incorporates clinical as well as statistical reasoning during the sequential strategy of the procedure.

C. Comments and evaluations

The entire domain of multivariate analysis is much too young and still too underdeveloped for definitive conclusions to be formed about any of the procedures. Nevertheless, certain basic principles in the procedures seem clear enough to allow at least temporary evaluations.

1. The disadvantages of multivariate targets. In Hotelling's T², MANOVA, and canonical correlations, the analysis deals with several dependent (target) variables simultaneously. The disadvantage of using multiple variables as concomitant targets is that all the variables are given equal status, regardless of their clinical or biologic importance. Thus, a patient who dies of a sudden cardiac arrhythmia two weeks after starting a new drug for rheumatoid arthritis may appear to have an excellent "multivariate" result, because the other target data (absence of symptoms, no cutaneous side effects, normalization of laboratory tests, and low cost of treatment) showed such a good response.

One way of getting around this problem is to assign different weights to the individual target variables—a tactic clinicians have been using for centuries without quantitatively specifying the weights. The assignment of formal weights for the target variables would enable better use of the cited multivariate procedures, but the choice of weights is necessarily arbitrary and cannot be validated by the analysis itself. Furthermore, if such weights are chosen, they could be used to convert the target variable into a multidimensional or composite index. This composite index could then be analyzed with conventional multivariate procedures that depend on a univariate target.

If an investigator insists on a simultaneous analysis of multiple target variables, my own preference would be to convert them into a single, carefully selected, composite index. Since the construction of such composite indexes is difficult and since the methodology is still underdeveloped, each target variable should be analyzed separately before any combinations are formed.

2. The disadvantages of non-dependent associations. The procedures for factor analysis, principal component analysis, and cluster analysis have the major disadvantage that they cannot be well validated because the variables are interdependent. There is no target variable to be used for determining whether a "prediction" is right or wrong in the same people or in a new group of test people. All that can be done is to calculate the amount of statistical variance that is "explained" or left "unexplained" by the mathematical maneuvers, but the results cannot be tested against a target "criterion" variable. Furthermore, the results are entirely arbitrary, and may change considerably with the decisions made during arbitrary selection of choices for axis rotations, measures of "affinity," and techniques of aggregation. Finally, the importance of the variables is determined exclusively by statistical calculations. The various components, factors, or clusters have no direct biologic meaning and are not selected according to any biologic principles.

My own preference in these untargetted interdependent situations is to convert them into targetted dependent situations. The target variable(s) could then be used as a focus for selecting and validating the results that emerge. A system of classification or analysis, like a project in scientific research, requires an objective. Without a stated target, the work may seem aimless and may lend itself to protracted disputes about the merits of different arbitrary schemes, none of which can be really tested or proved superior to any other.

In most activities of medical classification,[41] the process can readily be aimed at such target variables as an etiologic diagnosis or a prognostic outcome. These goals are particularly hard to achieve with data for psychologic conditions, however, because etiologic agents are difficult to identify, and prognostic outcomes have not been well investigated and specified. The absence of suitable target variables is probably the main reason that the factor, component, and cluster analytic schemes have been popularly applied to psychologic data. (These interdependent techniques have also been popular for classifying taxonomy in lower biologic organisms, for which target variables are seldom available in the form of either prognostic outcomes or evolutionary "etiologic" concepts in phylogenesis.) The use of target variables may greatly improve the status of multivariate analysis in psychology. Target variables can be attained by getting improved information about outcome events, and by using, in certain circumstances, such newly

available outcomes as the response to modern psychotropic drugs.

3. *The problems of validation.* When a dependent variable is used as a target in the analysis, the results can be validated, since they produce a "prediction" about the target. This prediction can be checked internally by determining how well it "fits" each member of the group whose data were used in the analysis. Thus, in a regression-type of procedure, the probability of myocardial infarction for a particular person might be calculated as 0.2. In a discriminant function procedure, the person might be designated as being in the non-myocardial-infarction group. In a stratification procedure, the person might be placed in a group for which the rate of myocardial infarction is 15%. In all three of these results, we would probably "predict" that the person did not have an infarction. We can then test the accuracy of the "prediction" by checking, in that person's data, whether an infarction did or did not occur. We can then add up the number of "congruent errors" produced by these individual predictions, and use the result as an index of effectiveness for the technique.

A more cogent type of validation is performed *externally* by checking the predictions in a different group of people. Since the multivariate results can always be "tailored" to provide a "good fit" for the data from which they were derived, the real test comes when the results are applied to people who were not included in the underlying data. Validations of this type have almost never been performed in the many clinical and epidemiologic reports that have used multivariate analysis. When such external tests are reported,[23] the claims of the original analysis are not always confirmed.

Two other types of external validation can also be employed. In one type, the results of one multivariate procedure are compared with those of another. For example, in an earlier paper[15] in this series, I showed that multivariate stratification and multiple logistic regression yielded essentially the same degree of congruent accuracy when applied to an illustrative set of data. An intriguing comparison of multiple regression vs. "AID" stratifications of health survey data was recently published by Andersen, Smedby, and Eklund.[1] For the second additional type of validation, the target event is membership in one of several possible nominal categories (such as the diagnosis of a disease), rather than a dichotomous predictive endpoint, such as occurrence or non-occurrence of myocardial infarction. In this circumstance, the results of the discriminant function or other multivariate analysis can be checked against the diagnoses made (for the same patients) by a different clinical examiner.

Finally, an external-internal type of validation can be attempted with data for a single group of people containing N members. Remove the first member from the group; perform the multivariate procedure for the remaining N-1 members; use the results to predict outcome for the first member. Then remove the second member; perform the procedure again for a group consisting of the first member and the other N-2 members; apply the new results to predict outcome for the second member. Continue sequentially for the entire group. In each instance, the prediction will be external, because it arises from a group of people who did not include the person for whom the prediction is made. Because an enormous amount of computer time may be consumed in performing N sets of multivariate analyses for a large group of people, this type of validation can be done in a randomly selected smaller set. Alternatively, a large group can be randomly divided into two parts. The results obtained with one part can then be used predictively on the other.

Many alternative methods could be cited for conducting validations that involve an external component. The performance of an external, "real-world" validation is obviously an essential of scientific research. Such validations are unfortunately absent from many published reports dealing with either the theory or the application of multivariate analytic procedures.

D. The most useful forms of multivariate analysis

For the reasons that have been cited, I believe that only a few types of multivariate analysis will make significant contributions to clinical or epidemiologic research. These procedures involve predictive associations or reductions between multiple independent variables and a single target variable. The results can be expressed in the groups created by multivariate stratification procedures or in the coefficients produced by the different congeners of multiple regression and discriminant function analysis.

Earlier in this series, I discussed[13] my reasons for preferring the stratification processes. They are oriented toward finding combinations of important properties that emerge from the data, and they require no assumptions about linear, quadratic, interactive or other mathematical models for the data. The stratification process also demarcates groups of people with specific characteristics that are more amenable to scientific explanation than the results found in a series of algebraic coefficients. Nevertheless, the regression and discriminant techniques can be powerful tools in the exploratory analysis of data. The most effective types of multivariate procedures may ultimately be produced by some combination of the regression-discriminatory and stratification techniques.

Since all of the multivariate concepts are relatively new, many more ideas remain to be investigated, created, and developed in the future. These subsequent developments may demonstrate errors in some of my preliminary appraisals here. If so, we shall have another example of circumstances in which a conclusion based on multivariate analysis turned out to be wrong.

References

1. Andersen, R., Smedby, B., and Eklund, G.: Automatic interaction detector program for analyzing health survey data, Health Services Research 6:165-183 (Summer), 1971.
2. Anderson, T. W.: Introduction to multivariate statistical analysis, New York, 1958, John Wiley & Sons, Inc. (Fourth printing, 1964.)

3. Beale, E. M. L.: A note on procedures for variable selection in multiple regression, Technometrics **12**:909-914, 1970.

4. Bock, R. D.: Multivariate statistical methods in behavioral research. New York, 1971, McGraw-Hill Book Co.

5. Box, G. E. P.: Use and abuse of regression, Technometrics **8**:625-629, 1966.

0. Bradley, J. V.: Distribution-free statistical tests, Englewood Cliffs, N. J., 1068, Prentice-Hall, Inc.

7. Cattell, R. B.: Factor analysis: An introduction to essentials. I. The purpose and underlying models, Biometrics **21**:190-215, 1965.

8. Cooley, W. W., and Lohnes, P. R.: Multivariate data analysis. New York, 1971, John Wiley & Sons, Inc.

9. Cormack, R. M.: A review of classification, J. Roy. Statist. Soc. (Series A) **134**:321-367, 1971.

10. Draper, N. R., and Smith, H.: Applied regression analysis, New York, 1966, John Wiley & Sons, Inc.

11. Efroymson, M. A.: Multiple regression analysis, Article 17, pp. 191-203, *in* Ralston, A., and Wilf, H. S., editors: Mathematical models for digital computers, New York, 1962, John Wiley & Sons, Inc.

12. Feinstein, A. R.: Clinical biostatistics: XIII. On homogeneity, taxonomy, and nosography, CLIN. PHARMACOL. THER. **13**:114-129, 1972.

13. Feinstein, A. R.: Clinical biostatistics: XIV. The purposes of prognostic stratification, CLIN. PHARMACOL. THER. **13**:285-297, 1972.

14. Feinstein, A. R.: Clinical biostatistics: XV. The process of prognostic stratification (Part 1), CLIN. PHARMACOL. THER. **13**:442-457, 1972.

15. Feinstein, A. R.: Clinical biostatistics: XVI. The process of prognostic stratification (Part 2), CLIN. PHARMACOL. THER. **13**:609-624, 1972.

16. Feinstein, A. R.: Clinical biostatistics: XVII. Synchronous partition and bivariate evaluation in predictive stratification, CLIN. PHARMACOL. THER. **13**:755-768, 1972.

17. Feinstein, A. R., and Landis, J. R.: A computer program for finding multivariate prognostic clusters, Clin. Res. **21**:725, April, 1973. (Abst.)

18. Fleiss, J. L., and Zubin, J.: On the methods and theory of clustering, Multivariate Behavioral Res. **4**:235-250, 1969.

19. Freeman, L. C.: Elementary applied statistics, New York, 1965, John Wiley & Sons, Inc.

20. Goodman, L. A.: The multivariate analysis of qualitative data: Interactions among multiple classifications, J. Am. Statist. Assn. **65**:226-256, 1970.

21. Honigfeld, G., Klein, D. F., and Feldman, S.: Prediction of psychopharmacologic effect in man: Development and validation of a computerized diagnostic decision tree, Computers Biomed. Res. **2**:350-361, 1969.

22. Hope, K.: Methods of multivariate analysis, London, 1968, University of London Press, Ltd.

23. Hyde, T. A.: Discriminant function in lung cancer, Lancet **1**:107, 1973. (Letter-to-Editor.)

24. Kendall, M. G.: A course in multivariate analysis, London, 1968, Charles Griffin & Co., Ltd.

25. Kendall, M. G.: The history and future of statistics. Article 12, *in* Bancroft, T. A., editor: Statistical papers in honor of George W. Snedecor, Ames, Iowa, 1972, Iowa State University Press.

26. Kendall, M. G., and Stuart, A.: The advanced theory of statistics, London, 1961 (vol. 2) and 1966 (vol. 3), Charles Griffin & Co., Ltd.

27. Klein, D. F., Honigfeld, G., and Feldman, S.: Prediction of drug effect by diagnostic decision tree, Dis. Nerv. Syst. **29**(Suppl.):159-187, 1968.

28. Kowalski, C. J.: A commentary on the use of multivariate statistical methods in anthropometric research, Am. J. Phys. Anthropol. **36**:119-132, 1972.

29. Lawley, D. N., and Maxwell, A. E.: Factor analysis as a statistical method, London, 1963, Butterworth & Co., Ltd.

30. Mainland, D.: A medical experimenter looks at factor analysis. Note 27, *in* Notes on biometry in medical research, Monograph 10-1, Supplement 4, August, 1968, Department of Medicine and Surgery, Veterans Administration, Washington, D. C.

31. Morrison, D. F.: Multivariate statistical methods, New York, 1967, McGraw-Hill Book Co.

32. Rao, C. R.: Advanced statistical methods in biometric research, New York, 1952, John Wiley & Sons, Inc.

33. Roy, S. N.: Some aspects of multivariate analysis, New York, 1957, John Wiley & Sons, Inc.

34. Seal, H. L.: Multivariate statistical analysis for biologists, London, 1964, Methuen & Co., Ltd.

35. Searle, S. R.: Matrix algebra for the biological sciences (including applications in statistics), New York, 1966, John Wiley & Sons, Inc.

36. Siegel, S.: Nonparametric statistics for the behavioral sciences, New York, 1956, McGraw-Hill Book Co., Inc.

37. Sokal, R. R., and Sneath, P. H. A.: Principles of numerical taxonomy, San Francisco, 1963, W. H. Freeman & Co.

38. Sonquist, J. A., and Morgan, J. N.: The detection of interaction effects: A report on a computer program for the selection of optimal combinations of explanatory variables,

Monograph No. 35, Ann Arbor, Mich., 1964, Survey Research Center Institute for Social Research, University of Michigan.

39. Snedecor, G. W., and Cochran, W. G.: Statistical methods, ed. 6, Ames, Iowa, 1967, Iowa State University Press, pp. 271-275.

40. Tatsuoka, M. M.: Multivariate analysis. Techniques for educational and psychological research, New York, 1971, John Wiley & Sons, Inc.

41. Temkin, O.: The history of classification in the medical sciences, pp. 11-19, *in* Katz, M. M., Cole, J. O., and Barton, W. E., editors: The role and methodology of classification in psychiatry and psychopathology, Washington, D. C., 1968, U. S. Government Printing Office.

42. Walker, S. H., and Duncan, D. B.: Estimation of the probability of an event as a function of several independent variables, Biometrika **54:**167-179, 1967.

CHAPTER 26

The purposes of prognostic stratification

When two or more treatments are randomly allocated to a population of patients whose different outcomes will later be tested for "statistical significance," a fundamental assumption is that the population was initially homogeneous.[9] The act of randomization divides a homogeneous population into homogeneous groups. The effects of the treatment assigned to each group can then be associated with any differences in the groups' post-therapeutic responses. If the population is *not* initially homogeneous, however, the groups created by the randomization will probably not be homogeneous, and the results will be difficult to evaluate. The initial differences within the heterogeneous groups, rather than the imposed treatments, may be responsible for differences in subsequent outcome.

A similar assumption about homogeneity is made whenever we analyze the results of any maneuver that has been imposed on the initial state of a population, regardless of whether the maneuver is a pathogenetic agent that may cause disease, a prophylactic agent that may prevent disease, or a treatment that may alter disease. When we compare the effects of the maneuver with the

effects of the comparative (or "control") maneuvers, we assume that the groups exposed to the compared maneuvers were initially homogeneous. Thus, when we draw conclusions about the alleged evils of cigarette smoking, our basic premise is that a homogeneous cohort has been divided into smokers and non-smokers and followed thereafter. When we decide that surgery is apparently superior to radiotherapy in the treatment of cancer, we assume that similar types of patients were exposed to both forms of therapy. If the initial cohorts are not homogeneous, our basic assumptions will be erroneous, and we must question the validity of our conclusions.

A discussion of the problems of homogeneity was begun in the previous paper of this series.[7] As noted in that discussion, the cohort members who are exposed to a maneuver and observed thereafter can be made initially homogeneous in that each person fulfills the eligibility criteria for admission to the cohort. According to these criteria, the members may be required to be similar in such variates as age, geographic location, health, or disease. The choice of suitable taxonomic denominations for these variates was the topic of the previous paper. Such denominations are needed to demarcate the different kinds of entities that will be nosographically regarded as "diseases," to indicate the pre-requisites of

Under the same name, this chapter originally appeared as "Clinical biostatistics—XIV." In Clin. Pharmacol. Ther. 13:285, 1972.

"health," or to define "similarities" in age or geography.

The main role of denomination in scientific research is to provide this specification for the entities that are subjected to the maneuver under investigation. If we wanted to study the effects of oxygen on premature infants, cigarette smoking on healthy adolescents, anticoagulants on myocardial infarction, or psychotropic drugs on schizophrenia, the diagnosis of *premature infant, healthy adolescent, myocardial infarction,* or *schizophrenia* is a fundamental necessity of the research. Regardless of the particular taxonomic strategies used to define those diagnostic categories, the population under study will be homogeneous for each diagnosis provided that the diagnostic criteria are clearly expressed and scrupulously maintained.

Despite homogeneity in denomination for the diagnosed initial state, however, the members of a cohort may still be heterogeneous in various features that determine susceptibility to the event that is the target of observation in the subsequent state. For example, if we wanted to compare the effect of different treatments in patients with breast cancer, and if the target event were survival at 5 years, we would want the compared groups to be alike not merely in having breast cancer, but particularly in their anticipated 5-year survival rate. We might therefore divide the patients according to different stages, histologic types, or other features that might affect prognosis for survival.

Among the diverse initial features that can affect general susceptibilities to a target event in cohort research[5] are psychic status and genetic background for maneuvers that are causes of disease; and the comorbidity, duration, and severity of the underlying disease for maneuvers that are used therapeutically. In order to remove or reduce the effects of prognostic heterogeneity, the original cohort can be divided into subgroups, or strata, of members who are similar in their prognostic expectations. The results of the therapeutic or other maneuvers are then compared within members of the same prognostic stratum.

The division of cohort populations into prognostic strata that have different susceptibilities for the target event is a scientific necessity of clinical epidemiologic research. Such prognostic stratifications are performed when we try to discern baseline "risk factors" for the development of a future disease, when patients are divided into "stages" for appraising the treatment of cancer, or when the "clinical course" or "natural history" of a group of diseased people is analyzed in search of prognostic distinctions. Regardless of whether the maneuver under scrutiny is pathogenetic, prophylactic, or remedial, and regardless of whether the cohort is investigated with prolective planning or with retrolective assemblies of data, a prognostic stratification is needed to improve the scientific quality and validity of the research. The rest of this discussion is devoted to the goals and achievements of prognostic stratification.

A. Reason for prognostic stratification

Like any other activity in science, a prognostic stratification can be performed for reasons that are analytic, predictive, or explicative.

1. Analytic. The analysis of data in populational research can be distorted or impeded by disproportions in the strata that constitute a population, or by diverse effects of the same maneuver in different strata.

a. Avoidance of "false positive" results. Suppose we found that a group of 100 men with disease D had a 10-year survival rate of 38%, whereas the rate was 62% for a group of 100 women with the same disease. We might conclude that the disease had distinctly different effects in men and in women.

Now suppose, however, that patients with this disease could be divided into a "good risk" prognostic stratum, with 80% 10-year survival, and a "poor risk" stratum with 20% 10-year survival. Suppose further that the male population contained 30 members from the good-risk stratum and 70 members from the poor-risk stratum, but that these distributions were exactly reversed in the female population. We would then find the following results for 10-year survival rates:

	MEN	WOMEN	TOTAL
GOOD RISK	24/30 (80%)	56/70 (80%)	80/100 (80%)
POOR RISK	14/70 (20%)	6/30 (20%)	20/100 (20%)
TOTAL	38/100 (38%)	62/100 (62%)	100/200 (50%)

On comparing results within the same prognostic strata, we would find that the disease had exactly the same effects in men as in women: 80% survival for good risks, and 20% survival for poor risks. Our original conclusion about the disparate effects of the disease in men and women would have been wrong because of the disproportionate distribution of the good-risk and poor-risk strata in the male and female cohorts. The male cohort was composed of 70% poor risks and 30% good risks, whereas the percentages were just the opposite in the cohort of women.

One of the main reasons for prognostic stratification is to avoid this type of "false positive" error in analysis. The error arises when the "significant difference" found in the total results is caused entirely by differences in the proportions of prognostic strata that constitute the compared populations. In an earlier paper[5] of this series, I cited several other examples of this type of error, which can be identified only from scientific considerations of prognosis, and which cannot be detected with the conventional mathematical reasoning used for concepts of α and β "errors" in statistical tests.

This type of difficulty has long been familiar to epidemiologists, who have devised various types of "adjustments" to compensate for disproportions in the age groups that compose the general populations used for comparisons of mortality and other epidemiologic rates. Because age is a distinct prognostic factor for death in a general population, the rates of death must be considered for different strata of age. In the "direct adjustment" procedure, the death rate for each age stratum receives its "correction" when multiplied by the proportionate amount of that stratum that is found in a "standard population" selected from census data. The sum of the "corrected" products for each age stratum is added together to convert the "crude death rate" into an "age-adjusted death rate."

Because the adjusted rate will depend on the proportionate distribution of strata in the selected "standard population," epidemiologists have now begun to recognize[8] that this type of "adjusted" rate can be just as misleading as the original "crude" rate. As a substitute, epidemiologists have proposed[8] that the individual death rates of diverse populations be compared within individual age-strata, without being "corrected and added together to form a single "adjusted" value for each population. In clinical therapy, this hazard of the adjustment procedure does not occur because a "standard population" of diseased people cannot be readily chosen from general census data. Besides, the good-risk and poor-risk groups of a clinical population represent different conditions in the "experiments of nature"[2] and should be contemplated separately rather than being combined into an "adjusted rate."

b. Avoidance of "false negative" results. An alternative type of problem occurs when the prognostic strata are similarly distributed in the compared cohorts but are affected differently by the compared treatments. Suppose we found that three cohorts, each containing 100 people, achieved an identical improvement rate, 50%, when treated, respectively, with agents A, B, and placebo. We might conclude that neither A nor B differed from each other or from the placebo. We might feel particularly secure in this conclusion if we knew that the three cohorts had a similar proportionate composition of prognostic strata—

each cohort containing 50% good-risk and 50% poor-risk patients.

Our confidence in this conclusion might be quite wrong, however. If we examined the results of treatment within each stratum, we might find the following data for improvement rates:

	PLACEBO	TREAT- MENT A	TREAT- MENT B
GOOD RISK	35/50 (70%)	45/50 (90%)	25/50 (50%)
POOR RISK	15/50 (30%)	5/50 (10%)	25/50 (50%)
TOTAL	50/100 (50%)	50/100 (50%)	50/100 (50%)

We now see that treatments A and B had exactly opposite effects in the two strata. Treatment A had good results in the good-risk patients and poor results in the poor-risk patients, whereas treatment B was poor for the good risks, but good for the poor risks. Although the two treatments were distinctively different from placebo and from one another, the differences were counterbalanced and cancelled out when the results were appraised only for the total population, without regard to prognostic distinctions.

Another important role of prognostic stratification, therefore, is to avoid this type of "false negative" conclusion. Without the stratified analysis of data, we would have erroneously decided that neither treatment was effective. In fact, however, both treatments were significantly different from placebo and significantly efficacious—but in different prognostic strata.

c. To improve efficiency in comparison. An additional role for prognostic stratification is to increase the efficiency of comparison by identifying those members of a cohort who are extremely likely or unlikely to achieve the target event.

For example, if we wanted to test the potency of a contraceptive agent in women,

we would certainly want to exclude anyone who has no chance of becoming pregnant. In post-menopausal women or in those who have had hysterectomy, the contraceptive will invariably be associated with "successful" results (i.e., no pregnancies). If we were to include such "non-fecundable" women in the trial, we would waste the time of the investigators and subjects, and we would reduce the efficiency of the research. Similarly, if we wanted to test an agent that enhanced the opportunity for pregnancy in people who have been infertile, we would want to identify and exclude women who are clearly non-fecundable. Because the agent will invariably be unsuccessful in such women, their inclusion in the trial would be wasteful and inefficient.

For these reasons, an important role of prognostic stratification is to identify the *polar* strata that have either nadir or zenith rates in prognostic expectations. For a nadir stratum, the anticipated rate of the target event is 0% (or close to 0%); for a zenith stratum, the anticipated rate of the target event is 100% (or close to 100%). Whenever polar strata can be clearly demarcated, they should be segregated for separate analysis since their admixture in the total data will "dilute" the results and produce inefficient statistical comparisons.

Suppose we find, in a randomized trial, that treatment X was associated with poor results in 16/100 (16%) of the patients, and treatment Y with poor results in 9/100 (9%). We might like to conclude that treatment Y is better than X, but we cannot do so because our statistical consultant tells us that the difference is not "statistically significant" ($\chi^2 = 2.24$; P < .1). When we ask our statistical consultant what would have been needed to attain the cherished goal of "significance," he calculates that χ^2 would become 3.91 and the results would become "statistically significant" (P < .05) if the percentages of 16% and 9% remained the same and if there were 170 rather than 100 people in each treatment group. Since four years were required to assemble the

200 people who entered the just-completed trial, we would not be particularly happy about spending an additional seven years to perform a new trial with 340 patients. Nevertheless, since "statistical significance" is so compellingly desirable, we see no alternative to the further efforts with a larger population.

Suppose, however, that the patients with the condition under treatment could be divided into two prognostic strata. Stratum A is an "excellent risk" group with the nadir target rate of 0% for poor results. Stratum B is a "poor risk" group, having an expected target rate of 63% for poor results. When the population is stratified in this manner for our existing data, we find that treatments X and Y each received 80 members from stratum A and 20 members from stratum B.

The occurrence of a poor result in the clinical trial can then be tabulated as follows:

	TREAT-MENT X	TREAT-MENT Y	TOTAL
STRATUM A ("Excellent Risk")	0/80 (0%)	0/80 (0%)	0/160 (0%)
STRATUM B ("Poor Risk")	16/20 (80%)	9/20 (45%)	25/40 (63%)
TOTAL	16/100 (16%)	9/100 (9%)	25/200 (12%)

We thus find that treatments X and Y were equally effectual (or ineffectual) in stratum A because none of the "excellent risk" patients had a poor result. All of the poor results that were noted in this trial occurred for patients in stratum B, where the rate was 80% for treatment X and 45% for treatment Y. This difference in rates for stratum B is "statistically significant" ($\chi^2 = 5.23$; $P < .05$).

We have therefore discovered that there was no need to perform a new trial. We have already convincingly demonstrated the value of treatment Y, but we almost failed to recognize the demonstration because our original design was inefficient (when we included patients from stratum A), and because our original analysis was inefficient (when we failed to separate the two prognostic strata).

By performing the stratification, we found a statistically significant difference that was previously undetected. The difference had been obscured by inclusion of a large proportion of stratum A patients, none of whom was destined to achieve the target event of a "poor result." We went to all the effort of admitting and following these patients in the trial, although their only real contribution was to obfuscate the results.

One of the major values of *post hoc* stratification, therefore, is to ensure that the results of a clinical trial have not been confused by admixing the members of zenith or nadir strata with patients having non-polar rates of prognostic anticipation.

2. Predictive. In the procedures just cited, the purpose of stratification was to increase the accuracy and efficiency of statistical analysis. A different reason for prognostic stratification is to enhance confidence in the predictive decisions of clinical practice and to improve planning for future choices or trials of therapy.

a. To increase prognostic accuracy. The way a clinician makes a prognosis for a new patient is to recall the results in a group of previous patients who "resemble" the current patient. Thus, when a particular patient's prognosis is expressed in such terms as *good, hopeless,* or *30% chance of 5-year survival,* those were the outcomes observed in similar groups of patients in the past. These groups of patients represent the prognostic strata that have been demarcated by previous clinical experience.

The types of prognostic expressions just cited, however, represent the prediction for a group rather than for an individual patient. Thus, when we say *30% chance of 5-year survival,* we have not made an individual prediction. We refer to the characteristics of a group. Since a particular patient will either survive or not survive, a prediction for that patient would consist of prognosticating either *yes* or *no* for 5-year survival.

If the patient belonged to a stratum with a 50% survival rate, we would be uncertain about which choice to make. If the survival rate for his stratum was 70% or 30%, we would feel more confident about predicting in the corresponding direction; and the closer the survival rate approached 100% or 0% in either direction, the more confident we might feel about a definite prediction of *yes* or *no*. Another important role of a polar stratum, therefore, is the increased assurance that it brings to clinical prognostication. The prediction is particularly likely to be correct if the patient belongs to a zenith or a nadir stratum that is clearly defined and that contains a large enough number of people for the previous results to be numerically meaningful.

For example, if previous clinical experience in a large series of patients with acute myocardial infarction had shown that death occurred for all of the 87 people who had both shock and pulmonary edema, we would surely predict death for a new patient who manifested these phenomena. On the other hand, if 132 people with no complications of any type had all lived, we would confidently prognosticate survival when encountering such a new patient.

b. To allow therapeutic choices. A prognostic stratification is also the basis for most choices of therapy. When we use phrases such as *operable, inoperable, Grade 1 carcinoma, insulin-dependent diabetes mellitus,* or *mild impairment of renal function,* we have described groups of patients with properties that enable therapeutic decisions to be made on the basis of prognostic distinctions. The clinician makes these decisions for a new patient by first determining an appropriate clinical stratum for that patient. After recalling the results obtained with the different treatments previously applied to that stratum, the clinician chooses the treatment that appeared to give the best results.

c. To improve design of therapeutic trials. The original planning as well as the subsequent analysis of an experimental therapeutic trial would be improved if the population could initially be divided into distinctive prognostic strata, and if the tested treatments were randomly allocated within the strata. This prolective strategy can be used, however, only when a satisfactory stratification has already been created for the main target event of treatment in the trial. As discussed later, a *single* type of stratification could not be used in a trial with multiple, equally important target events because different target events usually require different prognostic stratifications. Consequently, when multiple targets are to be investigated, the best investigative plan is to allocate therapy randomly regardless of strata, and to perform the analytic stratifications afterward (using techniques to be described later).

d. To test special therapeutic claims. In certain special circumstances, a knowledge of polar strata can enable the claims of a new therapy to be investigated easily and promptly, using "historical controls" as the comparison group. These special circumstances arise when a heralded new "cure" —such as Krebiozen for cancer or Vitamin C for the common cold—has aroused great public interest in the absence of satisfactory evidence of efficacy.

Because such "cures" are often advocated without adequate supporting data and because a suitable therapeutic trial may require extensive investigative effort, most clinical scientists are reluctant to become involved in the attempt to confirm or refute the claims. On the other hand, the taxpaying public, which sponsors so much medical research and which expects occasional investigative efforts to answer questions of major public interest, may wonder why a test of the new "cure" cannot be included among the many other experiments supported by public funds. The clinical investigator may merely increase the public's antagonism to "research" if he pleads that the potential "cure" has been left untested because the supporting evidence is not good and because an adequate test would require too much work.

In being reluctant to perform such a trial, the investigator recognizes the statistical difficulty of demonstrating that something is *ineffective*. The "null hypothesis" in statistical reasoning enables us to test the likelihood that two treatments are different (i.e., that treatment X is better than placebo), but there is no "non-null hypothesis" for testing whether they are similar (i.e., that treatment X is no different from placebo). Thus, when "statistical significance" is not found for the difference between two treatments, we cannot conclude that the difference is "insignificant." We can only say, in the terms of the old Scottish verdict, that "significance" was not proved. Since any difference can become "statistically significant" if the tested population is large enough, and since the touted new "cure" may fortuitously give somewhat better results than a placebo, the proponent of the "cure" may then claim that his agent was not fairly tested, and that the difference might have been "significant" if only more people had been included in the trial.

The problem can best be illustrated with some direct clinical data. The expected 6-month survival rate among patients with "inoperable" lung cancer is about 30%. According to the formula* for calculating the "standard error" of a percentage, we would expect that rate to have a standard error of 8.4% if we treated 30 patients with inoperable lung cancer. According to the method† used for estimating the "95% confidence limits" for the range of the true rate, we would assume that the boundaries of the survival rate could vary by chance from 13.2% to 46.8%. Consequently, with 30 patients divided into 15 who enter a "placebo" group and 15 treated with Krebiozen, we might find by chance that 2

survive for 6 months in the placebo group and that 6 survive in the Krebiozen group. Although this difference could readily arise by chance, the proponent of Krebiozen would certainly contend that his agent had shown favorable results.

If we increased the total number of patients to 60, the standard error of the rate would be reduced to 5.9%, so that the boundaries of "chance" would be reduced to a range of 18.2% to 41.8%. Thus we might find, by chance, 6 survivors among 30 "controls" and 13 survivors among 30 patients treated with Krebiozen. The Krebiozen proponent would again claim superiority for his treatment, and (using the same publicity techniques that he used before) would expostulate that his 7 extra survivors mean more than any tests of "statistical significance."

We got into this difficulty because patients with "inoperable" lung cancer are so prognostically vague. On the average 30% of them will survive for 6 months, thus creating the wide range of chance that permits the cited problems to occur. Suppose, however, that within the spectrum of "inoperable" patients we could demarcate a nadir stratum whose expected survival rate for 6 months was 0% or certainly no higher than 3%. For a 0% survival group, the expected standard error in rate is also 0%; for a 3% survival group, the standard error in rate for 30 people would be 3.1%, so that the upper boundary of survival would be 3+ (2×3.1) = 9.2%. Thus, we would expect at most 2 or 3 people of the 30 to survive by chance. We might therefore, without a specific clinical trial, use the nadir stratum as a "historical control" method for "screening" the claims of Krebiozen. We would give it to 30 people in a nadir stratum. If more than three people survived, we would decide that the proponent of Krebiozen has potential merits to his claim, and we could then plan a full scale clinical trial. If no more than three survived, the Krebiozen has not provided a convincing demonstration of the claims offered for it.

---

*If p is the value of the percentage, the "standard error" is $\sqrt{(pq)/n}$, where q = 100%−p, and n = the size of the group.

†If s is the standard error, the "95% confidence limits" extend from p−2s to p+2s.

Thus, with a "screening" test of 30 patients carefully chosen from a nadir stratum that acts as a "historical control," we could obtain more effective evidence than might be available from a full-scale therapeutic trial involving 60 patients who were selected only because they had "inoperable" cancer. A carefully chosen scientific clinical design, involving a precisely delineated nadir stratum, would once again be preferable to the clinically naive methods with which general statistical theories have so often been applied in the treatment of cancer.

3. **Explicative.** The third major purpose of prognostic stratification is to demarcate observed phenomena in a manner that allows them to receive a scientific explication, or explanation, of their mechanisms. This explicative purpose is not achieved with the theoretical statistical strategies that have currently become popular in predictive correlations.

These strategies, which can be called *regressive*, depend on such statistical techniques as multiple linear regression and discriminant function analysis. With the regressive techniques, an array of co-efficients is calculated for the observed variates in the background population. The co-efficients then act as "weights" that multiply the values for each of the corresponding variates of a new patient. The weighted products are then added together to yield a single result that becomes the predicted value for that patient.

For example, let us begin with a collection of data that describe the initial state and subsequent outcome of a large series of patients with lung cancer. With regressive techniques of analysis, we can arrive at an equation in which the probability of a patient's survival at 6 months might be expressed as $(0.063 \times \text{sex}) - (0.071 \times \text{age}) - (1.62 \times \text{size of tumor}) - (6.7 \times \text{degree of anatomic spread}) + \ldots$, etc. In contrast, with a stratification procedure, we would arrive at a designation of a group, such as Stage D, with a discrete set of characteristics such as *large, metastatic cancer* for which the 6-month survival rate is 20%.

The scientific disadvantages of regressive techniques of prediction have been discussed elsewhere[11] in clinical literature. A particularly cogent discussion of defects was presented in the statistical literature by Morgan and Sonquist.[11A]

One major flaw of the regressive strategy is its linearity. This type of statistical analysis is based on the addition of weighted values for isolated (linear) variates; it does not find the conjunctions of important biologic properties that define a group, such as Stage D. Instead of routinely examining the prognostic importance of such combinations as the properties cited in *tall old men*, the regressive analytic technique produces a separate numerical value for height, for age, and for sex, and adds these values together. In order to determine whether the simultaneous occurrence of *tall, old,* and *male* might be a prognostically significant conjunction of properties, some other procedure would have to be used to recognize the need for examining the conjunction. After it had been identified as important, the concurrence of *tall, old,* and *male* could then be entered into the statistical computations as though the three simultaneous characteristics were a separate "linear variable," but the co-existence of these attributes as an important combination could not be detected with ordinary activities* of multiple linear regression or discriminant function analysis.

A second flaw of the conventional statistical procedures is that the weighted linear addition is not based empirically on direct past experience. By suitable multiplications and additions of the appropriate statistical numbers, we might obtain a prognostic estimation for *short old men* or for *pregnant adolescent girls* even though no such patients had ever been observed in the population from which the statistical co-efficients were derived. Thus, because the population contained people of diverse heights, ages, sex, and pregnancy status, co-efficients could be calculated to allow prognostic predictions for short old men despite the absence of such men in the investigated population, and for pregnant adolescent girls even though the only observed pregnancies had occurred in older women. The regression model would be sufficiently ethereal and "imaginative" to be able to provide a prognosis even for pregnant men. In contrast, the stratification procedure makes its predictions only on the basis of the specific types of patients that were previously observed.

A third defect of the regressive techniques is the occasional production of major computational

---

*The regressive procedures can be specially programmed to examine every possible conjunction (or "interaction") of the variates, but the computation becomes horrendous if many variates are involved. For 30 variates, 2^{30} combinations must be appraised.

pecularities. Because the co-efficients emerge from prolonged "number-crunching" with complex matrix algebra, the results may sometimes seem bizarre. For example, in the multiple regression equation developed to predict the likelihood of a patient's death in the celebrated UGDP study,[14] the co-efficient for diastolic blood pressure emerged with a negative value. The implication is that the *lower* the blood pressure, the greater the likelihood of death. Because everything must be expressed in numerical forms, the regressive procedures often perform calculations of uncertain validity to provide co-efficients of uncertain meaning for numbers of unmeasurable dimension. This difficulty arises whenever a variate in the regression computations contains attributes such as nominal data (sex, occupation), existential data (presence or absence of chest pain), and ordinal data (stages of cancer). Another difficulty is the non-reproducibility of the calculations. The co-efficients that are produced by the computations will vary considerably according to the choice of certain arbitrary "parameters," the absence or presence of a "step-wise" procedure, and the upward or downward direction of the "steps." Finally, because the straightforward regression procedure often produces results— such as a negative probability of survival or probabilities greater than one—that are impossible for individual patients, certain arbitrary transformations have been necessary. The most popular of these, which is called the *logistic* transformation, adds increasing complexity and further computational increments of uncertain scientific validity to the basic procedure.

A fourth problem of the regressive tactics is intellectual. Most scientific investigators have difficulty enough in comprehending the theoretical aspects of relatively simple statistical procedures, but the regressive strategies are inscrutable. I have yet to encounter a clinical investigator (including myself) who fully understands all the nuances of the variance-covariance matrices, multivariate normality, and other theoretical assumptions of the computations. I have yet to encounter a statistician who could give a clear, crisp, scientifically meaningful account of the techniques. I have yet to find a statistical textbook or paper that gave a readable outline of the proceedings together with adequate illustrative data taken from clinical reality. The consequence of all this adumbration is that clinical epidemiologic investigators make use of regressive techniques without having the foggiest idea of how the procedures work and what they accomplish. The statistician tells the investigator to do a regressive analysis. The computer crunches the numbers. The investigator writes his paper. The editor accepts it for publication. The ultimate outcome is that the people who know what the results mean can not articulate them, whereas the people who might articulate the meaning do not know what it is.

Regardless of mathematical meaning and validity, however, the greatest and most overwhelming scientific flaw of the regressive procedures is that they do not produce strata. They create an array of additive numerical co-efficients. There is no specification of the particular properties that demarcate a group of people. When biologic scientists observe natural phenomena and attempt to explain those phenomena, however, the explanation begins with an observed discrete characteristic or a selected group of discrete characteristics. It does not begin with an additive array of numbers.

We first note that certain red blood cells become deformed into a sickle shape; and we then try to explain the mechanism of deformation. We first note the existence of a certain type of pulmonary abnormality called *pneumonia;* and we then look for microbial causes. We first note among patients with localized cancer that survival rates are better after a long duration of primary symptoms than after a short duration; and we then recognize the duration of symptoms as a manifestation of the cancer's rate of growth.[4] In all of these circumstances, the scientific search for explanation began with a phenomenon that had been noted in a demarcated group of entities, and that was characterized in a selective, discrete manner. We did not begin with an array of multiplicative co-efficients for values of hemoglobin, white blood count, bacterial colonies, roentgenographic density, and chronometric duration.

No matter how successful the regression or discriminant function procedures might be when used for analytic appraisals or when tested for predictive accuracy, the procedures cannot overcome their insurmountable defects for scientific explication. Since these statistical techniques do not demarcate the discrete characteristics of groups, the results are unsatisfactory for the type of scientific thinking that is used either in clinical denomination or in pathogenetic explanation.

Because of these inadequacies and because the massive, elaborate calculations are too oppressive to be frequently performed by hand or with a desk calculator, the regression and discriminant function procedures could have been expected to atrophy, like the investigation of "moments" around the mean, into interesting but impractical vestiges of statistical theory. With the advent of computers, however, the calculations could be performed easily and promptly; and with the general dissemination of "canned" computer programs, the procedures have become ubiquitously available, even for "users" who know nothing about the principles or assumptions that underlie the statistical strategy. Consequently, these tactics have become widely employed during the past few years, particularly when multiple variables are to be analyzed for predictive correlations with a target event.

Scientists who derive creative stimuli from real world data and concepts, however, have already begun to develop alternative approaches for using computers to improve, rather than merely automate, a defective status quo. Although most perceptive investigators can identify important prognostic properties without the need for automated analysis of data, a computer might be quite helpful in detecting features that have been overlooked. For the new techniques[1, 10-12] of data analysis, the computer expresses its results in the form of prognostic strata rather than regressive or discriminant co-efficients. Like the older procedures, these new approaches are phenetic in performance, because all the available data are investigated, but unlike the regressive tactics, the new techniques are phyletic in conclusion. They demarcate a selected group of properties that are distinct harbingers of prognosis. Developed by sociologic and clinical investigators, rather than by statisticians, the new techniques are still in their early stages of growth. The further improvement and implementation of these automated procedures for prognostic stratification offers a major creative challenge in modern data analysis, and a

further opportunity to use computers as a way of removing, rather than embellishing, the intellectual shackles of the past.

B. Preparation for prognostic stratification

After recognizing the importance of performing prognostic stratification, the investigator can begin to assemble the necessary scientific information and attitudes.

1. The population and data. The performance of a prognostic stratification (or, for that matter, of a regressive analysis), requires the availability of appropriate data from an appropriate population. The population is appropriate if it consists of an inception cohort,[6] in which the "baseline" condition (or "initial state") for each member is determined at zero time when the investigated maneuver was imposed. The data are appropriate if they contain an adequate description of the initial state and of a selected target event (such as *improvement of symptoms, development of coronary artery disease,* or *survival at 5 years*) that has been chosen as the focus for the prognostic stratification.

The goal of the stratification is to find the characteristics of the population's initial state that predictively correlate with the subsequent occurrence of the target event. The presence or absence of the cited characteristics, appearing alone or in various combinations, will demarcate strata (or groups) of people with distinctly different prognoses for the target event.

2. Choice of the target event. No population can be divided uniquely into a simple set of prognostic strata, because each target event that is under surveillance will require a separate prognostic stratification. Suppose we consider a population of people with acute myocardial infarction. The features that determine survival at one month are different from those that determine the persistence or disappearance of chest pain. The latter features will differ from those that determine the patient's subsequent susceptibility to pregnancy or satisfaction with the received medical care. Each of these different target events—one-month survival, persistence of chest pain, occurrence of pregnancy, and "consumer satisfaction"—would require a different stratification to list the particular characteristics that would prognosticate the likelihood or unlikelihood of the target's occurrence.

For this reason, a prognostic stratification often cannot be performed *before* a therapeutic trial begins. If the investigators have established a single target event as the major focus for the trial, a single stratification can be created for that target, and the therapy can be allocated randomly within those strata. But if equally important, multiple target events are to be evaluated, a single stratification is impossible. Even if adequate previous data were available to allow the several stratifications to be determined beforehand, the investigator still would not know which stratification to use when allocating treatment. In such circumstances, the randomization would be assigned without pre-stratification, and the stratified analysis would take place afterward.

In general, since no investigator can be certain in advance of all the targets he may want to analyze later, the best approach is to assemble suitable data with which a variety of stratifications can be performed *post hoc* after the trial is completed.

3. Establishment of the "nil hypothesis." In ideal circumstances, the analysis of prognosis would be limited to a "natural-history" population, whose members have received no therapeutic or other specific maneuvers that would intervene in the natural course of whatever condition is under investigation. These ideal circumstances cannot occur in the realities of clinical medicine. There never has been and never will be a true "natural-history" population.

Every person, sick or well, is constantly exposed to diverse stimuli that intervene in the course of daily life. Beyond the exposure to the particular maneuver under investigation, a person's family background,

occupation, place of residence, hobbies, habits, psychic state, and interaction with other people may affect the course of either health or disease. Even if deliberately assigned to "no treatment" or to a "placebo," in the hope of allowing "natural history" to occur, a patient is still exposed to the iatrotherapy provided by the personal interchange with a physician, and may still receive many other modes of pharmaceutical or non-pharmaceutical therapy for concomitant problems that may be transient or chronic.

The strategy of scientific investigation is to assume that certain interventions may be more potent than others in achieving (or preventing) the target event, but none of the many possible interventions that remain untested can be summarily dismissed as failing to influence "natural history." In clinical trials and surveys, we can therefore compare one specific form of treatment with another and (if everything else is equal) we can draw conclusions about their relative merits. But neither the intervention of a particular treatment nor its absence can guarantee that the investigated condition has evolved in a pattern of "natural history."

Scientists and statisticians engage in an act of self-delusion if they believe that the "natural history" of human ailments can be studied at all, and that the investigation should be restricted to an "untreated" or "placebo-control" group. This belief may have been valid for the agricultural plots, brewery vats, and fruit flies that were used as a basis for current theories of "biometry," but the belief is not true for a free-living human population. The first step of intellectual liberation for scientists who want to investigate prognosis, therefore, is to recognize that we can study a *clinical course*,[3] but not a *natural history*.

Once this liberation has occurred, the investigator can proceed to examine the clinical course for the combined population of the entire cohort, regardless of the therapeutic or other maneuvers to which the individual members may have been exposed. We thus form a "nil hypothesis,"* making the assumption that none of the interventional maneuvers have affected the clinical course. In the combined population, we then search for the initial state characteristics that demarcate prognostic strata. Having established those strata in an "unbiased" manner, without regard to therapy, we can then later examine (if we wish) the effects of therapy within each of the prognostic strata.

Our primary activity, however, was to find the prognostic strata for the initial state of the entire population, not for selected groups who had received specific modes of treatment. If certain factors are harbingers of prognosis before any therapeutic maneuvers are imposed, those factors should be discerned from the patient's state before treatment. Furthermore, by combining all the diversely treated patients into a single population, we can attain large numbers that can later be partitioned into smaller numbers of people with the different characteristics and combinations of characteristics for which the target event is correlated during the stratification process. If the analysis of prognosis is applied only within groups of people who received the "same" interventional maneuver, the available numbers within each group will be relatively small, and the opportunity to discern meaningful prognostic characteristics may be lost.

This type of therapeutic *nil hypothesis* is, of course, the reasoning that thoughtful clinicians have always used for making prognostic judgments. The decisions that a patient was a "good risk" or a "poor risk," that he was moribund or destined to recover, and that a situation was hopeless have traditionally been based on the total clinical spectrum and outcome of the observed condition, regardless of therapy. The intervention of therapy has been intended either to alter the anticipated outcome, or

to alter certain events that might accompany the anticipated outcome.

In many contemporary analyses of "risk factors" or other prognostic characteristics, however, the importance of the "nil hypothesis" has been neglected. The search for risk factors has been conducted not within the total population under surveillance, but within the groups exposed to similar interventions. What then emerges is a logical inconsistency: To demarcate a general characteristic that is independent of treatment, we examine the data of a selected group of people who received a specific form of treatment. This intellectual malady has been particularly rampant in certain statistically analyzed clinical trials, particularly when multiple linear regression was used as the method of searching for "risk factors" with each form of treatment.

4. Avoidance of statistical shibboleths about "retrospection." In order to discern either the strata of prognostic properties or the co-efficients of weighted regression, we must have data that describe the initial state of a cohort population and data that describe the subsequent target events. Such data are available only after the target events have occurred, and the analysis can be performed only in the "past tense," retrolectively. The data under investigation can be obtained from routine medical records or from a pre-planned research study, but the analysis of prognostic determinants cannot begin until the target events have had the opportunity to appear.

According to certain statistical ideologies about "experimental design," however, such *post hoc* analyses of data should be avoided. The statistical ideologists would permit us to appraise only the information that was organized according to a pre-designed plan of evaluation. The term "retrospective" has often been used (improperly, for reasons discussed elsewhere⁶) as a pejorative label that serves to discourage the *post hoc* appraisal of scientific data.

Clinical and epidemiologic investigators who follow advice from proponents of this

---

*The term *therapeutic nihilism* is often used for the assumption that treatment has not accomplished anything. The *nil* here is a contraction of *nihil*.

statistical doctrine are left unable to evaluate the past or to plan the future. In the absence of suitable retrolective analyses, the investigator can discern neither the prognostic strata needed for proper design of future prolective research, nor the particular types of data needed for suitable analysis after a prolective project has been completed. Lacking the information and instructions obtainable only from suitable retrolective studies, the investigators in a prolective project may discover, after concluding an elaborate, expensive, statistically designed, computer-monitored experimental trial, that they failed to collect large amounts of the fundamental evidence needed for a valid prognostic stratification.

An intellectual liberation for this shibboleth of statistical ideology has been offered by Tukey's[13] proposal of the term *data analysis* (rather than *statistical analysis*) to describe the necessary thoughts and goals of these scientific activities. With this orientation, we can proceed at our next meeting to consider the specific techniques used to achieve and evaluate a prognostic stratification.

References

1. Andrews, F. M., Morgan, J. N., and Sonquist, J. A.: Multiple classification analysis: A report on a computer program for multiple regression using categorical predictors, Ann Arbor, Mich., May, 1967, Survey Research Center, Institute for Social Research, University of Michigan.
2. Feinstein, A. R.: Clinical epidemiology. I. The populational experiments of nature and of man in human illness, Ann. Intern. Med. **69:**807-820, 1968.
3. Feinstein, A. R., Pritchett, J. A., and Schimpff, C. R.: The epidemiology of cancer therapy. II. The clinical course: Data, decisions, and temporal demarcations, Arch. Intern. Med. **123:**323-344, 1969.
4. Feinstein, A. R.: A clinical method for estimating the rate of growth of a cancer, Yale J. Biol. Med. **41:**422-433, 1969.
5. Feinstein, A. R.: Clinical biostatistics. X. Sources of 'transition bias' in cohort statistics, CLIN. PHARMACOL. THER. **12:**704-721, 1971.
6. Feinstein, A. R.: Clinical biostatistics. XI. Sources of 'chronology bias' in cohort statistics, CLIN. PHARMACOL. THER. **12:**864-879, 1971.
7. Feinstein, A. R.: Clinical biostatistics. XIII. On homogeneity, taxonomy, and nosography, CLIN. PHARMACOL. THER. **13:**114-129, 1972.
8. Fox, J. P., Hall, C. E., and Elveback, L. R.: Epidemiology. Man and disease, Toronto, 1970, The Macmillan Company.
9. Kempthorne, O.: The randomization theory of experimental inference, J. Am. Statist. Assoc. **50:**946-967, 1955.
10. Klein, D. F., Honigfield, G., and Feldman, S.: Prediction of drug effect by a successive screening decision tree diagnostic technique, *in* May, P., and Wittenborn, J., editors: Psychotropic drug response, Springfield, Ill., 1969, Charles C Thomas, Publisher.
11. Koss, N., and Feinstein, A. R.: Computer-aided prognosis. II. Development of a prognostic algorithm, Arch. Intern. Med. **127:**448-458, 1971.
11A. Morgan, J. N., and Sonquist, J. A.: Problems in the analysis of survery data, and a proposal, J. Am. Statist. Assoc. **58:**415-435, 1963.
12. Sonquist, J. A., and Morgan, J. N.: The detection of interaction effects: A report on a computer program for the selection of optimal combinations of explanatory variables. Monograph No. 35, Ann Arbor, Mich., 1964, Survey Research Center, Institute for Social Research, University of Michigan.
13. Tukey, J. W.: The future of data analysis, Ann. Math. Statist. **33:**1-67, 1962.
14. University Group Diabetes Program: A study of the effects of hypoglycemic agents on vascular complications in patients with adult-onset diabetes. Part I: Design, methods and baseline characteristics. Part II: Mortality results, Diabetes **19:** (Suppl. 2) 747-830, 1970.

CHAPTER 27

The process of prognostic stratification

As noted in the previous paper of this series,[6] the purposes of prognostic stratification are to improve the efficiency of research design and data analysis, to enhance confidence in prediction, and to demarcate phenomena for scientific explication. Without such stratifications, erroneous or distorted results will continue to be produced when conventional statistical "models" are applied to the data of medical cohorts. The statistical "models" are based on the analysis of response to the maneuver of a single experiment, but in most medical forms of cohort research, the investigator observes the results of a double experiment[2]: a maneuver arranged by man is imposed on the response to a previous maneuver arranged in essence by nature.

The different forms taken by those double maneuvers were outlined earlier[3] in this series of papers. In ontogenetic phenomena, nature's maneuvers provide a person with certain biologic capacities for growth and development; and man's maneuvers provide the environmental, nutritional, or other agents that may alter those natural events. In pathogenetic phenomena, nature's maneuvers provide a person with certain biologic qualities (in age, ancestry, psychic status,

etc.) that may affect susceptibility to disease; and man's maneuvers expose that person to the urban fumes, dietary indiscretions, infectious organisms, traumatic events, and other agents that may cause disease.

In the interventions with which doctors try to change nature's pathway, the imposed maneuvers can be remedial, contrapathic, or contratrophic. In remedial interventions, nature's maneuvers have created a diseased person with overt manifestations that are destined to evolve in a particular pattern; and the physician's maneuvers consist of treatment intended to alter the pattern. In the contrapathic form of prophylactic intervention, the maneuvers of nature or of man (or both) have produced people with different degrees of susceptibility to a particular disease and with different degrees of exposure to its cause(s). The physician's maneuvers consist of sanitation, vaccination, dietary changes, physical activities, or other efforts intended to thwart the development of the disease. In the contratrophic form of prophylactic intervention, nature's maneuvers have created a patient with an established disease that may become worse as it continues its clinical course; and the physician's maneuvers consist of various therapeutic tactics intended to keep the untoward events from happening. (Examples of contratrophic therapy are the use of anticoagulants to prevent thromboembolic phenomena after myocardial infarction, and glucose regulation to prevent vascular complications in patients with diabetes mellitus.)

Because traditional statistical models are based only on one type of "experimental" maneuver, rather than two, the activities

This chapter originally appeared as "Clinical biostatistics—XV. The process of prognostic stratification (Part I)." In Clin. Pharmacol. Ther. 13:442, 1972.

of man have received predominant and often exclusive attention in most statistical reports of cohort research. The underlying "experimental maneuvers" of nature have generally been neglected. The effects of nutrition on neonatal growth are frequently reported without regard to the infant's genetic or constitutional capacities for growth. The effects of smoking or high fat diets on longevity are studied without regard to the person's familial background, psychic status, or other features that may affect longevity. The results of remedial therapy may be cited without regard to the duration, severity, and other associated features that might affect the natural outcome of the treated manifestation. The results of contratrophic therapy may be cited without regard to the initial clinical severity and co-morbidity that can alter the natural course of future events for the disease under treatment.

Only in the past few years have clinical epidemiologic investigators begun to recognize the need for identifying the basic natural phenomena upon which the maneuvers of man are imposed. The scientific attempt to discern the face of nature beneath the maneuveral masks of man has been approached under several different names. Oncologists have developed "staging systems" to grade the prognostic severity of patients with cancer. Epidemiologists have searched for "risk factors" that might indicate increased susceptibility to developing certain diseases. Other clinical investigators have tried to find the various characteristics that would identify patients who were "good risks" or "bad risks" for the outcome of such diseases as myocardial infarction and ulcerative colitis.

The different groups of patients demarcated by these prognostic classifications represent "strata" of people in whom nature has performed different maneuvers. Since a cohort contains various proportions of these strata, the results of the maneuver to which a cohort is exposed will greatly depend on the proportionate distribu-

tion of the strata. Unless the different strata and their quantitative proportions are suitably identified and analyzed, major sources of bias[4] can enter the data of cohort research. The compared maneuvers may appear to give different results; but the real difference may arise only from disproportions in the strata that constitute the cohort.

A previous paper[4] of this series was concerned with the quantitative effects of the bias produced by those disproportions in strata. Our concern now is with the strata themselves. By what methods does an investigator search for them? How does he know when he has found them? How can he tell whether the arrangement he finds is worse or better than some other arrangement? In this paper and the one that follows it, we shall consider the process with which a prognostic stratification is created and evaluated.

A. Arrangement of data

The pre-requisite data for a prognostic stratification contain an account of the initial state and the subsequent occurrence (or non-occurrence) of a selected target event for each member of a cohort. The data are expressed as a series of individual values for different characteristics (sometimes called *properties* or *variables*) that will here be called *variates*. Thus, for a particular patient, the variate *sex* may have the nominal value, **male**; the variate *existence of chest pain* may have the existential value, **present**; the variate *loudness of systolic murmur* may have the ordinal value, **Grade 4**; and the variate *age* may have the metric[*] value **65 years**.

1. The target variate. Because a stratification refers to a particular target event, the target variate is usually expressed in an all-or-none form, such as **improved** or **not improved**, and **alive** or **dead**. The results of the stratification are expressed as rates (or percentages) with which

---

[*]The term *metric* is here used for data that are also called *dimensional, continuous,* or *interval*.

the target event did or did not occur in specified groups of the cohort.

2. *The predictor variates.* The variates that describe the initial state are called *predictor variates* when examined in relation to the target event. Since a stratification is based on categories, these predictor variates must be cited in categorical values. Nominal, existential, and ordinal variates are expressed categorically and need no alterations, but metric variates must be re-expressed in ordinal groups. Thus, the metric values for age might be converted to such ordinal categories as **newborn, young, middle-aged,** and **old.**

3. *Partition of a variate.* The particular array of categories in which a variate can be expressed is called a *partition*. A partition contains at least two categories, and in clinical research, rarely more than ten. The categories of the partition must be mutually exclusive, so that an individual person's value for that variate can be cited in only one of the categories. Thus, the partition for the nominal variate *sex* would usually have the categories **male and female.** To cover the scope of medical data, the values of **unknown** (for missing data) and **uncertain** (for equivocal or ambiguous data) may be included as categories of a partition.

The people who possess each of the categorical values cited in a partition form a group, or *stratum,* of the corresponding population. When the rates for the target events in that population are associated with each of the strata, the result is called a *prognostic stratification.*

4. *Composition of variates.* Before the stratification process begins, each predictor variate is expressed in univariate categories, based on the particular single feature that was characteristic of that variate. These single features may be simple or compound. A single variate is called simple if its values are based on elements from only one type of data. Such variates as *age* and *sex* are simple. Variates such as *size of heart* and *existence of rheumatic valvular murmur* are also simple if their

values are determined directly from roentgenography or auscultation, respectively. A single variate is called compound if it contains elements from more than one type of data. For example, the variate *physical complexion* is compound because it usually depends on such constituent features as color of skin, color of hair, and color of eyes.

To create compound variates, a set of operational rules or criteria must be established to specify the pattern in which the combined elements are demarcated. Thus, by establishing appropriate criteria in patients with acute rheumatic fever, we can form a compound variate, called *severity of carditis,* that is expressed in such categories as **none, possible, mild, moderate,** and **severe.** The criteria for assignment of these categories would depend on the values found in such simple variates as *existence of rheumatic valvular murmur* and *size of heart.* When appropriate criteria have been established, such categories as **Stage I, Stage II, Stage III,** and **Stage IV** would constitute a compound variate for patients with cancer.

5. *Criteria of gradation.* Regardless of whether a variate is simple or compound, its scientific usage requires suitable *gradation criteria* for the ranked categories. (Analogous criteria are required if the categories are nominal or existential, rather than ordinal.) For example, suppose the variate *age* was partitioned as **young, middle-aged,** and **old** without indications of the boundaries that demarcate these groups; or suppose *functional status* was partitioned into categories of **excellent, good, fair,** and **poor** that were not further described. The investigators who originally applied these ratings, and any other investigators who want to repeat the work in the future, could not achieve either consistency or reproducibility.

To be satisfactory, a complete set of "gradation criteria" must contain at least three distinct types of specification: a list of the elements that are included; a citation of the observational evidence required to designate each element; and a pattern of demarcation for the elements. For example, in an anatomic staging system for cancer of the breast, **lymphadenopathy** and **fixation** might be cited as elements in the staging. Designation criteria would be necessary to indicate the particular kinds of evidence (in size, shape, texture, etc., of lymph nodes and in physical mobility of the breast) that would be regarded as **lymphadenopathy** or **fixation.** Finally, as part of the "demarcation criteria," lymphadenopathy and fixation would each be assigned a ranked location such as **Stage II, Stage IV,** etc.

If a variate is simple and metric, such as *age,* the formation of gradation criteria is easy. The designation criteria would indicate the method of expressing age (measured from most recent birthday, nearest birthday, etc.) and the demarcation criteria would indicate the boundaries that might delineate **young** as 0-35 years, **middle-aged** as 36-60 years, etc. The criteria are more difficult and complex when the categories contain subjectively graded ranks—such as **excellent, mild, worse,** or **Grade 3**—and particularly when the ranks represent categories of a compound variate. Despite the obvious necessity for scientific reproducibility of research methods, such criteria are often omitted in whole or in part from published reports. A report may contain no gradation criteria of any type; or may include designation criteria without demarcation criteria (or vice versa); or the cited designation and demarcation criteria may be incomplete or inadequate.

6. *Alteration of a partition.* Since the categories of partition were chosen before the associated target events were noted, the investigator may want to alter the partition after the stratified results are examined. The two basic forms of alteration—elimination or refinement—can be accomplished in at least four different ways: consolidating, expanding, re-arranging, and conjoining.

a. Consolidation. Two or more strata that are individually undesirable can be eliminated by the process of consolidation. The several strata are combined to form a single stratum. Thus, the two groups **21-30** and **31-40** in an age partition might be consolidated to form a single group **21-40.** Such consolidations are usually performed if the strata contain too few members or not enough distinction to warrant retention of the individual categories. As discussed later, the number of members is "too few" if below an established minimal value, and the strata lack "distinction" if the difference in their target rates is too small to be important biologically or statistically.

Several combinations can occur during a single act of consolidation. Thus, if *age* has been partitioned into the ten categories **0-10, 11-20, 21-30, . . . , 91 and older**, a consolidation might create a new partition of four categories **0-30, 31-50, 51-70,** and **71 and older.** Although most consolidations will combine categories that are adjacent neighbors in an ordinal partition, the extreme categories can sometimes be combined for contrast with those in the center. Thus, the age group **0-20** and **71 and older** might be joined to form a new category called **extremes of age,** and the remaining groups **21-70** might be called **middle** or **other** age groups. Such consolidated arrangements of ends versus middles are often prompted by finding that the target rate shows a high-low-high or low-high-low pattern that produces similar rates at the extremes of the partition.

b. Expansion. The expansion of a partition is the reverse of a consolidation. The categories are "refined" by additional demarcations that divide an original category into two or more new categories. Thus the four-category age partition that was cited earlier (**0-30, . . . , 71 and older**) could be expanded into six categories (**0-10, 11-30, . . . , 71-80, 81 and older**) or into eight categories (**0-1, 2-10, 11-20, 21-30, . . . , 71-80, 81 and older**), or even more.

c. Re-arrangement. A partition is rearranged if the constituent elements received different demarcations while the number of categories remains unchanged. Thus, the cited four-category partition of age might be re-arranged as **pre-pubertal** (0-12 years), **adolescent** (13-20), **younger adults** (21-50), and **older adults** (51 and older). The process of re-arrangement, which consists of both elimination and refinement, is usually employed to strengthen a stratification's biologic or numerical distinction, as described later.

d. Conjunction. In all of the three alterations just described, the partition remained univariate. We changed it by changing the demarcation boundaries of the original constituents in its single variate. In the fourth type of alteration, we refine a partition by introducing additional categories from a different variate. Thus, the **male** and **female** categories of the variate *sex* could be conjoined with the foregoing four-category partition of *age* to form an eight-category bi-variate partition: **prepubertal female**, **prepubertal male**, **adolescent female**, **adolescent male**, and so on.

In the example just cited, we performed a *complete* conjunction of the partitions for the two variates. Since the two partitions contained four and two categories, respectively, the complete conjunction contained eight categories. Because an undesirably large number of categories may be created, some or many of the strata in a complete bi-variate conjunction are often consolidated. The consolidation, performed with techniques to be described later, produces a new variate with its own partition of composite categories. These bi-variate categories can subsequently be conjoined with additional variates if desired.

Alternatively, conjunctions may be performed in an isolated manner, by combining only selected single categories from two or more variates, without producing and examining the complete conjunction of partitions. In the example just cited, we might have left the first three age groups unchanged as **prepubertal**, **adolescent**, and **young adult**, but the **older adult** category could have been conjunctively divided into **older man** and **older woman**. In another arrangement, we might have divided the population into **adolescent boys, old women**, and **all others**.

B. Basic procedures in stratification

7. Formation of clusters. The conjunctions just described produced multivariate refinements of the basic categories of a univariate partition. Multivariate categories can also be formed as *clusters*, consisting of aggregates or unions. An *aggregate* is a combination of groups that are mutually exclusive, without overlapping membership. We can form an aggregate category called **young boys or old women** by combining the two categories **young boys** and **old women.** A *union* is a combination of groups that may have overlapping membership. The union of **old** and **male**, which is expressed as **old and/or male**, includes people who are old or male or both. The union would thus contain the aggregate of **old but not male, male but not old,** and **old male.**

This type of clustering has regularly been used for the categories combined in staging systems for cancer. Thus, **Stage IV** in certain classifications of breast cancer may include patients who have one or more of the following manifestations: fixation to chest wall, satellite skin nodules, supraclavicular metastasis, axillary fixation, or distant metastasis. The cluster technique is also used to consolidate the categories formed when two partitions are conjoined, as described in the preceding section. For example, if *age* were partitioned as **child, adolescent** and **adult,** and *sex* as **male** and **female,** the conjunction of these two partitions would create six bi-variate categories. The bi-variate partition could be reduced to four categories by forming the two clusters of **male or female children** and **male or female adolescents** while preserving **adult males** and **adult females.**

Since a stratification can be inspected for each of the many predictor variates that can be associated with the target event in a cohort population, the stratification process is intended not merely to examine the diverse partitions of predictor variates but particularly to find an optimal partition among the many that can be noted or created. The readily noted stratifications are produced by the original partitions of the individual predictor variates. The created stratifications are produced by alteration of those variates, and particularly by the combinations that join two or more variates into a *multivariate* partition. Thus, the categories contained in an anatomic staging and a symptomatic staging for cancer are each univariate partitions, but a conjunction of the two types of stages, forming a symptomatic-anatomic staging system,[1] would be a multivariate stratification. The categories formed in such deliberate combinations are obviously compound, and they can be called *composite* to denote their formation during the process of stratification rather than beforehand.

The stratification process will require decisions about optimity (to choose whether one partition is better than another) and decisions about alteration (to choose when and how a particular partition should be changed). The choice of optimity is illustrated in the following example:

Suppose a cohort contains 300 members of whom 150 (50%) have achieved the target event of survival at some specified serial duration. The predictor variates A and B have the respective categories a_1, a_2, a_3 and b_1, b_2, b_3. When we stratify the population for these two variates, we note the following results for survival rates in the partition for A:

a_1: 52/100 (52%)
a_2: 50/100 (50%)
a_3: 48/100 (48%)

The results in the stratification for B are:

b_1: 60/80 (75%)
b_2: 70/140 (50%)
b_3: 20/80 (25%)

Comparison of these two stratifications of data for the same population indicates that partition B is obviously better than partition A.

In the situation just cited, the superiority of one of the two partitions was readily apparent. In many other circumstances, however, the comparative merits of a particular pair of partitions may not be so clear. We shall therefore need some standards of judgment to decide what is a *good* partition, and what makes one partition *better* than another. The standards should also deal with decisions about eliminating or refining the strata of a particular partition.

The rest of this paper is concerned with the development of such standards. Some of the standards are purely qualitative, reflecting scientific concepts of biology that cannot be described numerically. Other standards will be arbitrarily quantitative, reflecting scientific ideas that can be expressed numerically, but that cannot be appraised with statistical tests of "inference." A third type of standard can be described in statistical terms, and appraised with concepts of "statistical significance."

A partition becomes "evaluated" when it is assessed according to these standards. Because a partition consists of a series of individual strata, the standards must provide methods for evaluating at least three functional components of the partition: the individual strata, the relationships among adjacent strata, and the accomplishments of the partition as a whole.

C. The evaluation of an individual stratum

A stratum is demarcated qualitatively by the taxonomic characteristics that define its members. These characteristics can be expressed in verbal terms (such as **men with chest pain**) or in numbers (such as **age 40-65**) or in both. The stratum is described quantitatively by the number of members it contains, and by the associated target rate. If the i-th stratum of a partition contains n_i members of whom t_i achieved the target event, the target rate is $p_i = t_i/n_i$. For the number of members, d_i who do not achieve the target event, the complementary "non-target rate" is $q_i = d_i/n_i$. According to the definition of these terms, $n_i = t_i + d_i$ and $q_i = 1 - p_i$. If we express the target rates in percentages, $p_i = (t_i/n_i) \times 100$ and $q_i = 100 - p_i$.

1. Qualitative standards. The two most

important qualitative features of a stratum are biologic homogeneity and scientific reproducibility.

a. Homogeneity. As noted in an earlier discussion,[6] the qualitative homogeneity of a stratum depends on the types of categorical elements that designate its members. A stratum whose elements are derived from a single simple variate, such as *age* or *sex*, will be homogeneous for the particular category, such as **adolescent** or **female**, that defines it. If the variate is compound (or clustered) the homogeneity of the stratum depends on the biologic relationships of the constituent elements. For example, the stratum **mild carditis,** as defined earlier, seems reasonably homogeneous because all of its elements represented certain characteristics of cardiac structure or function. The stratum **poor risk** for patients with acute myocardial infarction might be biologically homogeneous or heterogeneous according to the types of ailments it comprises. If the rating of **poor risk** depends exclusively on such cardiac abnormalities as shock, pulmonary edema, or a major arrhythmia, the poor-risk group would be relatively homogeneous. On the other hand, a patient with an uncomplicated infarct might still be regarded as a poor risk because of co-morbidity due to an associated cerebral hemorrhage or hepatic decompensation. In the latter situation, the poor-risk stratum would be biologically heterogeneous.

The clustering of heterogeneous biologic elements into a single stratum can be justified if the individual elements are shown to have similar target rates. The cluster would then be homogeneous in its quantitative aspects, if not in its biologic taxonomy. On the other hand, even if the biologic elements seem similar, their combination into a single stratum would be unwarranted if they had substantial differences in target rates. For example, the individual categories of **prolonged P-R interval** and **cardiac enlargement** might seem biologically similar because both refer to cardiac abnormalities, but their combina-

tion into a single stratum would be undesirable for predicting outcome of acute rheumatic fever because the two elements have distinctly different prognostic implications.[7]

In evaluating a clustered stratum, therefore, we would examine the biologic features and associated target rates of the constituent elements that are joined in the stratum. In optimal circumstances, the constituents would be homogeneous for both the biologic characteristics and the target rates. The next best arrangement, if the constituent elements are biologically heterogeneous, is for their individual target rates to be similar. The combination of elements with dissimilar target rates would be undesirable regardless of whether or not the elements are biologically homogeneous.

To distinguish between qualitative homogeneity in biologic characteristics and quantitative homogeneity in numerical target rates, the term *concordant* will be used for the biologic similarity of elements in a stratum, and the term *isometric* will be used for similarity of target rates. Thus, a clustered stratum is most desirable when its constituents are isometric and concordant; it is acceptable if isometric but discordant; and it is unacceptable or at least highly undesirable if poikilometric (i.e., constituents with diverse target rates) even though the constituents seem concordant.

The decisions about quantitative homogeneity in target rates can be made with numerical standards that will be described later, but the decisions about biologic concordance require scientific judgment and cannot be expressed in a mathematical formula. Thus, if we form a composite cluster as a "union" that contains people who are either musically talented or hypokalemic or both, the mixture of elements seems distinctly heterogeneous. If we form a cluster composed of people who have metastasis to the liver or metastasis to the lungs, or both, the mixture seems reasonably homogeneous. The decisions that made us ascribe *homogeneity* to a mixture of two types of metastasis and *heterogeneity* to a mixture of musical talents and serum potassium depended entirely on biologic or taxonomic concepts rather than statistical principles.

Although biologic concordance is obviously desirable when composite categories are formed, a purely biologic appraisal of homogeneity can be applied only when the categories are few and closely related, so that the combined categories are biologically meaningful. Thus, in patients with lung cancer, we can unite such diverse clinical manifestations as dysphagia, the superior vena cava syndrome, and paralytic vocal-cord hoarseness into a single category. The composite cluster is biologically homogeneous because all three manifestations have a common pathogenetic mechanism that can be used to give the cluster a name: **mediastinal metastasis.** The biologic concordance of other combinations may arise from common features of anatomy, physiology, or biochemistry.

In many other circumstances, however, particularly when multiple variates are combined, the resultant clusters may not have any immediate biologic correspondence. In such circumstances, a clustered stratum can be biologically evaluated according to the principle of "ordered neighbors." To illustrate this principle, let us assume that renal function and hepatic function have each been individually ranked in a four-category scale of **1** = *normal;* **2** = *mildly impaired;* **3** = *moderately impaired;* and **4** = *severely impaired.*.If we want to construct a composite mixture of categories for renal-and-hepatic function, the most obvious biologic similarities are found in the extremes of each scale. Thus the **1-1** elements and the **4-4** elements would yield two new categories that could be described respectively as *normal in both* and *severely abnormal in both.* As intermediate categories, we might have a cluster that consisted of a mixture of the **1-2, 2-1,** and **2-2** elements; another cluster containing the **2-3, 3-2,** and **3-3** elements; and possibly another containing the **3-4** and **4-3** mixtures.

The elements that formed these combinations can be regarded as "ordered

neighbors" because they are topographically adjacent to each other when conjoined in a cross-tabulation that resembles a "tic-tac-toe" grid. Such an arrangement is illustrated by the elements of the following table:

Rank of Renal Function	*Rank of Hepatic Function*			
	1	*2*	*3*	*4*
1	1-1	1-2	1-3	1-4
2	2-1	2-2	2-3	2-4
3	3-1	3-2	3-3	3-4
4	4-1	4-2	4-3	4-4

The elements of this table are indicated with two numbers that denote the contribution from the row and column categories of each combining variate. The elements that were not accounted for in the previously cited categories of clustering for ordered neighbors are those marked **3-1, 4-1, 4-2, 1-3, 1-4,** and **2-4.** These elements might conceivably be united in a single group, or, among several alternatives, they might be combined with other elements that were their "neighbors" in the table. An entire "neighborhood," extending for considerable topographic distance in the table, can be combined if all the adjacent members have a similar biologic characteristic and similar rates. For example, if the target rates are essentially identical for all elements of the group with normal hepatic function, regardless of renal function, the four categories **1-1, 2-1, 3-1,** and **4-1** could be combined into a single cluster.

The "ordered neighbor" principle would be violated if the combined elements had no biologic feature in common, and were not adjacent in the cross-tabulation of biologic rankings. Thus, the **1-4** and **4-1** groups possess, as a common feature, their junction of high and low extremes; the elements of the mixture **1-1, 2-1, 3-1** and **4-1** share the common columnar property of –1; the elements **2-3, 3-2,** and **3-3** are topographic "neighbors" in the table. But a mixture of the **1-1** and **4-4** elements would be a biologically heterogeneous combination of distant rather than neighboring categories, as would be such mixtures as the **1-2**, **3-1**, and **2-4** elements.

Thus, by noting the ordinal array of combined categories and by contemplating their ordered biologic locations in a cross-tabulation, we can determine the neighboring groups that would seem biologically concordant.

b. Reproducibility. An important scientific feature of a stratum is its reproducible definition. As noted earlier, such a definition requires gradation criteria that specify the elements of the stratum, the designation of their observational evidence, and an indication of their demarcation. When such criteria are omitted, a stratification is scientifically unacceptable even though its biologic and quantitative results may seem highly appealing. A major defect of current activities in clinical biostatistics, as repeatedly noted in these papers, is the failure to create such criteria for "soft data." Because criteria can easily be specified for the "hard data" of metric variates, the analysis of research may be confined to such data, ignoring the "soft data" that are often far more significant in biologic clinical importance.

2. Quantitative standards. A stratum can be assessed quantitatively according to its variance, its congruent fit, its ancestral fit, its isometry, and the confidence induced by its target rate and size.

a. Variance. The variance of the target rate for a stratum is the product, $p_i q_i$, of the target rate multiplied by the non-target rate. Thus, if a stratum has the target rate of 20% or .20, the variance of the rate is $(.20)(.80) = .16$. As either p (or q) approaches 100% (or 0%), the variance of the rate will approach zero. The smaller the variance, the more quantitatively homogeneous is the stratum for the target rate.

The total amount of variance contained within a stratum can be called the *group variance*, which is the product, $p_i q_i n_i$. Thus, in a stratum with 80 members, and a target rate of 25%, the group variance is $(.25)(.75)(80) = 15$. The concept of group

variance* will be of considerable value later when we compare results among different strata.

b. Congruent fit. The congruent fit of a stratum is a particularly important concept when the stratified results are to be used for future predictions. The congruent fit, which indicates the way that the stratum "predicted" the past events on which it is based, is determined from the number of errors that would be created if all members of the stratum were regarded as having (or not having) had the target event, according to the direction indicated by the rate of the stratum. If p_i is higher than 50%, we could regard the target event as having occurred for all n_i members of the stratum. This retrospective "prediction" would then be correct for t_i members and wrong for d_i members. Thus, for a stratum with a target rate of 60/80 (75%), we would predict occurrence of the target in all members. This prediction would be correct in 60 instances and wrong in 20. If p_i is below 50%, we would predict non-occurrence for everyone. The prediction would be right for d_i members and wrong for t_i. If the target rate is exactly 50%, a prediction of either occurrence or non-occurrence will be congruently right (or wrong) in half the members of the stratum.

The rate of congruent fit (which will be either p or q for an individual stratum) is not particularly valuable when applied individually, but can be a useful index of appraisal when applied to the "errors" of an entire partition. If e_i, the congruent error of the stratum, is the smaller value of t_i and s_i, its contribution to the rate of congruent error for a partitioned cohort containing N members is e_i/N. The con-

---

*Readers who are familiar with the technique for calculating variance in metric data will recognize that *group variance* for the types of proportions (or rates) under examination here is equivalent to the sums of the squared deviations from the mean—a term that is often called the *sum of squares* in the analysis of variance. When group variance is divided by n we get the variance, which is pq. If we take the square root of this variance and divide by $\sqrt{n}$, we get the familiar $\sqrt{pq/n}$, the standard error of a proportion.

gruent error rate for the entire partition will be $(\Sigma e_i)/N$, i.e., the sum of congruent errors in the individual strata, divided by the number of members in the cohort population. The smaller this value, the better is the congruent fit of the stratification.

The values for group variance of a stratum and its error in congruent fit are closely related. Since group variance is $p_i q_i n_i$, it can also be expressed either as

$$\left(\frac{t_i}{n_i}\right)\left(\frac{n_i-t_i}{n_i}\right)(n_i) = t_i - \frac{t_i^2}{n_i}$$

or as

$$\left(\frac{s_i}{n_i}\right)\left(\frac{n_i-s_i}{n_i}\right)(n_i) = s_i - \frac{s_i^2}{n_i}$$

Since the congruent error is either t_i or s_i, the group variance is always smaller than the congruent error by an amount that is the square of the number of "errant" members, divided by the total membership of the stratum. The largest congruent error rate that can be attained for an individual stratum is 50%, and the largest variance that can be attained for the rate of the stratum is 0.25. Both of these situations occur when $p = q = 0.5$ or 50%. The smallest congruent error rate and variance are 0, when p or q is either 100% or 0%.

c. Ancestral fit. If a single stratum has been created by the combination of two or more existing strata, the new stratum can be evaluated for the "goodness" with which it fits the results of the previous "ancestral" strata. Suppose two strata, with the respective target rates of 8/30 (27%) and 3/13 (23%) have been consolidated to form a new stratum with the rate 11/43 (26%). At the new rate of the consolidated stratum, we would expect to find that the target event occurs in 7.7 members ($= .26 \times 30$) of the old first stratum and in 3.3 members ($= .26 \times 13$) of the old second stratum. The target event should correspondingly be absent in 22.3 members of the old first stratum and in 9.7 members of the old second.

The goodness of ancestral fit can then be quantified with one of the many applications of the chi-square formula: (observed-expected)^2/expected. Thus, the chi-square score for goodness of fit here would be $(8-7.7)^2/7.7 + (3-3.3)^2/3.3 + (22-22.3)^2/22.3 + (10-9.7)^2/9.7 = 0.12 + .027 + .004 + .009 = .052$. This is a better fit than would have been created if our new stratum, with the same rate of 11/43, were produced by consolidating two previous strata with the target rates 10/30 and 1/13. This consolidated stratum would not provide as good a fit for its "ancestral" strata because the value for the χ^2 score would be 3.13.

The chi-square score in this situation merely indicates how well a consolidated stratum fits the ancestral strata that compose it: the smaller the value of χ^2, the better is the fit. If the χ^2 value is sufficiently large amid other considerations to be cited later, the two strata may be distinctive enough so that they should not be combined.

Another way of quantifying ancestral fit is to add the absolute values of |observed–expected| scores for the occurrence of the target event in each ancestral stratum. Thus, if the stratum 11/43 is combined from the ancestral strata 8/30 and 3/13, the ancestral error score is $|8 - 7.7| + |3 - 3.3| = 0.6$. If the stratum 11/43 is combined from the ancestral strata 10/30 and 1/13, the ancestral error score is $|10 - 7.7| + |1 - 3.3| = 4.6$. The first combination, having a lower ancestral error score, provides a better ancestral fit than the second.

d. Isometry. As we have just seen, the two strata 8/30 and 3/13 have rates that are close together: 27% and 23%. The isometry of their combination is reflected in the low scores for chi square and ancestral error of the combined stratum. The two strata 10/30 *(33%)* and 1/13 *(8%)* have rates that are much more widely separated. Their poikilometric combination was indicated by the high scores for chi square and ancestral error.

In the foregoing example, the relative closeness or distance of the difference in target rates was readily apparent. For general decisions, we must establish a boundary for the maximum difference that is permitted by the term *similar target rates* or *isometry*. The choice of this boundary will be discussed in a later section.

e. Size and predictive confidence. The closer that the target rate of a stratum approaches a *polar* value of either 0% or 100%, the fewer are the errors that will be made in the past congruence or future prediction of *yes* or *no* for the target event in all members of the stratum. (The errors increase as the target rate approaches the *meridian* value of 50%.) This same reasoning applies to small values of variance in the target rate of the stratum. The lower the variance, the more quantitatively homogeneous are the members of the stratum.

For congruence, predictive accuracy and quantitative homogeneity, therefore, we would prefer to have a polar target rate in the stratum. An ideal partition of a cohort would be a polarization that divides it into two strata—one with the *nadir* polar rate of 0%, and the other with the *zenith* polar rate of 100%. If such a partition has not been attained, we could explore some other partition, or we might consider further refinements of the strata in an effort to achieve the ideal.

The unlimited continuation of these refinements would be hampered, however, by at least two problems. One of these problems relates to the use of a stratum in intervention, rather than prediction. Despite the predictive advantages just cited, a polar stratum is not well suited for therapeutic trials because the stratum contains no variance to be affected by the therapeutic maneuver. All of the patients are destined to have essentially the same result. If this result is favorable, there is no need to test a new treatment that can only be deleterious. On the other hand, if the outcome of the stratum is universally unfavorable, the condition of the patients may be so bad that no treatment can affect it. Such a nadir stratum of patients might be quite valuable,

however, for the previously discussed[1] special investigation of a widely heralded "cure" for an "incurable" disease. If the new agent can produce any good results in a nadir stratum, it will warrant further therapeutic tests; otherwise, the agent may be merely the product of intense publicity and sparse data.

In general, however, a polar stratum would be excluded in planning therapeutic trials and segregated in reviewing data for a completed trial. As noted previously,[6] the polar strata can be either eliminated, or identified and analyzed separately, so that they do not obfuscate the results or create inefficiency in the statistical analyses. Such obfuscation can occur with favorable as well as unfavorable polar strata. For example, using multivariate prognostic stratification, Charlson and I[8] have identified a stratum of women who have a 96% 5-year survival rate with breast cancer. When a surgeon performs "careful selection" of patients to receive a new operation for breast cancer, he can attain splendid results—no matter what the operation may be—if his cohort is carefully selected to contain mainly patients from this almost-zenith stratum.

The hazards of an unrecognized polar stratum can be avoided during the stratification process by performing the diverse multivariate refinements that will be described later. The continuing addition of variates would be hampered, however, by an obvious second problem: the size of the stratum. Despite our intuitive confidence in predictions associated with a target rate of 0% or 100%, our quantitative certitude would be markedly reduced if the 0% represented a ratio such as 0/2 or the 100% represented a ratio such as 3/3. In both these instances, we would recognize that the stratum provides perfect congruence for its existing members, but the number of members is too small to warrant confidence about using the results in future predictions. On the other hand, if the 0% and 100% values represented such ratios as 0/93 and 75/75, we would feel quite confident about our subsequent estimates of *no* or *yes* for the target events.

We thus reach another decision that requires scientific clinical judgment and that cannot be made with any statistical theories. The strategies described statistically with the word "confidence" can not be applied to a polar stratum. If the rates of either p or q are at a polar value of 0% or 100%, the "standard error" of the rate ($\sqrt{pq/n}$) is zero, and we are left with a zero value for an anticipated "confidence interval" around the polar rate.

Instead of relying on this statistical type of confidence, we must therefore choose a minimum size of population that will give us clinical confidence when we go to use the stratum's rate predictively. In the previous examples, we felt clinically confident with a populational size of 75 and insecure with a size of 3. The choice of a minimum size, which will presumably lie somewhere between these two values, will vary according to each investigator's judgmental decisions. In a currently unpublished new method for using a computer to perform multivariate prognostic stratification, J. R. Landis and I selected 20 as the value for what might be called the *modicum:* the minimum population required in a stratum from which predictions are to be made. The size of the modicum will obviously vary with the magnitude of the analyzed cohort and the purposes of the analysis.

A stratum would thus be quantitatively acceptable if it contained at least the modicum number of members. A particular partition would then be acceptable only if each of its strata fulfilled the modicum requirement. If the strata of a partition do not fulfill the modicum requirement, we can either select some other partition for the final stratification, or consolidate one or more strata within the first partition. For example, working with a modicum value of 20, we might find that the survival rates for a population partitioned according to age are as follows: **below age 21**, 25/28; **ages 21-30**, 7/10; **ages 31-40**, 20/31; **ages 41-65**, 16/33; and **above age 65**, 13/80.

Since the second of these strata is below the modicum size of 20, we can combine it with an adjacent "neighbor" stratum to create a new stratum with above-modicum size. In this case, the ancestral fit will be better[*] if we choose the adjacent higher age group *(31-40)* rather than the adjacent lower group *(below age 21)* for the combination. By consolidating the second and third strata, we would attain the following partition: **below age 21**, 25/28; **ages 21-40**, 27/41; **ages 41-65**, 16/33; and **above age 65**, 13/80.

Conversely, if the target rate is non-polar in a stratum that contains more than a modicum of members, we might want to refine the stratum by dividing it into smaller strata, one or more of which will more closely approach a polar target rate. Thus, in the partition described in the preceding paragraph, we might be able to refine the last stratum by univariate expansion as follows: **age 66-85**, 12/59; and **above age 85**, 1/21. An alternate method of refinement would be to conjoin categories of an additional variate. Thus, by conjoining categories of sex, we could create composite strata consisting of **women above age 65**, with a rate of 8/45; and **men above age 65**, with a rate of 5/35.

D. The evaluation of two adjacent strata

The strata of a partition can always be arranged in a ranked order. If the categories of strata are themselves ordinal (ranked according to different age groups, or with such ratings as **none**, **mild**, **moderate**, **severe**), the partition is arranged according to the ascending or descending order of categories that form the "independent variate." If the categories are nominal or existential (when they express values for such variates as *birthplace, occupation,* or *existence of chest pain*) the partition can be arranged according to the target rates that form the "dependent variate."

---

[*]If we combine 7/10 with 25/28 to form a new category with 32/38, the χ^2 value is 2.06. If we combine 7/10 with 20/31 to form a new category with 27/41, the χ^2 value is 0.10. The lower value of χ^2 gives the better fit.

We can then inspect the relationships of target rates in adjacent paired strata of this ordered arrangement. If the target rates of a particular pair are not substantially different, we might question the merits of maintaining the two adjacent strata as separate entities. Assuming that each of the adjacent strata has satisfied our individual standards for biologic homogeneity and modicum size, we now need some new "pair-wise" standards for decisions about a "substantial difference" in the target rates of adjacent strata. All of the procedures described here can be applied to evaluate not only adjacent pairs in a partition containing more than two categories, but also partitions producing a "dichotomous split" into only two strata.

1. Scientific judgment. We now become confronted once again by decisions about a type of "significance" that is regularly ignored in textbooks of statistics and "experimental design." We must choose Δ—the amount of difference that makes a difference.

This decision cannot be accomplished by tests of "statistical significance." The tests are valuable for determining whether small groups contain enough members to make the differences numerically cogent, but the statistical procedures are generally useless in the "large-sample" situations where the groups contain an abundance of members. If the compared populations are large enough, any difference in target rates—no matter how tiny or trivial—can become "statistically significant." For example, the difference in target rates of two strata can be as small as 1%, and yet the chi-square score can be "statistically significant" if the strata contain enough people.*

As an act of scientific judgment, therefore, we must choose a value for the minimum difference that will be meaningfully significant between two target rates. If the actual increment exceeds this minimal dif-

ference, we proceed with tests of other statistical distinctions in the rates. If the increment does not exceed the chosen difference, we will assume that the two strata are essentially isometric and that they have not produced an important distinction. We might then decide to combine the two strata, to refine them by univariate or multivariate alterations, or to investigate some other variate that might yield a better stratification.

The choice of a value for this minimum difference in rates will depend on the data and on the purpose of the stratification. In some real-life circumstances—such as the interest rate on loans—a change of a fraction of a per cent might be quite significant. In other circumstances, a much higher increment will be required for the percentage differences to be accepted as important. For most clinical purposes, the minimum value for this limiting increment would be no lower than 5%, and often not less than 10%.

2. Statistical judgment. If the difference in rates exceeds the minimum required increment, we next want to know whether the two rates are based on numbers substantial enough to make the difference unlikely to have arisen by chance. Thus, the 50% difference between the target rates of 75% and 25% is obviously important, but would be unconvincing if based on the numerical values of 3/4 vs. 1/4. On the other hand, if the numbers associated with these rates were 60/80 vs. 20/80, we would have few doubts about the statistical distinctions.

The classical, generally accepted statistical procedure that we can use for evaluating the numerical distinctiveness or "significance" of a difference in two rates is the conventional chi-square test. Having chosen this test for our statistical inference, we must now make four further judgmental decisions:

1. Should the calculations of chi-square be corrected or uncorrected with the adjustment proposed by Yates?

2. Under what conditions should the

---

*If strata s_1 and s_2 have the target rates of 9% and 10%, the χ^2 score will be 3.85 (P < .05), if each stratum contains 6,620 members.

chi-square test be abandoned in favor of the Fisher exact probability test?

3. At what α level of probability do we want to declare "significance"?

4. Will α depend on one-sided or two-sided "tails" of the probability distribution?

The problems involved in the answers to these statistical questions are multiple, complex, and involve many more arbitary judgments than the judgmental decisions described previously. A discussion of the problems can be found in most good textbooks of statistics, and is beyond the scope of the current dissertation, although certain issues will be reserved for a later paper in this series. For the moment, let us assume that we have arrived at satisfactory answers to the questions and that we can employ the fourfold (i.e., 2×2) χ^2 test or its Fisherian counterpart as a way of testing numerical distinctions in two rates.

3. *Chi-square score.* If we choose an α level of .05 and a two-tailed test, we will declare the difference in rates to be "significant" whenever the chi-square score exceeds a boundary of 3.84. For other choices of α, or for a one-tailed rather than two-tailed test, we will need other χ^2 boundaries for this standard of numerical distinction. (If the Fisher test is used, the results emerge as direct probabilities to be compared with a chosen boundary of α, rather than chi-square.)

Having made these decisions, we calculate the value for the chi-square statistical score and we use the results as we did before in evaluating the size of the inter-stratum gradient. If the χ^2 score exceeds the chosen boundary, the inter-stratum gradient is "statistically significant" and the two strata can be left intact if we so desire. If the score does not exceed the chosen boundary, the result is not "significant." We might then condense the two strata, attempt to refine them further, or abandon the variate under survey. Alternatively, however, if the gradient itself is impressive but the chi-square score is not (because the number of patients is too small), we might be scientifically reluctant to discard the two

strata as "indistinct" until a larger case series has been investigated.

4. *Variance reduction score.* Because the χ^2 score depends so strongly on the size of the compared populations, an alternative statistical procedure can be used to get a result that is quite similar to the chi-square procedure, but relatively independent of population size. For an unpartitioned cohort containing N members with target rate P and non-target rate Q, the group variance is NPQ. After partition, the corresponding group variance of each stratum is $n_i p_i q_i$. The act of partition thus reduces group variance by the amount $NPQ - \Sigma n_i p_i q_i$. The proportionate reduction in group variance (which can be called the *variance reduction score*) is $(NPQ - \Sigma n_i p_i q_i)/NPQ$. By suitable algebraic manipulation, it can be shown that the formula for calculating χ^2 is $(NPQ - \Sigma n_i p_i q_i)/PQ$. The proportionate reduction in group variance is thus equal to χ^2/N.

Since this variance reduction score is not associated with any concepts of "degrees of freedom" and need not be converted according to concepts of probability, it can be used as a straightforward numerical index for comparing the merits of different pairs of strata, particularly when the pairs create different dichotomous splits of the same population. An arbitrary level of the variance reduction score must be chosen for determining whether a particular pair of strata has created a "substantial" effect on the group variance of their collective group. If this level is selected to be .01, the strata will be regarded as "distinctive" if their variance reduction score *exceeds* .01.

5. *Improvement in congruent fit.* Another aspect of numerical comparison in deciding whether two strata are separately better than their collective combination is to determine their effect on congruent fit. The congruent fit of a collective stratum is improved only when it is divided into two strata that "span" the meridian target rate of 50%, i.e., if one stratum has a rate above 50%, and the other has a rate below 50%.

Suppose a group with a target rate of 27/80 (34%) can be divided into two strata with rates 14/35 (40%) and 13/45 (29%). Since all of these rates are below 50%, we would "predict" non-occurrence of the target in all members. In the original group, our "prediction" would be correct in 53 members. In the two strata, we would also be correct in 53 (= 21+32) members, so that the stratification would not have improved the overall congruent fit. On the other hand, if we could divide the original group into two strata with rates 14/25 (56%) and 13/55 (24%), we would now "predict" occurrence of the target in the first stratum, and non-occurrence in the second. Our "predictions" would be correct in 56 (= 14+42) people, so that the congruent fit would have been improved by the stratification.

For this reason, a pair of "meridian-spanning" strata may sometimes enhance congruent fit sufficiently to warrant their preservation as separate strata even though their numbers are not large enough to achieve "distinction" in the chi-square score.

6. The direction of stratification.

In certain types of stratification the process is performed as a sequential series of isolated dichotomous conjunctions. The entire original population is first divided into two strata according to the presence or absence of a single category, such as **male**. One of the two new strata is then divided into two additional parts by the conjunction of another single category from another variate, such as **age above 65**. One of the three strata that have just been formed is then divided into two parts by the conjunction of another single category, such as **presence of chest pain**. At this point, we might have the four strata: **men with chest pain; men without chest pain; women above age 65;** and **women age 65 and below.** Alternatively, according to the way the splits were performed, we might have: **men; women age 65 and below; women above age 65 without chest pain; women above age 65 with chest pain.**

This sequential technique of partition can be used as the basis for an automated form of stratification, performed by digital computer. A discussion of some of the computer programs that have been developed for this procedure will be reserved for a later paper in this series. The main point to be noted now is that each of the programs must incorporate a decision-making strategy to choose, at each step, the "best" of a series of possible dichotomous splits (or pairs of strata) for the same population.

The strategy for choosing this "best" split will vary with the direction in which the stratification is oriented. This direction can be toward a goal of maximal reduction in group variance, closest approximation of a polar stratum, or greatest improvement in congruent fit.

For example, let us consider three different dichotomous splits of the same data for a population with the target rate of 60/300 (20%). This group has a congruent fit of 240 and a group variance of 48.

For partition A, we have
a_1: 12/150 (*8%*)
a_2: 48/150 (*32%*)

For partition B, we have
b_1: 0/20 (*0%*)
b_2: 60/280 (*21%*)

For partition C, we have
c_1: 48/280 (*17%*)
c_2: 12/20 (*60%*)

Partition C improves the congruent fit (from 240 to 244), but the congruence is unaffected by A and B, because their rates do not span the meridian of 50%. Partition B produces a polar stratum, but A and C do not. Because the group variance for partition A is 43.7, compared with 47.1 for B and 44.6 for C, partition A creates the greatest reduction in group variance.

Each of these three partitions therefore has one specific but different merit that makes it superior to the other two partitions. Consequently, at this juncture in an automated stratification technique, the population could be dichotomously divided in three different ways, according to whether the strategy incorporated in the algorithm for the computer program was directed toward the goal of variance reduction, polarization, or improved congruence. In the "AID" program of Sonquist and Morgan,[10] the strategy is based on variance reduction; in the program developed by Klein and co-workers,[9] the goal is improved congruence; and in a program that J. R. Landis and I have not yet published, the goal is polarization.

• • •

Our efforts thus far have been devoted to the accomplishments of the components of a partition. We have developed methods for deciding about the preservation of individual strata and the distinctiveness of adjacent pairs of strata. Having completed the evaluation of the parts, we can now consider what is accomplished by the partition as a whole. The standards needed for that purpose, together with some other important decisions in the stratification process, will be discussed at our next meeting.

References

1. Feinstein, A. R.: A new staging system for cancer and a reappraisal of "early" treatment and "cure" by radical surgery, N. Engl. J. Med. **279:**747-753, 1968.
2. Feinstein, A. R.: Clinical epidemiology. I. The populational experiments of nature and of man in human illness, Ann. Intern. Med. **69:**807-820, 1968.
3. Feinstein, A. R.: Clinical biostatistics. II. Statistics versus science in the design of experiments, CLIN. PHARMACOL. THER. **11:**282-292, 1970.
4. Feinstein, A. R.: Clinical biostatistics. X. Sources of 'transition bias' in cohort statistics, CLIN. PHARMACOL. THER. **12:**704-721, 1971.
5. Feinstein, A. R.: Clinical biostatistics. XIII. On homogeneity, taxonomy, and nosography, CLIN. PHARMACOL. THER. **13:**114-129, 1972.
6. Feinstein, A. R.: Clinical biostatistics. XIV. The purposes of prognostic stratification, CLIN. PHARMACOL. THER. **13:**285-297, 1972.
7. Feinstein, A. R., Stern, E., and Spagnuolo, M.: The prognosis of acute rheumatic fever, Am. Heart J. **68:**817-834, 1964.
8. Feinstein, A. R., and Charlson, M. E.: A new staging system for breast cancer and a reappraisal of therapy, Clin. Res. In press. (Abst.)
9. Klein, D. F., Honigfeld, G., and Feldman, S.: Prediction of drug effect by diagnostic decision tree, Dis. Nerv. Syst. **29:**159-187, 1968.
10. Sonquist, J. A., and Morgan, J. N.: The detection of interaction effects: A report on a computer program for the selection of optimal combinations of explanatory variables. Monograph No. 35, Ann Arbor, Mich., 1964, Survey Research Center, Institute for Social Research, University of Michigan.

CHAPTER 28

Evaluation of a prognostic stratification

At our two previous sessions,[9, 10] we considered the scientific necessity for prognostic stratification and we began discussing the process with which an investigator can explore the merits of different partitions used for the stratification.

A *partition* consists of the array of categories that express the values of a variate. The categories can be demarcated with verbal specifications (such as **men**), with numerical boundaries (such as **above age 65**), or with both (**men above age 65**). The groups of people delineated by the categories of a variate are called *strata*. When the rates of the subsequent target event in a cohort are associated with the initial strata, the variate is called a *predictor variate,* and the result is called a *prognostic stratification.* Since the data of clinical epidemiology are expressed in many individual variates, and since stratifications can be formed for each of the observed variates as well as for diverse multivariate combinations, we needed to establish methods for determining the effectiveness of a partition and for deciding when and how to alter it.

A partition can be changed in several ways. If the number of members in certain strata is below a modicum size (such as 20), the strata can be either eliminated by rearrangement of the partition's demarcation boundaries, or enlarged by combination with other strata. The strata chosen for combination should preferably have two types of homogeneity: They should be isometric in the similarity of their target rates, and concordant in the similarity of their biologic characteristics. Decisions about isometry will depend on the establishment of a maximum difference, such as 5%

or 10%, below which two rates will be regarded as essentially similar. Decisions about biologic concordance will depend on the underlying anatomic, biochemical, pathogenetic, or other features of the categories under scrutiny. When a clustered stratum is formed by combining categories from a conjoined partition of two ordinal variates, the previously discussed[10] concept of "ordered neighbors" can be used to help maintain biologic concordance in the cluster.

If a single stratum is above modicum size and does not have a polar target rate (i.e. 0% or 100%), an attempt is made to refine the stratum by dividing it according to additional characteristics. These characteristics can be added in a univariate manner by changing the boundaries of the partition. Thus, the age category **60-79** might be refined as **60-69** and **70-79**. The characteristics can also be added in a multivariate manner by conjoining from one or more separate variates. Thus, the age category **60-79** might be refined as **men aged 60-79** and **women aged 60-79**. Two univariate strata that appear isometric may show striking differences in rates when additional variates are conjoined. Thus, the target events might show similar rates for **men** and **women**, but may become sharply distinctive for **young men, young women, old men,** and **old women.**

The individual strata of an ordinal partition (such as **small, medium, large,** or **Stage I, . . . , Stage IV**) can be arranged in an "independent" ranked order according to the graded rating of their demarcating categories. The individual strata of a nominal partition (for such variates as *occupation* or *nationality*) have no inherent ranking of grades but can be arranged in a "dependent" rank order according to the associated rates of the target event. After a ranking is prepared by using either the independent or dependent variate, the pairs of adjacent strata in the ranked partition can be evaluated for "distinctiveness"

This chapter originally appeared as "Clinical biostatistics— XVI. The process of prognostic stratification (Part 2)." In Clin. Pharmacol. Ther. 13:609, 1972.

in such quantitative features as their difference in the target rates, the chi-square score, the reduction in group variance, and (in certain circumstances) the improvement in congruent fit. If a pair of adjacent strata does not fulfill certain minimal standards for distinctiveness, the two strata can be combined or altered in some other manner.

At this point in the proceedings, which is where we stopped at our last session,[10] we will have attained one or more partitions that are acceptable in the size of their individual strata and in the distinctiveness of adjacent strata. We now can turn to evaluating the accomplishments of each partition as a whole.

A. The evaluation of an entire partition

The standards of "holistic" assessment to be cited here apply to partitions with three or more strata, but the concepts are readily adaptable to partitions that contain only two.

1. Qualitative standards. An important scientific requirement of a partition is that it have enough scope and detail to account for all members of the population to which it is applied. As an example of inadequate scope, consider the partition of **5-20 years, 21-50 years,** and **51-85 years** for *age* of a general population. This partition does not provide strata for people who are below 5 or above 85 years of age. As an example of inadequate detail, consider the TMN staging system[2] that is popularly used in prognostic stratification for breast cancer. In the partition that forms the stages, different strata are assigned for such elements as *axillary lymphadenopathy* and *distant metastases*, but the topographic boundaries of the term *distant* are not specified. Consequently, if supraclavicular lymphadenopathy is encountered, we would not know whether to regard it as equivalent to *axillary* or to *distant* metastases.

2. Quantitative judgments. Four of the quantitative characteristics that help indicate the achievements of a stratified partition are monotonicity, total gradient, isometry of clusters, and distribution of population.

a. Monotonicity. The associated target rates for a graded ordinal partition are called *monotonic* if they also follow a ranked order, whose direction can be similar or opposite to the ordinal trend of the strata. In the survival rates associated with the following ordinal partition, the trend decreases monotonically: **young,** 90%; **middle-aged,** 75%; **old,** 50%. In the rates of subsequent myocardial infarction associated with the following electrocardiographic categories, the target trend increases monotonically: **normal,** 2%; **slight abnormalities,** 6%; **moderate abnormalities,** 11%; **major abnormalities,** 18%. In the survival rates associated with the following staging system for a particular cancer, the trend is not monotonic: **Stage I,** 76%; **Stage II,** 54%; **Stage III,** 59%; **Stage IV,** 20%.

If the ordinal ranks of a partition depend on an aspect of biologic severity, we would expect the associated target rates to be monotonic, since the idea of "severity" presumably reflected an anticipated effect on the target. If such a partition fails to have a monotonic target rate, we can conclude either that the partition was not effectively arranged, or that our ideas about "severity" were wrong. If we had correctly chosen and demarcated the categories of severity, the target rate should have shown a consistent relation to those categories.

Since the staging of a cancer is intended to reflect its adverse effects, the survival rates would be expected to decrease monotonically with higher grades of staging. In the illustration of the preceding paragraph, however, the downward trend was slightly reversed between Stages II and III. Since the general trend of the target rates followed our expectations, we might conclude that Stages I and IV were well demarcated but that Stages II and III were not. We might then explore various revisions of the contents of Stages II and III in the effort to restore monotonicity. On the other hand, if the cancer survival rates showed the following results, we might reject the entire staging system as having chosen ineffectually: **Stage I,** 20%; **Stage II,** 76%; **Stage III,** 31%; **Stage IV,** 54%.

If a partition has been ranked according to a biologic quantity that does not necessarily denote *severity,* we need not expect to find a monotonic trend in the target rates. Consider the following array of survival rates for an ordinal age partition of patients with a particular disease: **below age 31,** 30%; **age 31-54,** 65%; **age 46-60,** 67%; **above age 60,** 29%. In this nonmonotonic sequence of survival rates, the curve is trapezoidal (rising and falling), with survival rates worst in the two extreme age groups, and best in the middle groups. Since we had no advance beliefs about the prognostic distinctions of advancing age (particularly below age 60), the absence of monotonicity is not surprising or contradictory to what had been expected.

The property of monotonicity can be determined by simple inspection of the array of target rates in the ordinally arranged strata. Alternatively, the values for adjacent target rates can be subtracted from one another. In a monotonic stratification, the increments will be all positive or all negative, and a reversal in sign will denote a non-monotonic partition. Thus, for the three stratifications cited in the first paragraph of this section, the increments of rate were, respectively: −15% and −25% for the monotonically decreasing partition; 4%, 5%, and 7% for the monotonically increasing partition; and −22%, +5%, and −39% for the one that was non-monotonic.

A test for monotonicity of gradient is particularly important when a metric variate, such as *age, height,* or *blood pressure,* is partitioned into dichotomous strata. With a dichotomous split, any substantial difference in rates will create a gradient, and the investigator may draw a spurious conclusion about monotonicity unless the gradient has been specifically checked in a polychotomous rather than dichotomous partition.

For example, suppose the target rate in a population is 30/200 (15%). Suppose we now divide the population dichotomously according to height and find the rates of 10/40 (25%) for the **shorter** group and 20/160 (13%) for the **taller** group. We might then conclude that the target rate declines with an increase in height. If we had specifically checked for monotonicity

of the gradient, however, we would have divided the population into at least three ordinal strata, and preferably more than three. Had we performed such a polychotomous partition we might have found the following results: **short,** 10/40 (25%); **below medium,** 8/120 (7%); **above medium,** 7/20 (35%); and **tall,** 5/20 (25%). Our idea about a falling gradient would have been erroneous. Therefore, to avoid misleading conclusions about the existence of gradients, a metric variate should always be checked for its polychotomous partition before it is expressed in dichotomous form.

A striking example of unsatisfactory dichotomous partitions for metric variates is contained in the report[14] of the UGDP study of diabetes mellitus. The stratifications for "risk factors" in Table 8 (pages 802-803) of the UGDP report included seven metric variates (age, blood pressure, cholesterol, fasting blood glucose, relative body weight, visual acuity, and serum creatinine). All of these variates were split dichotomously, according to "cutting points" that were "arbitrarily selected." The target rates were listed for the two strata of each variate, but no data were presented to show whether the rates rose or fell monotonically in the manner expected of the biologic gradient for a "risk factor." In the absence of a test for monotonicity in these variates, the reader (and possibly the investigators) can have no idea of the true effect that would be discerned with a scientifically adequate polychotomous partition.

b. Total gradient. The *total gradient* in the target rate for a partition is the difference between the highest and lowest rates found in the individual strata. Assuming that all other numerical requirements have been fulfilled (for modicum size, statistical distinctiveness, and, when appropriate, monotonicity), we would prefer a partition with a large total gradient to one with a smaller gradient.

If a partition contained a dichotomous split performed in search of single "risk factors," the two strata would be regarded as essentially trivial—with neither stratum demarcating a significant risk factor—unless the gradient between them was sufficiently high. The choice of a "sufficiently high" value for this gradient is arbitrary, but a value of at least 10% seems reasonable.

The UGDP report[14] also provides an obvious example of the inappropriate application of the term "risk factors" to dichotomous partitions of strata that produced only minor or even trivial gradients in their target rates. Because the UGDP's Table 8 did not list the numbers of patients involved in the numerators or totals of the cited death rates, the actual "risk" of the "risk factors" is not apparent in that table. Using the method of calculation described elsewhere,[8] I have determined* the appropriate numbers and target rate percentages for the "selected baseline characteristics" reported by the UGDP. The results are shown here in Table I.

If we regard a gradient of 10% as indicative of a distinct risk factor, the data of Table I indicate that two of the strata labelled by the UGDP as "cardiovascular risk factors"—**definite hypertension present** and **serum cholesterol ≥ 300 mg./ 100 ml.**—were essentially trivial in this population, being associated with cardiovascular death gradients of only 7.1% and 7.4%. In forming a cluster designated as **one or more cardiovascular risk factors**, the UGDP data analysts created a union of five strata: hypertension, digitalis, angina pectoris, ECG abnormality, and elevated cholesterol. The results of this cluster were also trivial, producing a cardiovascular death gradient of only 9.0%. Omitted from this cluster were two strata that are shown in Table I to be more substantial cardiovascular risk factors: **arterial calcification** (gradient 14.2%) and **serum creatinine ≥ 1.5 mg./100 ml.** (gradient 10.3%). Another omission from the UGDP's combination of "cardiovascular risk factors" was **Age ≥ 55**, which also had a higher cardiovascular risk gradient (9.5%) than the selected cluster.

With one exception, all of the strata that have just been described as producing significant or trivial gradients for rates of cardiovascular death produced correspondingly significant or trivial gradients when the target event was total deaths. The exception was **visual acuity ≤ 20/200**, which had a gradient of 4.9% for cardiovascular deaths, but 11.4% for total deaths. The latter gradient for the relationship of visual acuity and total deaths was higher than the corresponding gradient for hypertension, elevated cholesterol, and the UGDP's cardiovascular cluster.

In a subsequent report,[4] the UGDP group extended its cardiovascular risk cluster to a union of eight rather than five "risk factors." This union included the previous five strata and three addi-

tional ones: **age ≥ 55 years, relative body weight ≥ 1.25,** and **arterial calcification.** The first and third of these augmented "risk factors" were reasonable additions to the cluster since they were associated with respective gradients, as shown in Table I, of 9.5% and 14.2%. The body weight "risk factor," however, was bizarre. Its gradient was only 3.9% and besides, the rate of cardiovascular deaths, as well as total deaths, was lower in the stratum with the higher body weight. The UGDP's carefully selected cluster of eight "baseline risk factors" for cardiovascular death thus included four strata that were significant risk factors (digitalis, angina pectoris, significant ECG abnormality, and arterial calcification), one stratum that was borderline significant (age ≥ 55), two strata that were trivial (hypertension and elevated cholesterol), and one stratum (relative body weight ≥ 1.25) that was actually beneficial rather than detrimental in this population.

c. Isometry of clusters. As noted in our previous discussion,[10] the strata combined in a multivariate cluster should have essentially similar target rates. Without this attention to isometry, a cluster would be an indiscriminate conglomerate of heterogeneous groups, rather than a scientifically meaningful aggregation.

An excellent example of scientific attention to isometry in clusters is provided in the staging system for breast cancer developed by Cutler and Myers.[5, 6] These authors stratified patients according to a large number of diverse risk factors, and then formed "stages" by clustering the groups that had similar survival rates.

An excellent example of the neglect of this scientific principle is provided in the "cardiovascular risk cluster" formed in the UGDP reports.[14] The original UGDP cluster of five strata contained an admixture of factors with cardiovascular death rates that can be noted in Table I to range from 33.3% (ECG abnormality) to 12.2% (hypertension). In the augmented cluster of eight strata, the corresponding death rates range from 33.3% to 5.7% (relative body weight ≥ 1.25). The indiscriminate manner in which the "risk factors" were originally selected was magnified when the cardiovascular risk cluster was later stratified, in a subsequent UGDP report,[4] for patients who had **0, 1, 2, 3, 4, 5,** or **6** of the cited eight "risk factors." With this type of stratification—based neither on biologic concordance nor on target rate isometry—a patient with the single negative risk factor of elevated body weight would be placed in

---

*The values for *arterial calcification* have been listed according to the correction later reported by the UGDP group.[1a]

Table I. *Stratification of "risk factors" in the UGDP report**

Variate	Partition	No. of Pts.	Total deaths Number and rate	Gradient	Cardiovascular deaths Number and rate	Gradient
Age	< 55	449	22 (4.9%)	13.0%	14 (3.1%)	9.5%
	≥ 55	374	67 (17.9%)		47 (12.6%)	
Sex	Male	229	38 (16.6%)	8.0%	25 (10.9%)	4.8%
	Female	594	51 (8.6%)		36 (6.1%)	
Race	White	435	59 (13.6%)	5.9%	41 (9.4%)	4.2%
	Nonwhite	388	30 (7.7%)		20 (5.2%)	
Definite hypertension	Absent	552	48 (8.7%)	6.3%	28 (5.1%)	7.1%
	Present	254	38 (15.0%)		31 (12.2%)	
History of digitalis use	No	762	69 (9.1%)	30.0%	46 (6.0%)	24.4%
	Yes	46	18 (39.1%)		14 (30.4%)	
History of angina pectoris	No	765	74 (9.7%)	20.1%	50 (6.5%)	14.8%
	Yes	47	14 (29.8%)		10 (21.3%)	
Significant ECG abnormality	Absent	777	74 (9.5%)	29.9%	48 (6.2%)	27.1%
	Present	33	13 (39.4%)		11 (33.3%)	
Cholesterol	< 300	697	71 (10.2%)	4.6%	45 (6.5%)	7.4%
	≥ 300	108	16 (14.8%)		15 (13.9%)	
Cluster of CV risk factors	None	411	27 (6.6%)	8.6%	13 (3.2%)	9.0%
	One or more	361	55 (15.2%)		13 (4.8%)	
Fasting blood glucose	< 110	272	21 (7.7%)	4.5%	48 (8.8%)	4.0%
	≥ 110	547	67 (12.2%)		44 (12.2%)	
Relative body weight	< 1.25	365	52 (14.0%)	5.9%	35 (9.6%)	3.9%
	≥ 1.25	458	37 (8.1%)		26 (5.7%)	
Visual acuity	> 20/200	725	76 (10.5%)	11.4%	53 (7.3%)	4.9%
	≤ 20/200	41	9 (21.9%)		5 (12.2%)	
Serum creatinine	< 1.5	781	74 (9.5%)	12.7%	50 (6.4%)	10.3%
	≥ 1.5	18	4 (22.2%)		3 (16.7%)	
Arterial calcification	Absent	665	54 (8.1%)	17.2%	34 (5.1%)	14.2%
	Present	134	34 (25.3%)		26 (19.3%)	

*Table adapted from data reported as Table 8, pages 802-803, reference 14.

the same stratum as a patient with the highly significant risk factor of ECG abnormality. The stratum of people with three risk factors would take one patient who had the "trivial" three factors of elevated body weight, elevated cholesterol, and hypertension and rank him in the same group as a patient who had the three most important factors: ECG abnormality, use of digitalis, and angina pectoris.

The peculiar biologic science of the UGDP stratification procedure can be quantitatively checked by noting the actual rates of cardiovascular death associated with the ordinal array of clustered "risk factors." Although neither the total results nor the numerators are listed in the reported tabulations, the data cited in Table 1 (page 1677) and Table 7 (page 1681) of the subsequent UGDP report[4] contain enough information to allow calculation of the actual risks associated with the UGDP's "risk factors."

The 756 patients reported in those two tables incurred 57 cardiovascular deaths, a rate of 7.5%. The gradient rose monotonically as follows: **1 factor**, 4/248 (1.6%); **2 factors**, 12/234 (5.1%); **3 factors**, 19/124 (15.3%); **4 factors**, 10/39 (25.7%); **5 factors**, 7/18 (38.9%); and **6 factors**, 2/3 (66.7%). From this apparently monotonic gradient, one might conclude that the UGDP partition, despite its biologic peculiarity, was quite satisfactory. The conclusion becomes promptly refuted, however, by noting the rate found among patients with none of these "risk factors." In the

0 factor group, the cardiovascular death rate was 3/90 (3.3%) a value higher than what was found in the **1 factor** group. The patients with no cardiovascular risk factors thus had a *higher* death rate than the patients in whom one of the cited factors was present.

Although a distinctly monotonic gradient appeared in the remainder of the partition, the clusters were formed without regard to the obvious poikilometry of the individual risk factors. Each cluster was allocated the same number of "risk factors," regardless of the target-rate distinctions that might have been noted in the different pairs, triplets, quadruplets, etc. of "risk factors" that were conjoined. Having performed the multivariate stratification improperly by assigning the same importance to all "risk factors," the UGDP group then analyzed the multivariate data in a different manner, with a "multiple logistic function." This technique "does not treat all risk factors as of equal importance" and is regarded by Cornfield[4] as "the most useful method that has emerged . . . after 15 years of cardiovascular epidemiology."

With the logistic function technique, a numerical "probability of cardiovascular death" was calculated for each patient according to the various characteristics present at baseline. As shown in Table 8 (page 1681) of the Cornfield report,[4] the population was then stratified into five ordinal groups having ascending values of these baseline probabilities: <.0065, .0065-.0140, .0141-.0295, .0297-.0665, and ⩾.0673. This type of stratification thus provides the attention to isometry that was ignored in the clustered "risk factors."

An interesting contradiction can be noted in the results for these two different methods of stratifying the same data. The term "low risk group" can be applied to those patients who had 0 or 1 risk factor according to the UGDP's cluster technique, and to those patients whose calculated probability of cardiovascular death was ⩽ .0140 according to the UGDP'S logistic technique. The observed cardiovascular mortality for the patients receiving placebo and tolbutamide in the two types of "low risk groups" was as follows:

Cluster Method
      Placebo   1/88 (1.1%)
      Tolbutamide 5/75 (6.7%)

Logistic Method
      Placebo   1/86 (1.2%)
      Tolbutamide 1/74 (1.3%)

The two methods of stratification produced about the same number of patients in the denominators of both sets of "low risk groups." With the cluster method, however, the tolbutamide group appeared to have a fatality rate six times higher than the placebo group, whereas with the logistic method applied to exactly the same data, this six-fold difference vanishes and the fatality rates for tolbutamide and placebo are essentially identical.

d. Distribution of population. In contemplating monotonicity, gradient, and isometry, we were concerned about the array of individual values for the target rates $p_i = t_i/n_i$, of the strata. Another important feature of a stratification is the way the population is proportionately distributed among the strata. This proportion for each stratum can be expressed as $k_i = n_i/N$ where $N = \Sigma n_i$, the number of people in the cohort population.

Suppose our original population contained 300 people, of whom 150 achieved the target event, and suppose we divide this population into strata with the rates of 75/102, 30/48, 33/75, and 12/75. The successive values for p_i (the target rates) are 73.5%, 62.5%, 44.0%, and 16.0%. The successive values for k_i are 34% (102/300), 16% (48/300), 25% (75/300), and 25% (75/300).

Because each k_i represents a proportion of the cohort population, the sum of the k_i values will always be 1 if expressed in fractions, or 100% if expressed in percentages. Furthermore, if we know the populational proportions and target rate in each stratum, we can determine the target rate $P = T/N$, for the entire population. If k_i are the proportions in each stratum and p_i are the rates in each stratum,

$$\Sigma p_i k_i = \Sigma \left(\frac{t_i}{n_i} \right) \left(\frac{n_i}{N} \right) = \Sigma \frac{t_i}{N} = \frac{T}{N} = P.$$

Thus, in the example of the preceding paragraph, we could recapitulate the target rate for the entire population (50% = 150/300), by adding the products of each stratum's proportionate distribution and target rate. (.735) (.34) + (.625) (.16) + (.44) (.25) + (.16) (.25) = .2499 + .1000 + .1100 + .0400 = .4999 ≅ 50%. [The minor deviation from 50% is due to the earlier rounding of percentages.]

Although certain statistical formulas, based on "moments around the mean," can be used to characterize the shape and symmetry of frequencies in a distribution of metric data, no corresponding formulas have been established for characterizing distributions when the data are assembled in the categories of a partition. Accordingly we can derive certain "visual" judgments about shape and symmetry of the distribution in a partition, and we can develop another numerical score for use in comparing distributions.

(1) VISUAL CHARACTERISTICS. The distribution of a population can be described as "uniform" or "flat" if all the k_i values are essentially equal. In a partition containing 4 strata, the k_i values of 51%, 49%, 48%, and 52% would indicate a uniform distribution. If the k_i values successively rise and then fall, the distribution is centripetal, with the majority of the population located in the inner or central strata. Such distributions can have a trapezoidal shape for four strata (e.g., 15%, 35%, 35%, 15%) or a pyramidal shape for three strata (e.g., 20%, 60%, 20%). If the k_i values successively fall and then rise, the distribution is centrifugal, with the majority of the population located in the extreme strata. Such distributions would be U-shaped for four strata (e.g. 35%, 15%, 15%, 35%) or V-shaped for three strata (e.g. 40%, 20%, 40%).

All of the patterns of distribution just cited were essentially symmetrical around the middle or middle-two strata. A distribution would be less desirable if it is asymmetrical. Thus, a populational distribution of 5%, 65%, and 30% in three strata, or 70%, 15%, 10%, 5% in four strata would be asymmetrical.

No single pattern of distribution can be regarded as optimal because different patterns may be preferable for different purposes of stratification. In general, a centripetal pattern of symmetry is desirable because it approximates the Gaussian curve in which so many populational phenomena are distributed. Thus, we would ordinarily expect the "middle" rates for a target event to occur in more people than the "extreme" rates. We can calculate whether or not a distribution is centripetal by noting the sum of the percentages of the population located in the middle or middle-most categories. If this sum of percentages exceeds 50%, the population has an essentially centripetal distribution. Thus, the two partitions with proportionate distributions of 10%, 35%, 45%, 10% and 5%, 15%, 60%, 12%, 8% are both clearly centripetal.

(2) DISTRIBUTION SCORE. With recourse to the mathematics of probability theory, we can create a *distribution score* to characterize the numerical dispersion of members in a partition. The total number of permutations of N things taken all at a time is equal to $N! = 1 \times 2 \times 3 \times \ldots \times N$. If those N things are divided into c classes, the total number of permutations is $\dfrac{N!}{n_1! n_2! \ldots n_c!}$, where n_1, n_2, ..., n_c are the number of things in each class. The value obtained with the latter formula can be used as the basis for a distribution score for the strata of a partition. Because the "factorial" numbers are unwieldly for ordinary calculations, their logarithms can be used in creating the distribution score. Thus, the distribution score would be $\log N! - \log n_1! - \log n_2! - \ldots - \log n_c! = \log N! - \Sigma (\log n_i!)$. (The values of the logarithms can be found in an appropriate mathematical handbook.)

For example, suppose a cohort containing 100 members is divided into four strata, each containing 25 members. The distribution score will be $157.97000 - (4 \times 25.19065) = 57.207$. If the same cohort is divided into groups of 19, 23, 27, and 31, the score will be $157.97000 - 17.08509 - 22.41249 - 28.03698 - 33.91502 = 56.520$. The more equally divided the cohort, the higher will be the distribution score.

The distribution score can be used to choose the better proportionality of two distributions when each appears essentially symmetrical and centripetal. Thus, suppose a cohort of 200 people can be distributed as 19, 77, 82, 22 or as 20, 84, 72, 24. The distribution score is 100.9 for the first partition and 102.4 for the second. If all other factors were equal, we would regard the second partition as having a better distribution.

3. Statistical scores. At least five specific types of statistical score are available to provide numerical ratings for the effectiveness of a partition.

a. Linear trend. Even when a ranked partition does not have a completely monotonic series of associated target rates, the rates may still show a basically linear trend in the way they rise or fall. One of the many variations of the chi-square procedure has been adapted to quantify the trend noted in an ordered sequence of rates (or proportions). The details of the strategy and calculations can be found in several textbooks.[1b, 13b] The basic idea is to assign a set of numerical weights to each of the strata, and then to calculate, by a least-squares technique, the regression equation for the data. The slope of this equation is found as a chi-square score that represents the linear trend of the target rates. If the slope is "significantly" different from zero, a distinctively linear trend has been demonstrated.

The formula for the linear trend score of this slope is

$$\chi_L^2 = \frac{N(N\Sigma w_i t_i - T\Sigma w_i n_i)^2}{T(N-T)\ [N\Sigma w_i^2 n_i - (\Sigma w_i n_i)^2]}$$

In this formula for χ_L^2, T represents the the number of people attaining the target event in a cohort of N members, and the t_i and n_i represent the corresponding values in each stratum. The w_i values are arbitrarily assigned to each stratum, and are generally chosen in a pattern that is symmetric around zero. Thus, the w_i values might be assigned as follows: for three strata, −1, 0, +1; for four strata, −3, −1, +1, +3; and for five strata, −2, −1, 0, +1, +2. The linear trend score is interpreted like a χ^2 test with one degree of freedom, so that a result exceeding 3.84 is associated with P < .05.

A particularly useful aspect of this linear trend procedure is in comparing the scores for several partitions of the same data. The higher the value of the score, the more distinctive is the linear trend produced by the partition.

b. Congruent fit. When all the members of stratum are "predicted" to have attained or not attained the target event, the stratum will produce either t_i or d_i ($= n_i - t_i$) errors in congruent fit. The number of congruent errors in fit produced by an entire partition can then be determined as described previously.[10] If e_i is the number of errors in each stratum, the congruent error rate is $\Sigma e_i/N$. The smaller this rate, the more congruent is the fit of the partition. The total

improvement in congruent fit can be expressed as the proportionate reduction in errors. Thus, if E is the number of congruent errors in the unstratified data (where E equals either T or D), the proportionate improvement in congruence is $(E-\Sigma e_i)/E$.

c. "Statistical significance." The "statistical significance" of an entire partition containing c categories is determined with the conventional version of the χ^2 test, applied in a 2×c manner, with the associated probability noted at c−1 "degrees of freedom."

Used in this way, the conventional χ^2 test has two roles. It can denote the numerical distinctiveness of the entire partition, according to the chosen α level of "significance." A partition that fails to achieve "significance" might either be rejected or subjected to various alterations intended to increase its distinction. The chi-square test can also be used to compare numerical distinctiveness among two or more "significant" partitions.

The direct comparison of chi-square values is convenient when the partitions contain the same number of strata. The partition with the highest chi-square score will be numerically the most distinctive. If the compared partitions do not have the same number of strata, however, the use of chi-square is difficult because the scores must be translated into probability values associated with the different "degrees of freedom" for each partition. In most tables of these associations, the chi-square value for different degrees of freedom is cited at specific levels of probability (such as .1, .05, .025, .01, and .001), but if the chi-square value lies between two of the cited points, the associated probability is not listed.

For example, if a four-stratum partition has a chi-square value of 11.5 and a five-stratum partition has a chi-square value of 13.5, their comparison requires that the chi-square values be translated into probability levels at 3 and 4 degrees of freedom, respectively. The usual tables of probability for chi-square scores would not include enough detail for us to get the exact values associated with the two cited scores, and in this instance, we could say only that the P value for each of the two partitions lies between .01 and .005. Without making special additional calculations or extrapolations, we would not be able to determine which of the two partitions is more distinctive.

d. Variance reduction. The variance reduction score that was previously described[10] for a two-stratum partition can be applied to any partition with more than two strata. The formula for calculation is based on the proportionate reduction in group variance, and is expressed as $(NPQ-\Sigma n_i p_i q_i)/NPQ$. Because this variance reduction score does not require interpretation with the "degrees of freedom" and probabilities needed for chi-square, it can readily be applied to compare results when the same population is stratified with different partitions, no matter how many strata they contain.

Since the original value of NPQ remains unchanged by partitions, only the value of $\Sigma n_i p_i q_i$ need be calculated to compare partitions. The smaller the value of $\Sigma n_i p_i q_i$, the greater is the reduction in variance. An even simpler calculational method is to recognize, after appropriate algebraic substitution, that $\Sigma n_i p_i q_i = T-\Sigma(t_i^2/n_i)$. Since the target rates are usually presented in the form t_i/n_i, the value of $\Sigma(t_i^2/n_i)$ can be quickly determined. The higher the value of $\Sigma(t_i^2/n_i)$, the greater is the reduction in variance created by the stratification.

e. The F score. In the analysis of variance for metric data, the "significance" of the results depends on the probability values associated with an F score, which is a ratio of two variances. The "mean" variance among (or between) the groups is divided by the "mean" variance within the groups. This same F score can be applied, if desired, to the rates of the strata in a partition.

The mean variance *among* the c strata is equal to the group variance among the strata divided by the c–1 degrees of freedom. The group variance among the strata is $\Sigma n_i(p_i-P)^2$, which can be algebraically converted into $NPQ-\Sigma n_i p_i q_i$. When this is divided by c–1, the result is the "mean" variance among strata. The mean variance *within* the strata is equal to the sum of group variances within each stratum, divided by the sum of degrees of freedom within each stratum. The sum of the group variance within each stratum is $\Sigma n_i p_i q_i$, and the corresponding value for degrees of freedom is $\Sigma(n_i-1) = N-c$. The mean variance within the strata thus becomes $(\Sigma n_i p_i q_i)/(N-c)$.

The F score can then be expressed as

$$\left(\frac{NPQ-\Sigma n_i p_i q_i}{\Sigma n_i p_i q_i}\right) \times \left(\frac{N-c}{c-1}\right)$$

If the variance reduction score noted in the previous section was actually calculated, and if we let θ be the value for this score, we have $\theta = (NPQ-\Sigma n_i p_i q_i)/NPQ$. Solving this equation for $\Sigma n_i p_i q_i$, and substituting the result in the formula for the F score, we get

$$F = \left(\frac{\theta}{1-\theta}\right)\left(\frac{N-c}{c-1}\right)$$

A simple computational form for θ is the following:

$$\theta = \frac{\Sigma\dfrac{t_i^2}{n_i} - \dfrac{T^2}{N}}{T - \dfrac{T^2}{N}}$$

Once we have calculated the value of θ for a particular partition, we are prepared to deal with all of the three statistical scores that have just been cited. The value for the variance reduction score is θ; the value for chi-square is $N\theta$; and the value for F is $(\theta/1-\theta) \times (N-c)/(c-1)$.

The F value can be used to appraise "significance" by searching appropriate tables for the level of probability associated with c–1 and N–c degrees of freedom. Because degrees of freedom are involved in converting the F score to values of probability, this score is not convenient for comparing partitions that contain unequal numbers of strata.

4. Illustration of evaluation procedures. These evaluation procedures can best be illustrated by demonstrating their use in several different partitions of the same data.

In a report of new techniques for staging rectal cancer,[7] a cohort of 221 patients whose rectal

Table II. *5-year survival rate according to three stratifications of same data**

Categories of staging	System of staging		
	Anatomic	Symptomatic	Composite
I	70/122 (57%)	43/83 (52%)	36/50 (72%)
II	12/46 (26%)	12/129 (33%)	40/85 (47%)
III	3/53 (6%)	0/9 (0%)	6/31 (19%)
IV	Not used	Not used	3/55 (5%)

*Table adapted from data reported in reference 7.

cancer had been resected was found to contain 85 (38%) members who survived five years. For these values, the number of congruent errors is 85, and the group variance is 52.3. The cohort of patients was then partitioned according to three different ordinally-ranked systems of staging: a 3-stratum anatomic staging, a 3-stratum symptomatic staging, and a 4-stratum composite staging containing bivariate clusters of the anatomic and symptomatic features. Since the details of classification, and the qualitative and biologic homogeneity of the partitions were discussed elsewhere,[9] only the quantitative aspects of the partitions will be considered here. Their numerical results are shown here in Table II.

For the individual strata of the partitions listed in Table II, the 3rd stratum of the symptomatic staging had a nadir rate of 0% (0/9), but would not fulfill the modicum requirement for a minimal size of 20. All other strata had sizes that exceeded the modicum value. The individual stratum that came next closest to a nadir value was Composite Stage IV, which had a group variance of 2.8, and a congruent fit of only 3 errors in 55, for a rate of 5%.

In the comparison of adjacent strata for the three partitions, the incremental differences in survival rates all exceeded 5%. The inter-stratum chi-square scores all exceeded 3.84, and so all of the differences in adjacent strata were "statistically significant," even though one of the strata did not fulfill the modicum requirement for size. All three staging systems thus appear to be distinctive.

The evaluations of the entire partitions are shown in Table III. All three systems had a monotonic trend, with the largest total gradient (67%) occurring in the composite staging. The populational distributions were centripetal for the symptomatic and composite stagings but not for the anatomic. The distribution scores were highest for the composite staging system and lowest for

the symptomatic staging. For all three staging systems, the linear trend scores and conventional chi-square scores were "statistically significant." The anatomic system of staging was superior to the symptomatic one in these two scores and also in the reduction of both congruent errors and group variance. The composite system of staging, however, was superior to both the anatomic and symptomatic systems in all of the quantitative indexes under appraisal. The composite system provided the largest gradient, the best distribution, the greatest linear trend score, the fewest congruent errors, and the greatest reduction in group variance.

We can therefore conclude that the anatomic staging system was superior to the symptomatic staging system, but that the composite anatomic-symptomatic system gave the best quantitative results in these three stratifications of the same data.

B. Illustration of composite stratification

In the illustration just cited, the composite (or multivariate) strata had already been formed before we evaluated them. In the illustration that follows, the formation of composite strata will be demonstrated.

1. The initial data. The data for this illustration are taken from a report[3] of results in the well known Framingham Study.[13] In the original tabulations of data, serum cholesterol had been partitioned into seven categories: < **200, 200-209, 210-219, 220-244, 245-259, 260-284,** and **285+.** Systolic blood pressure had been partitioned into eight categories: < **117, 117-126, 127-136, 137-146, 147-156, 157-166, 167-186,** and **187+.** The partitions of these two variates were then conjoined to produce a bivariate stratification, containing 56 categories. For each of those 56 categories, the values of n_i (the population initially "at risk") and t_i (the members who developed "clinically manifest coronary heart disease" during the next 6 years) were listed in Table 2 (page 60) of the report by Cornfield.[3] For Table 1 (page 59) of that report, the cholesterol and the blood pressure partitions were condensed to four categories each. The results of that cross-tabulation are re-arranged, augmented with percentages, and shown here as Table IV.

2. The discriminant function analysis. In reviewing the cited results, Cornfield stated, "The thinness of the data . . . imposes a clear limit to the conclusions . . . (The) coarse groupings . . . (are) hardly sufficient to indicate the way in which the effects of cholesterol and blood pressure combine to influence the risk of the disease." Cornfield's solution to this problem was to use discriminant

Table III. *Quantitative evaluation of total effectiveness for three stratification shown in Table II*

	System of staging		
	Anatomic	*Symptomatic*	*Composite*
Monotonicity	Yes	Yes	Yes
Total gradient	51%	52%	67%
Proportionate distribution			
Stage I	55.2%	37.5%	22.6%
Stage II	20.9%	58.4%	38.4%
Stage III	23.9%	4.1%	14.0%
Stage IV	—	—	24.9%
Distribution score	93.3	75.9	123.8
Linear trend score	45.1	13.3	55.8
Number of congruent errors	67	82	63
Conventional chi-square score	45.5	13.8	56.5
Group variance	41.5	49.0	38.9
Variance reduction score	.206	.062	.256

Table IV. *Rates of "coronary events" for members of the Framingham cohort*

Partition of serum cholesterol	*Partition of systolic blood pressure (mm. Hg)*				
	Below 127	*127-146*	*147-166*	*167 and Above*	*Total*
Below 200	2/119 *(1.7%)*	3/124 *(2.4%)*	3/50 *(6.0%)*	4/26 *(15.4%)*	12/319 *(3.8%)*
200-219	3/88 *(3.4%)*	2/100 *(2.0%)*	0/43 *(0%)*	3/23 *(13.0%)*	8/254 *(3.1%)*
220-259	8/127 *(6.3%)*	11/220 *(5.0)%*	6/74 *(8.1%)*	6/49 *(12.2%)*	31/470 *(6.6%)*
260 and Above	7/74 *(9.5%)*	12/111 *(10.8%)*	11/57 *(19.3%)*	11/44 *(25.0%)*	41/286 *(14.3%)*
Total	20/408 *(4.9%)*	28/555 *(5.0%)*	20/224 *(8.9%)*	24/142 *(16.9%)*	92/1329 *(6.9%)*

functions as a "mathematical model which summarizes the observations in a small number of disposable parameters." With the discriminant analysis, Cornfield arrived at two principal equations to describe the combination of effects. The first equation was

$$P = 1/[1+e^{(23.13-6.14x_1-3.29x_2)}]$$

where P was the rate of the target event, X_1 was $\log_{10}$ cholesterol, and X_2 was $\log_{10}$ (blood pressure-75). A second equation, suggested when P was below 20%, was

$$P = .0091 \left(\frac{Y_1}{100}\right)^{2.66} \left(\frac{Y_2-75}{100}\right)^{1.47}$$

where Y_1 and Y_2 were serum cholesterol in mg./100 c.c. and systolic blood pressure in mm. Hg.

From these equations Cornfield concluded that "no matter what the blood pressure a 1% differ-

ence in cholesterol is associated with a 2.66% difference in risk" and "a 1% increase in systolic blood pressure from 110 mm. Hg is associated with a 4.62% difference in risk no matter what the cholesterol level." Cornfield's discriminant function analysis of this information has become a classic reference for the many such analyses that have subsequently been applied to epidemiologic and clinical data.

To a biologic scientist, however, these discriminant equations—with their additive co-efficients or exponential superscripts—may seem inscrutable, and, besides, the scientist may want to think about the changes produced when the two variables change simultaneously, rather than separately. I shall therefore demonstrate the way in which these same data can be analyzed by the process of multivariate prognostic stratification.

3. Examination and consolidation of strata.

Table V. *Rates of "coronary events" after consolidation of univariate strata in Table IV.*

Partition of serum cholesterol	Partition of systolic blood pressure			
	Below 147 (Low)	147-166 (Medium)	167 & Above (High)	Total
Below 219 (Low)	10/431 (2.3%)	3/93 (3.2%)	7/49 (14.3%)	20/573 (3.5%)
220-259 (Medium)	19/347 (5.5%)	6/74 (8.1%)	6/49 (12.2%)	31/470 (6.6%)
260 and Above (High)	19/185 (10.3%)	11/57 (19.3%)	11/44 (25.0%)	41/286 (14.3%)
Total	48/963 (5.0%)	20/224 (8.9%)	24/142 (16.9%)	92/1329 (6.9%)

From examining the data of Table IV, we can immediately note an error in Cornfield's general conclusions. The conclusions seem essentially true for the gradients in rate from the second to fourth category of each variate, but not for the change from first to second category. The rates of coronary events show very little increase between the first and second cholesterol categories (from **below 200** to **200-219**), and also between the first and second blood pressure categories (from **below 127 to 127-146**). In total results for the four main cholesterol categories, the rates are 4.9%, 5.0%, 8.9%, and 16.9. The corresponding total results for blood pressure are 3.8%, 3.1%, 6.6%, and 14.3%. The same trends noted in these totals are also present for the rates within the bivariate strata of each category. (Since the rate percentages were not included in the original tabular report of these data, the distinctions may not have been evident in that table.)

The distinctions from the first to second category of each variate are so slight, in fact, that our initial step in the stratification process would be to consolidate the first two categories of each partition. We are then left with three strata in each partition, producing the 9-stratum bivariate cross-tabulation shown in Table V. The data of Table V now demonstrate the "double gradient" or "trend within a trend" that was mathematically suggested by the previous discriminant equations. For each stratum of blood pressure, the rate rises with increasing level of cholesterol, and for each stratum of cholesterol, the rate rises with increasing level of blood pressure. The rate for the group with highest levels of both blood pressure and cholesterol was 25.0%, which is about 12 times the rate (2.3%) in the group with the lowest values of both variates.

Since this bivariate cross-partition contains the cumbersome number of nine categories, and since some of the adjacent rates are relatively similar,

we would now like to consolidate some of the strata. The rate in the highest bivariate stratum (25.0%) is distinctively different from any of its neighbors, and so this stratum will be preserved. The bivariate stratum with the next highest rate (19.3%) is also sufficiently distinctive to warrant its intact preservation. The two next highest rates (14.3% and 12.2%) are close together quantitatively and occur topographically in "biologic neighbors" who are within the same blood pressure stratum at the upper right of Table V. Accordingly, these two "neighbors" will be consolidated to form a joint rate of 13.2% (= 13/98).

We are now left with five bivariate strata, having rates ranging from 2.3% to 10.3% on the left side of Table V. We might unite the 10.3% group with the composite stratum formed in the previous step, but a combination of the 8.1% and 10.3% strata, which are "diagonal neighbors," seems more appealing. With these two groups combined to form a 9.7% group (= 25/259), our last step is to combine the three lowest groups, having a joint rate of 3.7% (= 32/871).

The pattern of these consolidations can be shown as follows, with the letters indicating the newly formed composite strata:

Serum cholesterol	Systolic blood pressure		
	Low	Medium	High
Low	A	A	C
Medium	A	B	C
High	B	D	E

The target rates for the five bivariate consolidated strata are shown in Table VI. The joint mixtures of different levels of blood pressure and cholesterol produce steadily increasing rates from the low-low and low-medium mixtures, up to the medium-high and high-high mixtures. The distribution of population in this partition is highly skewed, as would be expected for data of this type, with 65.5% (= 871/1329) of the cohort located in stratum A and only 3.3% (= 44/1329) in stratum E.

The 3.6% difference in rate between stratum B and C is smaller than might be desired for "distinctiveness" of strata. The distinctions for these and other strata in the composite partition would probably be more sharply "refined" if we could augment the two variates of cholesterol and blood pressure with some of the other variates noted as "risk factors" in the Framingham study.

4. Comparison of discriminant and stratification results. To compare how well the basic data are fitted by the discriminant function analysis and by the multivariate stratification, we cannot use the previously described congruent-fit scores[10] because none of the rates spans the meridian value of 50%. As an alternative, we could calculate the number of "coronary patients" expected in each stratum on the basis of the two statistical approaches. We could then contrast the expected value with the observed value, using the ancestral fit score described previously.[10] This type of calculation is not particularly attractive clinically because it often produces fractions of patients for the "expected" values, but since the technique was sanctioned and applied in Cornfield's report, we shall make use of it here.

For each of the original 56 groups cited in Cornfield's Table 2 (page 60),[3] he has listed the actual number of target events that occurred in that group, together with the number that would have been expected according to the discriminant function calculations. By multiplying the membership of each original group and the target rate of the corresponding composite stratum, we can calculate the number of events that would have been expected in each group according to the composite stratification. (For example, in the original group that was based on **cholesterol 220-244** conjoined with **blood pressure 147-156**, there were 29 members of whom 3 developed the target event of coronary disease. According to discriminant function, 2.4 such people were expected, and according to the composite stratification, 2.8 such people (= 9.7% × 29) were expected.

If the expected values are compared with the observed values for each of the 56 categories, we find that on 26 occasions the "discriminant expectations" were closer to the observed result than the "stratified expectations"; on 24 occasions, the "stratified expectations" were closer; and there were 6 ties. For the ancestral fit score, the sum of the absolute values of |observed-expected| in the 56 categories was 57.1 for "stratified" and 60.8 for "discriminant" values. The sums of the corresponding squared deviations were 104.8 for the stratified and 115.7 for the discriminant techniques.

We can therefore conclude that the two techniques produce quite similar results for "goodness" of fit." The choice between the two procedures is then a matter of scientific "taste." Biologists who like to think about categorical groups, biologic trends, and concomitant variations will probably prefer the stratification; statisticians who like to think about mathematical coefficients and linear or exponential models will probably prefer the discriminant technique. The intellectual ecumenicism of science has room for both procedures.

Table VI. *Rates of "coronary events" within composite bivariate strata*

Pattern of constituents		Composite stratum	Rate
Serum cholesterol	Systolic BP		
Low Low Medium	Low Medium Low	A	32/871 (3.7%)
Medium High	Medium Low	B	25/259 (9.7%)
Low Medium	High High	C	13/98 (13.3%)
High	Medium	D	11/57 (19.3%)
High	High	E	11/44 (25.0%)

C. Decisions about termination

Our last main concern during the stratification process is to determine when it should stop. At what point do we decide that a stratification is "optimal" and that the probing should end?

We have already noted[10] that the process can be continued as long as any stratum can be further reduced in group variance or directed more closely toward a polar target rate. Since the continuation of the process usually involves conjoining categories from multiple variates, the process will obviously end when no further variates or categories remain available for conjunction. Another obvious endpoint is the modicum size limit for strata. A stratum might not be further refined if its division creates new strata that are below the modicum size. A more common endpoint in dealing with the complexities of multivariate medical data is the failure of additional refinements to produce substantial improvements either in the statistical scores or in other quantitative standards used for appraising the results. After diverse multivariate combinations have been tried and found to be ineffectual in improving these quantitative results, the data analyst may decide to stop.

A different set of endpoints can be based on biologic scientific judgment rather than statistical scores. As the existing strata are further refined into additional multivariate strata, the number of groups will become unwieldy, and besides, many of the strata will have relatively similar target rates. To reduce the number of groups, strata with similar rates could then be clustered into a single stratum. These isometric clusters, however, might be quite heterogeneous biologically because their constituent groups have diverse multivariate characteristics. Accordingly, the data analyst may often prefer to stop the process when he has reached a stratification that is relatively concordant in its biologic clusters, even though the quantitative scores of the partition might be improved with the conjunction of further variates.

Finally, for purposes of subsequent application as well as for scientific explication, an investigator would want the groups of strata to be demarcated in a manner that not only produces biologic concordance for each isometric stratum, but that also keeps the strata as non-multivariate as possible. When more and more different variates become conjoined into the strata, the problem of remembering and applying their distinctions in future clinical work can become formidable. A clinician might easily be able to recall the details needed to classify patients according to the separate cholesterol and blood pressure groups noted individually in the preceding section. When the individual groups are conjoined and then clustered into the composite array of cholesterol-blood pressure strata, however, the mnemonic task of remembering criteria for each composite stratum would be much more difficult. In a newly created system of staging for breast cancer, Charlson and I[11] developed a four-category partition (graded as A, B, C, and D) that contained composite elements from individual partitions of anatomic, chronometric, symptomatic, and co-morbid variates. Criteria for demarcating the array of these "Composite A-C-S-C Stages" are too complex to be used without the aid of a written pattern of demarcation.

This problem in clinical mnemonics can easily be solved when computers become readily accessible as adjuncts to clinical activities. The computer can be programmed to "remember" all the necessary criteria of classification, and it can promptly print out the patient's appropriate stratum as soon as the clinician records the patient's multivariate data.

The problem of scientific explication, however, is not amenable to this type of automated solution. On examining the different outcomes that occurred in different strata, a scientist will search for anatomic, functional, or other mechanisms that might explain the distinctions. This explanatory activity requires a type of scientific insight that cannot be delegated to mathematical reasoning. For example, many mathematical models have been developed to analyze the chronometric variate that cites the time elapsed from first manifestations of a cancer to the date of treatment. In some of these models, each cancer is assumed to have a constant rate of growth, and the time interval is usually ascribed to the patient's "delay in seeking treatment." An investigator with scientific insight, however, would recognize that cancers can grow at different speeds, and that this chronometric interval can also be a functional index of the cancer's rate of growth.

The scientific search for explication of group phenomena is one of the major reasons for demarcating the phenomena with prognostic stratification. The stratification process produces clustered multivariate groups, whereas the statistical procedures of linear regression and discriminant function analysis produce additive multivariate coefficients. The scientific advantage in identification would be lost, however, if the multivariate complexity of the stratified groups is so great that they defy any rational attempts at explicative analysis. For this reason, an investigator may want to restrict the multivariate conjunctions to just a few variates that seem most cogent and most likely to yield distinctive scientific meaning. After the original candidate variates have been selected, decisions about their individual "cogency" can be aided by the statistical scores found for their univariate partitions, but scientific wisdom will be required to recognize the variates that should be originally included as candidates, and to choose the conjunctive or other distinctions that may be biologically significant.

We thus return to the fundamental difference that separates creative scientific research from imaginative statistical theory: a sense of what is important. The scientist acquires this sense by observing the phenomena of the real world; the statistician determines "significance" by mathematical computations. The scientist's judgment is thus particularly crucial not for the analytic calculations, but for choosing the variates that should be analyzed. If the scientist allows important characteristics to be omitted or inadequately replaced, the subsequent calculations may provide an elaborate, intricately computed, "statistically significant" set of results that confuse or neglect the major realities.

The UGDP study[14] also provides an illustration of defects in the initial choice of variables for analysis. Although a diabetic patient's baseline risk for mortality would be affected by co-morbid disease[12] in lungs, liver, and sites other than the cardiovascular system, the UGDP group examined only cardiovascular co-morbidity. Although the baseline risks in cardiovascular co-morbidity would be affected by such previous events as strokes, cerebral ischemic episodes, severity of angina pectoris, clinical myocardial infarction, recency and severity of congestive heart failure, and severity of arrhythmias, the UGDP group examined only "a history of use of digitalis," "a history of angina pectoris," and certain electrocardiographic abnormalities.

No matter how the basic data of clinical research may be analyzed for prognostic association—by stratified biologic clusters or by computed statistical regressions—no amount of analysis can turn bad data into good. No amount of mathematical manipulation can compensate for crucial information that is absent or neglected. And no statistical tests of "significance" can provide biologic meaning for information that is trivial, confounded, or distorted. For the ultimate test that determines the value or importance of scientific research, statistical computations and "confidence" can never replace scientific prudence and credibility.

References

1a. Anonymous: "Errata," Diabetes **20**:238, 1971.
1b. Armitage, P.: Statistical methods in medical research, New York, 1971, John Wiley & Sons, Inc.
2. Berndt, H., and Titze, U.: TNM clinical stage classification of breast cancer, Int. J. Cancer **4**:837-844, 1969.
3. Cornfield, J.: Joint dependence of risk of coronary heart disease on serum cholesterol and systolic blood pressure: a discriminant function analysis, Fed. Proc. **21**:58-61, 1962.
4. Cornfield, J.: The University Group Diabetes Program. A further statistical analysis of the mortality findings, J. A. M. A. **217**:1676-1687, 1971.
5. Cutler, S. J.: Statistical exploration of prognostic factors, *in* Breast cancer: Early *and* Late, Chicago, 1970, Year Book Medical Publishers, Inc.
6. Cutler, S. J., and Myers, M. H.: Clinical classification of extent of disease in cancer of the breast, J. Natl. Cancer Inst. **39**:193-207, 1967.
7. Feinstein, A. R.: A new staging system for cancer and a reappraisal of "early" treatment and "cure" by radical surgery, N. Engl. J. Med. **279**:747-753, 1968.
8. Feinstein, A. R.: Clinical biostatistics. VIII. An analytic appraisal of the University Group Diabetes Program (UGDP) study, CLIN. PHARMACOL. THER. **12**:167-191, 1971.
9. Feinstein, A. R.: Clinical biostatistics. XIV. The purposes of prognostic stratification, CLIN. PHARMACOL. THER. **13**:285-297, 1972.
10. Feinstein, A. R.: Clinical biostatistics. XV. The process of prognostic stratification (Part

1), CLIN. PHARMACOL. THER. 442-457, 1972.

11. Feinstein, A. R., and Charlson, M. E.: A new staging system for breast cancer and a reappraisal of therapy, Clin. Res. **20**:635, 1972. (Abst.)

12. Kaplan, M. H., and Feinstein, A. R.: The importance of co-morbidity in the outcome of diabetes mellitus, J. Clin. Invest. **50**:52a, 1971. (Abst.)

13a. Kannel, W. B., Dawber, T. R., Kagan, A, Revotskie, N., and Stokes, J. III: Factors of risk in the development of coronary heart disease—six-year follow-up experience. The Farmingham Study, Ann. Intern. Med. **55**:33-50, 1961.

13b. Maxwell, A. E.: Analysing qualitative data, New York, 1961, John Wiley & Sons, Inc.

14. University Group Diabetes Program: A study of the effects of hypoglycemic agents on vascular complications in patients with adult-onset diabetes. Part I: Design, methods, and baseline characteristics. Part II: Mortality results, Diabetes **19**:(Suppl. 2) 747-830, 1970.

CHAPTER 29

Additional tactics in prognostic stratification

During the past few papers in this series,[5-7] two sets of strategies were developed for concomitant application in forming and evaluating a prognostic stratification. One set of strategies contained judgmental biologic principles that were addressed to scientific issues. The issues refer to concordant homogeneity, i.e., the biologic similarity of members in the same group; and to meaningful explication, i.e., the facility with which a biologic explanation can be provided for the mechanisms or pathogenesis of the phenomena that characterize a group. The other set of strategies contained quantitative mathematical principles that were addressed to statistical issues. These issues refer to isometric homogeneity, i.e., the quantitative similarity of target rates among components of a group; and numerical distinctiveness, i.e., the size and "statistical significance" of the gradient in target rates among different groups.

These strategies for a stratified arrangement of data from multiple biologic variables have two fundamental differences from the existing methods offered by the conventional "multivariate" statistical pro-

cedures used for prognostic (or predictive) correlations:

a. Formation of groups. The stratification process demarcates clustered groups of people, whereas the conventional "regressive" techniques of statistics produce additive co-efficients for multiple variables. Thus, a man who is 78 inches tall might be classified by stratification in a category called **tall men**. In regressive statistical procedures, his sex (coded as *2*) and his height (coded as *78*) would be multiplied by such co-efficients as 1.4 and 0.02, respectively, and he would be identified by the sum of their products as *4.36* ($= [2 \times 1.4] + [78 \times 0.02]$). He might then be classified in the category **4.0 – 5.0**.

b. Attention to biology. The stratification process incorporates biologic standards and values into the demarcations, whereas the statistical techniques are based exclusively on mathematical theories, without regard to the specific biologic significance or connotations of the numbers that emerge.

The incorporation of biologic thinking into the statistical management of multiple variables is a particularly important feature of the stratification process, and represents an effort to restore emphasis to the *bio*

This chapter originally appeared as "Clinical biostatistics—XVII. Synchronous partition and bivariate evaluation in predictive stratification." In Clin. Pharmacol. Ther. 13:755, 1972.

portion of *biostatistics*. To be a creatively productive intellectual domain in clinical medicine, biostatistics must be developed as a fusion of clinical and statistical principles, rather than as a mathematical application of statistical methods to data that happen to come from clinical sources. The intricate multiplicity of variables is one of the main characteristics that distinguish people from the simpler substances studied when current biostatistical theories were formed. For those theories to be suitable to the multivariate challenges of clinical activities, the ideas that may have been appropriate for agricultural crops, brewery vats, fruit flies, and caged animals cannot be merely transposed into the complexity of free-living human beings. Biostatistical principles for the proper study of mankind must emerge from the proper study of human phenomena.

Since the clinical decisions of prognostic stratification will be made most effectively by data analysts who are intimately familiar with clinical biology, the stratification process should not be performed *in vacuo* by a statistician to whom the data are abandoned. The clinical investigator should be an active participant and contributing collaborator to the analytic process—joining his clinical wisdom about biologic features of the data to the statistician's sagacity about the numerical techniques.

The previous discussions[6, 7] of statistical biology for multivariate prognostic stratification are neither complete nor definitive. They represent a suggested base from which further expansions or revisions can be developed by the statistico-clinical collaborators who do future work in this domain. In this paper, which concludes the current sub-series on predictive (or prognostic) stratification, I shall discuss two additional tactics that can augment the stratifier's analytic "armamentarium."

A. Synchronous partition

The rates cited in a stratification are expressed in the form of a numerator per denominator. The denominator contains the number of members in a defined cohort of people, and the numerator denotes the number of those people in whom a specified target event later occurred. For all of the procedures we have hitherto considered, the denominators depended on characteristics that were present at baseline, in the "initial state," before the members of the cohort were exposed to the investigated maneuver. The maneuver under surveillance could be an alleged cause of disease in pathogenetic studies; a pharmaceutical agent or surgical procedure in therapeutic studies; or the passage of time in studies of normal ontogenesis or of clinical courses of disease. The demarcated strata in the denominators were given such names as *risk factors* or *stages,* and the elements of demarcation were derived from such pre-maneuveral baseline features as age, sex, symptoms, and paraclinical data.

This type of stratification can be called *prochronous* because the entities in the denominator were noted in serial time *before* the maneuver was instigated. Another type of stratification that is particularly important in studies of pathogenesis or therapy can be called *synchronous*. In synchronous stratification, the denominator data depend on events that occurred *while* the maneuver was in progress.

Since the results of epidemiologic studies of pathogenesis can be greatly distorted by inequalities in "target detection,"[4] a synchronous stratification can be used to divide the population according to different degrees of intensity in the examinations used for diagnostic detection of the target event. Analogously, since inequalities in patients' compliance can produce misleading results in therapeutic studies of oral agents, the patients can be synchronously stratified according to the fidelity with which they maintained the prescribed regimen.

Thus, to investigate whether contraceptive pills increase the hazard of thromboembolism, we would stratify the cohort of pill-takers and the cohort of non-pill-takers according to their synchronous exposure to the frequent careful clinical examinations needed for detection of thromboembolic phenomena. The rate of thromboembolic events for each cohort would then be compared within strata of patients who received commensurate exposure to the diagnostic examinations. To investigate the effectiveness of a daily oral penicillin regimen versus monthly injections in preventing recurrences of rheumatic fever, we would stratify the two cohorts into patients who did or did not faithfully maintain the prescribed antibiotic regimens. The rates of rheumatic recurrence would then be compared for strata of patients who were good or not good in their compliance with therapy.

A synchronous stratification can also depend on an ancillary effect of the therapy (or maneuver) under investigation. For example, to determine whether rigorous regulation of blood sugar prevents vascular complications in the treatment of patients with diabetes mellitus, we would want to know how well the blood sugar was actually regulated during the synchronous administration of therapy. In the analysis of such data, the target event that enters the numerators is the occurrence of vascular complications after treatment. The prochronous stratification of denominators might depend on such baseline variables as age, metabolic severity of diabetes, and co-morbidity of vascular or other associated diseases before treatment is instituted, but the synchronous stratification would depend on the degree with which blood sugar was "controlled" during the course of the treatment.

A synchronous stratification requires a *synchronous partition* of the particular variable—such as detectability of target event, compliance with therapy, or regulation of blood sugar—that has been chosen for analysis. In the example just cited, the regulation of blood sugar might be classified as **excellent, satisfactory,** or **inadequate,** and the synchronous stratification would cite the rates of vascular complications in each of these three categories of patients. Another example of synchronous stratification for an ancillary therapeutic

effect would be an investigation to determine whether the lowering of serum lipids prevents myocardial infarction (or other adverse cardiac events) in patients with established coronary artery disease. In this situation, we would want to know the rate of the target cardiac events according to partitioned categories of the synchronous change in serum lipids after therapy is instituted.

1. Procedure for synchronous partition. The entities to be classified in a synchronous partition occur between the time that the maneuver was instituted and the occurrence (or non-occurrence) of the target event. Several types of categorical expression can be used for the classification. The category can be a simple, direct observation, such as **yes** or **no** for the variable *patient continued working full-time.* For variables that require a more complex judgment—such as *compliance with therapeutic instructions* or *regulation of blood sugar*—the expressions can appear in such terms as **good, fair,** or **poor.** Phenomena that are originally expressed in metric data, such as *amount of change in serum cholesterol,* may be partitioned into such "transition" categories as **rise, no essential change, slight decrease,** and **large decrease.**

The formation of a synchronous partition in data analysis thus requires several steps:

1. The synchronous phenomenon is defined in a variable that expresses either an occurrence (such as *fidelity of maintenance of treatment*) or a transition (such as *change in cholesterol*).

2. Categories of partition are established for the synchronous variable. If the variable relates to an occurrence, the categories of expression take such forms as **yes** and **no,** or **good, fair,** and **poor.** If the variable relates to a transition, the categories of expression take such forms as **higher, same,** and **lower.**

3. The patients are divided according to these categories, and the rates of the target event are cited for each category.

4. In addition, if the data are numerous enough and the analysis is pertinent, an ad-

ditional prochronous variable or variables can be added to the synchronous stratification. Thus, each category of prochronous partition (such as **old** and **young**) might be further divided into categories of synchronous partition (such as **good compliance** and **not good compliance**). In the example just cited, the combination of synchronous and prochronous partitions would produce a four-category stratification: **old and good, young and good, old and not good,** and **young and not good.**

2. *Retrograde citations.* All of the stratifications just noted produced a "prospective" citation for the data. To a question such as "What is the likelihood that a diabetic patient with good regulation of blood sugar will get a vascular complication?", our answer gave the occurrence rate of such complications in patients with good regulation of blood sugar. The rates in the stratifications express the "prospective" risk of occurrence for the target event in each "risk factor" group, because the number of patients in each "risk factor" group is placed in the denominator, and the number of target events among those patients is placed in the numerator.

In many statistical analyses of such data, however, our main question is answered in a retrograde manner. The denominators are chosen not according to the patients' "risk factors," but according to the occurrence or non-occurrence of the target event. The synchronous entity is then placed in the numerator, so that the result is expressed as a mean or reversed proportion, not as the rate we wanted to know.

For example, suppose we had determined the occurrence or non-occurrence of bleeding esophageal varices as a target event in a cohort of patients with cirrhosiss of the liver. Suppose we now wanted to relate this target event to the synchronous average level of serum bilirubin in those patients. The data might show that the rate of bleed-

ing was 1/37 (*3%*) in patients with bilirubin values **below 1.5;** 3/23 (*13%*) for bilirubin values of **1.6 – 2.5;** 8/30 (*27%*) for values of **2.6 – 5.0;** and 9/17 (*53%*) for values of **5.1 and higher.** Such data would tell us the risk of bleeding in each bilirubin group. In a retrograde citation, the data would be expressed as follows: in patients who did not bleed, the mean bilirubin was 3.68 ± 4.24; and in patients who bled, the mean bilirubin was 6.9 ± 5.9. This retrograde citation would denote the general idea that bilirubin was higher in bleeders than in non-bleeders, but it would not give rates of risk for bilirubin as a synchronous "risk factor."

Such retrograde citations are common in clinical literature. A recent example appeared in the report of two concurrent trials of clofibrate treatment of ischemic heart disease in the United Kingdom.[8, 12] These trials will receive a more detailed discussion in a later paper of this series. For the moment, we can note the way in which the investigators reported the data about lowering of serum lipids.

A transition variable, *cholesterol response*, was defined as shown in Formula 1. Thus, a patient with a pretreatment level of 275 and a subsequent mean value of 250 would have a response units value of 20 = $[(275-250)/(275-150)] \times 100 = (25/125) \times 100$.

To answer the "prospective" question whether adverse coronary events are less likely when cholesterol levels are reduced, we would partition the patients synchronously according to those "response units." The change in cholesterol for some patients could be classified as **rise** (a negative value in response units), and other changes could be classified as **little or no fall** and **substantial fall.** [The boundaries for the three categories in this partition would depend on the range and distribution of response-

$$\frac{\text{Response}}{\text{units}} = \frac{(\text{Pretreatment cholesterol level–mean of levels at all later visits}) \times 100}{\text{Pretreatment level} - 150} \qquad (1)$$

Chart 1

Treatment	Occurrence of adverse target events	Newcastle trial[8]		Scottish Trial[12]	
		No. of Pts.	Mean response	No. of Pts.	Mean response
Clofibrate	No "Incidents"	137	13.6	214	27.2
	"Incidents"	44	26.0	44	14.3
Placebo	No "Incidents"	126	-2.3	226	-7.1
	"Incidents"	63	-3.5	57	-1.8

unit values in the population.] We would then determine the rates with which the target cardiac events had occurred in the three synchronous strata of cholesterol response.

Instead, however, the investigators in the U. K. clofibrate trials presented a retrograde citation of their data. The patients were divided according to the occurrence or non-occurrence of target events; and for each of those event categories, the investigators listed the mean response units of serum cholesterol. The results can be adapted from the published Table XV of each report and summarized as shown in Chart 1.

These data clearly show that the cholesterol levels fell in the clofibrate patients and remained essentially unchanged in the placebo groups, but our main concern is whether adverse incidents occurred less frequently in the patients with large falls in cholesterol. This question cannot be answered from the data supplied in this table. We can note only that the mean fall in cholesterol in the Newcastle trial was greater for patients experiencing "incidents" than in patients who did not, and that this relationship was reversed in the Scottish trial—but our basic question about risk remains unanswered from this retrograde technique of citation.

The difficulty with the technique is that the different events occurring in different strata are rendered undistinguishable when everything is agglomerated to calculate the mean retrograde values. To illustrate this point, consider the synchronous stratification shown in Chart 2 for a hypothetical clinical trial.

In this situation, the rates of the target

Chart 2

Results in synchronous variable	Rate of untoward events	
	Treatment A	Treatment B
Rise	8/20 (40%)	24/60 (40%)
Same	8/40 (20%)	8/40 (20%)
Fall	0/60 (0%)	0/20 (0%)
TOTAL	16/120 (13%)	32/120 (27%)

events are exactly the same for each treatment in each of the three categories of synchronous response. In the total results, however, treatment A seems better than B. The reason is that a **fall** in the response variable occurred in substantially more members of the *A* group than the *B* group. Within similar categories of response, the results were the same for *A* and *B*.

Expressed in retrograde citation, these subtle differentiations would be obliterated. Let us assume, for the sake of calculations, that the average values for **rise, same,** and **fall** were +10, 0, and –10, respectively. The mean for the "events" group in treatment A would be +5.0. (This value is obtained as $[(10 \times 8) + (0 \times 8) + (-10 \times 0)] \div 16$.) The mean for the "non-events" group in *A* would be –4.6, obtained as $[(10 \times 12) + (0 \times 32) + (-10 \times 60)] \div 104$. For treatment *B*, using analogous calculations, the mean would be +7.5 for the events group, and +1.8 for the non-events group. The type of clear clinical distinctions that are evident in the stratified data would be lost.

3. The absence of synchronous analysis.

Although a retrograde citation may not be a particularly desirable method of expressing the relationship between target events and a synchronous variable, the citation provides the reader with at least a general idea of what happened. In many important therapeutic trials, however, the necessary analysis is wholly omitted from the published reports. The investigators do not provide either a synchronous stratification or a retrograde citation of the data.

Such an omission occurred in the published reports[1, 9, 10, 14] of the UGDP study of treatment for adults with maturity-onset diabetes mellitus. A prime question to be asked about such treatment is whether or not the rigorous control of blood sugar helps to prevent vascular complications. Although the UGDP investigators assembled data that might help answer this question, no appropriate analyses have been published.

In Table 10, page 805, of the main UGDP report,[14] the investigators listed the number of patients in each of the three categories (**good, fair,** or **poor**) of partition for the synchronous variable, *level of blood glucose control*. These listings would be the denominators for rates that could have given an answer to the question clinicians have long debated. All that was needed to get the rates was the associated numerator data (the corresponding numbers of patients with deaths or vascular complications), but neither the numerators nor the rates have been included among the many other statistical collections issued by the UGDP.

Nevertheless, a reader who makes the necessary effort can detect the missing numerator data from a different source of information in the main UGDP report.[14] In Tables B-1, B-2, B-3, and B-4 in Appendix B (pages 827-830), the investigators have provided a tabular "case history" for each of the deceased patients. By noting the cause of death and blood glucose control that are listed for each patient, we can assemble the numerators of cardiovascular deaths to be associated with the previous

Chart 3

Level of glucose control	Total no. of patients	No. and (percentage) of cardiovascular deaths
Good	307	16 (5.2%)
Fair	287	22 (7.7%)
Poor	216	22 (10.2%)
TOTAL	810	60 (7.4%)

numerator-less denominators. Combining all results regardless of therapy, we then find Chart 3.

When examined with the chi-square test, in an appropriately one-tailed interpretation at 2 d.f., this gradient in the rates of synchronous stratification is "statistically significant" at $P < .05$ ($x^2 = 4.62$). The patients with good control of blood glucose thus appeared to have distinctively lower rates of cardiovascular death than the patients with worse control.

B. Bivariate evaluation

A multivariate stratum contains a combination of categories that have been conjoined from their individual locations in univariate partitions. Thus, the multivariate stratum **tall old men** contains a conjunction of the category **tall** from the partition of *height*, **old** from the partition of *age*, and **men** from the partition of *sex*. A single multivariate stratum can contain one such conjunction or a cluster of several separate conjunctions. Thus, the category **poor risk** might contain the cluster of **tall old men** and **uremic women.**

When multivariate categories are formed during the stratification process, the original univariate categories are conjoined in a sequential manner. Two categories, such as **old** and **men**, are first conjoined to form a new composite category, **old men.** An additional category, **tall**, might then be conjoined to create the composite category **tall old men.** Another category, **uremic**, might then be conjoined to form **uremic tall old men.**

1. Strategies in sequential multivariate partition. At least two different types of basic strategy can be used for forming the conjunctions that are produced at each step in the sequential process. One such basic stretegy, which might be called the *dichotomous split* technique, is used in the procedure described by Sonquist and Morgan.[13] In the first step, the population is divided into two groups according to the "best" dichotomous division of a single variable. At each step thereafter, the data analyst explores the conjunction of existing groups with individual categories of all other candidate variables. The "best" of these conjunctions is then split off to become a new group. This new group and the residue of its ancestral group then join the other groups eligible for exploratory conjunction and selective separation in the next step of the proceedings.

For example, in the first step, we might split the population into **men** and **women**. In the second step, the split might produce **old men, young men** and **women**. The third step might produce **old men, tall young men, non-tall young men,** and **women**. The fourth step might produce **old men, tall young men, non-tall young men, uremic women,** and **non-uremic women.** At the end of the process, the individual groups can be aggregated into clusters of strata that have similar target rates.

(A separate sub-strategy is needed for choosing the "best" dichotomous split at each sequential step. In the Sonquist-Morgan procedure, the strategic principle is maximum reduction of group variance. In other analogous procedures that were briefly noted in an earlier paper in this series,[6] the principle is maximum polarization of target rate or maximum reduction of error in congruent fit.)

Although an effective method for producing multivariate predictive strata, the "dichotomous split" technique does not allow constant attention to biologic homogeneity. At each step, isolated categories from individual variables are used to demarcate a group of people from the rest of the population under analysis. The successive groups are formed on the basis of the associated target rates, without specific regard to biologic concordance in the constituent elements.

Attention to biologic concordance is permitted in a different basic strategy, which might be called *bivariate conjunctions*. At each step of the bivariate conjunction technique, the entire population is included in the new partition. The opportunity to examine the entire population, rather than separated groups, is the main tactic that allows a data analyst to apply principles of biologic concordance throughout the stratification process. The methods used for those biologic judgments were described earlier in in this series.[6] The rest of this discussion is concerned with some additional principles that can be used for statistical decisions at each step in the sequence of bivariate conjunctions.

2. Formation of bivariate partitions. A bivariate partition is a cross-tabulation of the partitions for two individual variables. The resulting arrangement resembles the perpendicular intersections of the tabular structure seen in a game that is called "tic tac toe" in the United States and "naughts and crosses" in the United Kingdom. The categories of one variable become the rows, and the categories of the other variable become the columns of this cross-tabulation. If the row variable contains r categories and the column variable c categories, the cross-tabulation contains $r \times c$ cells, each of which is a bivariate stratum.

When the associated data are entered, each of these cells, unless devoid of members, will contain two numbers: a denominator comprising the patients who belonged to that bivariate stratum, and a numerator comprising the number of those patients who attained the target event. A third number, the target rate of numerator per denominator, is also entered in each cell. The row totals and column totals will show the way the population had previously been stratified in the individual univariate partitions. The grand totals will show the results for the unpartitioned original population.

For the cell in the i-th row and j-th column, these results can be symbolically written as $t_{ij}/n_{ij} = p_{ij}$. The totals of the i-th row can be written as $U_i/N_i = P_i$. The totals of the j-th column can be written as $V_j/N_j = P_j$. The grand totals are $T/N = P$. In more sophisticated statistical nota-

$$\text{tion, } U_i = \sum_{j=1}^{c} t_{ij} = t_{i.}; \ V_j = \sum_{i=1}^{r} t_{ij} = t_{.j}; \text{ and}$$

$$T = \sum_{i=1}^{r} \sum_{j=1}^{c} t_{ij} = t_{..} \text{. (Numerical ex-}$$

amples of such cross-tabulations were presented earlier in this series,[6,7] and other examples will be shown here later on.)

Our next step in the process is to reduce the number of bivariate strata by consolidating the cells into clusters. The consolidation is performed according to the principles of biologic concordance and target-rate isometry that were discussed previously.[6] These consolidated clusters will be the partitioned strata of a new composite variable, containing elements from both of the two previous variables. If k "predictor" variables were initially considered in the analysis of data, we will have removed two old variables, leaving k-2 of the original univariate partitions. These k-2 variables now receive bivariate cross-tabulation with the new composite variable. The "best" of these cross tabulations (selected by methods described later) is then consolidated to form the clusters of another new composite variable that will contain elements from three of the original variables. The process then continues sequentially until it is ended for one of the diverse reasons cited previously,[7] or until all of the original variables are exhausted.

3. Choice of univariate "contenders." In any investigation of a human cohort, an enormous number of variables can be chosen for use as predictor variates. For K such variates, there will be $(K)(K-1)/2$ cross tabulations of bivariate pairs to consider when the first composite variable is formed. To reduce the number of bivariate conjunctions that require inspection, the data analyst can initially choose a smaller subset, containing $k(k<K)$ original variates that appear particularly promising as "contenders" for producing "optimal" stratifications. The analysis will then be restricted to these k variates, and the bivariate analysis will begin with the $(k)(k-1)/2$ cross-tabulations formed from those k variates.

The principles to be used in selecting those "contender" variables were discussed previously.[6,7] Some of the major principles were that each stratum should contain enough members to warrant predictive confidence, and that the stratified target rates should show distinctive gradients from highest to lowest values and from one category to the next. Furthermore, the distinctiveness in number of members and size of gradients should be confirmed by a "significant" result in such statistical appraisals as the variance reduction score or the chi-square test.

4. Evaluation of bivariate partitions. From the k univariate "contenders," a total of $(k)(k-1)/2$ bivariate stratifications will now require evaluation and the "best" of these bivariate groupings will be chosen for consolidation into the new composite variate. (The display and evaluation can be considerably aided by a computer program that automates production of the cross-tabulations, target rates, and other necessary calculations.) Some of these cross-tabulations can be immediately dismissed as unsatisfactory because of their biologic "discord." Other cross-tabulations will reveal that certain individual variables were deceptively distinctive, acquiring their gradients not from predictive importance of the strata, but from disproportions in distribution of members. The choice of a "best" bivariate grouping will then be made from the bivariate partitions that remain after removal of those that are unsatisfactory in features of either bivariate biology or univariate gradients.

For these activities, the data analyst will require two statistical strategies: to determine bivariate loss of distinction in an apparently distinctive univariate partition, and to choose the "best" of a group of bivariately distinctive partitions. These two strategies will be discussed separately.

a. Bivariate distinction and the "double gradient." Each of the univariate "contenders" was associated with a distinctive gradient in target rate. If this gradient is an "independent" feature of the categories of that variable, we would expect the gradient to persist within the categories of a conjoined variable. A gradient that vanishes during the conjunction was probably not an inherent feature of the associated variable, and arose for other reasons. Therefore, if two variables each have an independently distinctive gradient, we would expect their bivariate conjunction to show a "double gradient." The gradient of each variable should be essentially maintained within the categories of the other variable.

To illustrate this principle, let us consider a population in which the total survival rate is 103/200 (52%). In a univariate partition of *sex*, the stratified rates are 62/100 (*62%*) for **women** and 41/100 (*41%*) for **men**. In a univariate *stage of disease* partition, the stratified rates for the same population are 86/110 (*78%*) for **mild** and 17/90 (*19%*) for **severe**. Each of these gradients (21% for *sex* and 59% for *stage of disease*) is large enough to be biologically regarded as distinctive. In chi-square tests of statistical distinctiveness, we find that for sex, $x^2 = 8.8$, $P < .01$; and for *stage of disease*, $x^2 = 69.7$, $P < .0001$. (The x^2 tests were interpreted as two-tailed, although, as discussed later, *stage of disease* should have been one-tailed.)

We have thus established that the *sex* gradient and the *stage of disease* gradient are each distinctive, from both a biologic and statistical viewpoint. We now want to determine whether the gradients are *independent*. Does each gradient persist within the context of the other? To answer this question, we examine the bivariate cross-tabulation of data and find Chart 4.

From direct visual inspection, we now see that the *sex* gradient essentially vanishes within the context of the *stage* gradient, but

Chart 4

	Men	Women	TOTAL
Mild	30/40 (*75%*)	56/70 (*80%*)	86/110 (*78%*)
Severe	11/60 (*18%*)	6/30 (*20%*)	17/90 (*19%*)
TOTAL	41/100 (*41%*)	62/100 (*62%*)	103/200 (*52%*)

not vice versa. Thus, the sex gradient between **men** and **women** is only 5% (= 80% − 75%) within the **mild** stage and only 2% (= 20% − 18%) in the **severe** stage. On the other hand, the stage gradient between **mild** and **severe** is 57% within **men** and 60% within **women**.

To confirm the statistical aspects of this point, we can perform intracategorical chi-square tests. Such tests are based on comparing results of the cells of a particular row or column versus the marginal totals for that row or column. The formula for such calculations in the i-th row category would be

$$x^2 = \left(\Sigma \frac{t_{ij}{}^2}{n_{ij}} - \frac{U_i{}^2}{N_i} \right) \div P_i Q_i$$

and for the j-th column category, we would have

$$x^2 = \left(\Sigma \frac{t_{ij}{}^2}{n_{ij}} - \frac{V_j{}^2}{N_j} \right) \div P_j Q_j$$

For simplicity of computations with a desk-top calculator, the division by $P_i Q_i$ in the formula for a row category can be expressed as multiplication by

$$\left(\frac{N_i}{U_i} \times \frac{N_i}{N_i - U_i} \right) = \frac{N_i{}^2}{U_i (N_i - U_i)}$$

A corresponding adaptation is used in the formula for column categories.

Applying these formulas to the foregoing bivariate tabulation, we find the following results. Within the row category of **mild**, chi square is

$$\left(\frac{30^2}{40} + \frac{56^2}{70} - \frac{86^2}{110} \right) \times \frac{110^2}{86 \times 24} = 0.37$$

Within the row category of **severe**, chi square is

$$\left(\frac{11^2}{60} + \frac{6^2}{30} - \frac{17^2}{90}\right) \times \frac{90^2}{17 \times 73} = 0.04$$

Neither of these values is "statistically significant." On the other hand, the chi square results within the columns—31.9 within the **men** category and 32.1 within the **women** category are both highly "significant" (P < .001). These results provide statistical confirmation for what we had previously noted during our "eyeball" test of the data.

We can therefore conclude that the *sex* gradient in this cohort was unimportant and actually illusory. It arose, as do many types of distortion in cohort statistics, from a disproportionate division of the cohort among prognostically important strata. In the cohort just described, the *stage* stratification was prognostically important, but the men and women were distributed in a highly disproportionate manner among the **mild** and **severe** strata. In the male cohort, only 40% of the population (40/100) was in the **mild** stratum compared with 70% (70/100) in the female cohort. This disproportionate distribution then created the spurious gradient noted in the total results for men and women.

Thus, in selecting "contenders" with which to form a composite stratification for the entire population of 200 people, we would preserve *stage* as an important univariate partition. We would discard *sex*, however, and explore other univariate partitions instead.

b. Inter-categorical distinctions. In the tests that were just performed, we examined the intracategorical distinctions for each row and column of the cross-tabulation. Since the bivariate stratification has produced a new array of bivariate categories for the entire population, we can also examine the inter-categorical distinctions of the entire array. This procedure can be performed with an "overall" chi-square test of all the bivariate categories. The computational formula for this calculation would be

$$\chi^2 = \left[\Sigma\Sigma\frac{t_{ij}^2}{n_{ij}} - \frac{T^2}{N}\right] \times \left[\frac{N^2}{T(N-T)}\right]$$

[The double $\Sigma\Sigma$ sign in the preceding formula indicates that we have summed the results for all rows and columns of cells in the bivariate partition.]

The application of this inter-categorical strategy can best be demonstrated with some real-world data. This information is taken from research, previously reported in preliminary form,[3] that is now being prepared for final publication. One of the main purposes of the research was to develop an improved system of prognostic staging for patients with cancer of the rectum.

In these patients, partitions and prognostic stratifications were examined for five-year survival rates in relation to such individual variables as *sex, age, anatomic stage, symptomatic stage, prognostic co-morbidity* (of associated ailments), and *co-morbid gastrointestinal disease.* The illustrations here are concerned only with the last three of those variables and with the three bivariate paired tabulations that could be formed from them.

The total five year survival rate for the entire population was 29% (91/318). For the partition of the variable *symptomatic staging,* the categories and survival rates were as follows:

Indolent:	44/103	*(43%)*
Obtrusive:	47/187	*(25%)*
Deleterious:	0/28	*(0%)*

For partition of the variable *prognostic co-morbidity,* the corresponding results were:

Absent:	85/264	*(32%)*
Present:	6/54	*(11%)*

For partition of the variable *co-morbid gastrointestinal disease,* the results were:

Concurrent:	33/85	*(39%)*
Antecedent:	19/61	*(31%)*
None:	39/172	*(23%)*

In each of these three individual univariate partitions, the overall chi-square tests were statistically significant at P < .05. (The respective chi-square values were 22.4, 9.8, and 7.5.) Accordingly, the next step was to explore the bivariate cross-tabulations of these three partitions, as listed in Table I.

Table I. *Illustration of three pairs of bivariate cross-tabulations*
[Data for 5-year survival rates according to different classifications of patients with cancer of the rectum.]

		Symptom stage			
		Indolent	*Obtrusive*	*Deleterious*	*Totals*
Co-morbid G.I. Disease	*Concurrent*	18/38 (47%)	15/41 (37%)	0/6 (0%)	33/85 (39%)
	Antecedent	9/20 (45%)	10/36 (28%)	0/5 (0%)	19/61 (31%)
	None	17/45 (38%)	22/110 (20%)	0/17 (0%)	39/172 (23%)
Totals		44/103 (43%)	47/187 (25%)	0/28 (0%)	91/318 (29%)
Prognostic Co-morbidity	*Absent*	40/84 (48%)	45/160 (28%)	0/20 (0%)	85/264 (32%)
	Present	4/19 (21%)	2/27 (7%)	0/8 (0%)	6/54 (11%)

		Co-morbid G.I. disease			
		Concurrent	*Antecedent*	*None*	*Totals*
Prognostic Co-morbidity	*Absent*	31/72 (43%)	18/48 (37%)	36/144 (25%)	85/264 (32%)
	Present	2/13 (15%)	1/13 (8%)	3/28 (11%)	6/54 (11%)
Totals		33/85 (39%)	19/61 (31%)	39/172 (23%)	91/318 (29%)

The results of Table I show, with two exceptions, that all of the survival gradients previously noted for the individual variates are essentially maintained during their intra-categorical separations in the paired tabulations. One exception is in the **deleterious** symptom stage, where no intra-categorical gradient would be expected because the initial target rate had a nadir value of 0%. The other exception occurs in the last of the three tabulations shown in Table I. When the **present** category of *prognostic co-morbidity* is cross-partitioned against the three categories of *co-morbid G.I. disease*, the latter variable loses the monotonic gradient previously noted in its totals. The loss of this gradient would suggest that one of the other two variable-pairings is a preferable bivariate partition, but before reaching this conclusion we can examine

the diverse chi-square calculations for the three bivariate stratifications, as shown in Table II.

For the results within rows and columns, Table II confirms that the cited gradient in Row 2 (the **present** category) of *prognostic co-morbidity* vs. *co-morbid G.I. disease* becomes not only lost, but also statistically indistinctive ($P > .4$). In addition, in the bivariate stratification of *co-morbid G.I. disease* vs. *symptom stage*, the total gradient for co-morbid G.I. disease becomes statistically indistinct ($P > .35$) when tested within the category **indolent**, which is Column 1 of that table.

From these results, we would suspect that the most biologically effective of the three bivariate stratifications is the one containing *prognostic co-morbidity* vs. *symptom stage*. This suspicion is supported by

Table II. *Chi-square results* for stratifications shown in Table I*

		Co-morbid G.I. disease vs. symptom stage			Prognostic co-morbidity vs. symptom stage			Prognostic co-morbidity vs. co-morbid G. I. disease		
		x^2 Value	d. f.	P	x^2 Value	d. f.	P	x^2 Value	d. f.	P
Total		27.53	8	<.0005	32.57	5	<.00025	18.42	5	<.0025
Within rows										
	Row 1	11.29	2	<.0025	19.86	2	<.0025	7.92	2	<.0125
	Row 2	4.24	2	<.1	3.28	2	<.1	0.40	2	>4
	Row 3	5.06	2	<.05	— — —			— — —		
Within columns										
	Col. 1	0.83	2	>.35	4.47	1	<.025	3.55	1	<.1
	Col. 2	4.53	2	<.1	5.27	1	<.0125	4.24	1	<.1
	Col. 3	0	2	—	0	1	—	2.73	1	<.15

*All P values are interpreted as one-tailed.

the total chi-square results in the inter-categorical comparisons, as shown at the top of Table II. Although the total chi-square tests were highly "significant" statistically for all three bivariate stratifications, the highest value of x^2 and correspondingly lowest value of P occurred for *prognostic co-morbidity* vs. *symptom stage*. Accordingly, the latter stratification would be the best one to choose from the three under examination if we wanted to consolidate two univariate conjunctions into a new composite partition.

The data of the cited bivariate stratification lend themselves quite readily to forming a new array of composite categories that would seem reasonably homogeneous in both biologic concordance and target-rate isometry. The composite results would be as shown in Chart 5.

c. The interpretation of chi-square results. Because the chi-square test is an

Chart 5

Category from symptom stage		Category from prognostic co-morbidity	New composite category	Survival rate
Indolent	and	Absent	A	40/84 (48%)
Indolent Obtrusive	and and	Present; or Absent	B	49/179 (27%)
Obtrusive Deleterious	and and	Absent; or Either	C	2/55 (4%)

invaluable aid in the foregoing decisions, the interpretation of the test requires careful attenion to two fundamental issues in using a table* of chi-square values: the degrees of freedom and the one-sided vs. two-sided tails of distribution for probability in the P values.

The determination of degrees of freedom simply requires that we note the values for *r*, the number of row categories; and *c*, the number of column categories. The degrees of freedom will then be as follows: *c-1*, for a test within a row category; *r-1* for a test within a column category; and *rc-1* for an intercategorical test of the entire bivariate partition.

The problem of one vs. two tails in the probability values for P is not so easily resolved. Although fundamental to any use of statistical tables for tests of "significance," this problem receives little or no attention in most statistical books intended for medical readers. The clearest discussion I have seen is contained in an excellent (non-medically oriented) paperback book by Langley,[11] who advocates the routine use of two-sided probabilities in order to avoid introducing subjective judgments into the analysis. Since the stratification pro-

*My own preference, because of extensiveness in degrees of freedom and attention to one-tail vs. two-tail distinctions, is the tabulation contained in the Geigy Scientific Tables.[2]

cesses discussed here are deliberately intended to allow the use of biologic judgment, I shall admire Langley's exposition while disagreeing with his conclusions.

I suspect that the reason for the disagreement is the different approaches used by a statistician and a scientist in the analysis of data. A statistician usually regards the "test of significance" as a way of investigating a mathematical null hypothesis that is created as a theoretical necessity for performing the test. A scientist uses the test as a way of determining whether his numbers are large enough to reduce the possibility that the observed difference may arise by chance. If the observed difference is trivial, the scientist will usually be uninterested in the statistical test, even if its results are "significant."

Furthermore, a statistician begins with no previous beliefs about what the results should show, and is willing to accept even-handedly the possibility that the results can go in either direction. The scientist, however, often has some strong beliefs about the direction of the results. If the results go in a direction opposite to what he expects, he is unconcerned about "statistical significance." He wants to find out what went wrong, and he will either re-design the experiment, or plan different arrangements in the analysis of data.

In many situations in which the chi-square test is applied during predictive stratification, the preferred procedure is a one-sided, rather than two-sided, interpretation of the probability values. For example, if patients with metastatic cancer have higher survival rates than patients with localized cancer, we would immediately want to know why this peculiarity occurred. Was there something wrong with the methods of diagnosis, classification, or treatment? The answer to that question would be our main concern—not the level of probability in the statistical test.

Similarly, when a stratification has been prepared on the basis of severity of disease, we expect the associated target rates to follow a corresponding direction. Thus, for a particular ailment, we might have no advance expectations that **men** will fare better than **women,** or vice versa, but we would anticipate better results in **good risk** than in **bad risk** patients. Consequently, the interpretation of the chi-square test for a nominal variable, such as *sex*, might be two-tailed, whereas the interpretation for an ordinal variable, such as *severity of disease*, might be one-tailed.

After a gradient has been shown in the categories of a univariate partition, we would expect that gradient to be maintained for intra-categorical partitions with another variable. Thus, after we have noted that **men** have a substantially lower survival rate than **women** for a particular disease, we would expect **men physicians** to have lower rates than **women physicians,** and **men lawyers** to have lower rates than **women lawyers** in the bivariate stratifications of *sex* and *occupation*. Consequently, most of the chi-square tests done for intra-categorical stratifications should be one-tailed. The tests used for inter-categorical stratifications may occasionally be two-tailed (particularly if the marginal totals gave us no *a priori* expectations), but will also usually be one-tailed. For this reason, all of the P values shown here in Table II were derived from the one-sided results listed in the Geigy tabulations.[2] Readers who do not have access to these tabulations can attain the one-way results by taking half of the P value listed in conventional citations of the chi-square test data.

It should be noted that "significant" values of P are more likely to be obtained from a one-tailed rather than two-tailed interpretation because smaller values of chi-square are accepted as "significant." Thus, to attain a P value of $< .05$ at one degree of freedom, the chi-square score must exceed 3.841 in a two-tailed interpretation, and 2.706 in a one-tailed interpretation.

•   •   •

Another important set of decisions in the stratification process deals with the basic choice of "cutting points" or demarcation boundaries in the univariate partition of a metric variable, such as *age, blood pressure,* or *serum cholesterol.* These decisions, which can be greatly aided with the appropriate use of a computer, will be deferred for discussion at a later date.

This sub-series of papers on the biostatistical process of prognostic stratification is now concluded. Some of the principles and problems in the stratification process will be especially pertinent to the topic discussed at our next session: an appraisal of the recent trials of clofibrate in coronary artery disease.

References

1. Cornfield, J.: The University Group Diabetes Program. A further statistical analysis of the mortality findings. J. A. M. A. **217**:1676-1687, 1971.
2. Documenta Geigy. *In* Diem, K., editor: Scientific tables, ed. 6, Ardsley, N. Y., 1962, Geigy Chemical Corp.
3. Feinstein, A. R.: Symptoms as an index of biologic behaviour and prognosis in human cancer, Nature **209**:241-245, 1966.
4. Feinstein, A. R.: Clinical biostatistics. VII. The rancid sample, the tilted target, and the medical poll-bearer, CLIN. PHARMACOL. THER. **12**:134-150, 1971.
5. Feinstein, A. R.: Clinical biostatistics. XIV. The purposes of prognostic stratification, CLIN. PHARMACOL. THER. **13**:285-297, 1972.
6. Feinstein, A. R.: Clinical biostatistics. XV The process of prognostic stratification (Part 1), CLIN. PHARMACOL. THER. **13**:442-457, 1972.
7. Feinstein, A. R.: Clinical biostatistics. XVI. The process of prognostic stratification (Part 2), CLIN. PHARMACOL. THER. **13**:609-624, 1972.
8. Five-year study by a group of physicians of the Newcastle upon Tyne region. Trial of clofibrate in the treatment of ischaemic heart disease, Br. Med. J. **2**:767-775, 1971.
9. Goldner, M. G., Knatterud, G. L., and Prout, T. E.: Effects of hypoglycemic agents on vascular complications in patients with adult-onset diabetes. III. Clinical implications of UGDP results, J. A. M. A. **218**:1400-1410, 1971.
10. Knatterud, G. L., Meinert, C. L., Klimt, C. R., Osborne, R. K., and Martin, D. B.: Effects of hypoglycemic agents on vascular complications in patients with adult-onset diabetes. IV. A preliminary report on phenformin results, J. A. M. A. **217**:777-784, 1971.
11. Langley, R.: Practical statistics, London, 1968, Pan Books Ltd., pp. 143-148.
12. Report by a research committee of the Scottish Society of Physicians. Ischaemic heart disease: A secondary prevention trial using clofibrate, Br. Med. J. **2**:775-784, 1971.
13. Sonquist, J. A., and Morgan, J. N.: The detection of interaction effects: A report on a computer program for the selection of optimal combinations of explanatory variables. Monograph No. 35, Ann Arbor, Mich., 1964, Survey Research Center, Institute for Social Research, University of Michigan.
14. University Group Diabetes Program. A study of the effects of hypoglycemic agents on vascular complications in patients with adult-onset diabetes. I. Design, methods and baseline results; and II. Mortality results, Diabetes **19**: (Suppl. 2) 747-830, 1970.

INDEXES

The index is divided into three parts. The first (pp. 447-452) indicates the authors cited in the text and references. The second (pp. 453-464) indicates the methodologic topics discussed in the text. The third (pp. 465-468) indicates the clinical and other practical examples mentioned during the discussions.

Index of Authors*

See also INDEX OF METHODOLOGIC TOPICS and INDEX OF CLINICAL AND OTHER PRACTICAL EXAMPLES

A

Abbey, H., 255
Abrams, M., 87, 184
Acheson, R. M., *182*, 185
Ad Hoc Committee, 52, 269, 367
Adams, L. L., 284
Adelstein, A. M., 284
Ahmed, F., 349
Amador, E., 254
American Medical Association, 367
Andersen, R., *382*
Anderson, D. O., 184
Anderson, T. W., 382
Andrews, D. F., 349
Andrews, F. M., 397
Anscombe, F., 68
Apgar, V., 241
Apley, J., 103
Armitage, P., 68, *308*, *315*, 319, 428
Aronow, L., 270
Arthes, F. G., 213
Arthur, R. J., 255
Atkins, H., 319
Auerbach, O., 195

B

Bailar, J. C., *102*, 103
Bailey, N. T., 87
Baird, D. C., 26
Bakan, D., 68
Baker, F. B., 303
Baker, L. A., 213
Ballard, G. P., 213
Bangdiwala, I., 213
Barnett, R. N., *188*, 195, *232*, 241, 253, 254
Baron, D. N., 367
Barrett-Connor, E., 184
Barron, S. S., 254

Barsky, A. J., 132
Beadenkopf, W. G., 87, 184
Beale, E. M. L., 383
Beckman, H., 269
Beecher, H. K., 269, 270
Beer, R. J., 367
Bellotti, C., 284
Benjamin, B., 87
Bennett, B. M., 226
Bennett, G. A., 270
Benson, E. S., *253*, 254, 255
Bergeson, P. S., *219*, *220*, 226
Berkley, C., 368
Berkson, J., *43*, 52, 68, *80*, *84*, 87, 103, *179*, 184, 226
Bernard, C., *137*, *144*, 152
Bradford Hill, A., 87, *94*, 103, *184*, 283, *315*, 319
Bradley, J. V., 26, 68, *301*, 303, 383
Brady, K., 241
Branscomb, L. M., *345*, 349
Brooks, S. H., 255
Bross, D. J., 68
Bruce, R. A., 120
Brugsch, H. G., *245*, 254
Buckland, W. R., *171*, 184, *186*, *188*, *191*, 196
Burgen, A. S. V., 270
Buros, O. K., 241

C

Callow, A. D., 88
Cameron, J. M., 152
Campbell, R. C., 87, *315*, 319
Caron, H. S., 133
Carr, C. J., 270
Casey, A. E., 254
Cattell, R. B., *379*, 383
Chai, H., 241
Chalmers, T. C., 88, 120, *127*, 132, 283, 284
Chapin, F. S., 26
Charlson, M. E., *408*, *427*, 429
Church, C. N., 241
Cicchetti, D. V., 226

---

*Italic page numbers refer to authors mentioned in text. All other page numbers indicate a bibliographic citation.

447

Index of Methodologic Topics

See also INDEX OF AUTHORS and INDEX OF CLINICAL AND OTHER PRACTICAL EXAMPLES

A

Ablative risk ratio, 207-208
Abnormal, medical meaning of, 244
Acceptance of research proposals, 39
Access to medical care, effect on disease rates, 42, 43
Accuracy
  prognostic, increase in, through prognostic stratification, 389-390
  rates of diagnostic test, 218
Actuarial analysis, 62
Additive scores of indexes, 47
Adherence; *see* Compliance
Adverse drug reaction, 109, 268, 271-272
  identification of, in pharmaceutical surveillance, 274-275
  lack of diagnostic algorithm for, 274-275
Age standardization; *see* Age-adjusted rate
Age-adjusted rate, 56, 94
  direct method, 94, 387
  indirect method, 94
  substitution of age-specific rate for, 387
Age-specific
  cohort, 93
  rate, 93
  strata, 93
  substitution of, for age-adjusted rate, 387
Aggregate, as type of cluster in prognostic stratification, 402
Aggregation of indexes, 47
  additive scores, 47
  Boolean clusters, 47
  taxonomic, types of, 359
Alcohol, ascertainment of effect of, in surveys, 55
Algorithm, 257
Allocation
  of maneuvers to populations, 54-59, 105-120
  of treatment in therapeutic trials, 106-120
  problems in, 109-111
    experiments, 56-59
    surveys, 54-56
  random
    advantages of, 111

Allocation—cont'd
  random—cont'd
    cardinal defect of, 118-120
    clinical objections to, 111-112
    disadvantages of, 112-114
    intrinsic problems of, 114-118
α error, 67, 322
α level
  and "diagnostic specificity," 321-322
  of "significance," 11, 290, 316
ANOVA (analysis of variance), 376
Architecture of research, 26, 28-37, 38-52, 54-68
Ascertainment of maneuvers in surveys, 54-55
Assignment of subject to maneuvers, method of, 58-59
Association(s)
  measures of, 376-378
    for dependent variables, 380-378
    for independent variables, 376
    for interdependent variables, 376
  non-dependent, disadvantages of, 380-381
  of data, 373
Assumptions, statistical, underlying principles of probability, 291

B

Bad risk, 24, 30, 110, 387
Baseline condition; *see* Initial state
Berkson's fallacy, 43, 80, 179
β error, 67, 343
  calculation of, 325-327
  importance of, 330
β level of significance, 11, 325
Bias
  assembly, 163
    measurement of, 165
  calculations of, in a trohoc, 208-209
  chronology
    in cohort statistics, 74, 103
    sources of, 89-102
    in trohoc research, 203
  "compliance," consequences of, 122-132
  examples of "rancid" sampling, 172-175

Index of Clinical and Other Practical Examples

See also INDEX OF AUTHORS and INDEX OF METHODOLOGIC TOPICS

465